PERIMETRY
With and Without Automation

PERIMETRY

With and Without Automation

Douglas R. Anderson, M.D.
Professor of Ophthalmology, Bascom Palmer Eye Institute,
University of Miami School of Medicine, Miami, Florida

Second Edition

With 308 illustrations
Illustrated by **Leona M. Allison**

The C. V. Mosby Company
ST. LOUIS • WASHINGTON, D.C. • TORONTO 1987

MOSBY

A TRADITION OF PUBLISHING EXCELLENCE

Editor: Eugenia A. Klein
Manuscript Editor: George B. Stericker, Jr.
Book Design: Kay M. Kramer
Cover Design: Liz Fett
Production: Terry Silvey and Ginny Douglas

Second Edition

Printed in the United States of America

The C.V. Mosby Company
11830 Westline Industrial Drive, St. Louis, Missouri 63146

Library of Congress Cataloging-in-Publication Data

Anderson, Douglas R., 1938-
Perimetry with and without automation.

Rev. ed. of: Testing the field of vision. 1982.
Bibliography: p.
Includes index.
1. Perimetry. 2. Perimetry—Automation.
I. Anderson, Douglas R., 1938- . Testing the field of vision. II. Title. [DNLM: 1. Perimetry. 2. Vision Disorders—diagnosis. 3. Visual Fields. WW 145 A546t]
RE79.P4A53 1987 617.7'5 86-21791
ISBN 0-8016-0208-4

AC/W/W 9 8 7 6 5 4 3 2 1 01/A/095

To Wirtley

Preface

This book is intended to provide practical guidance to the use of visual field testing in clinical practice. I hope it will be helpful to practitioners switching from manual to automated perimetry, and also valuable for ophthalmologists and technicians in training. Much of this edition stems from *Testing the Field of Vision,* published in 1982, which emphasized the manual field examination performed with the Goldmann perimeter. However, this edition expands into the areas of automated perimetry and the interpretation of the results.

The sequence of chapters is reorganized. Information pertinent to both automated and manual perimetry has been retained and, with the new material, constitutes Part I. Information pertinent only to the practical aspects of manual perimetry has been extracted and placed in Part II. In Part I the relationship between kinetic and static field examinations is illustrated and the two are discussed side by side, for two reasons: Both methods are in common usage at present; thus specialists in professional and technical training need to be familiar with both and to understand their relationship. Practitioners changing to automated perimetry will want to use their prior knowledge of kinetic methods as a base on which to build their understanding of static perimetry.

Most visual field testbooks, while covering glaucoma, dwell on neuroophthalmic diagnosis—in keeping with the interest of the authors. This book concentrates more heavily on glaucoma—in keeping with my prime interest, and also as seems appropriate for the needs of the typical clinical office, in which patients with glaucoma outnumber those with neuroophthalmic conditions. All the essential elements of visual field testing in the context of neuroophthalmic diagnosis are contained in this book. However, to make use of these findings in combination with other clinical findings for diagnosis, the reader will have to consult the neuroophthalmic literature. Indeed, the same is true of glaucoma, for this book covers only the perimetric component of the art and science of glaucoma diagnosis and management.

The book is designed to be used for individual reading or self-teaching, perhaps supplemented by some guidance from an experienced person. It is also designed for use as a textbook in perimetry courses (see Appendix A).

Douglas R. Anderson

Contents

PERIMETRY
With and Without Automation

PART ONE

PRINCIPLES OF VISUAL FIELD TESTING

CHAPTER 1

Introductory concepts

THE VISUAL FIELD

With our eyes directed straight forward, we pay attention to the details of the object at which we are looking. While looking at an object, we are able to detect the presence of other objects above, below, and to the sides of the object of regard—though we may not be able to discern the details or even say what the objects are.

FIG. 1-1. Field of vision of the right and left eyes. Note that the fields of view of the two eyes overlap. There is a broad area where objects are seen by both eyes but to the extreme right or extreme left objects are seen by only one eye. In this way the field of view with both eyes open is greater than with either eye alone. (Illustration by George E. Schwenk.)

To see for yourself that you cannot discern details of an object without looking right at it, look at a spot 2 feet to the side of a visual acuity chart and see if you can read the small letters (the details of the chart) while your eyes are directed at the spot.

When an object in the peripheral field catches our attention, perhaps because it is moving or flashing, we reflexly turn our eyes toward it so we can see its details and identify it. Visual function, then, includes both the ability to detect the presence of objects in a field of vision and the ability to discern the details of an object as we turn our eyes to look directly at it. Without both of these components of visual function, we are handicapped.

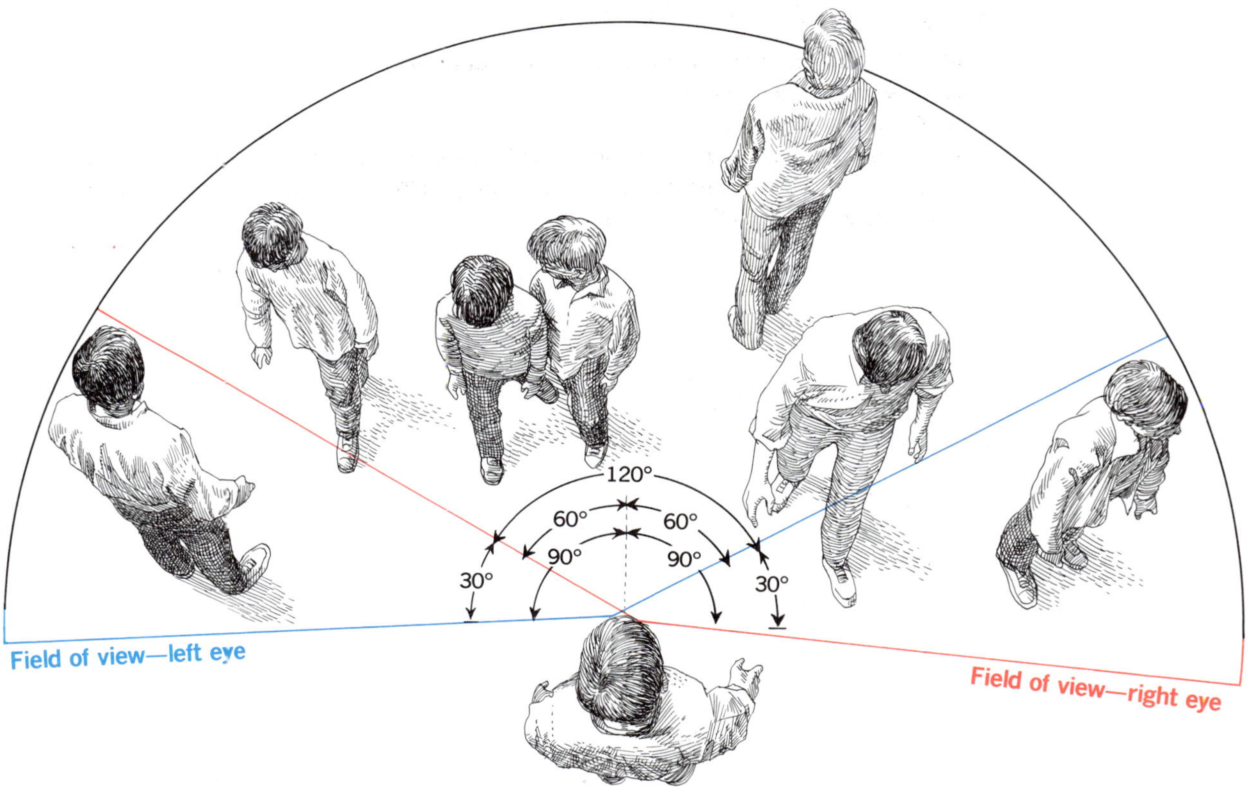
120°
60°
60°
90°
90°
30°
30°
Field of view—left eye
Field of view—right eye

FIG. 1-1

BOUNDARIES OF THE VISUAL FIELD

The boundaries of the field of vision, measured in degrees from the point of fixation (the object at which the eye is directed), are approximately

60 degrees superiorly (above)
75 degrees inferiorly (below)
100 degrees temporally (to the right for the right eye, to the left for the left eye)
60 degrees nasally (to the left for the right eye, to the right for the left eye)

The extreme boundary of the visual field could be determined by bringing a large object from behind around the head of an individual who is looking straight ahead and asking when the object first becomes visible to him. If a disease state has contracted the peripheral boundary of his visual field, it may be necessary to bring the object quite far around before it is seen.

FIG. 1-2. Limits of the average normal visual field.
A, Upward and downward.
B, Temporal and nasal.
C, Plot of the limits for the right eye. Note that the field is standardly plotted on the field diagram "as the patient sees it"—the border of the visual field to his right being plotted to the right on the field diagram.

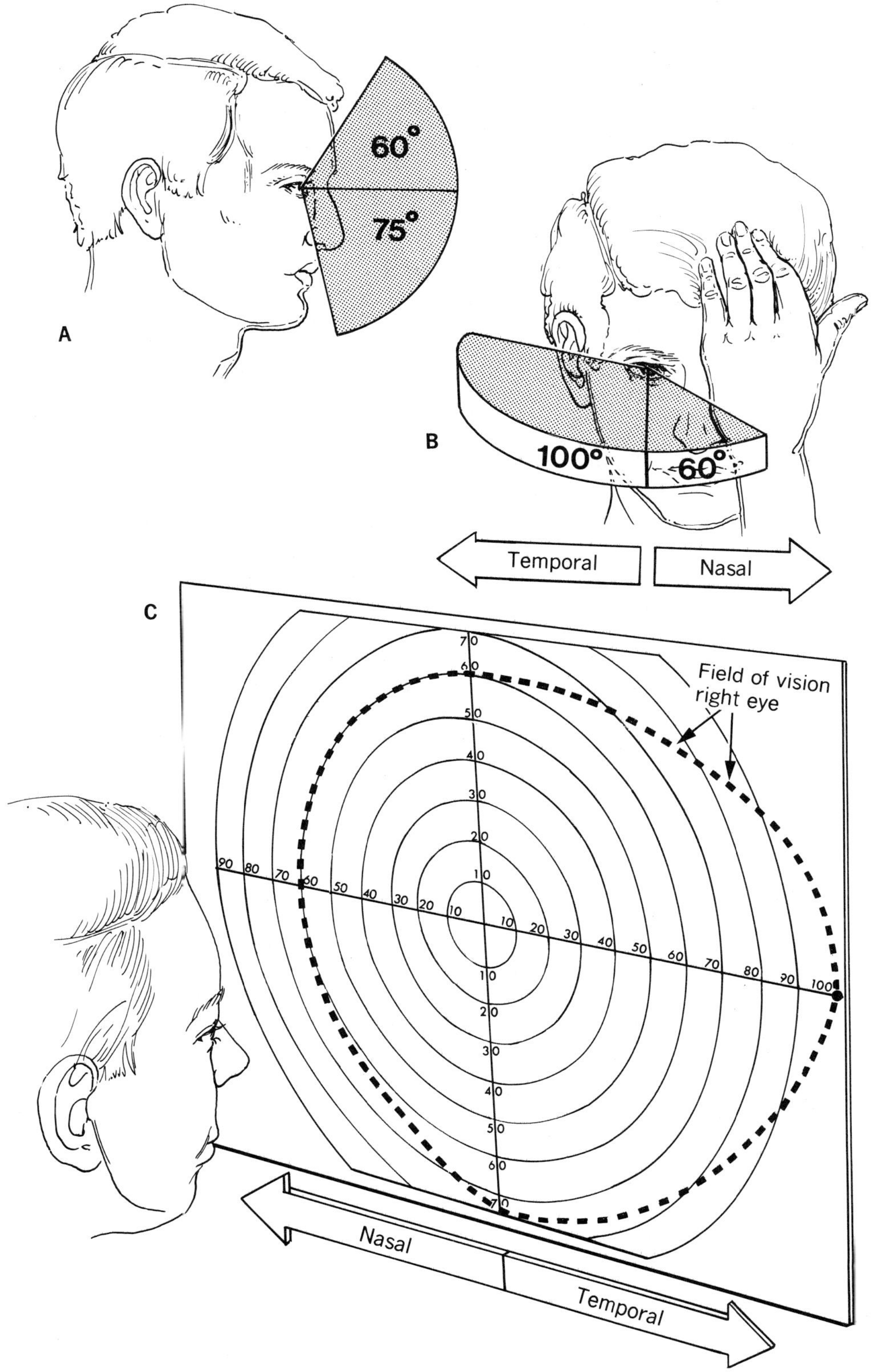

60°
75°
A
B
100°
60°
Temporal
Nasal
C
Field of vision right eye
Nasal
Temporal

FIG. 1-2

VISUAL CHARACTERISTICS WITHIN THE VISUAL FIELD

Determining the outside boundary of the visual field is one aspect of testing the field but is not really the aspect that is of greatest diagnostic importance. More important is the fact that within the boundary every point in the visual field has certain characteristics of visual function.

For example, as already noted, the ability to discern details (i.e., visual acuity) is greatest at the point of fixation. Clinically, we ask the patient to look at letters so we can determine the visual acuity at the point of fixation in terms of the smallest letters that can be identified when the person is looking directly at the letter (Fig. 1-3, *A*).

If we wished, we could determine the visual acuity at all other points in the visual field by having the person look at a certain spot, placing a letter chart at selected locations (e.g., 10 degrees to the nasal side), and determining the smallest letter that could be correctly identified (Fig. 1-3, *B*). We could do this for many points scattered throughout the visual field (e.g., 10 degrees temporally, 10 degrees superiorly, 20 degrees nasally, 30 degrees nasally) and thereby document or quantify the functional ability (or visual acuity) in each region of the field of vision in that individual. It would be found that the acuity was best at the point of fixation and became less and less as the chart was placed farther from fixation.

FIG. 1-3. Determining visual acuity.
A, Usual method, for testing at the point of fixation.
B, Hypothetical method for testing at 10 degrees from fixation.

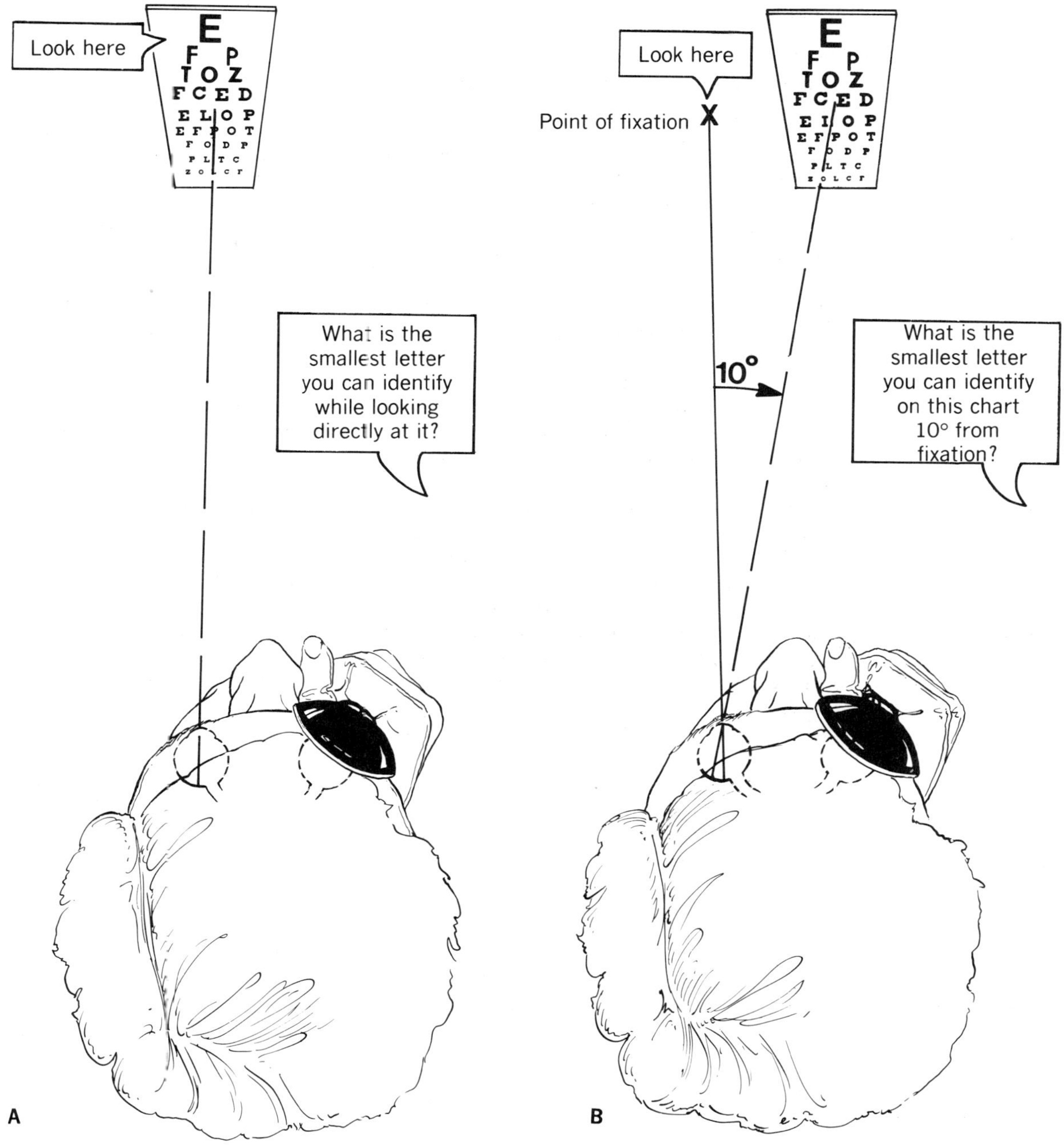
Look here
What is the smallest letter you can identify while looking directly at it?
A
Look here
Point of fixation
10°
What is the smallest letter you can identify on this chart 10° from fixation?
B

FIG. 1-3

In clinical practice we do not quantify the functional ability within the visual field in terms of the smallest letters that can be identified. Instead, we quantify in terms of the weakest white spot that can be seen in each region of the field. With the tangent screen technique of field testing (p. 27), these test stimuli consist of white beads or disks of standard diameter (e.g., 1, 3, 5, and 10 mm). With projection perimeters (p. 30) the stimuli typically consist of projected white spots that can be adjusted in both size and intensity.

It is important to know what factors enter into the visibility of a white spot:

APPARENT SIZE (DIAMETER OR AREA) OF THE SPOT is an important factor. The apparent size depends on the real size and the distance of the spot from the eye. Thus a 3 mm spot 1 meter from the eye is equivalent to a 6 mm spot that is 2 meters from the eye or a 1 mm spot that is 0.33 meter from the eye. With perimeters the distance is fixed, and relative visibility relates to the real size of the spot. With the tangent screen, which can be used at varying distances, both the size of the spot and the distance are considered.

INTENSITY OF THE SPOT is important, too. In a reciprocal relationship two spots may be roughly equivalent visual stimuli if one is 0.5 log-unit more intense but half the diameter (one fourth the area) of the other. The exact equivalency relationship of size and intensity is different in different parts of the visual field.

BACKGROUND ILLUMINATION is the third factor to which we pay special attention in quantitative perimetry. It has two effects on stimulus visibility. First, the background is important because a stimulus of certain intensity will be less visible against a light background than against a dark one. Second, the background intensity also determines the degree of light or dark adaptation of the retina (photopic, mesopic, or scotopic), which of course influences whether or not dim stimuli are seen.

OTHER FACTORS are also important. These include color, movement of the stimulus, duration of the stimulus, attentiveness of the person, and refractive state of the eye. Throughout most of the field, a moving stimulus is somewhat more visible than a nonmoving one. The duration of a stimulus is important for a brief flash (e.g., 1/100 second vs. 2/100 second), but duration does not change the visibility of a stimulus after a certain critical time—approximately 1/3 second or longer. After this length of time, duration does not matter because maximum temporal summation has occurred.

VISUAL THRESHOLD: DEFINITION

Every point within the visual field has a visual threshold, which can be defined roughly as the weakest test stimulus that is just visible in a particular location under the specific test conditions. (A more accurate detailed definition is given in Chapter 14.)

Also visible at each location are all test stimuli that are stronger (larger or more intense) than the threshold stimulus. Such a stimulus, stronger than the threshold stimulus, is a *suprathreshold* (or *supraliminal**) *stimulus*.

An object is *not* seen if it is weaker (smaller or less intense) than the threshold stimulus—that is, if it is an *infrathreshold* (or *subliminal*) *stimulus*.

> Visual field testing—which is what this book is all about—involves testing the visual threshold throughout the field of vision, not simply making a determination of the extreme outside boundary of the visual field.

---

*More common in European usage, from the Latin word *(limen, liminis)* for connecting timber or support of a doorway (i.e., threshold, limit).

METHODS FOR TESTING VISUAL THRESHOLD

Static threshold perimetry

For visual field testing, the patient's eyes should be held in a steady position by having him look at a specific point—the fixation target or point of fixation. At some other place within the field of vision a spot stimulus of light is presented and the patient communicates whether or not he can see it.

With a typical projection perimeter this would be a projected spot of white light of a selected size and intensity on a background of a certain standard intensity. The size of the spot and the background illumination are kept the same. The dimmest stimulus that can be seen is determined by trial and error and is recorded as the threshold stimulus for that location in the field.

FIG. 1-4. Diagram of the visual field within 40 degrees of fixation. The visual threshold at twenty locations is tested with five different stimuli (*A, B, C, D,* and *E*). At each location the weakest stimulus that can be seen is indicated, i.e., the threshold at that location.

Note the similarity between recording the weakest white spot that is visible (determination of visual threshold) and recording the smallest letter that can be identified (determination of visual acuity).

In *static threshold perimetry,* then, a location is chosen and the stimulus is presented in that location without moving it. The white spot is presented at various intensities so it can be determined which intensities are visible at that location and which are not. The process is repeated at other representative locations of interest.

In the example (Fig. 1-4), *D* represents a weak (dim) stimulus and *E* is the weakest. Wherever stimulus *D* is visible as a threshold stimulus, stimuli *A, B,* and *C,* being stronger, are also visible. They are suprathreshold (supraliminal) for that location. In the places marked with a *C* the two stronger stimuli, represented by *A* and *B,* would also be visible and would be supraliminal for that location. The weaker stimuli, represented by *D* and *E,* would not be visible, meaning that they are infrathreshold (subliminal) for that location. In the center portion of the field, near the point of fixation, the eye is very sensitive, able to see the weakest stimulus. However, toward the periphery of the field, stronger illumination is needed for the stimulus to be seen.

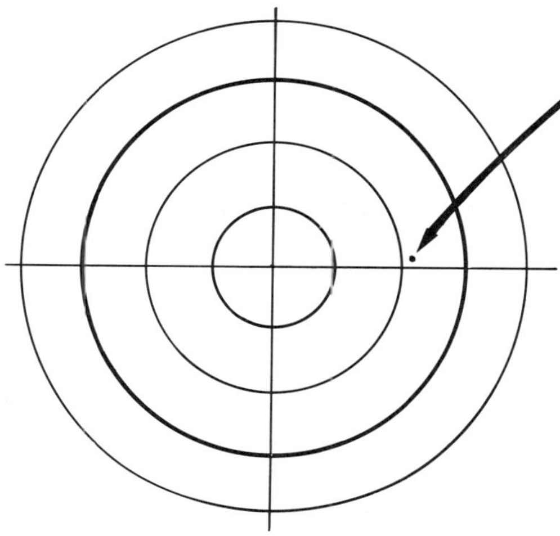

Question:	Answer:
Can you see stimulus A here?	Yes
Can you see stimulus B?	Yes
How about C?	Yes
Can you see D?	No
How about E?	No

Conclusion: Stimulus C is threshold (weakest stimulus seen)

A is the weakest stimulus seen here (threshold)

B is the weakest seen here

C is threshold here

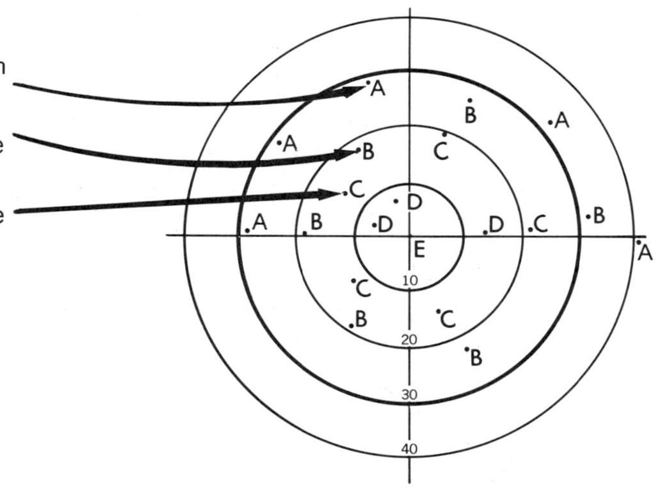

FIG. 1-4

Kinetic threshold perimetry

The line connecting all points where *C* is the threshold is called the *isopter* for stimulus *C*.

FIG. 1-5, A. The isopter for stimulus *C*.

An important characteristic of an isopter is that its stimulus (*C* in this instance) cannot be seen anywhere outside the isopter, because everywhere outside the isopter the stimulus is infrathreshold. The *C* stimulus, however, is seen everywhere inside the region surrounded by the isopter, being threshold at the line and suprathreshold closer to the center. It is important to note that near the isopter the stimulus is threshold and that it becomes more and more suprathreshold for locations closer to fixation.

Because the isopter is a boundary between a region where the stimulus is visible and where it is not visible, the location of the isopter for a given stimulus can be determined by moving the stimulus from the periphery toward the center of the field. As long as the stimulus is in a region where it is infrathreshold, it will not be seen, but it becomes visible as soon as it reaches the isopter where it is threshold. It remains visible after it enters the region surrounded by the isopter where it is suprathreshold.

FIG. 1-5, B. Determining the isopter for stimulus *C*.

In *kinetic perimetry,* then, a selected stimulus is moved from an area where it is not seen toward an area where it is seen, and the location where it becomes visible is recorded as just described (Fig. 1-5, *B*). This process is repeated from all directions toward the center (fixation) until the isopter can be drawn by connecting the points where the stimulus first becomes visible. Several isopters can be drawn by repeating the process with several stimuli of differing intensity or size.

The exact location of the kinetic isopter for a stimulus depends on the rate of movement of the stimulus. It is not *exactly* the same as the location of the isopter for the static stimulus. However, within the limits of accuracy of static and kinetic methods used clinically, the two are sufficiently equivalent if careful technique is used (Chapters 17 and 23), except when the Riddoch phenomenon is prominent (Chapter 9).

FIG. 1-5, C. The isopters for *A, B, C,* and *D.* Note that the weak stimulus *(D)* is seen only inside the region enclosed by its isopter, a small area near fixation, the most sensitive part of the field. In contrast, a stronger stimulus (such as *B*) is seen over a larger area, the area enclosed by its isopter.

Thus

> Kinetic perimetry asks, "Where is stimulus x threshold?"
> Static perimetry asks, "What is threshold at location x?"

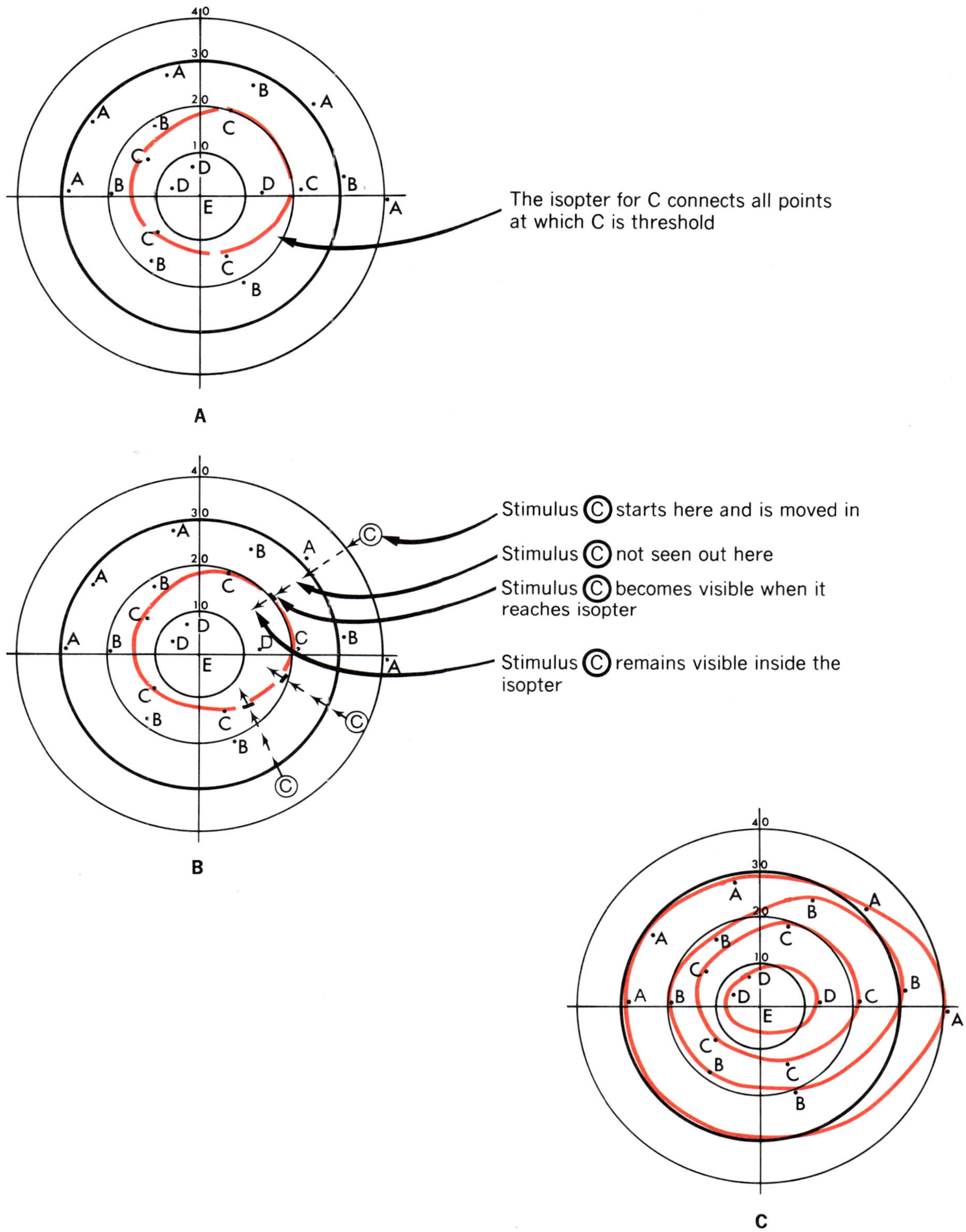
The isopter for C connects all points at which C is threshold
A
Stimulus C starts here and is moved in
Stimulus C not seen out here
Stimulus C becomes visible when it reaches isopter
Stimulus C remains visible inside the isopter
B
C

FIG. 1-5

Nonquantitative field testing

Not all methods for visual field testing quantify the visual threshold at representative locations in the field. For certain diagnostic purposes, quantified threshold determination may not be necessary or desirable.

Examples of such techniques, to be covered in greater detail later in this book, include

SUPRATHRESHOLD (AS OPPOSED TO THRESHOLD) STATIC PERIMETRY, in which a stimulus is presented at a location where it should be visible (i.e., it should be suprathreshold). If the stimulus is seen, the location is considered to have a normal sensitivity without a determination being made of the exact threshold. This is equivalent to showing an individual the 20/40 acuity line in a driver's license examination and if he can see it he is judged to have visual acuity that is sufficiently normal for driving, without bothering to determine if the acuity might be 20/25, 20/30, or 20/15.

COMPARISON TECHNIQUES, in which the quality of vision (brightness, color saturation, etc.) is compared in two equivalent locations of the field. Thus, if an object is duller or dimmer 5 degrees to the right than it is 5 degrees to the left, somehow the visual quality is poorer to the right of fixation than it is to the left, which constitutes an abnormality in the visual field.

SUBJECTIVE RECOGNITION OF A REGION OF POOR VISION when looking at a grid of lines (Amsler grid). This may suffice to demonstrate the presence of the diagnostic abnormality without the need to quantify the defect.

All these techniques are important in perimetry, even though they are not quantitative.

REPRESENTATION OF QUANTITATIVE TEST RESULTS
Isopter plot

In kinetic threshold perimetry, the traditional manual method of testing the visual field, the location is marked when the stimulus is first seen as it moves from the nonseeing to the seeing area for that stimulus. A line is drawn connecting the points to form the isopter for that stimulus.

FIG. 1-6, A. Isopter for stimulus I-3e of the Goldmann perimeter. Note that the threshold is known only at points where the stimulus first becomes visible.

The threshold is not known in the region more peripheral than the isopter. The stimulus was infrathreshold along the path approaching the isopter, but you do not know how much infrathreshold. (In other words, you do know how much stronger the stimulus would have to be to become visible at various points along the path.)

Similarly the threshold is not known in the region inside the isopter. If the stimulus is moved further inward, it should remain visible if the visual field is normal. However, you do not actually know whether or not the field is normal and the stimulus is indeed visible within the isopter unless the stimulus is actually placed inside the isopter and you ask the patient if, in fact, it is visible. Even when you determine that the stimulus is visible everywhere within the isopter, you do not know how much dimmer the stimulus can be made and still be seen; so threshold has not been determined.

Finally, even along the isopter, the threshold is known only at the spots actually tested. The line joining the tested spots is an interpolation but is likely to represent the true isopter if the spots are sufficiently close.

When several isopters are plotted, the diagram resembles a contour map.

FIG. 1-6, B. Plot of several isopters. Note that the locations at which threshold was determined blanket the entire field of vision.

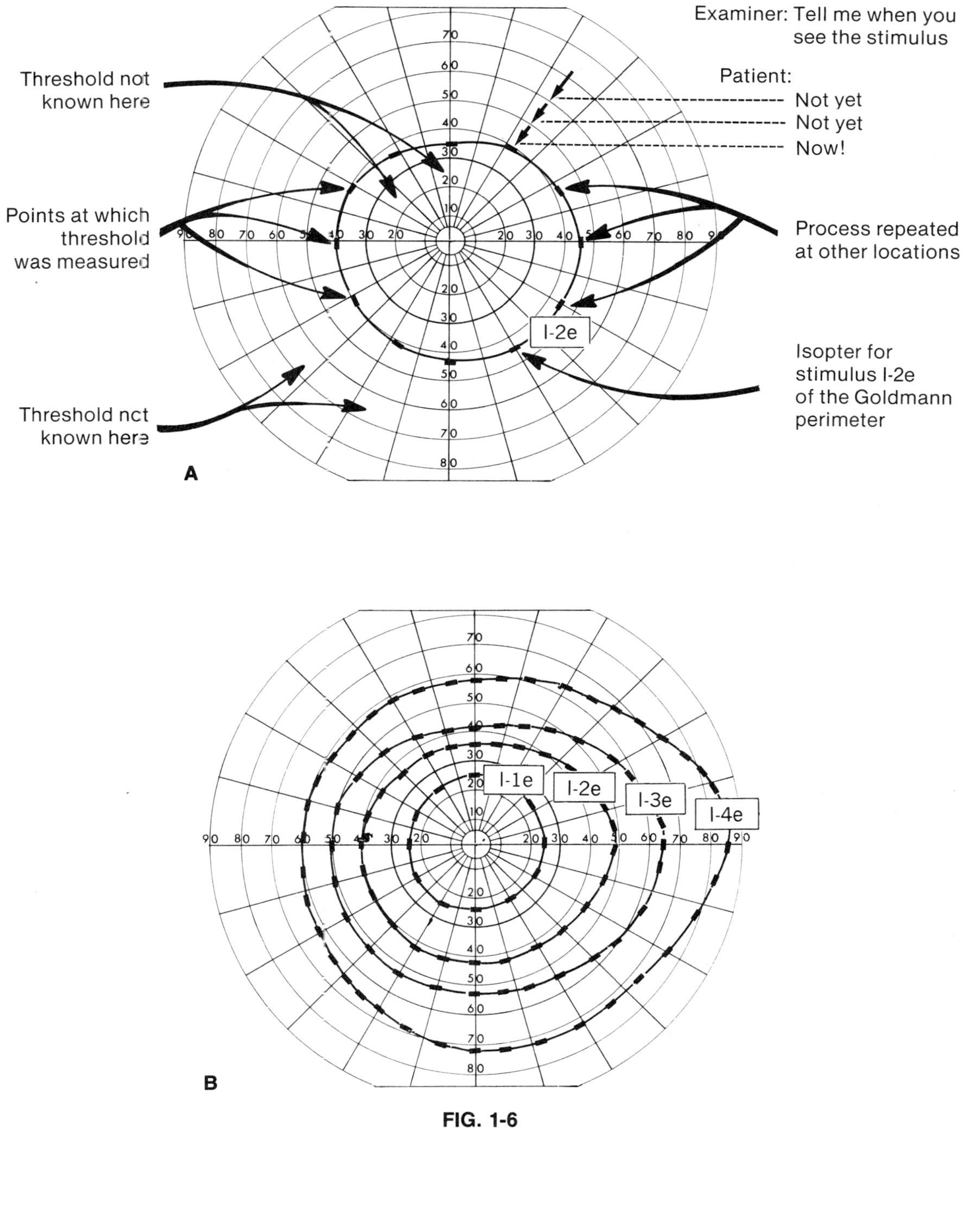
Examiner: Tell me when you see the stimulus
Patient:
Not yet
Not yet
Now!
Threshold not known here
Points at which threshold was measured
Process repeated at other locations
I-2e
Isopter for stimulus I-2e of the Goldmann perimeter
Threshold not known here
A
I-1e
I-2e
I-3e
I-4e
B

FIG. 1-6

Numeric and greyscale (greytone) printouts

When static threshold perimetry is performed at numerous locations, as is typically done in full thresholding programs of automated perimeters, the results may be reported as threshold values printed on a map of the visual field (Fig. 1-7, *A*). To aid in perceiving a diagnostic pattern at a glance, as a prelude to studying the numeric values in detail, a greyscale is often also provided (Fig. 1-7, *B*). Each grey level represents a certain small range of threshold values (e.g., 21 to 25 decibels). The boundary between the grey levels is equivalent to an isopter. For example, consider the boundary between the greyscale symbols for 21 to 25 dB and the symbols representing 26 to 30 dB. It encloses all the points where the 26 dB stimulus is seen, and the boundary can be thought of as the isopter for the 26 dB stimulus.

In some printouts not all the locations with a greyscale symbol are tested. Untested locations may be assigned at presumed threshold values (calculated by interpolation from neighboring points that actually were tested) to shade in the greyscale plot and make the contour of the isopters easier to appreciate. As with kinetic perimetry, the threshold is known only at the points tested and the threshold at other locations is either estimated or assumed.

It is worth emphasizing that in both kinetic perimetry and static perimetry the threshold is known quantitatively only at the spots where the patient indicates that the object is visible. The number of places tested with either method depends on the time available to do the field testing. Given a practical limit on the number of places where threshold can be determined in the time available, the diagnostic value of the information depends on whether or not the examiner has chosen wisely the places within the field where such quantitative information is obtained (Chapter 11).

FIG. 1-7. Greyscale and numeric printouts of automated static threshold perimetry. This normal field of a right eye was tested out to 60 degrees in a pattern of points that was more closely spaced within 30 degrees. The numeric values are in decibels of sensitivity.

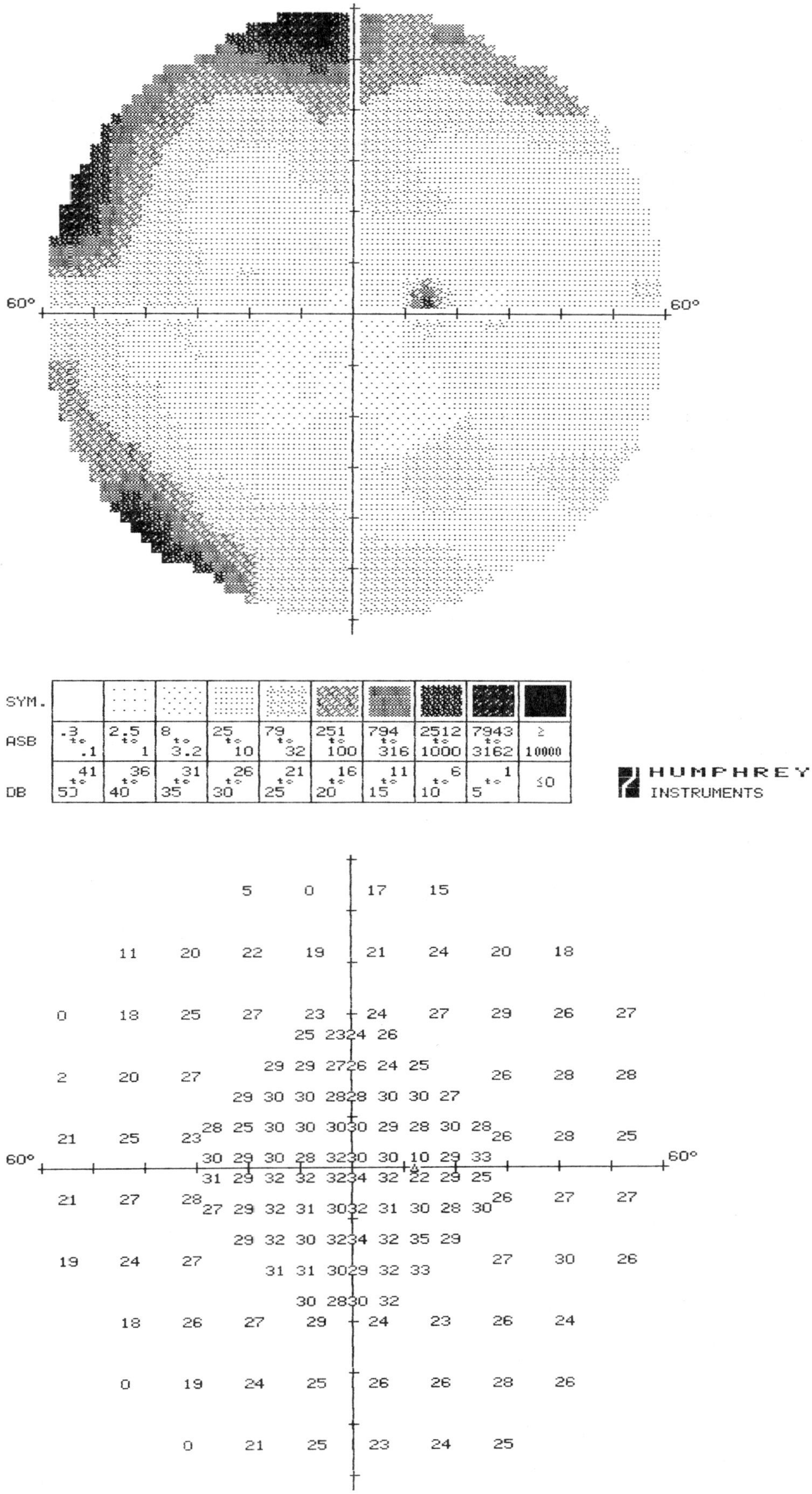
60°
60°
SYM.
ASB
.3 to .1
2.5 to 1
8 to 3.2
25 to 10
79 to 32
251 to 100
794 to 316
2512 to 1000
7943 to 3162
≥ 10000
DB
41 to 50
36 to 40
31 to 35
26 to 30
21 to 25
16 to 20
11 to 15
6 to 10
1 to 5
≤0
HUMPHREY
INSTRUMENTS

FIG. 1-7

Profile plot

Rather than perform static threshold determination at scattered points in the visual field, it is sometimes useful to determine the threshold at points along one of the meridians. Such a test is known as meridional static threshold perimetry or a *static cut*. The results can be represented as a graph.

FIG. 1-8. Static threshold perimetry performed along an oblique meridian. In this case it is performed from the upper nasal quadrant, through the point of fixation, into the lower temporal quadrant. The points where threshold was tested are indicated on the field diagram, and the thresholds at some of these points are indicated by letters *A, B, C, D,* or *E.* The results are also indicated on the graph, which shows greatest sensitivity at the point of fixation.

Note, once again, that visual threshold is determined only at the points tested and not at any other places within the field of vision. Thus in the static cut shown in Fig. 1-8 the visual threshold is not known for any points in the lower nasal and upper temporal quadrants but only for the positions along the line where visual threshold was tested.

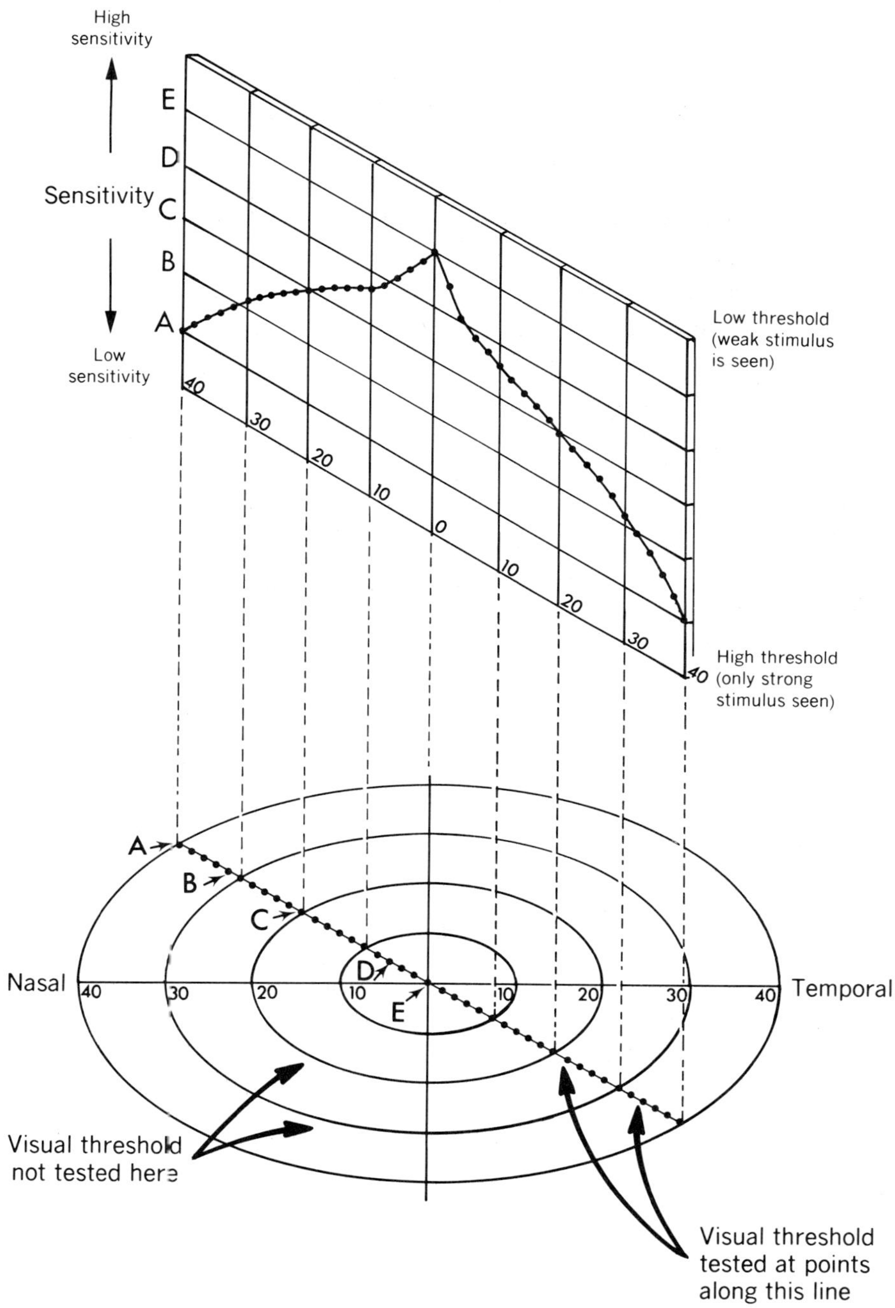
High sensitivity
E
D
Sensitivity
C
B
A
Low sensitivity
40
30
20
10
0
10
20
30
40
Low threshold (weak stimulus is seen)
High threshold (only strong stimulus seen)
A
B
C
D
E
Nasal
40
30
20
10
10
20
30
40
Temporal
Visual threshold not tested here
Visual threshold tested at points along this line

FIG. 1-8

Hill of vision

The "island of vision" or "hill of vision" is a three-dimensional graph of visual sensitivity. The horizontal axis represents location in the visual field. The altitude of the hill (vertical direction) at any location represents the visual sensitivity at that location.

FIG. 1-9. Hill of vision. The hill (graph) is highest where dim small objects of low contrast are visible. It is lower where an object must be more intense or larger or have more contrast to be seen.

The hill of vision can be considered as a contour map (isopter plot) representing horizontal slices through the visual field. This is usual in kinetic perimetry. The numeric and greyscale printouts of automated devices provide equivalent views of the hill from above. The hill can also be represented as a vertical slice (profile plot). This is usual in meridional static perimetry done manually or with an automated device.

Sensitivity is the inverse of *threshold*. The point of fixation in the center is highly sensitive and has low threshold in that a very weak stimulus is visible. Thus a low visual threshold means high sensitivity to light. Inversely, the peripheral regions have a high threshold because only a strong stimulus is visible. Thus a high visual threshold means low sensitivity to light. The hill of vision and graphs of static perimetry are in terms of sensitivity rather than threshold. Therefore the most sensitive areas of the field show up as the highest points on the graph.

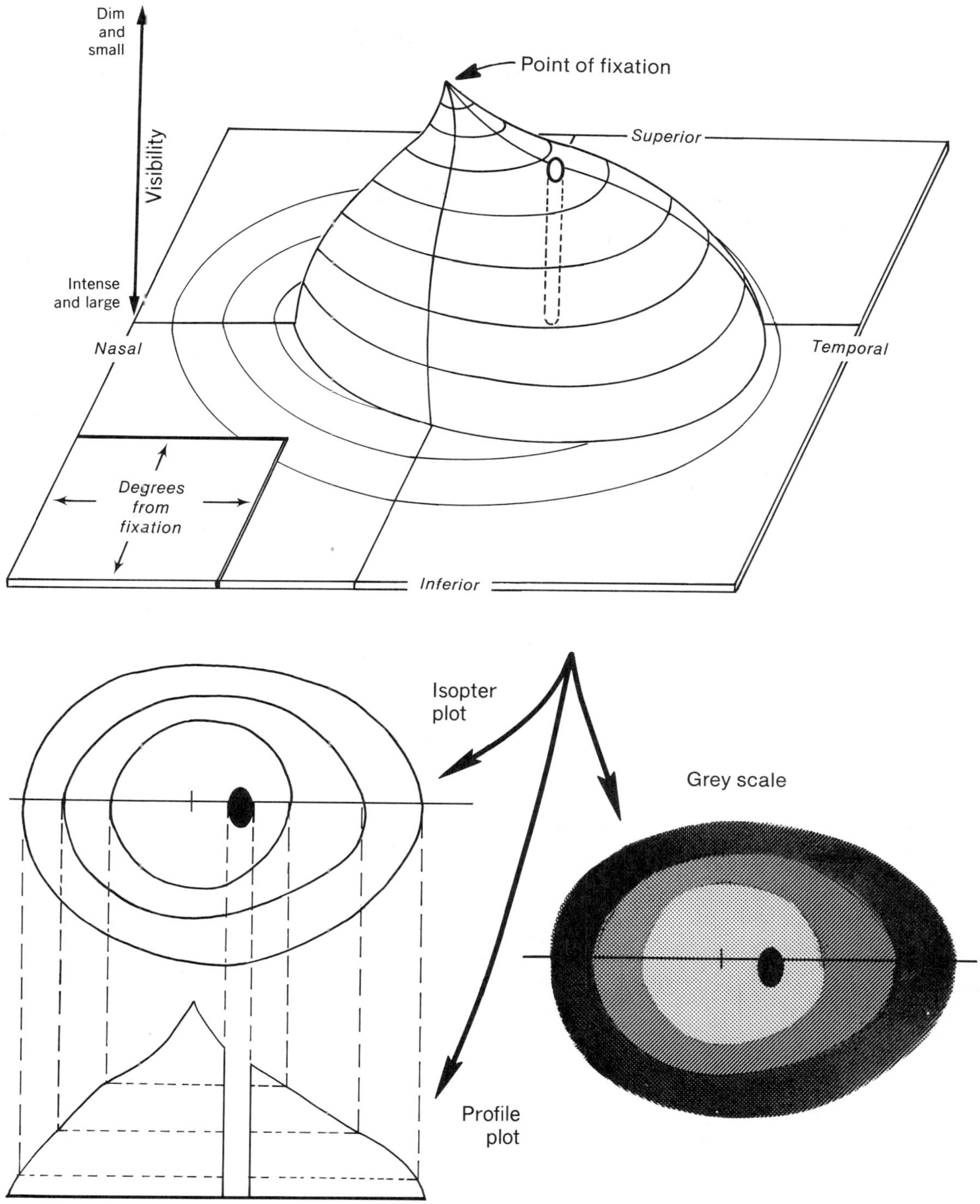
Dim
and
small
Visibility
Intense
and large
Point of fixation
Superior
Nasal
Temporal
Degrees
from
fixation
Inferior
Isopter
plot
Grey scale
Profile
plot

FIG. 1-9

SUMMARY

Every point in the visual field has a certain visual threshold, defined for practical purposes as the weakest stimulus visible in that location. Visual field testing consists of determining the visual threshold (or the inverse, visual sensitivity) at selected points throughout the field of vision, as well as determining the outside boundary of the field of vision.

In *static* perimetry a *stationary test stimulus* in a given location is intensified (or enlarged) until it is seen, thereby enabling the examiner to determine the visibility threshold at that location. In *kinetic* perimetry a selected test stimulus is *moved* until it crosses its isopter, which is the location where it is threshold.

Both methods, static and kinetic, demonstrate visual threshold at one location where the stimulus is just barely visible. By repeated testing with various stimuli it is possible to determine threshold at numerous locations. In static threshold perimetry the results are presented as a numeric or greyscale scatterplot or as a graph or profile representing a slice through the hill of vision. In kinetic perimetry the results are recorded as isopters representing horizontal slices through the hill.

CHAPTER 2

Instruments and strategies (programs)

A number of methods are in common use to test visual function throughout the visual field (i.e., to test visual function away from the point of fixation). This chapter presents an overview of the instruments in common use. Some have particular features that make them more suitable for particular clinical purposes. Every practitioner should have several methods available to use in different clinical situations (discussed in Chapter 11).

TANGENT SCREEN

The tangent screen has been in use since the turn of the century and is still used skillfully by some practitioners. White discs or spheres (test objects) are moved across a black screen with a black wand. The luminous intensity of the test objects is held constant from one occasion to another by keeping the room light constant (classically, 7 footcandles of daylight) and by keeping the test object clean. Several isopters are plotted kinetically with white or colored test objects of different sizes. Static suprathreshold testing is accomplished by placing the test object in various locations and asking the patient if it is visible.

The tangent screen is simple and inexpensive and, when used with skill, can provide entirely adequate screening, diagnostic, and quantitative field examinations. With a good room arrangement (i.e., with the screen on the wall 1 meter away from a rotating examining chair), a field examination can be performed by the clinician quickly and with almost no fuss or bother. The practical convenience may be a definite advantage in clinical offices where quick diagnostic examinations predominate (e.g., in neuroophthalmic practice) and quantitated field examinations are less often needed. Moreover, a skilled perimetrist will find the ability to change the testing distance from 1 to 2 meters helpful in the diagnosis of functional (hysterical) visual loss or in plotting details of small defects in the central 15 degrees.

The Bausch & Lomb Auto-Plot, a device that projects a white spot of light onto a grey (instead of black) tangent screen, is a useful but not essential modification. Indeed, if done skillfully, a focused spot of light projected onto any flat wall with a hand-held flashlight can be used for certain diagnostic purposes that do not require strict quantitation (see Chapter 11).

In plotting several isopters, the stimuli are not varied in intensity. The variables are size of the object (1 mm, 2 mm, etc.), color of the object (white, red, etc.), and distance of the screen (1000 mm, 2000 mm, etc.). When a 1 mm white test object is used at 1 meter (1000 mm), the isopter is labeled "1w/1000," which is more or less equivalent to an object twice the size at twice the distance (2w/2000). Almost always the test objects used are white, the testing distance is 1 meter, and only the size is varied. When a 2-meter distance is used, remember that the circle on the screen representing 30 degrees at 1 meter is a 15-degree circle for 2 meters.

FIG. 2-1. Using the tangent screen. To plot an isopter, the examiner asks the patient to look at the fixation spot at the center of the screen and then moves the test object from the edge of the screen toward fixation. The patient reports when the test object first becomes visible. It is important that the patient report when he first sees the white test object, not when he first sees the wand. The examiner monitors fixation directly by watching the patient's eyes. He should watch the patient's eyes, not the wand, while moving the wand. In this way, he can know that the patient's eye is steadily fixed at the instant when the patient reports seeing the stimulus.

The tangent screen is flat; and no matter how big it is, it does not come around the patient's side as far as 90 degrees. With the usual method, only the central 30 degrees is tested. Fortunately, the central field is diagnostically more important than the periphery. When the more peripheral field must be tested, an arc or bowl perimeter should be used to supplement the tangent screen.*

---

*For more details on the use of tangent screens, see Harrington, D.O.: *The Visual Fields: A Textbook and Atlas of Clinical Perimetry,* ed. 5, St. Louis, 1981, The C.V. Mosby Co., pp. 26-42.

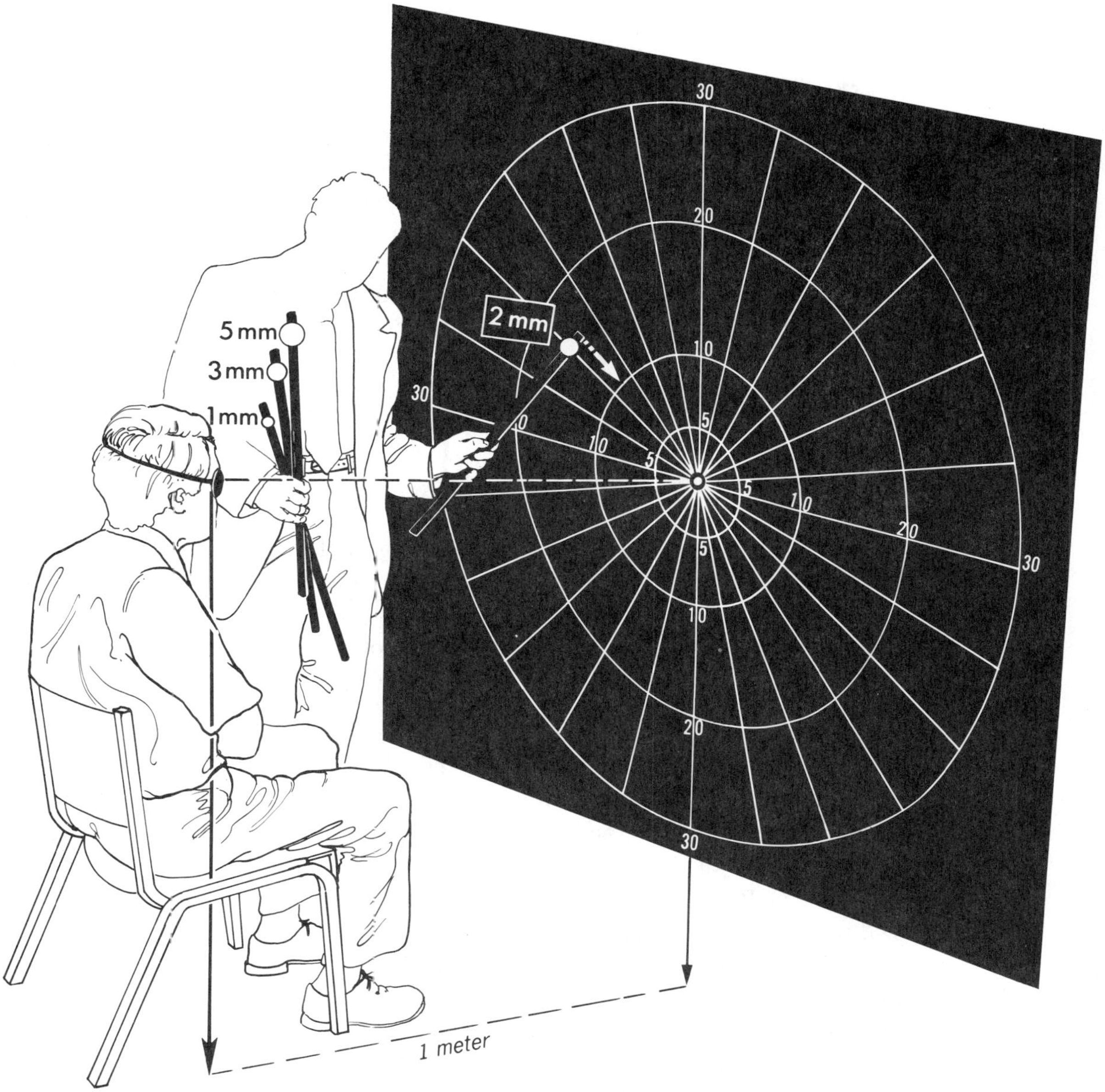

FIG. 2-1

ARC PERIMETER

To test the visual field beyond 30 degrees from fixation, an arc perimeter can be used. A semicircular band of white background about 0.33 meter (330 mm) in radius is tilted at various angles of inclination to test all meridians in the field. A hand-held test object or a projected spot of light is moved along the arc and the isopters are plotted. The isopter for a 3 mm white test spot would be labeled 3w/330, similar to the notation used for the tangent screen.

FIG. 2-2, A. The arc perimeter.

The arc perimeter shares with the tangent screen the difficulty of achieving appropriate background illumination. Nonetheless, the combination of a tangent screen and an arc perimeter may be of advantage when dealing with feeble or neurologically ill patients, because with both instruments the patient and the examiner are in full view of each other, giving less sense of isolation to the patient than occurs when a bowl perimeter like the Goldmann is used. However, with the bowl perimeter, voice contact is usually sufficient, and the bowl perimeter offers the ability to perform both central and peripheral field tests with the same instrument, as well as the confidence of standardized quantitation.

MANUAL BOWL PROJECTION PERIMETER
The perimeters of Goldmann and Harms

The bowl projection perimeter (Fig. 2-2, *B*) enables the examiner to test both central and peripheral fields with one instrument. The test stimulus is a white spot of light, whose size and intensity can be varied, projected onto an evenly illuminated white bowl. The position of the white spot is controlled manually.

FIG. 2-2, B. The bowl projection perimeter.

The Goldmann perimeter became widely used after it was introduced. The widespread usage of an instrument of standard design brought with it an era of uniform test conditions among clinical offices. The background illumination, test distances, stimulus sizes, and stimulus intensities were all standard. *Testing the Field of Vision,* the predecessor of this book, was aimed mainly at teaching the use of the Goldmann perimeter. Because this perimeter is still in wide usage, and will be for some time, the technical aspects of using it effectively are retained as Part II of this book. Haag-Streit manufactured the original instrument, but copies by other companies (Topcon, Inc., and Marco Equipment, Inc.) have maintained the standard conditions of background intensity, stimulus size, and stimulus intensity. These instruments have been used almost exclusively for kinetic visual field testing, usually augmented with suprathreshold static testing. The Goldmann perimeter can be employed for static *threshold* testing (e.g., as a meridional static cut) but is not used very often for this purpose.

The Harms or Tübingen perimeter (Oculus) is another manually operated projection bowl perimeter. It was designed more specifically to allow meridional static threshold perimetry (the "static cut") to be done in addition to kinetic perimetry. It has been used mainly in specialized academic centers.

A

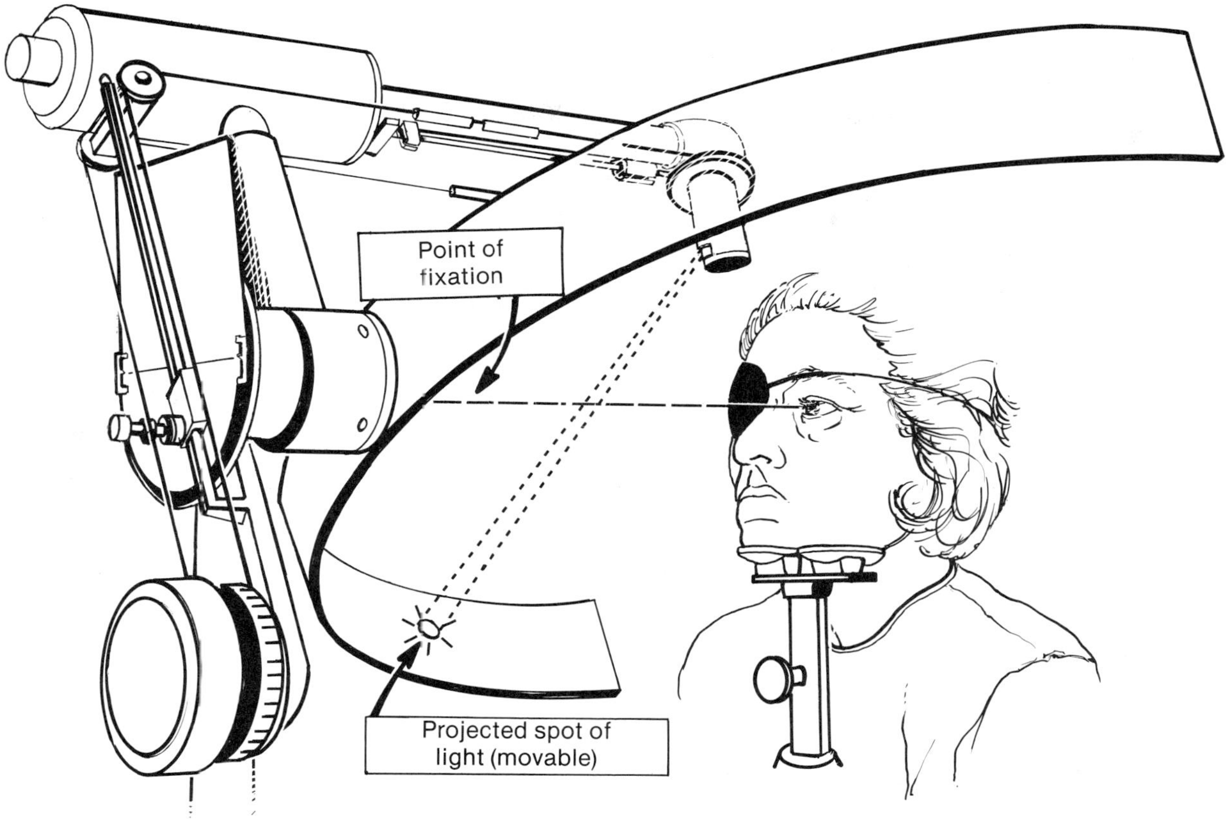

Point of
fixation
Projected spot of
light (movable)

B

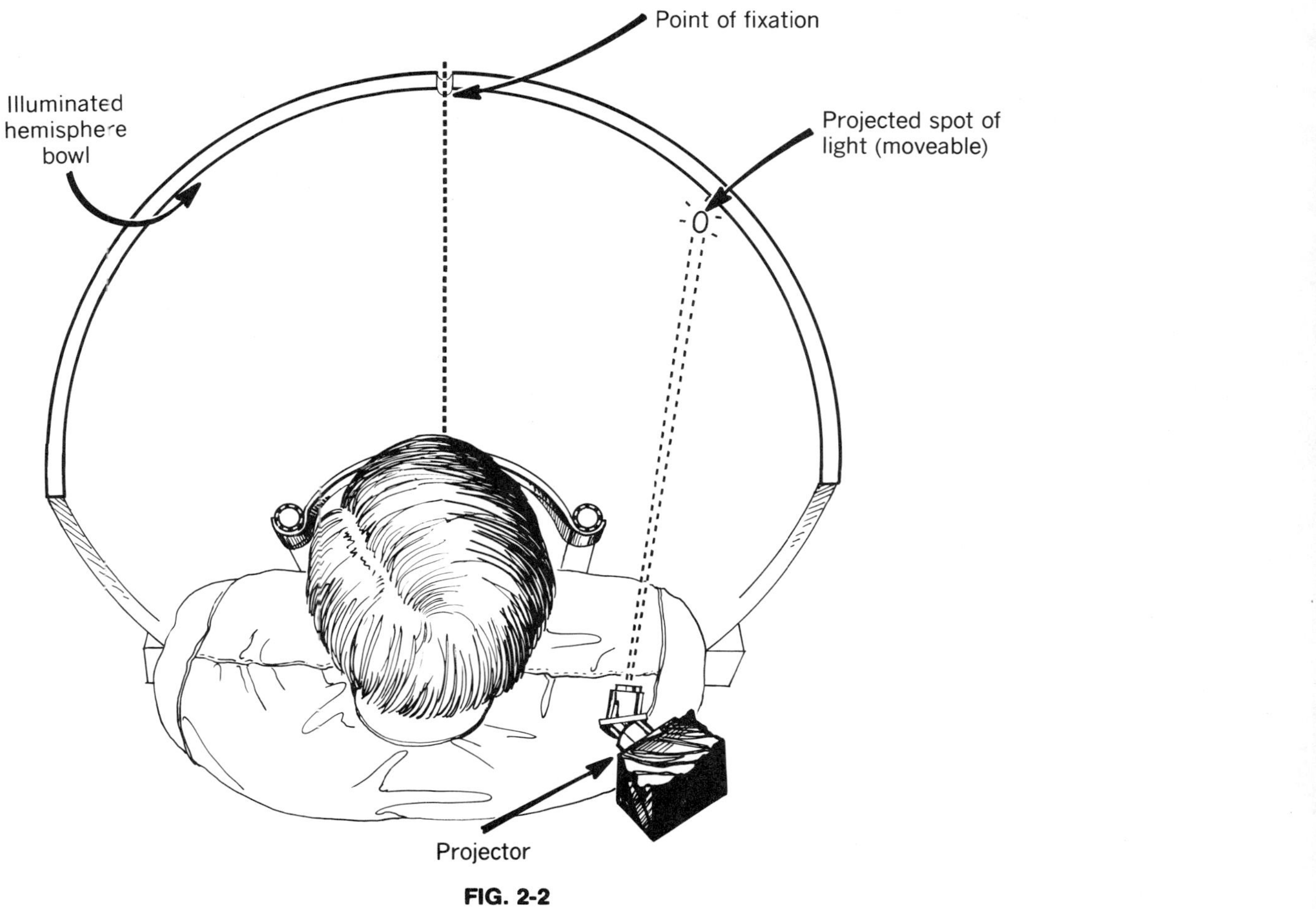

Point of fixation
Illuminated
hemisphere
bowl
Projected spot of
light (moveable)
Projector

FIG. 2-2

Stimulus intensity, the Goldmann standard

The properly calibrated Goldmann perimeter projects a stimulus with maximum luminosity (intensity) of 1000 apostilbs* (asb) onto a background of 31.6 asb. When a light stimulus of lesser intensity is desired, the projected spot is attenuated by neutral-density filters.

The attenuation of light is expressed in logarithmic units, or decibels (dB). One log-unit equals 10 dB (or 0.1 log-unit equals 1 dB). A 1.0 log-unit (10 dB) filter attenuates the light to 1/10 of its original intensity, reducing the stimulus from 1000 asb to 100 asb. Thus a 1.0 log-unit filter allows 10% of the light to be transmitted. A 2.0 log-unit (20 dB) filter reduces the intensity to 1/100 of its original value, from 1000 asb to 10 asb. In other words, it allows 1% transmission of light. Similarly a 3.0 log-unit (30 dB) filter reduces the intensity to 1/1000 of its original value, from 1000 asb to 1 asb (0.1% transmission).

A 0.5 log-unit (5 dB) filter reduces the intensity from 1000 asb to 316 asb (31.6% transmission). If a second 0.5 log-unit filter is placed in the pathway of light, the intensity is attenuated to 100 asb (31.6% of 316 asb). In other words, when two 0.5 log-unit filters are combined, the effect is the same as a 1.0 log-unit filter, attenuating the projected spot from 1000 asb to 100 asb.

---

*The apostilb (asb) is the unit of illuminance of European origin that has been used in quantitative clinical perimetry for decades. It corresponds to 1 lumen per square meter of incident surface. There are several other measurement systems for intensity of light. To achieve international standardization, the currently preferred unit is the candela per square meter (cd/m^2), or the nit. To convert asb to cd/m^2, divide by π (3.14159) or multiply by $1/\pi$ (0.31831). Thus the 1000 asb maximum stimulus intensity of the Goldmann perimeter corresponds to 318.3 cd/m^2, and the 31.6 asb background intensity corresponds to 10.1 cd/m^2.

Logarithmic units (instead of absolute units) of light intensity are used because visual perception seems to relate to ratios between light intensities rather than to differences between them. Thus the sensation related to doubling the intensity from 30 to 60 asb is equivalent to the sensation of doubling the intensity from 300 to 600 asb, even though the latter involves an increase of 300 asb while the former involves an increase of only 30 asb. A practical consequence of using logarithmic units is that graphs of a psychophysical phenomenon such as visual threshold can be made over a wide range (from 1 to 10,000 asb), with the ability to represent small changes of intensity in the low end of the scale (for example, from 10 to 20 asb). Moreover, as illustrated in the previous paragraph, the log values of filters can be easily added together in a meaningful way.

It is not necessary that the clinician or perimetrist be facile with converting asb to log-units or decibels. The reader should, however, recognize that

There is no direct conversion factor between apostilbs and log-units. The conversion between them involves logarithms and exponents.

A decibel is simply 0.1 log-unit (*deci* = tenth), no more, no less.

Apostilbs are absolute units of luminous intensity; thus 315 apostilbs on one instrument is the same as 315 asb on another.

Log-units and decibels are relative; they represent a certain attenuation from the maximum stimulus intensity on a particular instrument. For example, on the Goldmann perimeter the maximum stimulus is 1000 asb and a 5 dB attenuation results in 316 asb. On another instrument, with a 10,000 asb maximal luminous intensity, a 5 dB attenuation is 3160 asb (ten times as much light). **Thus 5 dB on one instrument is not the same as 5 dB on another.**

The reader who will be using the Goldmann perimeter (or an automated instrument that designates stimulus intensity by the Goldmann standard) should also understand the use of filter combinations.

The original Goldmann perimeter provided four stimulus intensities (numbered 1 to 4 respectively) in 0.5 log-unit steps: *stimulus 4,* the most intense, at 1000 asb; *stimulus 3,* attenuated 0.5 log-unit, its intensity at 316 asb; *stimulus 2,* attenuated 1 log-unit, its intensity at 100 asb; and *stimulus 1,* attenuated 1.5 log-units, its intensity at 31.6 asb. In addition, the Goldmann perimeter is now equipped with a series of filters (a to e) in 0.1 log-unit steps: filter *e,* providing no attenuation; filter *d,* 0.1 log-unit attenuation; filter *c,* 0.2 log-unit attenuation; filter *b,* 0.3 log-unit attenuation; and filter *a* 0.4 log-unit attenuation.

When the numbered and lettered filters are used in combination, attenuation in 0.1 log-unit steps up to 1.9 log-units is as follows (see Table 2-1):

Filter combination 4e gives 0.0 log-unit attenuation (1000 asb)
Filter combination 4d gives 0.1 log-unit attenuation (800 asb)
Filter combination 4c gives 0.2 log-unit attenuation (630 asb)
Filter combination 4b gives 0.3 log-unit attenuation (500 asb)
Filter combination 4a gives 0.4 log-unit attenuation (400 asb)
Filter combination 3e gives 0.5 log-unit attenuation (320 asb)
Filter combination 3d gives 0.6 log-unit attenuation (250 asb)
Filter combination 3c gives 0.7 log-unit attenuation (200 asb)
↗ ↖ ↑
(0.5 + 0.2 = 0.7)

. . .

Filter combination 1a gives 1.9 log-unit attenuation (13 asb)

For the rare occasion when more than 1.9 log-units of attenuation is required, some recent models of the Goldmann perimeter are equipped with a third set of filters, allowing an additional 2.0 or 4.0 log-unit light reduction. In these cases the notation used calls for a bar to be placed over the number-letter combination when the 2.0 log-unit filter is used and a double bar when the 4.0 log-unit filter is used. Thus $\overline{4e}$ represents 2.0 log-units of attenuation (10 asb), $\overline{4d}$ represents 2.1 log-units of attenuation (8 asb), and so on.

Table 2-1. Notation of stimulus intensity (Goldmann perimeter, maximum stimulus 1000 asb, background 31.6 asb)

Filter combination	Attenuation		Intensity (apostilbs)
	Log units	Decibels	
4e	0.0	0	1000
4d	0.1	1	800
4c	0.2	2	630
4b	0.3	3	500
4a	0.4	4	400
3e	0.5	5	320
3d	0.6	6	250
3c	0.7	7	200
3b	0.8	8	160
3a	0.9	9	130
2e	1.0	10	100
2d	1.1	11	80
2c	1.2	12	63
2b	1.3	13	50
2a	1.4	14	40
1e	1.5	15	32
1d	1.6	16	25
1c	1.7	17	20
1b	1.8	18	16
1a	1.9	19	13
$\overline{4e}$	2.0	20	10
$\overline{4d}$	2.1	21	8
$\overline{4c}$	2.2	22	6
$\overline{4b}$	2.3	23	5
$\overline{4a}$	2.4	24	4
$\overline{3e}$	2.5	25	3.2
$\overline{3d}$	2.6	26	2.5
$\overline{3c}$	2.7	27	2.0
$\overline{3b}$	2.8	28	1.6
$\overline{3a}$	2.9	29	1.3
$\overline{2e}$	3.0	30	1.0
$\overline{2d}$	3.1	31	0.8
$\overline{2c}$	3.2	32	0.6
$\overline{2b}$	3.3	33	0.5
$\overline{2a}$	3.4	34	0.4

Stimulus size, the Goldmann standard

The projected spot is not exactly circular, so the size of the stimulus is expressed primarily not in terms of diameter or arc of intercept but in terms of area. Of course, it is the apparent size as degrees of arc of intercept (not the real size) that relates to visibility; thus if comparison is made with stimuli on other instruments, the fixed viewing distance of 30 cm on the Goldmann perimeter must be taken into account. Professor Goldmann used a notation in Roman numerals to define six standard sizes:

0 = 0.0625 (1/16) mm^2 at 30 cm (average diameter, 0.05 degree)
I = 0.25 (1/4) mm^2 at 30 cm (average diameter, 0.11 degree)
II = 1 mm^2 at 30 cm (average diameter, 0.22 degree)
III = 4 mm^2 at 30 cm (average diameter, 0.43 degree)
IV = 16 mm^2 at 30 cm (average diameter, 0.86 degree)
V = 64 mm^2 at 30 cm (average diameter, 1.72 degrees)

The complete notation for the stimulus includes both the size (in Roman numerals) and the intensity (in terms of filter combination). Thus a stimulus may be represented as I-3e,* II-4e, V-4e, etc. The standard for manual perimetry (but not for automated perimetry, see p. 43) established by Goldmann is to use size I. Larger sizes (II through V) are used only when a I-4 is not a strong enough stimulus to quantify an abnormal region, and then the larger sizes are used only with intensity 4. At the other end of the scale, size 0 is used only when a I-1 stimulus is too strong for detailed testing near the fovea and the 2.0 log-unit filter is not available (see Chapter 23).

---

*Denoted verbally by saying "one-three-eee."

Goldmann selected these size-increment steps based on the fact that, in terms of visibility, quadrupling the area (doubling the diameter) is *roughly* the psychophysical equivalent of increasing the intensity by 0.5 log-unit. (The exact relationship between size and intensity is different in different parts of the retina.) Thus an intensity change from I-3e to I-4e is about the same as a size change from I-4e to II-4e, which keeps consecutive isopters about the same distance apart. Also an *increase* in size from I to II balances a *decrease* in intensity from 4e to 3e. Therefore I-4e is roughly the psychophysical equivalent of II-3e, and also of III-2e. However, as noted, the larger sizes are not standardly used with the weaker stimuli in manual perimetry.

FIG. 2-3. Standard sequence of stimulus strengths for the Goldmann perimeter.

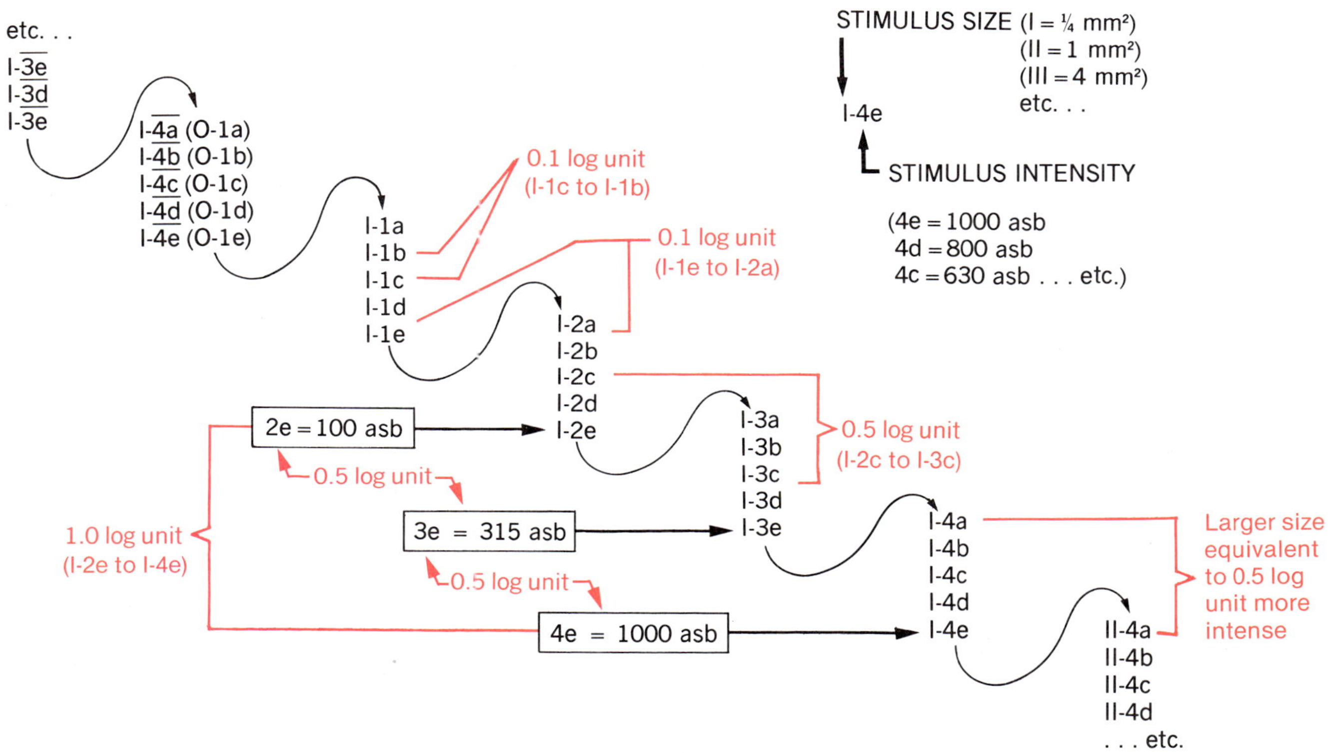
etc. . .
I-3e
I-3d
I-3e
I-4a (O-1a)
I-4b (O-1b)
I-4c (O-1c)
I-4d (O-1d)
I-4e (O-1e)
I-1a
I-1b
I-1c
I-1d
I-1e
0.1 log unit
(I-1c to I-1b)
0.1 log unit
(I-1e to I-2a)
I-2a
I-2b
I-2c
I-2d
I-2e
2e = 100 asb
0.5 log unit
I-3a
I-3b
I-3c
I-3d
I-3e
0.5 log unit
(I-2c to I-3c)
1.0 log unit
(I-2e to I-4e)
3e = 315 asb
0.5 log unit
4e = 1000 asb
I-4a
I-4b
I-4c
I-4d
I-4e
II-4a
II-4b
II-4c
II-4d
. . . etc.
Larger size equivalent to 0.5 log unit more intense
STIMULUS SIZE (I = ¼ mm²)
(II = 1 mm²)
(III = 4 mm²)
etc. . .
I-4e
STIMULUS INTENSITY
(4e = 1000 asb
4d = 800 asb
4c = 630 asb . . . etc.)

FIG. 2-3

ADDITIONAL READING

The original description of the bowl perimeters of Goldmann and Harms and the original scientific studies that form the basis of quantitative perimetry with these instruments are found in the following articles:

Goldmann, H.: Lichtsinn mit besonderer Berücksichtigung der Perimetrie, Ophthalmologica **158:**362-386, 1969.

Goldmann, H.: Demonstration unseres neuen Projektionskugel-perimeters samt theoretischen und klinischen Bemerkungen über Perimetrie, Ophthalmologica **111:**187-192, 1946.

Goldmann, H.: Grundlagen exakter Perimetrie, Ophthalmologica **109:**57-70, 1945.

Goldmann, H.: Ein selbstregistrierendes Projektionskugelperimeter, Ophthalmologica **109:**71-79, 1945.

Harms, H.: Die Technik der statischen Perimetrie, Ophthalmologica **158:**387-405, 1969.

Harms, H.: Die Bedeutung einer einheitlichen Prüfweise aller Sehfunktionen, Ber. Dtsch. Ophthalmol. Ges. **63:**281-285, 1960.

Harms, H.: Entwicklungsmöglichkeiten der Perimetrie, Albrecht von Graefes Arch. Klin. Exp. Ophthalmol. **150:**28-57, 1950.

Sloan, L.L.: Area and luminance of test object as variables in examination of the visual field by projection perimetry, Vision Res. **1:**121-138, 1960.

AUTOMATED (COMPUTERIZED) PERIMETERS
Suprathreshold and threshold testing

A number of rather different automated perimeters have emerged in the last decade. Some have already disappeared from the market place. Others are proving to be remarkably convenient and useful, and each year brings new instruments that may or may not prove practical.

Although some instruments have the mechanical ability to provide kinetic stimuli, none are now programmed to do so automatically. The instruments all utilize static stimuli and fall into two main classes: those capable of both static threshold and suprathreshold perimetry and those that utilize only suprathreshold static perimetry.

Instruments capable of static threshold perimetry (full thresholding) in addition to suprathreshold static perimetry include:

OCTOPUS, MODELS 201, 500, AND 2000. The Octopus (so named because the original model had a selection of eight programs) is a projection perimeter designed and updated by an expert Swiss group. It has an increasing selection of programs and improved capabilities.

HUMPHREY FIELD ANALYZER. This increasingly popular automated projection perimeter is updated periodically with replaceable chips as improved programs develop. Like the Octopus, it has an increasing selection of programs and capabilities.

DICON AUTOPERIMETER. The Dicon (CooperVision) differs from the Humphrey and the Octopus in that it uses light emitting diodes (LEDs) for stimulus presentation instead of a projected white spot. It is upgradable as new programs develop. The emphasis has been on screening programs, but the instrument now has a fully quantifying program for the central field. Its capability can be increased when programmed by the manufacturer to do so.

COMPETER. This is the Swedish Krakau instrument, with an imaginative and very rapid thresholding strategy. It uses LEDs mounted in a flat plane and tests only the central field.

DIGILAB 350. This is an authorized American copy of the Competer, with modifications.

DIGILAB 750. This new perimeter, based on the Competer's methodology, uses LEDs behind the diffusing surface of the perimeter bowl (''rear projection''). It is operated through an IBM personal computer.

FIELDMASTER 300. This instrument (the Squid) is an expensive projection perimeter marketed to compete with the original Octopus 201. It can be programmed by the user.

FIELDMASTER 275. This smaller and less expensive version of the Squid has just entered the market place.

FIELDMASTER 50. This unit presents stimuli with 262 LEDs. Suprathreshold screening is standard, and full threshold programs are optional.

Instruments that utilize suprathreshold static perimetry exclusively include the following:

FIELDMASTER 101R, 101PR, AND 200. The stimuli are delivered to the bowl surface from behind through a fiberoptic cable. This instrument is capable of one-level screening at 99 or 133 points.

FIELDMASTER 225. A similar perimeter with the ability to use threshold-related stimuli at 149 locations, this instrument has a limited threshold capability (static cuts along four meridians).

AUTOMATIC TANGENT SCREEN, MODELS 1, 1A, AND 2000. This very inexpensive instrument tests the central field with one-level screening.

DICON AP 200. Only slightly more expensive than the Automatic Tangent Screen, this unit has threshold-related strategy to test 196 locations.

PERIMAT 206. This unit (the Rodenstock) is capable of threshold-related screening at some or all of 206 locations served by LEDs.

TÜBINGEN AUTOMATIC PERIMETER (OCULUS). This unit has threshold-related screening capability, with stimuli delivered through fiberoptics to 249 locations.

TOPCON COMPUTERIZED PERIMETER SBP-1000. This unit presents stimuli by means of 257 LEDs.

To accomplish full thresholding, perimeters in the first category present stimuli of various intensities in specific locations. The patient pushes a button for the computer to record which stimuli are seen and which are not. The intensity of a stimulus presented at a given location is decreased from a previous presentation if the patient saw the previous stimulus at that location, and vice versa. This requires a computer decision based on the accumulated responses of the patient. When threshold has been determined at all locations, the results are printed out and, in some instruments, may be stored on a disk for future reference. Some instruments also make calculations of the patient's consistency of responses, average sensitivity, changes from one time to another, differences from normal values, and so on.

For static suprathreshold testing the task is easier. Stimuli of a selected intensity are presented in a prescribed sequence of locations, and the perimeter simply records for each location whether the stimulus was seen or not.

Background illumination

Not all the automated instruments use the same intensity of background illumination. For the Octopus a background of 4 apostilbs has been selected, which is less intense than used in either the Goldmann (32 asb) or the Harms (10 asb) manual perimeter. The reason for using the dimmer background is that a stimulus of a given intensity is more visible against a dim background than it is against a bright background. The enhanced perception, in effect, gives a stronger psychophysical value to the strongest stimulus that the machine is capable of producing, and this is of help in quantifying severe visual field defects. The disadvantage of a dimmer background is that the retinal illumination may no longer be in the photopic (light-adapted) range with smaller pupil size. If this happens, any variation in pupil size may affect visual threshold and responses may become more variable.

For most other automated instruments the Goldmann standard of a 32 asb background is kept. Some instruments use a standard 32 asb background but allow other intensities to be selected for special purposes.

Stimulus size

In kinetic perimetry both the size and the intensity of a stimulus are adjusted to achieve a range of isopters. Size I is used except when larger sizes are required to quantify severely abnormal regions.

In threshold static perimetry the size is kept fixed and only the intensity is changed. Most automated perimeters use a standard 4 mm^2 stimulus size, equivalent to Goldmann size III, because the smaller size I at maximum intensity is not a strong enough stimulus to quantify the depth of defects (although some perimeters allow use of sizes larger or smaller than size III for special purposes). Size III has the additional advantage that its visibility is less affected by refractive errors than that of size I. It has the disadvantage that light scatter is greater; thus a bright stimulus presented to a blind area of the retina may be perceived by an adjacent seeing area into which the excessive light scatters. This scatter is not so great a problem that it outweighs the advantages of size III. However, size V is not standardly used because it has an even greater scatter and because it is also larger than some of the scotomas one may wish to detect. (Stimulus size V intercepts about 1.7 degrees, a little less than half the horizontal diameter of the blind spot. Size III intercepts 0.43 degree, about ⅑ the diameter of the blind spot.) Note that in perimeters with a bowl radius other than 30 cm, the area (in square millimeters) of the projected spot must be adjusted to maintain equivalence with the Goldmann size III.

In perimeters that use light-emitting diodes (LEDs) or fiberoptic cables the stimulus size is not adjustable but is fixed by the size of the light source, which may not correspond exactly to one of the standard Goldmann sizes.

Stimulus intensity

In perimeters that use uncovered LEDs the stimulus intensity is simply the intensity of light produced by the LED.

In projection perimeters the total luminous intensity in the spot of light is the intensity of the background plus the additional light projected as a stimulus. However, the stimulus intensity is standardly expressed simply as the amount of light (in apostilbs) projected onto the existing background, because it is not the absolute intensity but the difference between the spot and the surrounding "background" that is relevant to the visual perception tested in perimetry.

When expressed in apostilbs, the measure of stimulus intensity is in absolute units. A 600 asb stimulus, for example, will be the same on all perimeters. However, decibels and log-units are relative units of measure. When the stimulus intensity is expressed in decibels (dB), stimuli of two perimeters of the same decibel value are identical only if the maximum stimuli of the two instruments are the same. Between two of the more popular existing instruments, for example, the Humphrey Field Analyzer has a maximum stimulus of 10,000 asb whereas the unattenuated stimulus of the Octopus is 1000 asb. Thus a 20 dB stimulus of the Octopus perimeter is 10 asb while a 20 dB stimulus on the Humphrey is 100 asb—ten times as much light.

Note, however, that when comparing the *visibility* of stimuli it must be kept in mind that the background is eight times more intense (32 asb vs. 4 asb) in the Humphrey instrument, reducing the visual effectiveness of the ten-times brighter stimulus.

Comparison of stimulus values

For the visual field to be quantified (i.e., the visual threshold to be measured at a selection of representative locations), it is necessary that the range of available stimulus values ("dynamic range" of the instrument) include (1) the normal range of threshold values from the fovea to the periphery and (2) a range of stronger stimuli with which the threshold can be determined in areas of defective sensation.

To avoid the problems associated with a stronger light bulb, Goldmann did not include stimuli more intense than 1000 apostilbs but instead provided larger sizes to be used when the I-4e stimulus was not adequately strong to quantify the threshold in a defective area. This solution was adequate for isopter plots, but for static threshold perimetry it is preferable to change only one variable (intensity) while keeping the other variable (size) constant.

Three methods to keep the size constant and yet provide strong visual stimuli in automated perimeters have been mentioned in the preceding three sections: use of a dim background (enhancing the contrast of the surround with the light stimulus), use of a larger standard stimulus size (with weaker stimuli being provided by a denser set of filters), and use of a stronger light source (a solvable engineering problem). Various designers and manufacturers have different reasons for selecting one or a combination of these three methods, with the result that the industry does not have a standard for the important stimulus variables in visual field testing.

It is unfortunate that no reliable conversion formula is possible for establishing the equivalence of stimulus values of the various perimeters. The conversion factor to correct the intensity values for a difference in size depends on retinal location (and other factors) and may not be the same in defective areas as it is in normal areas. A given ratio of stimulus intensity to background intensity has a fixed visibility (Weber's law) only if the background is sufficient to provide photopic retinal adaptation; thus an equivalence established at one pupil size may not hold for a different pupil size if the background is dim. The stimulus intensity of an uncovered LED is expressed as the total light intensity of the LED stimulus; but for projection perimeters the stimulus is expressed as intensity of light added to the existing background, not as the total intensity of the stimulus. LED instruments also differ from projection perimeters by having a nonwhite color and by the fact that in some instruments when the stimulus is off the test site is dark rather than like the surrounding bowl illuminance. In addition, the threshold values obtained are affected to some degree by the details of the bracketing strategy used to determine threshold. For all these reasons, it is not possible to make a completely accurate conversion of threshold values between two instruments.

Suprathreshold testing

In its simplest form, suprathreshold testing consists of presenting a test stimulus of a selected size and intensity at 75 to 150 points in various positions within the central 30 degrees. This method is the original Armaly screening method; and in manual perimetry one might, for example, spot-check specified locations with the I-2e or I-3e stimulus (see Chapters 21 and 22).

With an automated perimeter a test stimulus size and intensity might similarly be selected. Often this is a standard stimulus that should be comfortably visible over the region to be tested, perhaps taking into account the patient's age. It is important that the stimulus not be too strong, lest it be seen in a mildly defective region and the presence of an abnormality not be detected.

The task of an automated perimeter is simply to present the stimuli in selected locations and record to which presentation the patient responds. Everyone will occasionally fail to respond to a stimulus because of a blink, a lapse of attention, etc. Therefore it is routine whenever a person fails to respond to a stimulus presentation that its location be later tested again before the conclusion is drawn that the stimulus is not seen there. The confirmation with a second stimulus presentation is sometimes omitted if several adjacent points are missed, because the missed responses at adjacent points serve to confirm each other (see p. 418).

When the same stimulus is used everywhere in the region to be tested, the test is called a *one-level* suprathreshold screen. There are two important modifications of the one-level suprathreshold strategy with a standard stimulus. They are (1) use of a *threshold-related* stimulus instead of a standard stimulus and (2) use of *eccentricity compensation* instead of a one-level screening. Either or both of these modifications may be used in various automated programs.

The **threshold-related strategy** uses a stimulus appropriate to the overall height of the individual patient's own hill of vision. This is accomplished by an actual threshold determination at one or several points within the field. The stimulus to be used to spot-check the central field is selected to be slightly brighter than the threshold at the edge of the region to be tested. It is thus related to the threshold of the specific individual (i.e., "threshold related"). This strategy enhances the likelihood of detecting places where the sensitivity is mildly reduced. Also, if the field has a generalized depression, the use of a threshold-related stimulus allows a superimposed local defect to be detected and thereby enhances the diagnostic specificity of finding a field abnormality. If a standard-for-age stimulus were used in the presence of a generalized depression, possibly all points would be abnormal and a distinction could not be made between a pure generalized depression without localized defects and a generalized depression with superimposed localized defects. With the threshold-related stimulus a generalized depression (with or without additional local defects) is recognized by the threshold values obtained at the initial test location. In manual perimetry, use of a threshold-related stimulus is accomplished by plotting an isopter and testing within the isopter for scotomas (Chapter 18). Specifically, in testing the central field for glaucomatous defects the stimulus is selected by determining threshold (statically or kinetically) at 25 to 30 degrees temporally (Chapter 21).

When **eccentricity compensation** is used, the stimulus intensity is adjusted for different distances from fixation. The stimulus used near fixation is a certain amount brighter (e.g., 3 to 5 dB) than the anticipated threshold in the region around fixation. Further away a more intense stimulus is used, one that is the same amount (3 to 5 dB) brighter than the threshold anticipated at the more eccentric location. In the crudest form of eccentricity compensation the stimulus is adjusted into two broad regions: one for the central 30 degrees and one, 0.5 or 1.0 log-unit more intense, for the peripheral areas. Greater sensitivity is achieved if the field is subdivided into several concentric regions or the stimulus intensity is adjusted continuously at every eccentricity according to the normal shape of the hill of vision.

The reason for using eccentricity compensation is that a stimulus chosen to be clearly visible at 30 degrees (say, 4 dB brighter than threshold at 30 degrees) will be 14 dB brighter than threshold at fixation (which is about 10 dB more sensitive than the region near 30 degrees). Even if there is a shallow (say, up to 10 dB deep) local defect near fixation, the stimulus used in the one-level method may be seen, because it is 14 dB brighter than the normal threshold there and is thus 4 dB brighter than the threshold in the 10 dB deep defect. Eccentricity compensation is difficult to achieve in manual perimetry, but is easily accomplished by computerized machines, and can be used routinely because it does not add to the time of performing the test.

Static threshold perimetry

To measure visual threshold at a location in the field, a minimum of two stimulus presentations must be used. It is necessary to present one stimulus that can be seen and another slightly weaker one that cannot be seen. In this way the weakest visible stimulus (threshold) has been determined. This is equivalent to measuring visual acuity: to say that the visual acuity is 20/40, it is necessary to determine that the 20/40 line can be read *and* that the 20/30 line cannot. Of course, because we do not know in advance what the threshold value will be, it takes several stimulus presentations (six on the average) to find the limit between visibility and invisibility.

In traditional manual static perimetry, as with the Harms perimeter, threshold is determined by the *method of limits*. A stimulus too dim to be seen is presented. Subsequently, stimuli in 0.1 log-unit steps of increasing intensity are presented until one is seen. The first one seen is recorded as the dimmest stimulus visible (the lower limit of visibility). Some of the technical details of accomplishing this test are touched on in Part II of this book (Chapter 23).

In automated perimetry a bracketing or "staircase" strategy is used. Stimuli are first presented in large steps (e.g., 0.4 log-unit) until the boundary from invisibility to visibility (or vice versa) is crossed. This brackets the general range of luminosity that contains the threshold value. Then, going back and forth with smaller increments of luminous intensity, the threshold is more accurately determined. The various automated strategies differ with regard to how it is determined when the end point has been reached and with regard to the interval of luminosity (2 dB to 5 dB) used in the final steps. These details affect how long the test takes, as well as the precision of the threshold value obtained and its reproducibility on retesting. However, the strategy used is beyond the control of the user and he must depend on the manufacturer for a reasonable compromise between accuracy and the time required to perform the test.

The threshold is not necessarily completely determined at one location before moving on to another. Rather, consecutive stimulus presentations are made at different locations. However, when the sequence returns to a given spot, the stimulus presented is either brighter or dimmer than the previous one shown at that location depending on the previously recorded responses at that spot.

The number of stimulus presentations required at a given location to come in on the threshold value depends partly on how close to threshold the stimulus is at first presentation. Several methods are used to reduce the time required for the visual field test by anticipating the threshold at each spot as well as possible. One estimate is the normal threshold value for the age of that person. This method provides a good estimate for nearly normal fields, but not so good for those with more severe defects. Another estimate is the threshold determined on the previous visual field examination in that individual. This method is particularly useful for abnormal fields but depends on the instrument's having the capability of storing and retrieving the previous test results. Another method (called *prethresholding*), effective for both normal and abnormal fields, is to determine threshold completely at one point in each quadrant and then use the value obtained at each spot as a starting point for determining threshold at the several immediately adjacent points; the values at those spots are then used as starting points for the next series of surrounding spots, and so on. This method utilizes the fact that an abnormal spot is likely to be surrounded by other abnormal spots while normal spots are likely to have other normal spots adjacent.

Interactive strategies

One of the things a skilled manual perimetrist does is use information about the seeming nature of the visual field as it is being revealed in an individual to modify the technique as the test proceeds. Thus, seemingly abnormal areas may be outlined in more detail than normal regions and responses may be rechecked if out of keeping with responses at adjacent points.

Some automated perimetric programs have begun similarly to make use of information as it unfolds. The simplest is the semiquantitation or quantitation of abnormal points in suprathreshold testing. For semiquantitation, if a suprathreshold stimulus is not seen the spot is retested with a maximum stimulus. A rough degree of relative or absolute abnormality is thus quantified. By way of analogy with visual acuity testing, a person who could not see the 20/40 line might be shown the 20/400 line. Depending on his responses, his acuity might be classified as normal (20/40 or better), moderately abnormal (between 20/40 and 20/400), or severely abnormal (worse than 20/400).

Some automated threshold programs do a more careful quantitation of abnormal points. At any point where the suprathreshold stimulus is not seen, threshold is determined accurately by the visual bracketing method, not just semiquantified. Thus points are first classified as normal or abnormal by suprathreshold testing, and then threshold is determined at the abnormal points (but not at the normal ones). Such a program takes more time than the usual suprathreshold program if there are many abnormal points, but it remains quicker than a full thresholding program if many of the points have a normal threshold.

Another interactive strategy in suprathreshold testing is the automatic testing of a closer grid of points within an apparently abnormal area. Thus, if one or two points are missed, additional locations between and around these points may be tested.

For full threshold programs one interactive strategy has already been described, namely the prethresholding of selected points to have a more accurate starting point for thresholding of the next series of spots to be tested. Another is the routine retesting of any point whose threshold values are out of keeping with the threshold of surrounding points; this helps to confirm small or shallow scotomas and nasal steps. A future advance that can be expected in automated perimetry is the further use of interactive strategies to examine areas of interest in the field more accurately and more rapidly.

Pattern of test points

Already it is apparent that the use of an automated perimeter may have many choices with regard to the field test. First, there is a choice of suprathreshold or threshold strategies. For the former the choice may be subdivided into the use or nonuse of threshold-related stimuli, eccentricity compensation, or both. The use of interactive strategies is another option. There may be the option of using a nonstandard background intensity, stimulus size, or (for suprathreshold testing) stimulus intensity for special purposes. The number of possible combinations is quite large and is increased by still other program options.

Among these other options are several (sometimes too many) choices with regard to the number and location of points to be tested, but not all patterns are available on every machine.

A frequently used pattern is an evenly spaced grid of points 6 degrees apart (6-degree resolution) that blankets the central 30 degrees of the field. Sometimes the grid is so aligned that it includes the point of fixation (program 31 or 33 of the Octopus, 30-1 or 30-3 of the Humphrey instrument). Alternatively, the grid may be offset 3 degrees horizontally and vertically, which is more useful because it allows points above and below the horizontal meridian to be compared when looking for a nasal step, and for points to the right and left of the vertical meridian to be compared when looking for a hemianopia.

The number of points to be tested is an important consideration, because it relates to the length of time the test takes. A grid of points 6 degrees apart may seem to leave too much space between the points tested; but to perform a full static threshold determination on a pattern of points only 3 degrees apart would take twice as long, without doubling the number of defects that would be detected and effectively quantified. Moreover, such a test performed on both eyes would often exceed the test time that could be tolerated by the usual elderly glaucoma patient.

The consensus seems to be that for threshold tests about 75 points in the central field is both acceptably thorough and acceptably brief (20 to 25 minutes per eye) for the typical clinical needs. For suprathreshold tests the same number of points gives a nicely rapid (5 minutes per eye) and accurate test. The number of points tested could be doubled, which would only double the test time and perhaps add a useful percent to the detection rate (but *not* double it). If more than 150 points are tested by the suprathreshold method, the return per additional test time diminishes even more and the question can be raised whether it might not be a better investment of time to test fewer points (75) more thoroughly by full thresholding.

An intermediate approach is to test the entire central field with a wide (6 degrees apart) grid and then test any confirmed suspicious or uncertain areas with a closer grid. Perhaps even better is to use from the onset a specifically designed pattern of points—for example, a pattern for glaucoma that has more closely spaced stimuli around fixation (where defects may be small and, in any event, are of more serious import) and around the nasal meridian (where defects are most frequent) but more widely spaced test points elsewhere in the field.

Other components of test program

Automated programs may also (routinely or as an option) perform "catch trials." To catch false-positive responses (in which the patient responds to a light he did not see), the machine may make all the sounds of presenting a stimulus but not actually do so, ultimately reporting the proportion of times the patient responds to a nonpresentation. To catch false-negative responses, a bright stimulus is presented in a known seeing region of the field and the number of times the patient fails to respond to it is recorded.

Another maneuver is to repeat the threshold determination at a selected number of points and record the variability of threshold measurements in the individual. Some programs (used to test a small region very carefully) determine threshold more than once at a limited number of test spots, recording the average of the measurements as threshold and also recording the variability of measurement at each location (as the standard deviation). (See Figs. 11-1 and 14-1 for some examples.)

All told, there are dozens of combinations of program options. Most practitioners eventually come down to using one or two programs or combinations routinely and a handful of others occasionally. Among all the available combinations, only half a dozen end up in the repertoire of a given office. (For further discussion, see Chapter 11 and p. 340.)

Printouts

The results of the field test are presented in various forms, related to the type of test performed.

For suprathreshold testing, the points are indicated with one symbol if the stimulus was seen and with another if the stimulus was not seen. If defective points are semiquantified, symbols are used to show which locations have relative abnormality and which have absolute loss (to the maximum stimulus available). If full threshold quantitation is performed on points missed with suprathreshold testing, then the defective points may be marked with the depth of the defect (number of decibels below the expected threshold value) or the numeric value of the stimulus found to be threshold. (Sometimes, as in programs 33 and 34 of the Octopus, the presumed normal points on suprathreshold testing are assigned a threshold value that is normal for that person's age. In such a printout the examiner must think carefully to distinguish points where threshold was actually measured from points that were artificially assigned the normal value without full testing.)

FIG. 2-4. Examples of suprathreshold test results.
A, Semiquantified field. Different symbols show normal points, those that are relatively defective, and those that have absolute defects (are insensitive to the maximum stimulus).
B, Suprathreshold test with quantitation of abnormal points. Each point is labeled as normal, or else a numeric value is given that represents the sensitivity expressed as the number of decibels below the expected value. The higher the number, the more abnormal is the point.

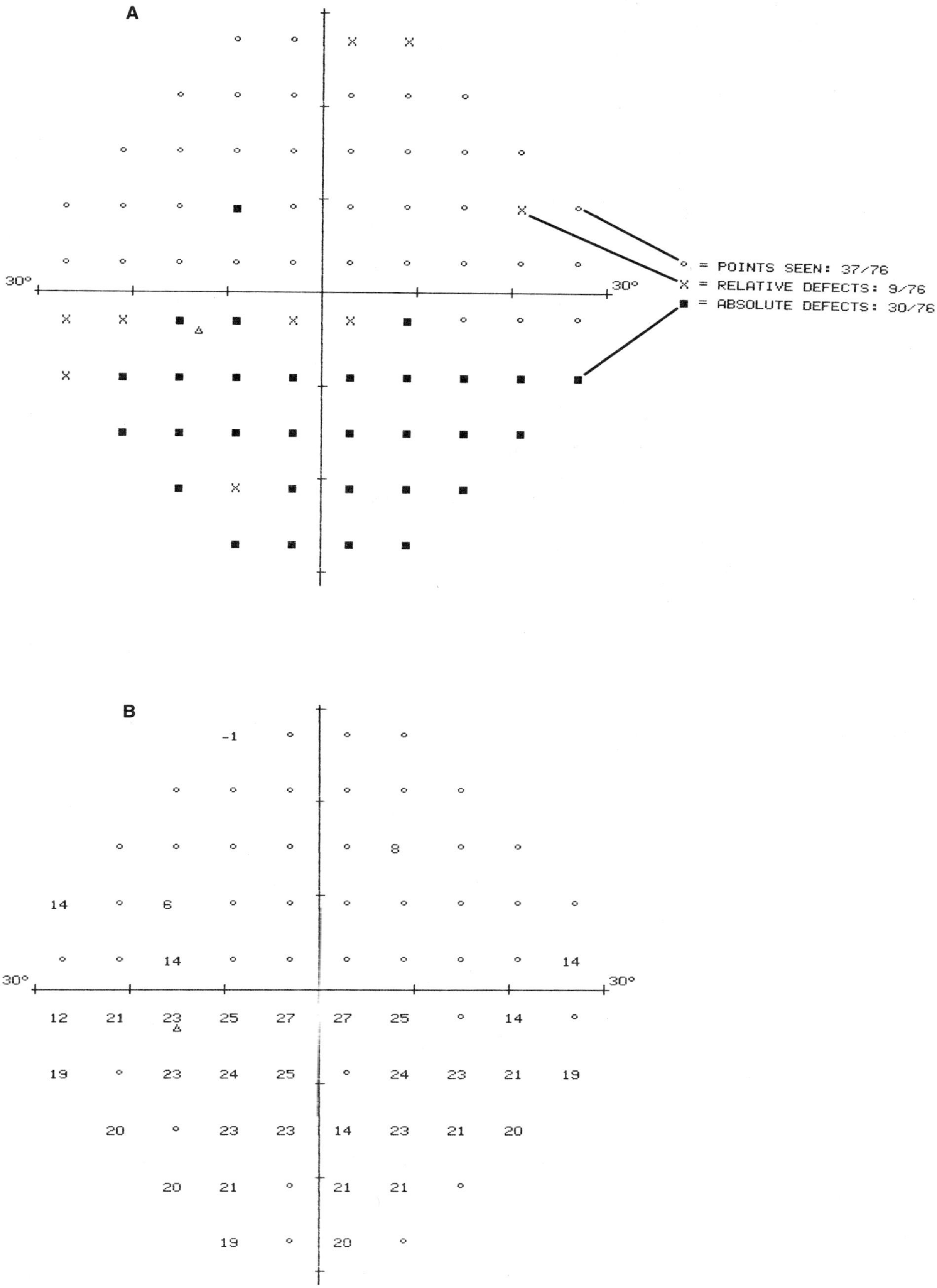
A
30°
30°
= POINTS SEEN: 37/76
X = RELATIVE DEFECTS: 9/76
■ = ABSOLUTE DEFECTS: 30/76
B
30°
30°

FIG. 2-4

For threshold quantitation a typical printout displays a map of the field on which are printed the threshold values in decibels. Both numbers may be given in places where the threshold was measured twice. To supplement this basic report, a greyscale printout is provided in which symbols of differing size are printed according to the threshold value. In most common greyscale printouts many more spots are represented than were actually tested. For the purpose of the printout, intermediate points are assigned values interpolated from nearby points that were actually tested. In such diagrams the contour of the hill of vision and the presence of any defective areas are often obvious at a glance, but they are not a substitute for the record of actual threshold values.

The printout also shows other information obtained during the test, such as the proportion of false-negative and false-positive catch trials, the variability of duplicate threshold measurements, and the proportion of time that fixation was not maintained (see Fig. 13-12).

FIG. 2-5. Report of threshold values and corresponding greyscale. The central 30 degrees was tested. To show the variability of threshold determination in this particular patient, two numeric values appear at locations that were tested twice. A threshold value of 0 indicates that the strongest stimulus was not seen, and the corresponding points are entirely black on the greyscale printout. The arrows denote the meridian along which a static cut is shown in Fig. 2-6.

Instruments with threshold capabilities will also provide some kind of graphic representation of a meridional static cut, representing a vertical slice through the hill of vision.

FIG. 2-6. Static cut printout of the 135- to 315-degree meridian in Fig. 2-5. See Fig. 5-4 for another example.

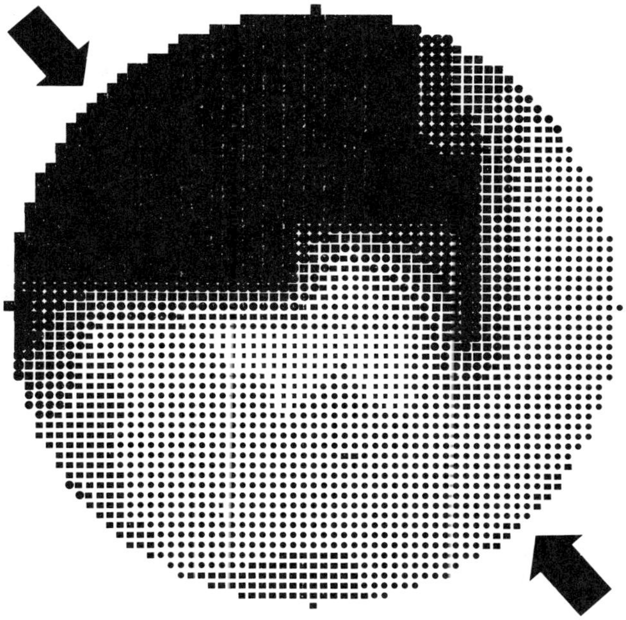

0 0 0 0
0 0

0 0 0 0 0 8

0 0 0 0 0 0 0 18
0

0 0 0 0 0 0 0 0 21 21
0

0 0 0 0 0 24 12 0 22 23

0 21 22 27 26 26 26 0 24 23
6 25

12 19 23 24 25 26 27 19 25 24
27 25

20 22 23 25 20 22 23 23
25

23 26 23 23 25 24
22

20 19 19 24

Symb.	::::	::::	::::	::::	::::	::::	::::	::::	■
dB	51–36	35–31	30–26	25–21	20–16	15–11	10–6	5–1	0
asb	0,008–0,25	0,31–0,8	1–2,5	3,1–8	10–25	31–80	100–250	315–800	1000

1 asb = 0,318 cd/m²

OCTOPUS®

FIG. 2-5

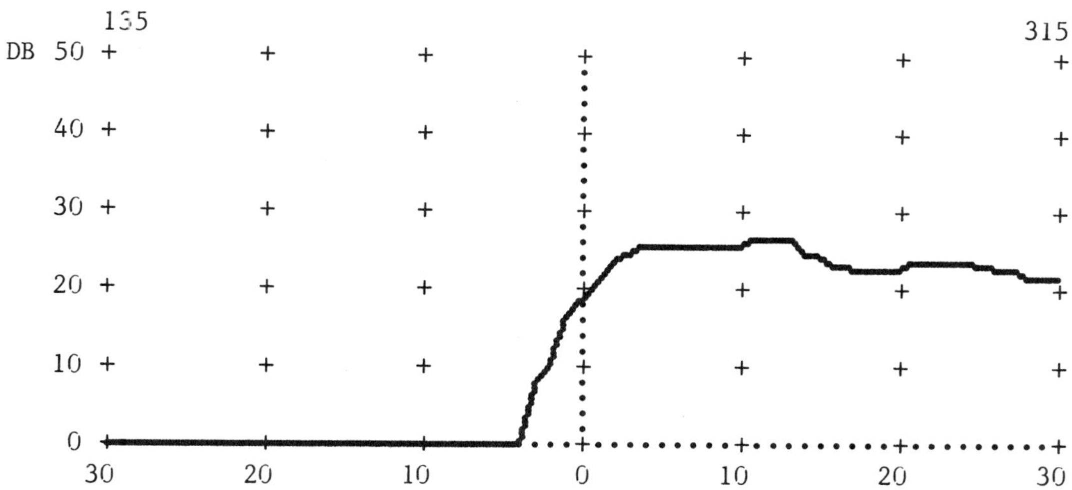

FIG. 2-6

To allow study of the depth of defects, another numeric printout provides a field map on which is printed the degree of abnormality at each point. The Humphrey Statpac Total Deviation and Octopus CO printouts show the degree of abnormality given as the difference from the normal value for age, which in the Octopus is printed only if sensitivity is reduced at least 5 dB from the normal value. The Humphrey instrument also provides a map of values obtained as the difference between actual threshold and an expected value (Pattern Deviation). The expected value is determined from the normal shape of the hill of vision and the actual threshold at the most normal or supranormal regions of the field (but ignoring the outlying best points), provided the points are not severely depressed (in which case a certain lower normal limit of sensitivity is assumed). The difference-from-normal method indicates all abnormalities whereas the difference-from-expected method calls greater attention to localized defects.

FIG. 2-7. Difference-from-normal printout (Octopus). The actual values on the left correspond to the threshold values in Fig. 2-5. The normal values are given on the right, and the difference is shown in the center box if the actual value is at least 5 dB less than normal.

FIG. 2-8. Difference-from-expected printout. At the top are shown the greyscale and actual threshold values. Below is the difference-from-expected printout. Based on the threshold in the second best quadrant (in this case the upper temporal and lower nasal quadrants), the predicted height of the hill of vision is 29 dB at the point of fixation ("central reference level"). All other points are assigned an expected value based on the normal shape of the hill of vision, and the difference-from-expected value is shown. The lower temporal quadrant is better than expected (as indicated by the negative numbers). The most defective region, in the upper nasal quadrant, is denoted with positive numbers. (See Fig. 10-8 for an example of how localized loss is highlighted in a field that also shows generalized loss.)

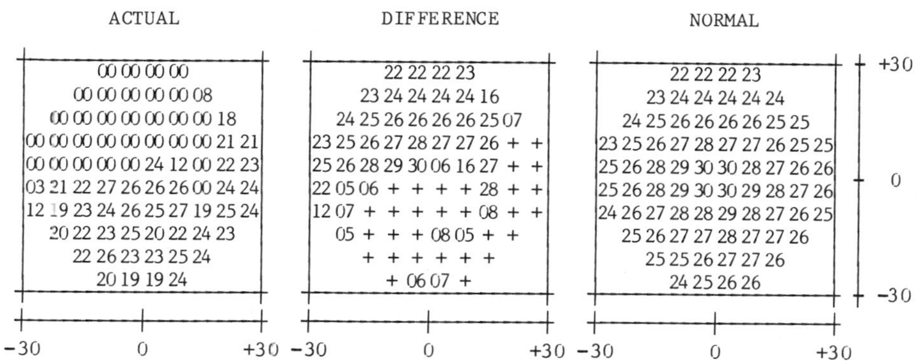
ACTUAL
DIFFERENCE
NORMAL
+30
0
-30
-30
0
+30

FIG. 2-7

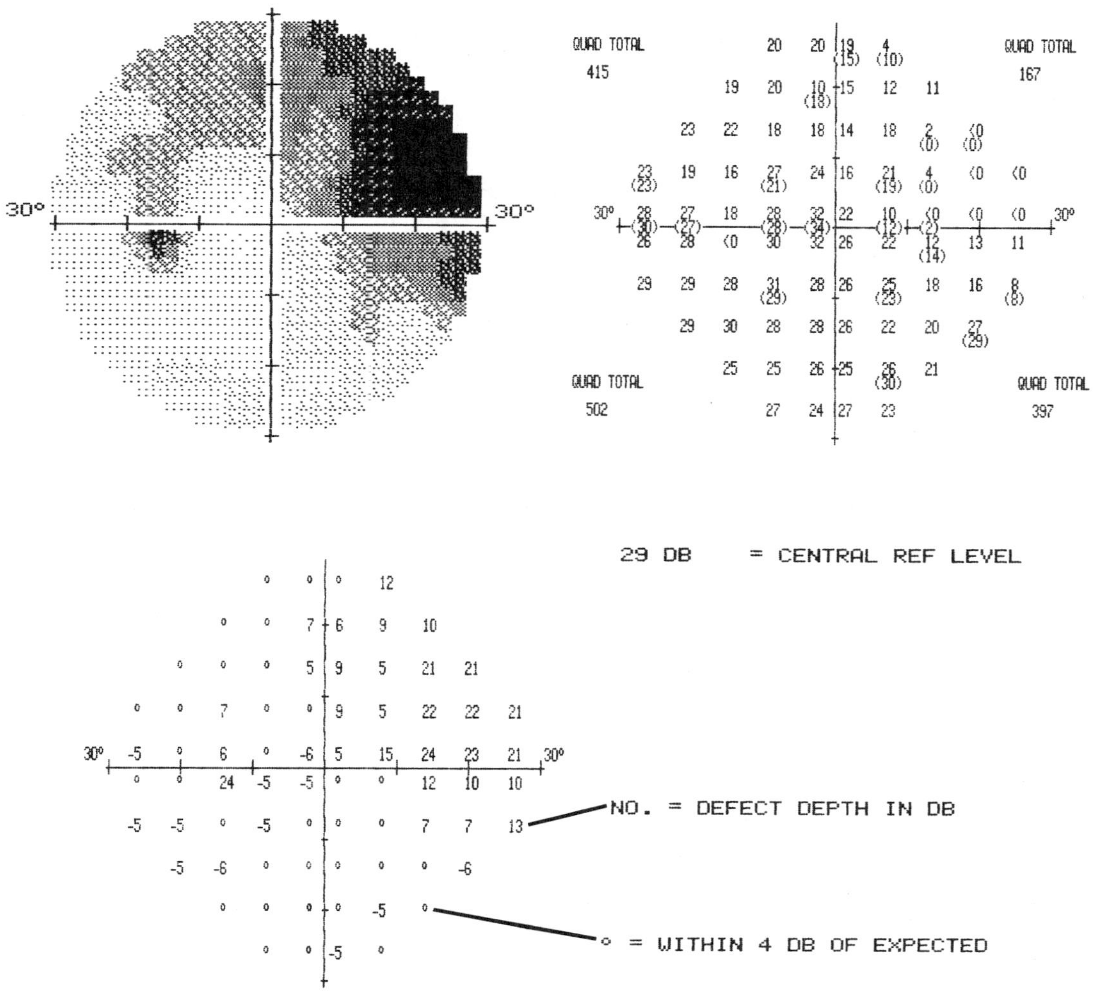
30°
QUAD TOTAL
415
QUAD TOTAL
167
QUAD TOTAL
502
QUAD TOTAL
397
29 DB = CENTRAL REF LEVEL
NO. = DEFECT DEPTH IN DB
o = WITHIN 4 DB OF EXPECTED

FIG. 2-8

When two fields done some time apart are compared, the change in threshold over time at each location may be indicated as well as a table of calculated values on the two occasions that can be compared.

FIG. 2-9. Comparison of visual fields done on the right eye of a patient 2 days apart. A point-by-point comparison of the actual thresholds on the two occasions (above) is tedious. In the lower left hand corner is a printout showing a subtraction of the sensitivity values on the first occasion from those on the second occasion. For some points there is no change (0); for others there is a higher sensitivity (plus numbers) from 1 to 5 dB; for still others a deterioration of sensitivity occurs (minus numbers) from 1 to 5 dB. The average change is an improvement of 0.7 decibel, which by the t-test is statistically significant (see the discussion on p. 310 concerning long-term fluctuation).

The table of sensitivities shows the mean value for the whole field to be 19.2 decibels on June 4, with a 0.7 decibel improvement to 19.9 decibels on June 6. Both values are depressed compared to the normal mean sensitivity of 26.1 decibels. When each of several zones of the visual field is examined separately, a small but consistent improvement in sensitivity becomes apparent. The number of abnormal points fell from 66 to 63. On both examinations the intratest variability (RMS fluctuation) is very small (1.5 decibels). See Figs. 13-50 and 13-51 for another example of these printouts.

The aforementioned types of data report are the ones most commonly encountered at the present time. Each of the many less frequently used programs gives results in a format appropriate to the special test. Additionally, as new programs are developed, new report formats must be developed to go with them—for example a greyscale to indicate the probability that a given point is abnormal. This book is too short to go into a discussion of every type, but each should be easily understood by those who comprehend the basic printouts described and illustrated.

			16	17 20	14 14	11			
		18	18	19	19	20	18		
	21	20	17	15	19	20	17 22	20	
20	19	19	19 21	20	20	21	21	20	19
19	20	20	20	21	20	19	17	20	20
19 20	20	20	22	23	22	19	0	20	21 20
17	16	18	21	21 20	21 22	20	21	18	21
	17	19	19	15	20	20	20 19	22	
		17 17	18	16	21	21	20		
			20	19	20	22			

			17	16 17	13 17	12			
		19	20	17	19	18	19		
	20	21	21	20	20	21	22 22	21	
19	19	20	21 20	19	22	21	21	20	19
19	23	23	21	22	23	22	18	23	19
19 22	19	20	22	23	24	19	1	21	22 23
15	17	20	23	22 20	22 21	17	22	17	23
	19	20	20	19	21	22	19 21	21	
		19 22	17	20	22	20	21		
			15	19	20	19			

			1	- 2.	1	1			
		1.	2.	- 2	0	- 2.	1		
	- 1:	1.	4	5	1	1	3.	1.	
- 1:	0	1	0	- 1	2	0	0	0	0
0	3.	3	1	1	3	3		3.	- 1
1	- 1	0	0	0	2	0		1	2.
- 2	1	2	2	1	0	- 3	1	- 1	2:
	2	1	1	4	1	2	1	- 1.	
		3	- 1	4	1	- 1	1		
			- 5.	0	0	- 3.			

	6.04.84	6.06.84
MEAN SENSITIVITY		
WHOLE FIELD (N: 26.1)	19.2	19.9
QUAD.UPP.NAS.(N: 25.4)	18.9	19.8
LOW.NAS.(N: 26.4)	18.7	19.4
UPP.TMP.(N: 25.5)	18.9	19.8
LOW.TMP.(N: 27.1)	20.4	20.7
ECC. 0 - 10 (N: 28.9)	20.6	21.6
10 - 20 (N: 26.9)	19.2	20.6
20 - 30 (N: 25.0)	18.9	19.2
NO. OF DISTURBED POINTS	66	63
R.M.S. FLUCTUATION	1.5	1.5

FIG. 2-9

Additional features of automated perimeters

Various methods are used to monitor the steadiness with which the patient maintains visual function on the central target.

The Heijl-Krakau method consists of presenting a test stimulus in the known position of the physiologic blind spot. The patient can see it only if the eye has wandered from the center position of gaze. The result of the monitoring may be simply to report the proportion of time that fixation has been lost, or it may be assumed that whenever fixation is lost the most recent stimulus presentations are inaccurate and need to be repeated. Unfortunately, the latter approach can greatly prolong the testing session.

In other instruments fixation is monitored by the image of the pupil or a corneal reflection. This method is continuous whereas the Heijl-Krakau method is an intermittent sampling of fixation steadiness. With the continuous method the test may be interrupted and an alarm sounded whenever fixation wanders. Unfortunately, the monitor may be affected not only by a drift in gaze direction but also by blinks or slight lateral shift of the entire head, which is of no consequence to the field test.

Neither of these automatic methods is completely satisfactory for fixation monitoring. The best method is direct observation by the perimetrist, either through a telescope or on a video monitor. The latter has the definite advantage that the operator does not have to sit uncomfortably at the scope for long periods and thus the monitoring of fixation is far more likely to be done continuously, with encouragement and reminders to the patient as necessary.

The time needed to print out the results of a field test may be longer than the perimetrist or patient wants, causing a delay before the next field test begins. Especially for machines in continuous use, a buffer that accepts the data and feeds them to the printer (perhaps in an adjacent room to cut down on the noise level) will allow the perimeter's computer to be free to begin the next test while the report of the previous one is being printed.

The ability to store the test data on a disk is an advantage that allows previous data to be used as a starting point for subsequent threshold tests, and for computerized assistance in comparing a series of two or more visual field examinations. It may also be of help if the perimetrist wishes to proceed to other patients before taking the time to print out the results from the previous patient. This may be an alternative to rigging up a print buffer, provided the office routine is such that the report of the field test is not needed right away.

SELECTION OF PERIMETRIC EQUIPMENT FOR THE OFFICE

In a broad sense, perimetry is part of the evaluation of visual function. A method to test the visual field is needed in every clinical office, just as every office needs to be equipped to test acuity and to perform refraction (and perhaps also to screen for defective color vision, test for contrast sensitivity, and test for glare).

For visual field examinations every practitioner needs to be facile with (and have available) confrontation methods and the Amsler grid. These methods are quick and *often* useful.

The office also needs some provision for quantitative testing of the central field and the peripheral field. The tangent screen and an arc perimeter are a combination that has satisfied this need in many offices. An alternative is the projection bowl perimeter (Goldmann), which has been a standard in recent decades.

Automated instruments are becoming a popular way to satisfy the need for field examination. They are less dependent on the skill and experience of the technician and through the years can provide a reproducibly standard examination despite changes in office personnel. There are two viable plans. One is to use an automated instrument that performs only suprathreshold spot checking for screening and diagnosis but to use a manual method (e.g., the Goldmann) for refined diagnosis and for following the progress of patients with progressive disease such as glaucoma. The alternative is to rely only on automated methods, in which case the instrument must be capable of quantitative threshold determinations and should test not only the central field but also the peripheral field (unless one plans to rely on confrontation methods or a manual perimeter for occasions when evaluation of the peripheral field is helpful). As the practitioner becomes conversant with the use of automated perimetry, he will gradually feel the need for a program that allows more detailed examination of a particular region in the field and programs that assist in the interpretation of the field (more of which will undoubtedly develop in the next few years). The latter will require that the data be stored on a disk for future reference. If a practitioner does not wish to buy a second, more capable, perimeter in the future as his needs grow, he will do well to buy one that already has these advanced features or can be easily upgraded.

For community screening programs an automated machine that conducts single suprathreshold testing may be appropriate. For research studies a machine must be selected by careful consideration of the data that will be needed for the study. In any event, it is necessary to consider the types of examination called for by the purposes at hand (see Chapter 11).

ADDITIONAL READING

Details of the capabilities of available automated instruments can be gleaned from three references:

Drance, S.M., and Anderson, D.R.: Automatic perimetry in glaucoma, Chapters 7 through 12, Orlando, Fla., 1985, Grune & Stratton, Inc.

Keltner, J.L., and Johnson, C.A.: Comparative material on automated and semiautomated perimeters—1985, Ophthalmology, vol. 92 (Instrument and book supplement), pp. 34-57, August 1985.

Silverstone, D.E., and Hirsch, J.: Automated field testing: techniques of examination and interpretation, Chapter 5, Norwalk, Conn., 1986, Appleton-Century-Crofts, pp. 53-87.

CHAPTER 3

Alternate and supplemental methods of field evaluation

Chapter 2 dealt with the methods and instruments used in formal quantitative testing of the visual field. To know these methods is not enough. There are qualitative methods that are advantageous for particular purposes. Certain clinical situations will, in fact, *require* other methods either instead of or in addition to quantitative perimetry.

AMSLER GRID

The Amsler grid is a method of testing the inner approximately 10 degrees of the central visual field. The standard chart consists of a grid of white lines on black paper held at a reading distance of 28 to 30 cm. The size of each square is 5 mm, which occupies 1 degree of the field. The complete set of Amsler grids has six other patterns useful in special situations in which the standard chart does not suffice.* The patient is asked to look at a grid of squares and describe the areas where the lines are either missing or distorted. It is a qualitative test but one that is quite useful in detecting central or paracentral scotomas as well as areas where the vision is distorted even if there is no reduction in light sensitivity. Distortion (as opposed to absence) of the grid squares (or metamorphopsia) suggests a retinal lesion rather than a central scotoma caused by an optic nerve lesion.

Because of its ease, rapidity, and sensitivity the Amsler grid is useful in settings where one does not want quantitative information but wants simply to know quickly and accurately whether or not a central scotoma is present. It is particularly useful as an adjunct to the Goldmann perimeter because the central 2 degrees cannot be adequately tested on the Goldmann without a special projection device.

*For more details on the Amsler grid, see the following:
Amsler, M.: L'Examen qualitatif de la fonction maculaire, Ophthalmologica **114:**248-261, 1947.
Amsler, M.: Quantitative and qualitative vision, Trans. Ophthalmol. Soc. U.K. **69:**397-410, 1949.

FIG. 3-1. The standard Amsler grid. The patient is asked if he sees the white dot at the center. Then, while he continues to stare at the dot, he is asked if all four corners of the grid are visible, there are absent areas in the pattern, or the squares are distorted or blurred anywhere.

CONFRONTATION TECHNIQUES

Confrontation techniques for evaluating the visual field are often very useful in a variety of situations:

1. To screen for the presence of unsuspected field defects as part of a routine eye examination that would not ordinarily include formal field testing (We include a quick confrontation finger-counting field in every complete eye examination but of course do not do formal perimetry on every patient.)
2. To educate the patient about field testing before performing perimetry (see p. 182)
3. To determine approximately the type and extent of a field defect to be expected on perimetry
4. To confirm or deny perimetric findings (For example, extreme contraction of the field detectable by perimetry may or may not be present on confrontation and the perimetry may be wrong. Likewise, confrontation comparison tests may suggest a hemianopia not discovered by perimetry or may confirm the perimetric findings.)
5. As the only type of field examination that is feasible for some patients (One should not underestimate the amount of valuable information obtainable by a careful confrontation method, even for patients who cannot perform well on the perimeter.)

The basic confrontation techniques to be described on the following pages are (1) the finger-counting method and (2) the comparison method.

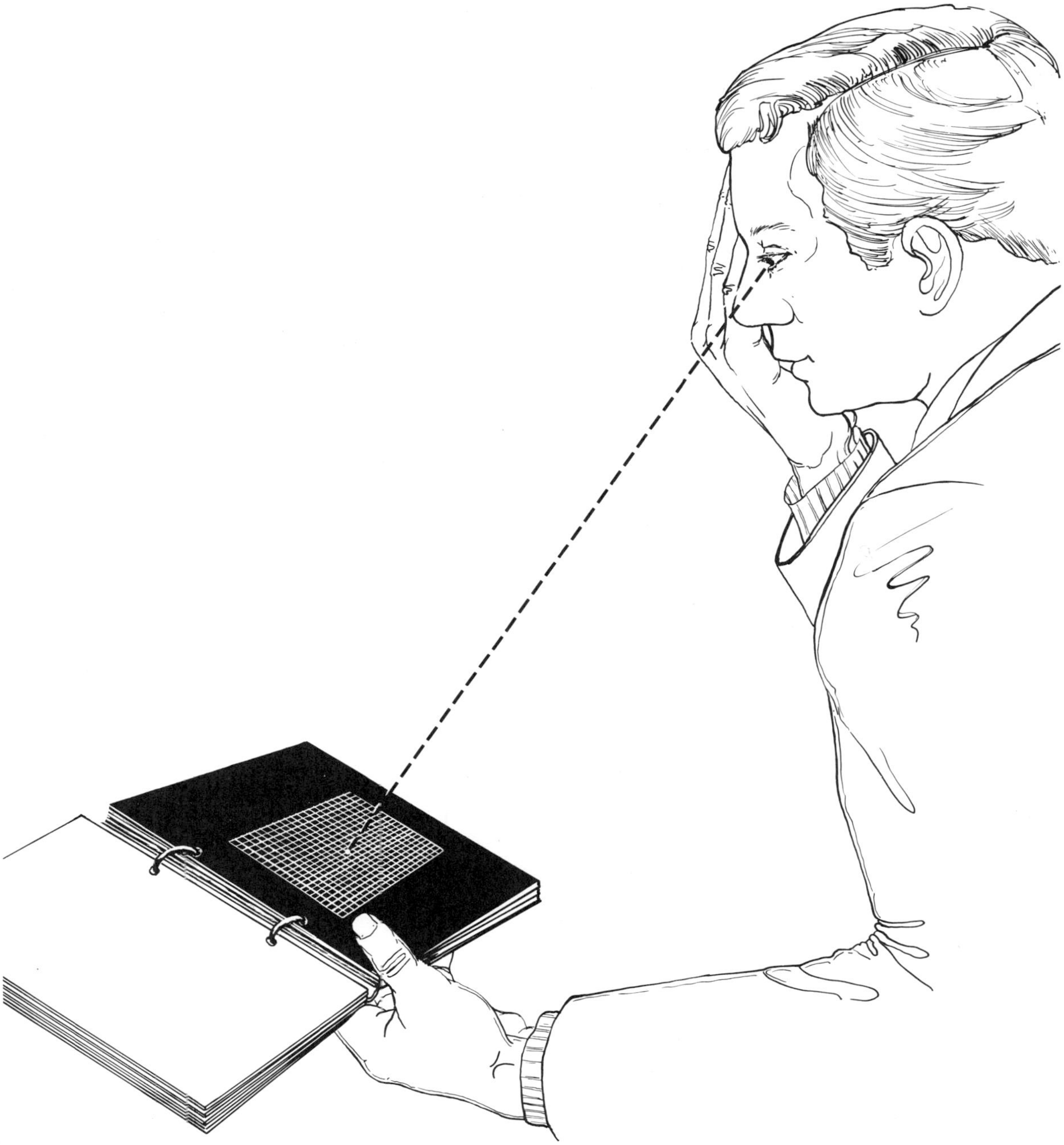

FIG. 3-1

Finger-counting method: screening

The finger-counting method of screening was originally described by Welsh.* As in all field testing, each eye is tested separately. The patient should use his palm, not his fingers, to occlude the other eye. The palm is used to ensure that he does not peek between fingers and does not exert pressure on the covered eye, blurring his vision and making subsequent testing of this eye difficult. There should be no glare, but the examiner's back, ideally, should be toward a blank evenly illuminated wall without windows or other bright sources of light.

The patient is asked to fixate on the examiner's face (usually the nose) and report how many fingers the examiner holds up in the peripheral field. Each quadrant is tested separately by placing the hand 3 or 4 feet away from the patient, about 45 degrees from fixation. Normally a person with a normal pupil size and without opacity in the media or other visual abnormality should be able to count fingers at 6 to 10 feet away, out to 60 degrees temporally and 45 to 50 degrees nasally. Therefore, counting fingers 3 to 4 feet away at 45 degrees should be achieved comfortably if the visual field is normal.

The examiner can hold up either one finger or two and the patient can report how many fingers he sees. The examiner can also present four fingers or a whole hand so the patient has a choice of one, two, or all. A closed fist (no fingers) can also be used. Never use three fingers because three is exceedingly difficult to differentiate from two or four.

Especially if the patient is having trouble fixating, you can hold up both fists in a manner that will not allow him to tell which hand you will be using. Then, elevate one, two, or four fingers of one hand or the other and lower them again before the patient shifts his fixation to look directly at them.

FIG. 3-2. Finger-counting confrontation field.

---

*Welsh, R.C.: Finger counting in the four quadrants as a method of visual field gross screening, Arch. Ophthalmol. **66:**678-679, 1961.

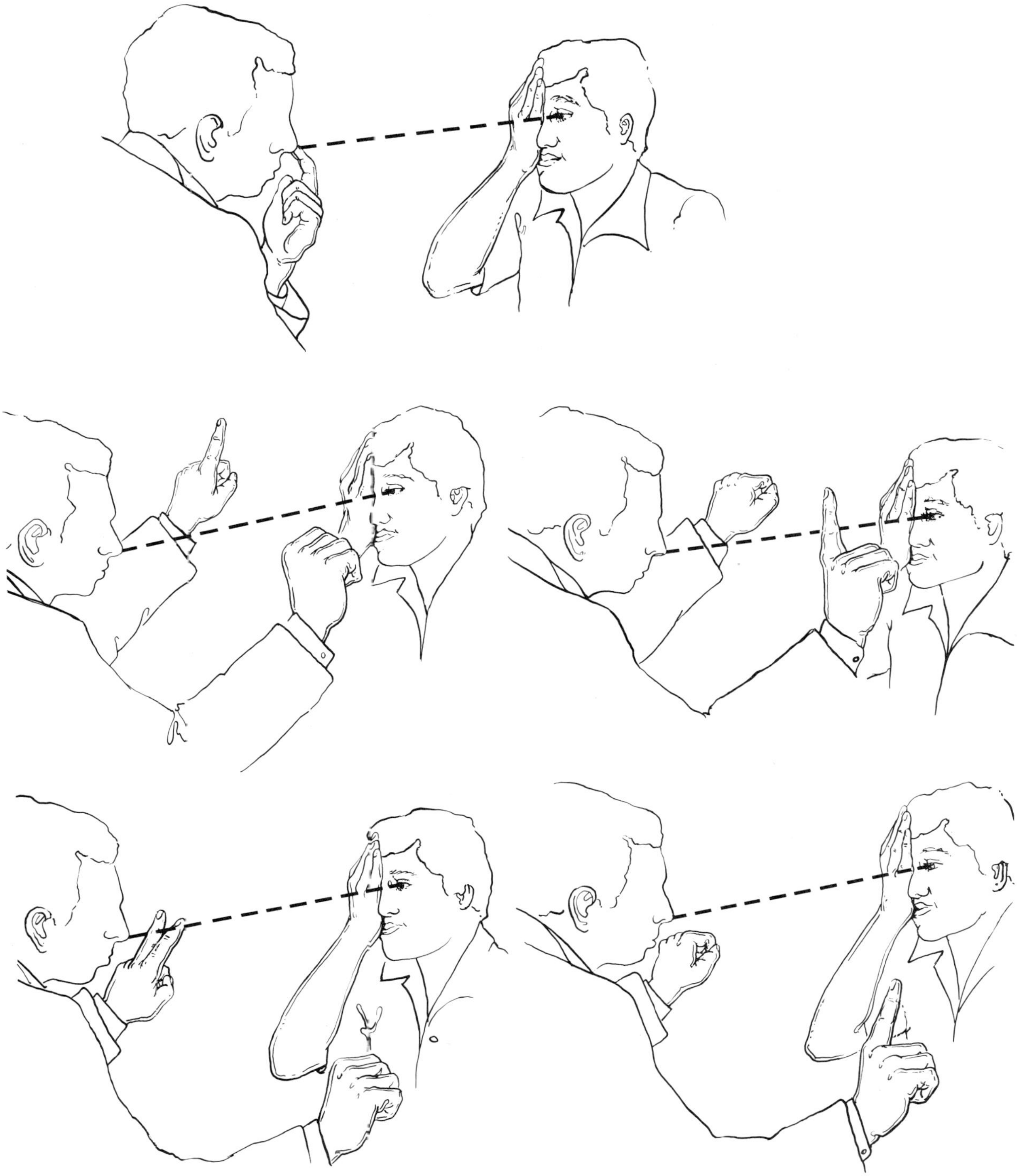

FIG. 3-2

Finger-counting method: quantitation

If the fingers cannot be counted in a given quadrant at 45 degrees, there are two helpful maneuvers.

FIG. 3-3. Quantitation by confrontation.
A, In the first quantitative maneuver the hand with upheld fingers can be moved transversely in an arc toward fixation, staying 2 to 3 feet from the patient. The procedure resembles kinetic perimetry and the idea is to determine how close to fixation the hand must be before the fingers can be counted. Similar to the technique when plotting an isopter, the direction of movement need not be toward fixation. For example, if there is marked difference between two quadrants, it may be possible to confirm dramatically the presence of a hemianopia or a nasal step if the patient is suddenly able to count the fingers as the hand crosses the vertical meridian or the horizontal meridian nasally.
B, In the second quantitation maneuver the hand is moved toward the patient along the line 45 degrees from fixation until the fingers can be counted (or start at 6 feet away and back away until the fingers cannot be counted) and the minimum closeness required to count fingers is compared among the four quadrants. This maneuver resembles static perimetry.

In the segments of the field where fingers cannot be counted, it should be determined whether or not the patient can distinguish if the fingers are wiggling or holding still. If he cannot make that distinction, it should be determined whether or not with correct projection he can detect the presence or absence of a light. This will help make the distinction between a severe depression and a contraction of the field, which is an absolute defect (p. 130).

When the visual sensation is so poor that you are looking for the presence or absence of light perception in different areas of the field, it is important to make note of whether or not the patient can accurately tell you where the light is located. Only then can you be sure that this area of the field is intact to light perception. For example, suppose a patient has a contracted field with only a temporal island of vision remaining from glaucoma and also has a cataract (which diffuses light within the eye). When you place a light in the nasal field, the patient may be able to tell you correctly that the light is on as a result of diffusion of the light by the cataract onto the seeing retina. He may also tell you either that he sees there is light temporally or that he sees the light but is not sure where it is located. However, with the light on the temporal side, he may be able to tell you where the light is located and report that he now sees it brightly whereas when the light was on the nasal side he was aware only of a dim glow. Sometimes it is quite striking that, as you move the light around, the patient can suddenly localize the light accurately, letting you know that you have crossed the boundary into the seeing portion of the field. In a patient with cataract and glaucoma, it may be encouraging that he can project light not only on the temporal side but in a region around fixation as well, even though he cannot accurately localize light seen in the nasal quadrant. The finding of accurate projection around fixation suggests that there is an intact central island of vision, perhaps with the potential of good acuity when a cataract is removed. The outlook is not so good if accurate light projection exists only in the temporal field, or if the patient reports that the light is dimmer at fixation than it is in the temporal field.

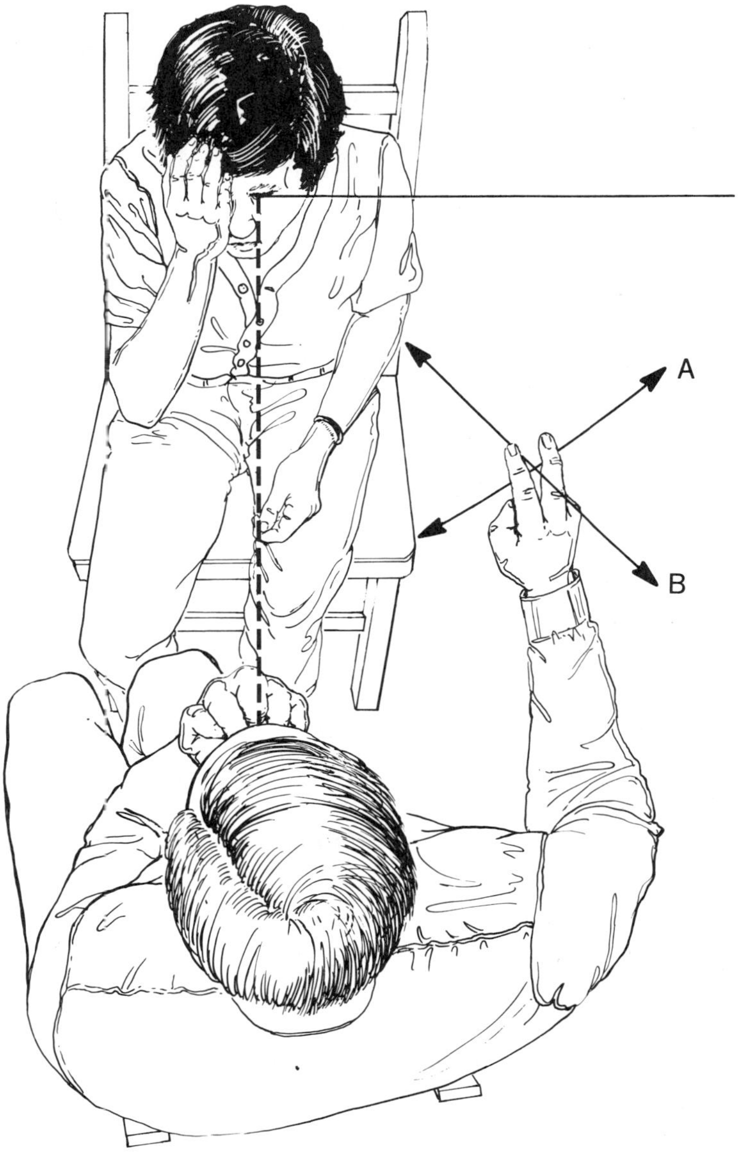

FIG. 3-3

Diagramming confrontation fields

The conventional method of diagramming all visual fields is "as the patient sees it"—the right eye to the right, the left eye to the left, the nasal side of the field toward the center, and the temporal side toward the edge. This diagramming is easy to accomplish with a technique such as the tangent screen and the perimeter, but with confrontation methods it is necessary that the examiner invert right and left from his perspective so it ends up on the paper "as the patient sees it." In doing so, it is well to label the diagram with an "N" between the two eyes and a "T" on the two edges, marking the right and the left eye, so there is no ambiguity. This is particularly important because some experienced individuals intentionally diagram their confrontation findings in the unconventional manner, "as the examiner sees it."*

FIG. 3-4. Diagram of hypothetical visual fields by confrontation. In the first example, as might occur in a patient with both glaucoma and cataract, there is generalized depression and reduced acuity, especially in the left eye, and, additionally, a localized depression in the upper nasal quadrant. In the second example, as might occur in the presence of retinal detachment, there is very localized visual loss. *HM* indicates the region where the vision is limited to the detection of hand movements. *FC* indicates the region where fingers can be counted at the indicated distance.

Considerable qualitative and even semiquantitative information can be obtained from a carefully performed finger-counting confrontation field with quantitation of abnormal areas. With care, you may be able to determine whether there is a central scotoma or not or whether a patient with glaucoma has a central island of vision remaining or only a temporal island. This can be done even when the vision is so poor (because of cataracts) or fixation is so poor (because of reduced vision) that an adequate examination with a perimeter or tangent screen cannot be accomplished. For such occasions, you need to be experienced in performing confrontation fields.

It is also useful to perform confrontation field testing as a matter of routine in conjunction with perimetry to confirm or deny the perimetric findings when there may be a fault in perimetric technique as well as to learn through experience how to do a better perimetric examination. For example, if the confrontation technique does not reveal a defect and the perimetric examination shows a reasonably dense defect in one quadrant, you should repeat the confrontation field, both to corroborate the presence of a defect and to learn why the defect was missed initially by confrontation. With such experience, the use of confrontation fields routinely on all patients seen in the office becomes a quick but reasonably accurate technique.

---

*Welsh, R.C.: How to quanti-tate and unconventionally diagram finger-counting confrontation visual fields, Ophthalmol. Times **5**(4):17, 19, 30, 34, 48, 53, 1980.

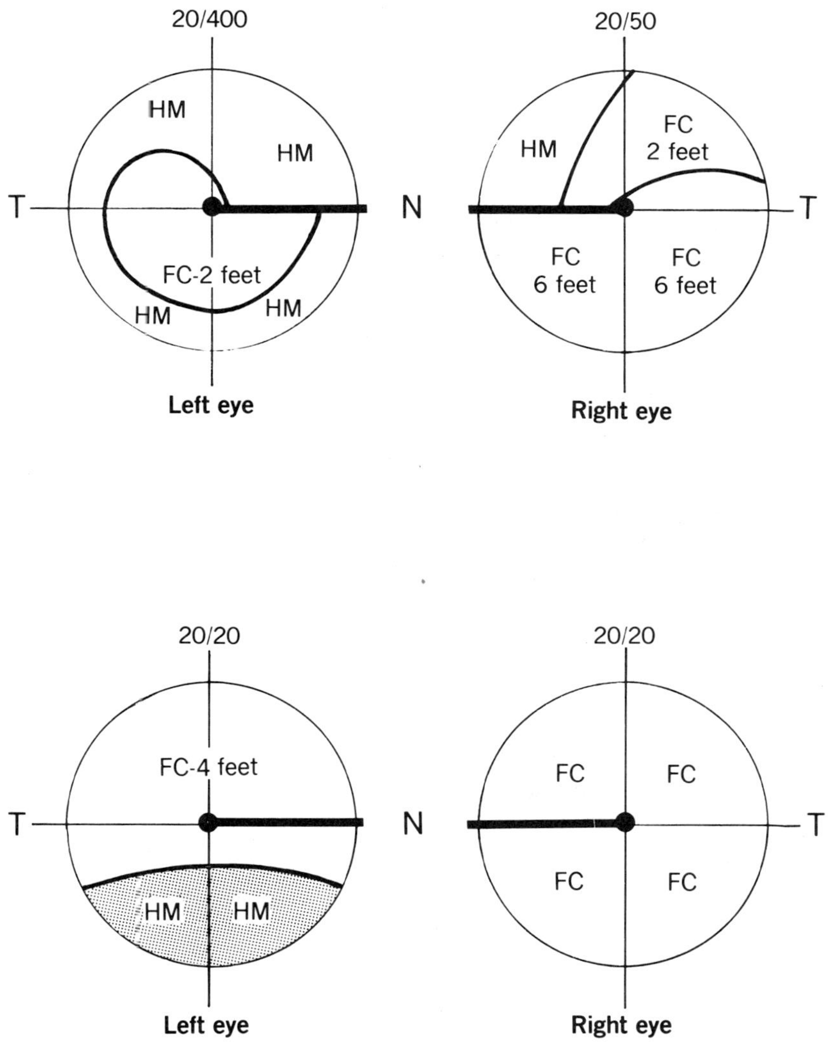

20/400
HM
HM
T
N
FC-2 feet
HM
HM
Left eye
20/50
HM
FC
2 feet
T
FC
6 feet
FC
6 feet
Right eye
20/20
FC-4 feet
T
N
HM
HM
Left eye
20/20
FC
FC
T
FC
FC
Right eye

FIG. 3-4

Comparison techniques

With all the techniques described so far, you should always ask the patient whether or not he is able to see a certain stimulus (e.g., a light or wiggling fingers). Even with the finger-counting technique, basically you are asking whether or not the patient is able to see the fingers; asking him to tell you how many fingers you have up is simply confirming that he can see them.

With a comparison technique, you are asking the patient a fundamentally different question: to compare a stimulus in two locations and to tell you whether they are the same or different. The usefulness of the technique depends on the fact that if visual sensation is reduced because of a change in visual threshold all stimuli are subjectively less bright in that region (p. 336). For example, visual sensation is depressed on one side of the vertical midline in hemianopias, whether bitemporal as a result of chiasmal lesions or homonymous as a result of postchiasmal lesions. Usual perimetric techniques detect this depression in terms of reduced light sensitivity (or reduced visual threshold). Finger-counting confrontation may also detect a depression in terms of acuity (sharpness of vision). However, the hemianopic depression is also reflected in the brightness of stimuli in that area and in color saturation. For many individuals it seems easier to appreciate differences in color saturation than to distinguish differences in brightness, so a colored object is often used in comparison testing by confrontation. A red object may, for example, seem maroon to the right and bright red to the left of fixation.

To detect this difference, you may take a red object of reasonable size, ½ to 2 inches in diameter (such as the cap off a cycloplegic bottle), have the patient fixate on your nose, and ask him if the red object has the exact same color 3 to 6 inches to the right of fixation as it does 3 to 6 inches to the left. This can be done somewhat above fixation and again somewhat below fixation.

You should pay the greatest attention to the patient's first response. The color difference should be instantly obvious to him. If he has to think about it, he may be reporting some subtle lighting difference or something else, and the test is unreliable.

FIG. 3-5. Searching for quadrant differences in color saturation.

You may ask the patient to compare the two sides with the red object shown in sequence, as illustrated, or you can hold up two red objects simultaneously, one on each side, and ask him to compare them.

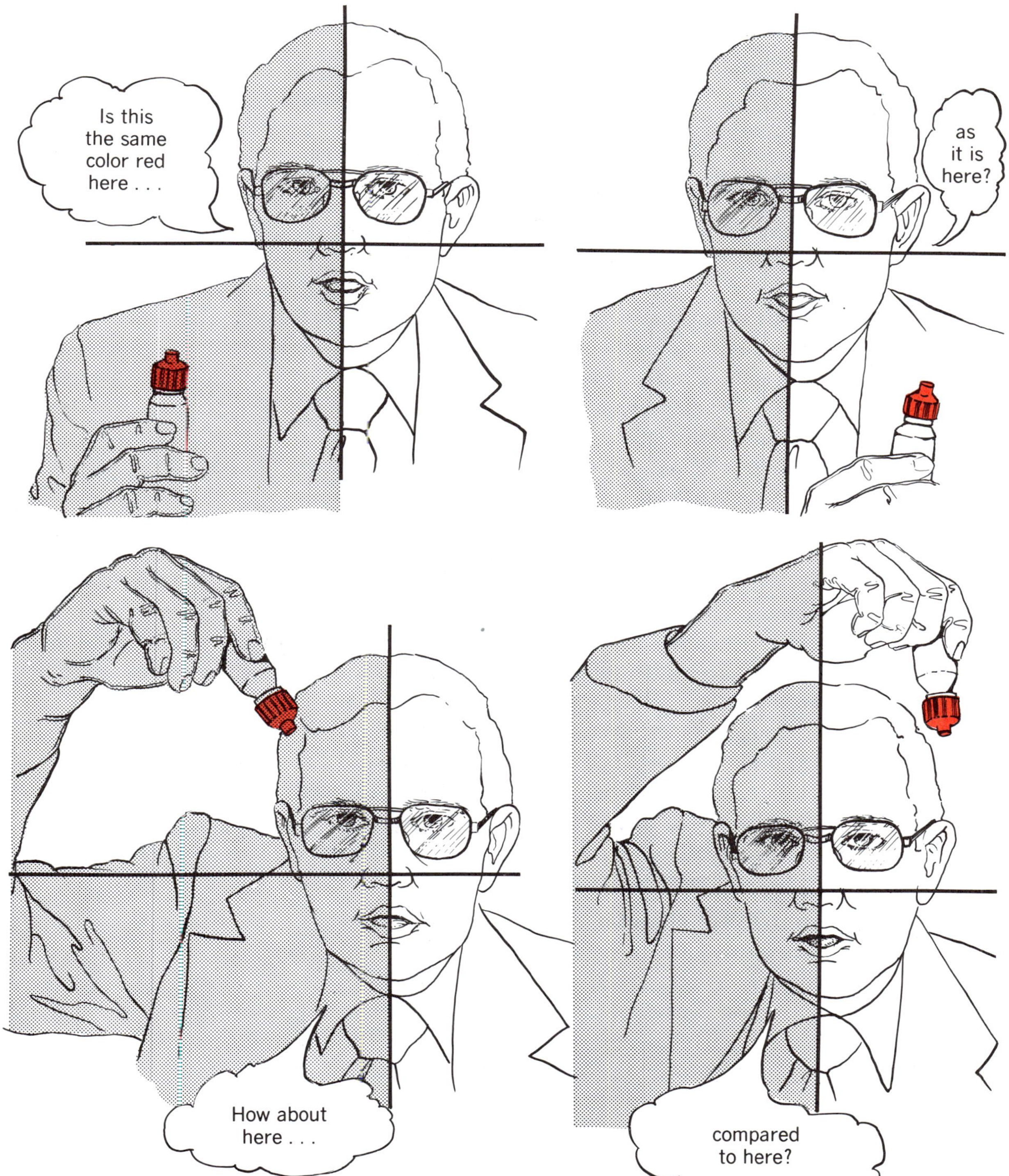
Is this the same color red here . . .
as it is here?
How about here . . .
compared to here?

FIG. 3-5

If the patient reports that the color is different (or to confirm in your own mind that there is no difference), you should move the object horizontally and ask the patient to tell you when it changes color, moving it across the vertical midline above fixation and then repeating below fixation.

FIG. 3-6. Confirming a hemianopia. If the patient reports that the object changes color exactly at the vertical midline, there is strong evidence that a hemianopia is present. A definite absence of a color difference is strong evidence that there is no hemianopia. This test is so sensitive that it should be done whenever a visual field examination is performed in search of a hemianopia, even if the perimetric or tangent screen examination has not revealed hemianopia. If hemianopia is not revealed by perimetry but is found by a color comparison test, do the perimetric testing again.

The same principle of having the patient compare the two sides of the vertical meridian can be used to compare the clarity with which the patient can see your two palms as you hold them on the two sides of fixation. He may be able to report that the two palms seem different after you ask him if they appear equally bright and equally distant.

This principle can also be used at the perimeter by asking the patient to compare the brightness of the test stimulus to the right and to the left. For example, the brightness 10 degrees from fixation along the 45-degree meridian can be compared to the brightness 10 degrees from fixation along the 135-degree meridian. This can also be done 10 degrees from fixation along the 225-degree meridian and the 315-degree meridian. If the patient detects a difference, the stimulus can be moved horizontally to see if the brightness changes just as the stimulus crosses the vertical midline. Application of the technique in neurologic testing is discussed on p. 176.

Comparison methods can also be used to check for central scotomas (p. 123). The patient may find that the red object has a duller color at fixation than it does to the side. In a normal field, color, brightness, and acuity are greatest at fixation.

FIG. 3-7. Checking for a central scotoma by color comparison techniques. A central scotoma is present if the patient reports that the color is brighter away from fixation than at fixation.

ADDITIONAL READING

Some additional information about confrontation testing can be found in:

Frisen, L.: A versatile color confrontation test for the central visual field: a comparison with automatic perimetry, Arch. Ophthalmol. **89:**3-9, 1973.

Glaser, J.S.: Neuro-ophthalmology, New York, 1978, Harper & Row, Publishers, pp. 12-20.

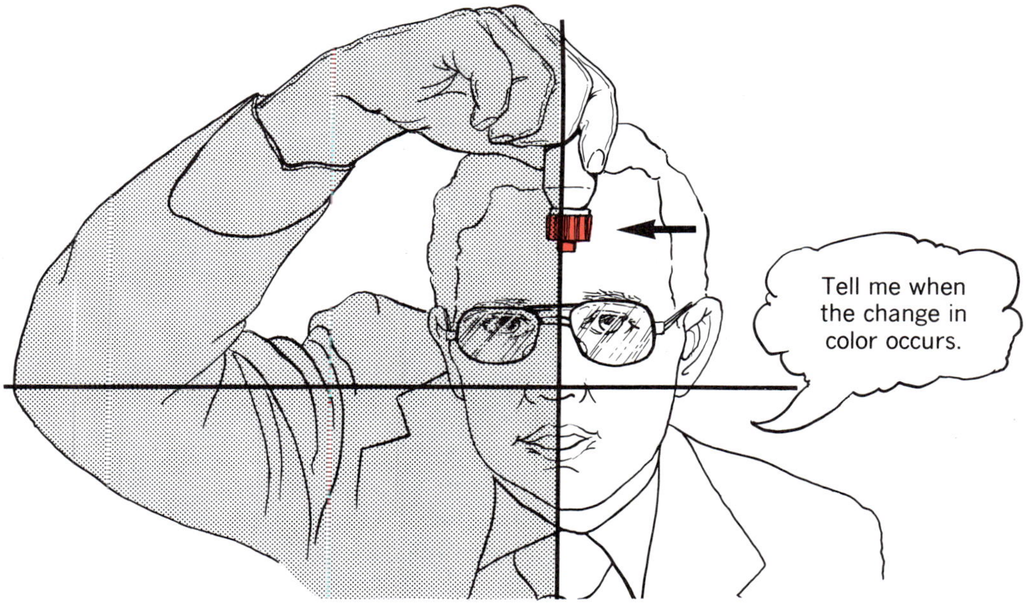
Tell me when
the change in
color occurs.

FIG. 3-6

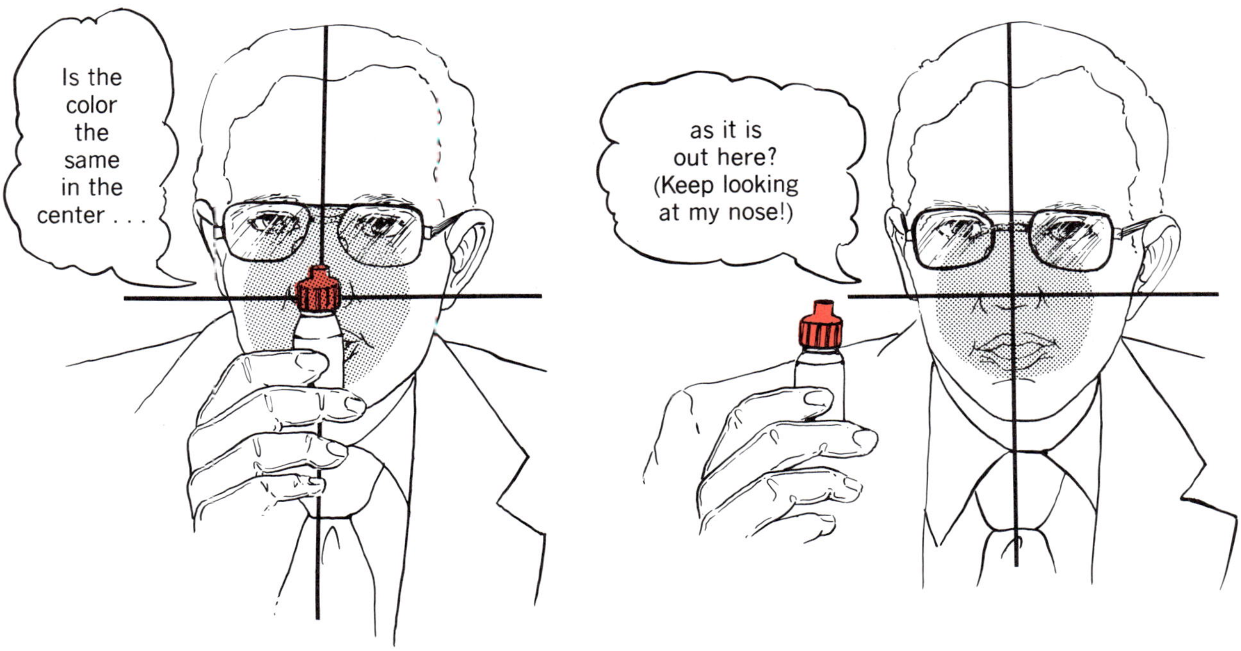
Is the
color
the
same
in the
center . . .
as it is
out here?
(Keep looking
at my nose!)

FIG. 3-7

CHAPTER 4

Anatomy and function

THE EYE

The wall of the eye is made up of three layers:

The outer layer consists of the *cornea,* which is clear, and the *sclera,* which is white. The region where the cornea and sclera join is called the limbus.

The second layer is the uveal tract, which has three parts—iris, ciliary body, and choroid. The *iris* has an opening, the pupil, and the root of the iris inserts into the ciliary body. The *ciliary body* lies within the anteriormost part of the sclera and contains the ciliary muscle, which is responsible for changing the shape of the lens. This allows the eye to focus on objects at varying distances, or to "accommodate." The ciliary body also produces aqueous humor. The third part of the uveal tract is the *choroid,* which lies under the retina and provides nutrition to the outer retina.

The innermost layer of the ocular wall is the *retina*. It receives and detects the light that has been focused into an image by the cornea and lens. Visual impulses are transmitted from the retina to the brain by the optic nerve.

Within the eye, the lens lies directly behind the pupil. It is suspended from the ciliary body by zonular fibers. As already noted, the lens shape (accommodation) is controlled by muscles in the ciliary body. In front of the iris and lens is the anterior chamber, filled with aqueous humor. Behind the lens is the vitreous cavity filled with vitreous humor.

FIG. 4-1. Cross section of the eye.

To reach the retina, light must pass through several normally transparent structures:

1. The cornea, which begins to focus the light (by virtue of its curvature)
2. The anterior chamber, filled with aqueous humor
3. The pupil, which can vary in size
4. The lens, which completes the process of focusing the light
5. The vitreous humor

If any of these structures is altered, blocking or scattering the light rays, or if the focusing is imperfect, then visual function will be disturbed. It is important to keep in mind these "preretinal factors" as well as disturbances in the neural "visual pathway" (Chapter 9).

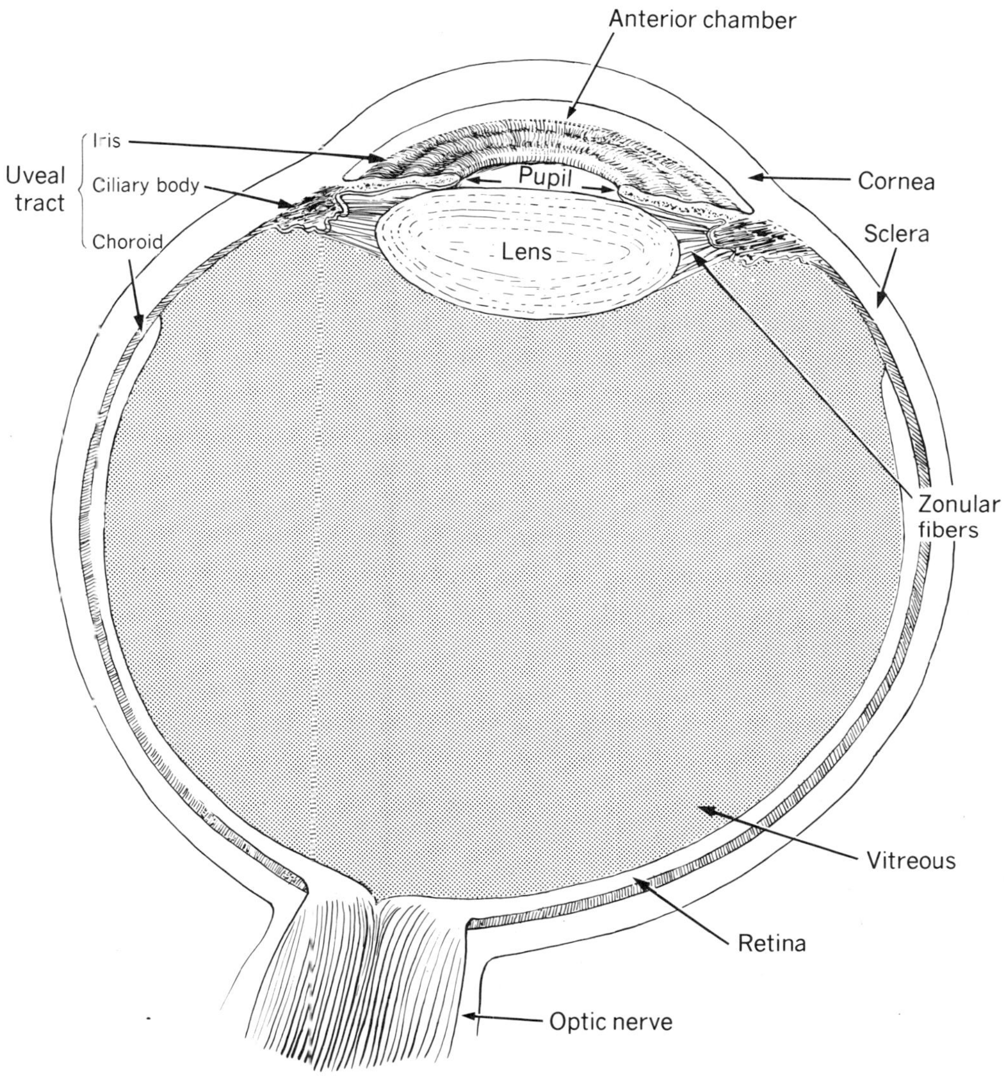
Anterior chamber
Iris
Uveal tract
Ciliary body
Choroid
Pupil
Lens
Cornea
Sclera
Zonular fibers
Vitreous
Retina
Optic nerve

FIG. 4-1

CORRESPONDENCE OF THE RETINA AND VISUAL FIELD

Every point in the retina corresponds to a certain direction in the visual field. For example, the fovea (centered at the back of the eye) corresponds to the point of fixation. The fovea is centered in the macula, a part of the retina specialized for sharp vision and for color discrimination. This area of the retina can discern detail, allowing one to read very small letters, and also has the highest sensitivity for detecting the stimuli used for visual field testing. Points in the peripheral retina, near the ciliary body, correspond to points in the peripheral visual field.

Because the image formed by the optics of the eye is upside down and backward, just as in a camera, the image is reversed; thus the nasal retina sees objects in the temporal visual field and vice versa. Also, points in the upper (superior) retina correspond to objects in the lower (inferior) visual field and vice versa.

From all points in the retina the visual information is converted to nervous impulses. These are collected by nerve fibers that course along the inner surface of the retina toward a spot 10 to 15 degrees on the nasal side of the fovea, a little above the horizontal. Here the nerve fibers collect together to become the optic nerve, which exits from the back of the eye and courses toward the brain. At the spot where these nerve fibers bundle together, which is called the optic nerve head or optic disc, there is necessarily an opening through the retina to allow the exit of the nerve fibers into the optic nerve. Because light cannot be detected where there is an opening in the retina, a corresponding region exists in the visual field 10 to 15 degrees from fixation where stimuli are not seen. This location in the visual field is called the physiologic scotoma or physiologic blind spot. Because the optic nerve exits from the nasal side of the eye, the blind spot is in the temporal portion of the visual field.

FIG. 4-2. Diagram of the left eye. In this view the eye is seen from above to show the relationship between retinal location and visual field location.

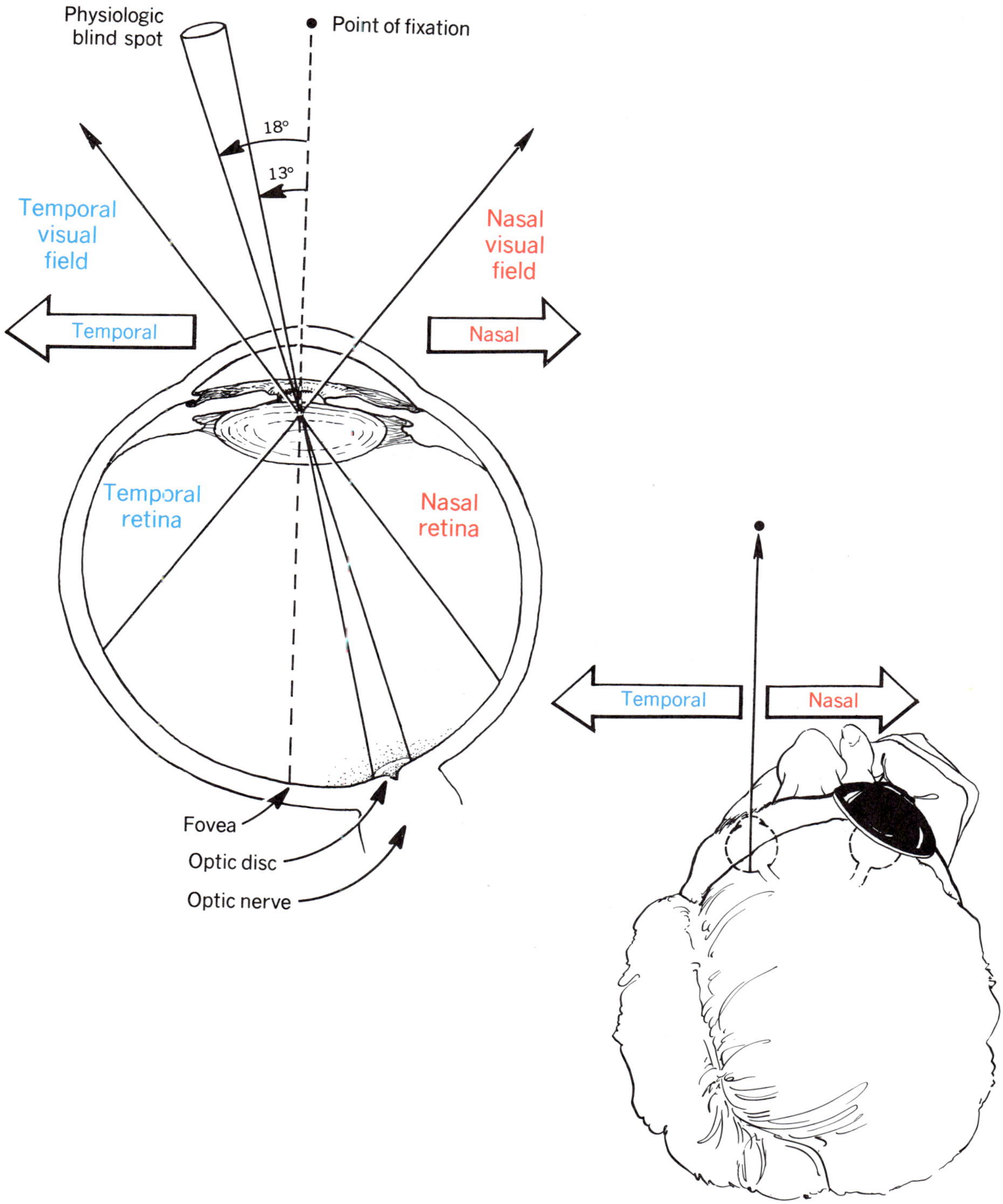
Physiologic
blind spot
Point of fixation
18°
13°
Temporal
visual
field
Nasal
visual
field
Temporal
Nasal
Temporal
retina
Nasal
retina
Fovea
Optic disc
Optic nerve
Temporal
Nasal

FIG. 4-2

CHAPTER 5

The normal visual field

In the more central region of the field it is possible to see smaller and dimmer objects (weaker stimuli) than in the peripheral visual field. Hence the I-2e test stimulus can be seen over a certain area but a more intense test stimulus, such as the I-4e can be seen over a larger area. The area within which each test stimulus can be seen is bounded by the *isopter* for that stimulus and may be mapped on a chart.

FIG. 5-1. A normal visual field (Goldmann). For progressively stronger stimuli the area surrounded by the isopter is progressively larger. Eventually, however, the absolute periphery of the visual field is reached and the field does not extend beyond the absolute periphery, no matter how large or bright the test stimulus becomes. Each isopter plotted here is 0.5 log-unit more intense than the previous.

The region inside the I-3e isopter is not equally sensitive everywhere. For example, in the region where the I-1e stimulus is visible (inside the I-1e isopter), the I-3e stimulus is at least 1.0 log-unit more intense than necessary for it to be seen (i.e., it is at least 1.0 log-unit suprathreshold) because I-1e is visible and the I-3e is 1.0 log-unit more intense than the I-1e. Similarly, in the region between the I-2e and I-1e isopters, the I-3e is 0.5 to 1.0 log-unit suprathreshold because the I-3e stimulus is 0.5 log-unit more intense than I-2e and 1.0 log-unit more intense than I-1e.

It should be noted that the apparent brightness of a stimulus relates to how much more intense than threshold it is. Thus the I-3e appears dim just inside the I-3e isopter, where it is just barely suprathreshold, and the I-1e appears dim just inside its isopter; however, the I-3e appears bright inside the I-1e isopter, where it is at least 1.0 log-unit more intense than threshold.

Isopter plot

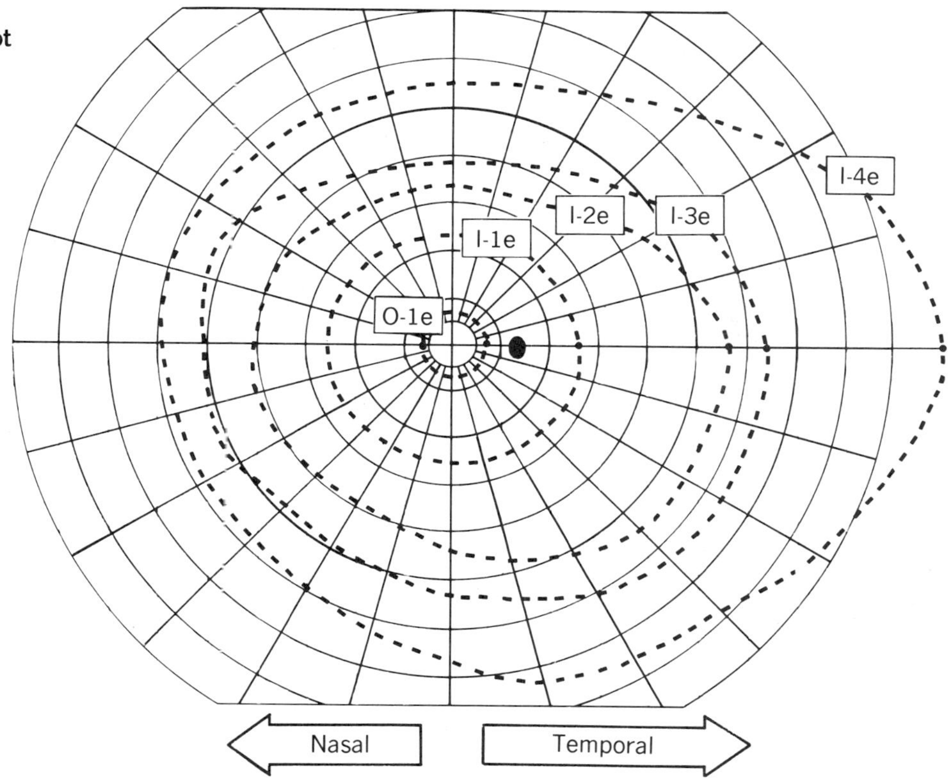

FIG. 5-1

FIG. 5-2. A normal visual field (Humphrey Field Analyzer). The visual field out to 60 degrees is represented on greytone and threshold value (decibel) printouts. Note that on the nasal side the absolute edge of the field is reached (zero values for some points at the upper left). See Fig. 1-7 for another example of a normal field.

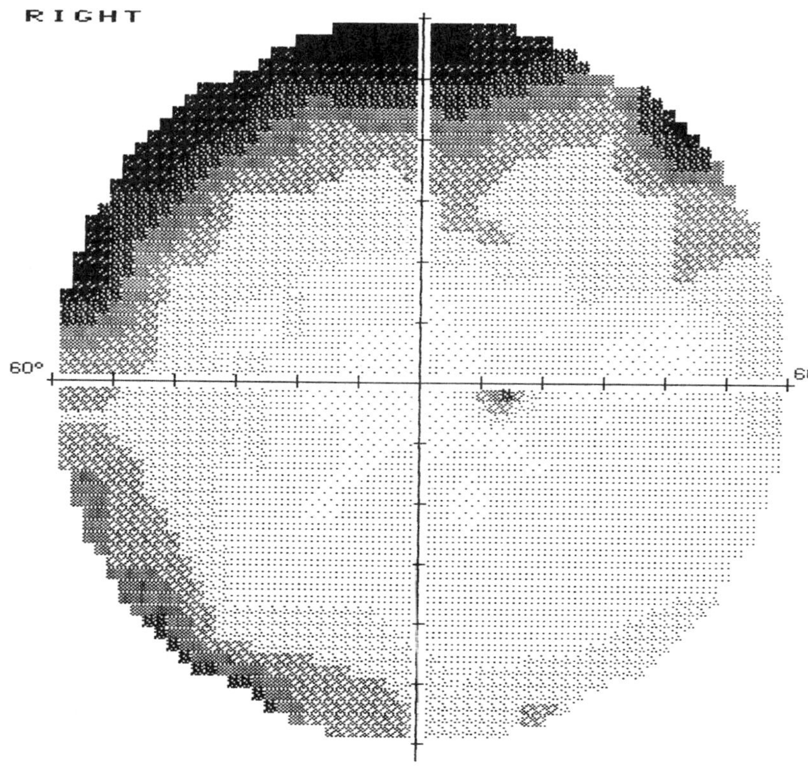

SYM.										
ASB	.8 to .1	2.5 to 1	8 to 3.2	25 to 10	79 to 32	251 to 100	794 to 316	2512 to 1000	7943 to 3162	≥ 10000
DB	41 to 50	36 to 40	31 to 35	26 to 30	21 to 25	16 to 20	11 to 15	6 to 10	1 to 5	≤0

HUMPHREY INSTRUMENTS

FIG. 5-2

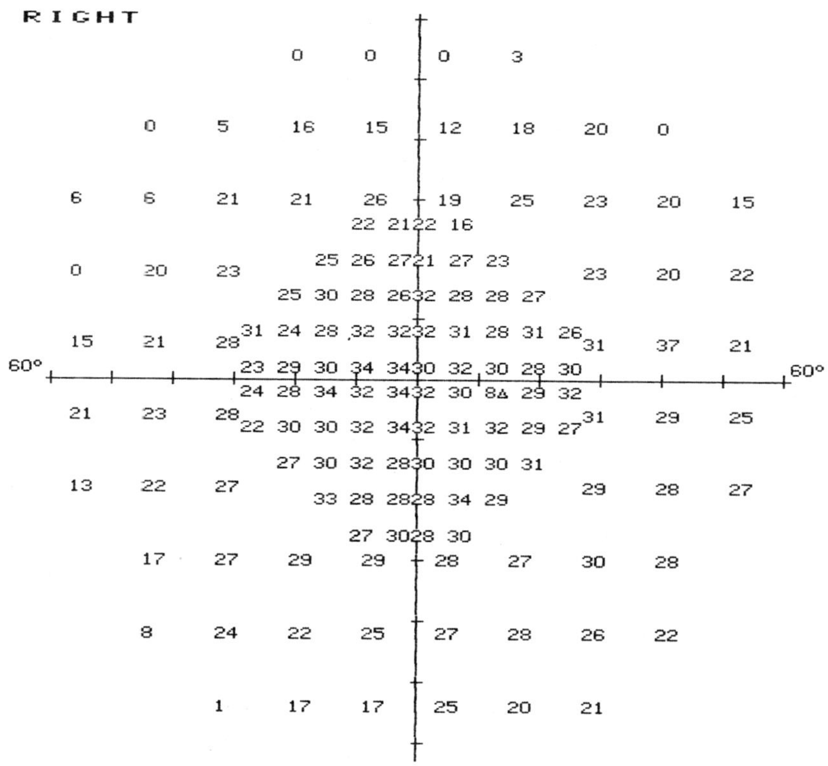

FIG. 5-2, cont'd

Another feature of the normal field to note is that the isopters are not round but bulge toward the temporal side and are flattened superiorly. This means that visual sensitivity is less (i.e., depressed) superiorly compared to inferiorly. Thus I-3e is threshold at 40 degrees superiorly but the dimmer stimulus, I-2e, is threshold at 40 degrees inferiorly. Similarly I-3e is threshold at 50 degrees nasally but the weaker stimulus, I-2e, is threshold at 50 degrees temporally.

In kinetic perimetry the stimulus is moved from a region where it is infrathreshold (invisible), across a boundary where it is threshold (barely visible), into a region where it is suprathreshold (easily visible). The point at which the stimulus first becomes visible is the place where the stimulus is threshold. The line connecting the points where the stimulus first became visible is a line connecting points with equal visual sensitivity.

Thus, along the isopter for I-1e the visual threshold is I-1e. Likewise, I-2e is threshold at the isopter for I-2e. At points in the zone between these two isopters the threshold is a light intensity somewhere between I-1e and I-2e, which is to say that I-2e is visible but I-1e is not. In the same way, between the isopters for I-2e and I-3e the threshold is somewhere between these two.

After several isopters are plotted, the points along a meridian can be plotted on a graph to represent a profile of the "hill of vision" because visual threshold is known at each isopter. Of course, static perimetry is the technique used to obtain a profile plot in actual practice, but a profile derived from kinetically determined points is shown here to emphasize the equivalence of an isopter plot and a profile plot (see p. 25).

FIG. 5-3. Isopter plot of a normal visual field and a profile plot along the horizontal meridian. Each isopter plotted here is 0.5 log-unit more intense than the previous. When the isopters are far apart, the 0.5 log-unit intensity change in the threshold occurs gradually as you proceed away from fixation along the meridian; and this is a flat region in a profile plot. When the isopters are close together, the threshold changes more rapidly as you proceed along the meridian between the two isopters; and this corresponds to a steep slope in the hill of vision. Thus the steepness of slope corresponds to the distance between two isopters that differ in intensity by a specific amount.

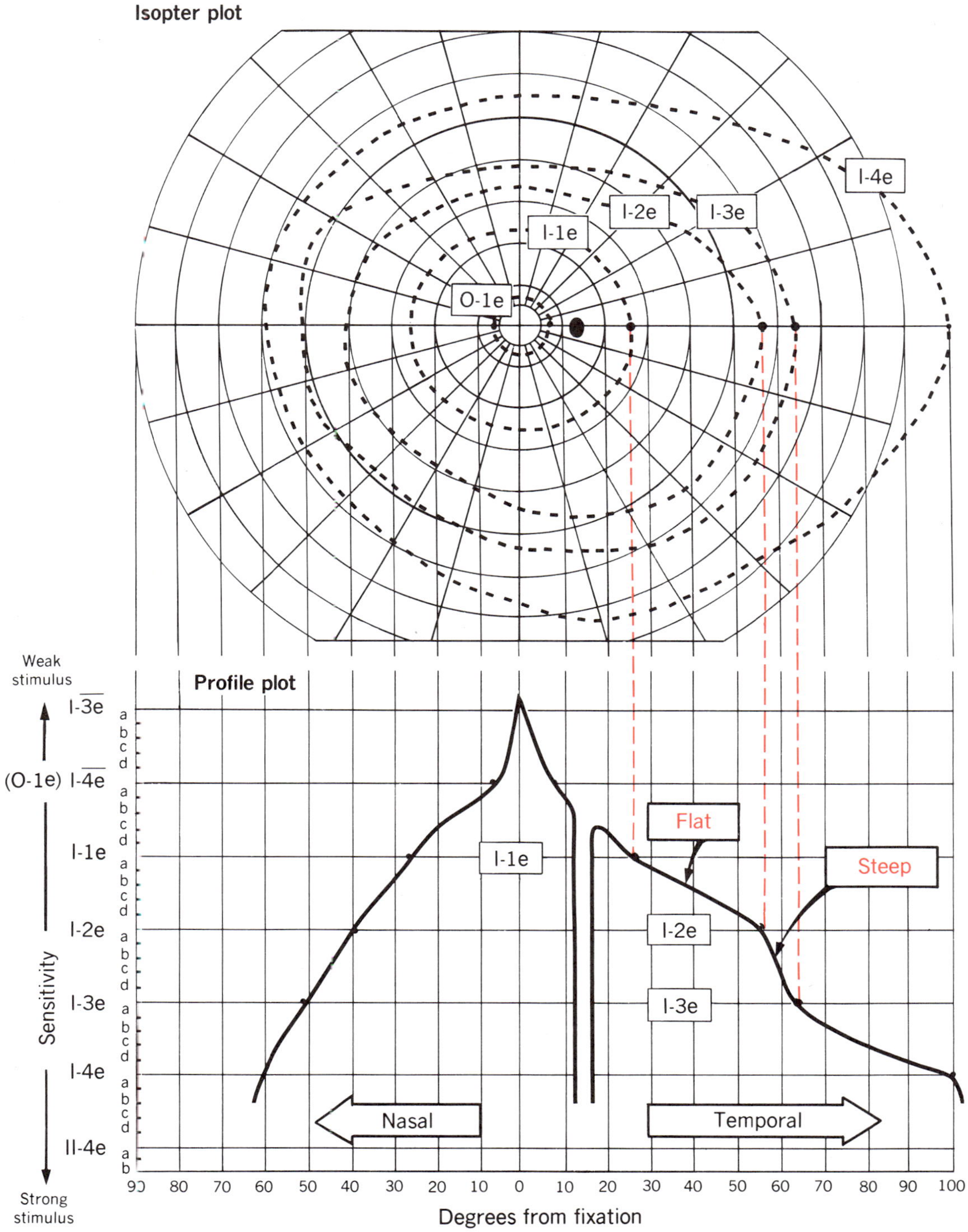
Isopter plot
I-4e
I-2e
I-3e
I-1e
O-1e
Profile plot
Weak stimulus
Strong stimulus
Sensitivity
I-3e
(O-1e) I-4e
I-1e
I-2e
I-3e
I-4e
II-4e
a
b
c
d
I-1e
Flat
Steep
I-2e
I-3e
Nasal
Temporal
90 80 70 60 50 40 30 20 10 0 10 20 30 40 50 60 70 80 90 100
Degrees from fixation

FIG. 5-3

In static threshold perimetry the superior field tends to be slightly less sensitive than the inferior field (corresponding to the flattening of isopters superiorly in Fig. 5-1).

FIG. 5-4. Central 30 degrees of a normal field (Humphrey Field Analyzer, program 31). The greyscale and actual threshold printouts are shown as well as a static cut along the 0- to 180-degree meridian.

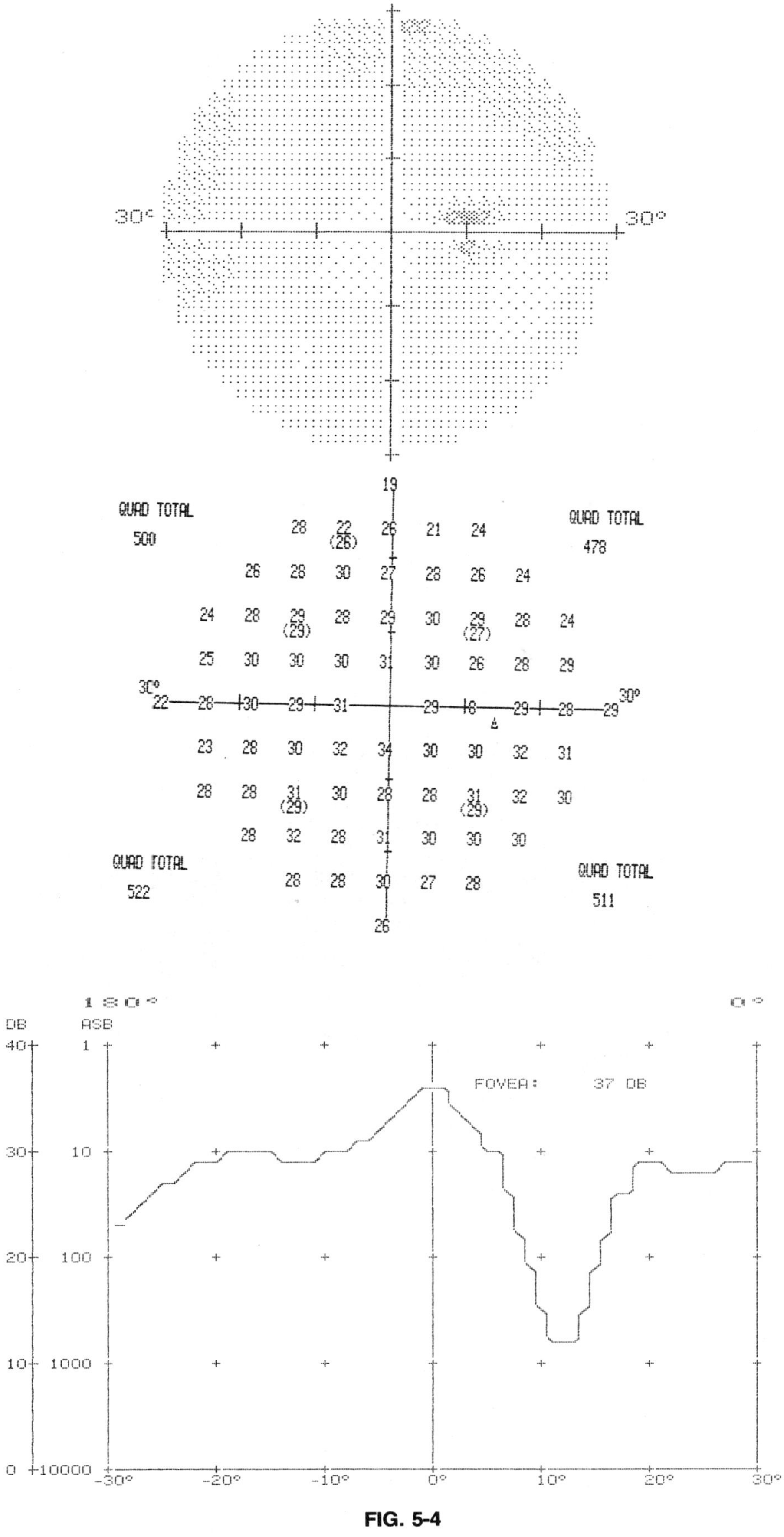
30°
30°
QUAD TOTAL
500
QUAD TOTAL
478
QUAD TOTAL
522
QUAD TOTAL
511
180°
0°
DB
ASB
FOVEA: 37 DB
40 1
30 10
20 100
10 1000
0 10000
-30° -20° -10° 0° 10° 20° 30°

FIG. 5-4

CHAPTER 6

Scotomas

NATURE OF A SCOTOMA

It is normal for a test stimulus to be seen everywhere within the region bounded by its isopter. A *scotoma* is an abnormal region of reduced sensitivity within the isopter. Here the test stimulus is not seen.

FIG. 6-1. Scotoma: an area of reduced visual sensation. The area within the scotoma is less able to perceive test objects than the region surrounding the scotoma.

Except for the physiologic blind spot, any scotoma is abnormal. Scotomas are described or named according to their location, size, or shape.

FIG. 6-2. Examples of scotomas.
A, Central—involving fixation.
B, Centrocecal—joining the blind spot to fixation.
C, Paracentral—near fixation, within 20 degrees.
D, Arcuate (Bjerrum's)—curving above or below fixation.

The boundary of a scotoma is essentially an isopter separating a region where the stimulus (I-2e in this case) is not seen from a region where the stimulus is seen. The isopter marking the boundary of a scotoma differs from the usual isopter in that it encloses an area where the stimulus (I-2e) is *not* seen. By contrast, the usual isopter encloses an area where the stimulus *is* seen. To avoid confusion, we refer to the former as "the I-2e boundary of a scotoma" and the latter simply as "the isopter for I-2e."

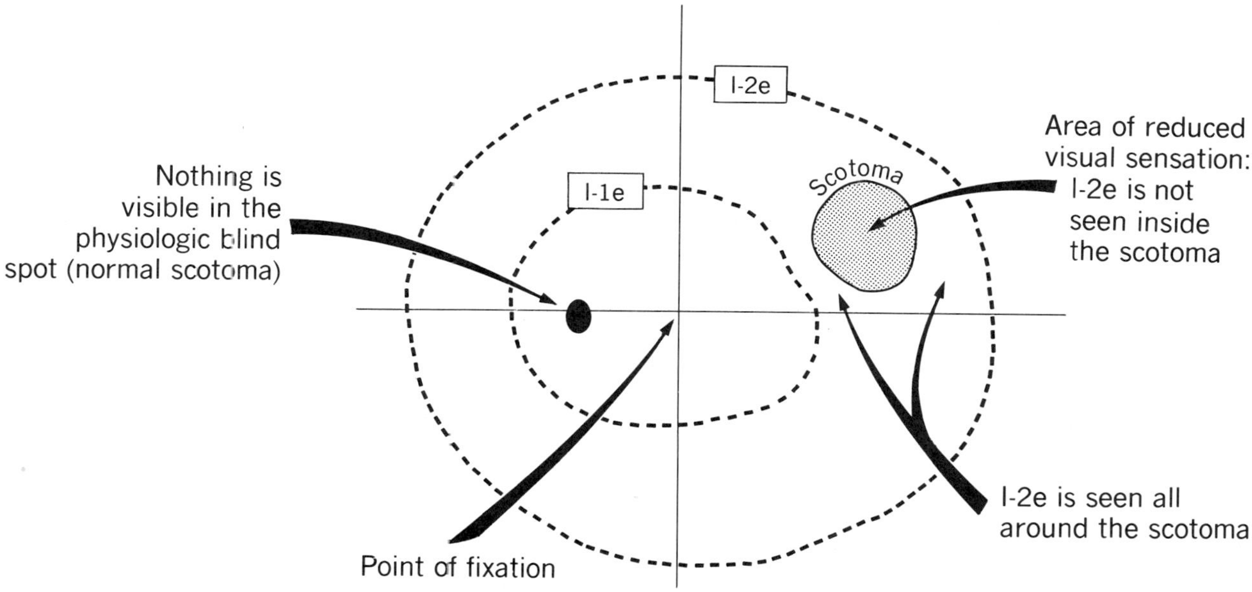
I-2e
I-1e
Scotoma
Nothing is visible in the physiologic blind spot (normal scotoma)
Area of reduced visual sensation: I-2e is not seen inside the scotoma
Point of fixation
I-2e is seen all around the scotoma

FIG. 6-1

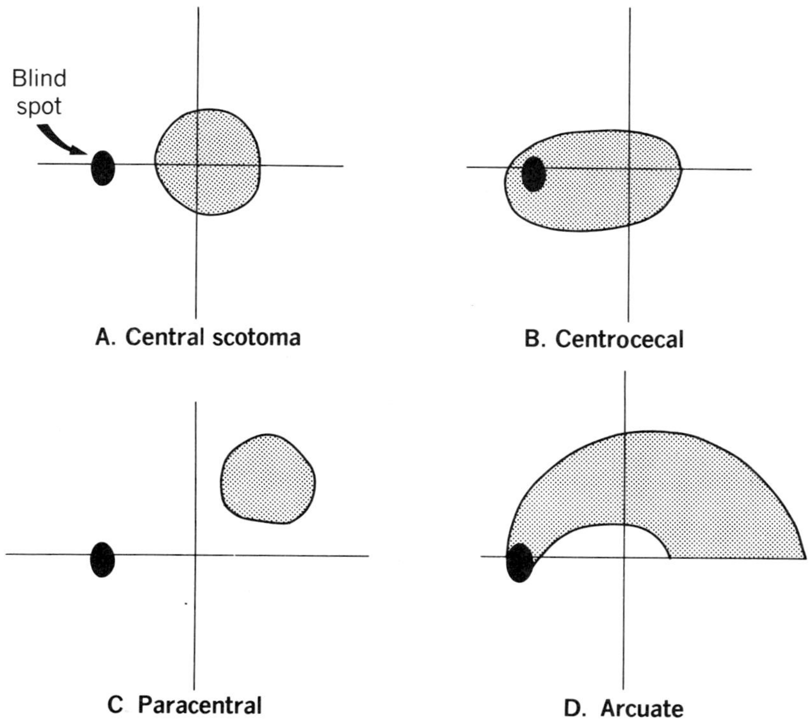
Blind spot
A. Central scotoma
B. Centrocecal
C Paracentral
D. Arcuate

FIG. 6-2

DETECTING SCOTOMAS

To detect scotomas in a visual field, you need to search for areas within an isopter where the stimulus should be seen but is not.

FIG. 6-3. Detecting scotomas in an isopter plot.
A, After the isopter is drawn, the stimulus is presented at several points within the isopter and the patient is asked whether or not he sees it. The stimulus is presented at each location for about 1 second without moving.
B, After a stronger stimulus is used to plot a larger isopter, the region between the isopters is checked for visibility of the stronger stimulus. It is not necessary to check within the smaller isopters with the stronger stimulus because if the weaker stimulus was seen it is certain that the larger one will be seen too.

In these figures you ask a question and the patient responds "yes" or "no." In actual practice you simply flash the light (in essence, asking the patient if he sees it) and the patient responds with the buzzer when he sees the light, which means "yes." The lack of a response means "no." There is no actual conversation (see p. 190).

We can call this procedure for detecting scotomas **static suprathreshold spot-checking.** The procedure is "static" because the patient is asked if he can see a nonmoving object. It is not "threshold" because the threshold is not determined: the test stimulus is expected to be "suprathreshold" (because it is being presented *inside* its isopter). In this procedure you are "spot-checking" in areas where the object should be suprathreshold (visible) so as to be able to detect a scotoma where, in fact, the stimulus is infrathreshold (not visible).

The technique for detecting scotomas in conjunction with kinetic perimetry is described in Chapter 18.

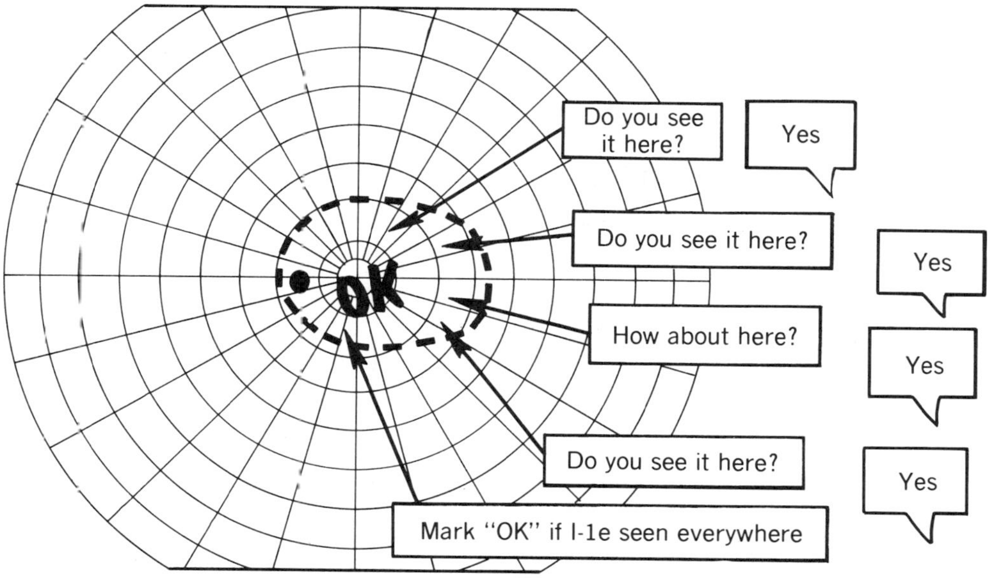

A. Static suprathreshold spot checking

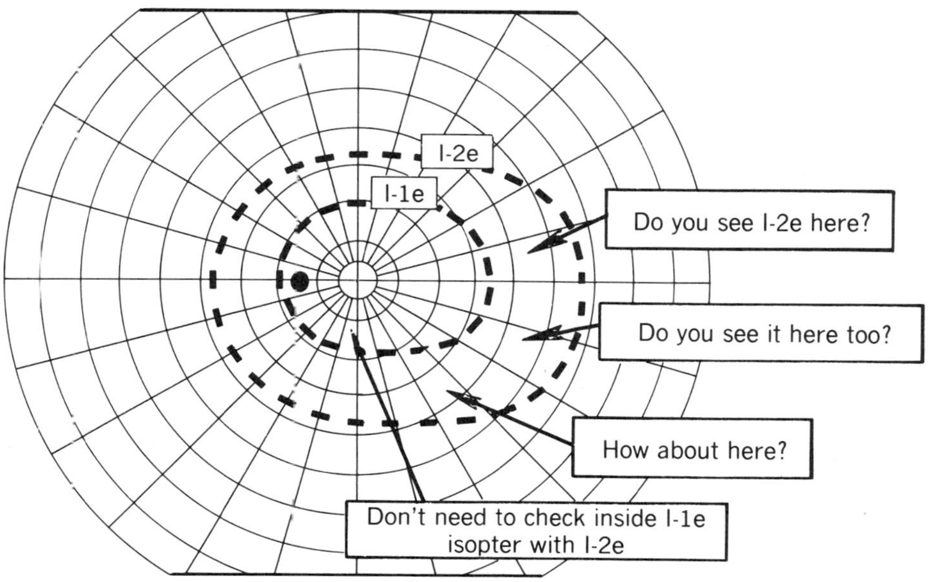

B. Static suprathreshold checking with larger object

FIG. 6-3

The isopters need not always be plotted. It may be assumed (without plotting the isopters) that the I-1e stimulus should be visible everywhere within 15 degrees of fixation and that the I-2e stimulus should be visible everywhere within 30 degrees of fixation (see Fig. 6-3, *B*, for an example of this). A suprathreshold spot check of 75 to 150 locations within 30 degrees of fixation with the I-2e stimulus constitutes a quick and simple one-level method for detecting scotomas in the central visual field. A refinement, with very little extra effort, is to spot-check inside 15 degrees with the I-1e stimulus and between 15 and 30 degrees with the I-2e stimulus. Such compensation of the stimulus intensity for eccentricity allows shallower scotomas near fixation to be detected than if the I-2e stimulus is used everywhere (see p. 404).

This is exactly what automated perimeters do. No isopters are plotted. Stimuli that are normally somewhat suprathreshold are presented over the region of interest. The stimulus intensity may or may not be compensated for eccentricity. Eccentricity compensation adds no time to the test and, for optimum results, should be used.

FIG. 6-4. Scotoma detected by automated suprathreshold testing. The stimulus was not seen at four locations but was at surrounding points.

Scotomas are also detected by threshold static perimetry. A scotoma is recognized when the sensitivity at one or several adjacent points is less than at surrounding locations.

FIG. 6-5. Scotoma in an automated static threshold test. The sensitivity is less than at surrounding points. In particular, it is better at points more peripheral than within the scotoma.

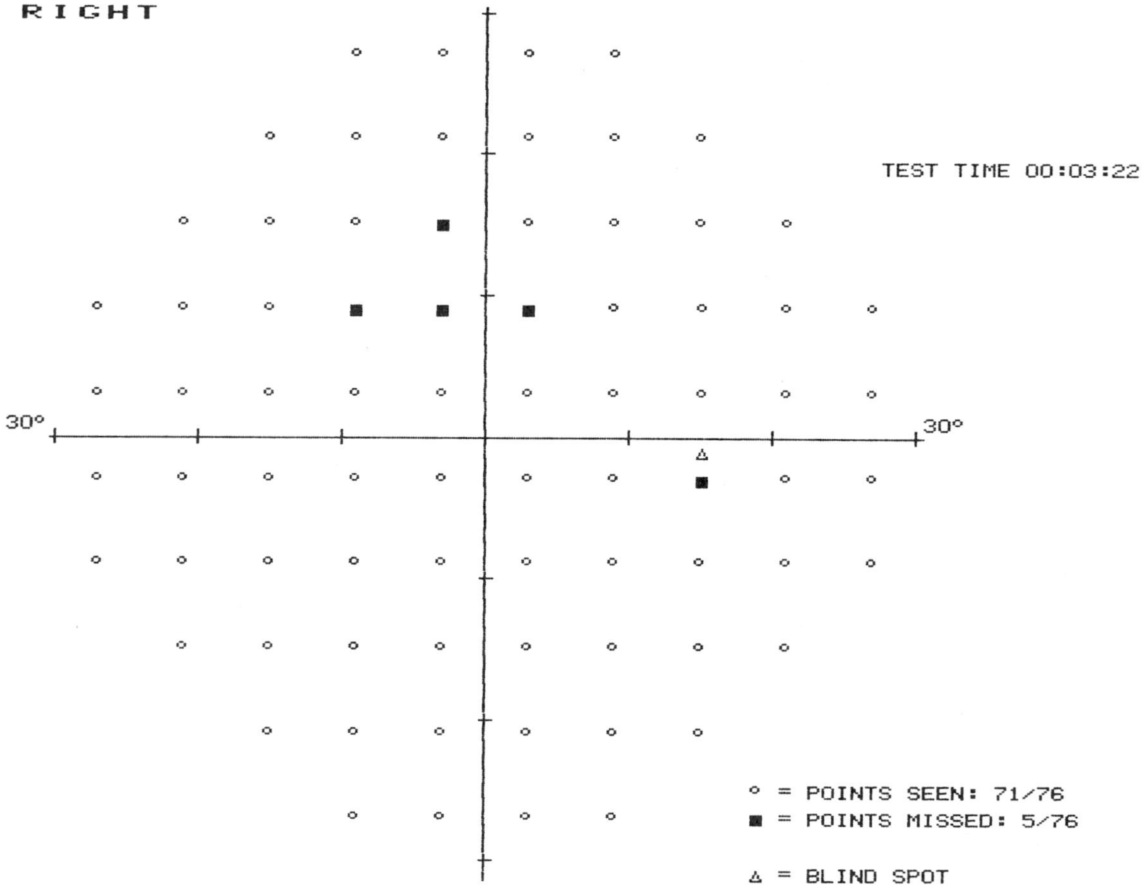
RIGHT
TEST TIME 00:03:22
30°
30°
○ = POINTS SEEN: 71/76
■ = POINTS MISSED: 5/76
△ = BLIND SPOT

FIG. 6-4

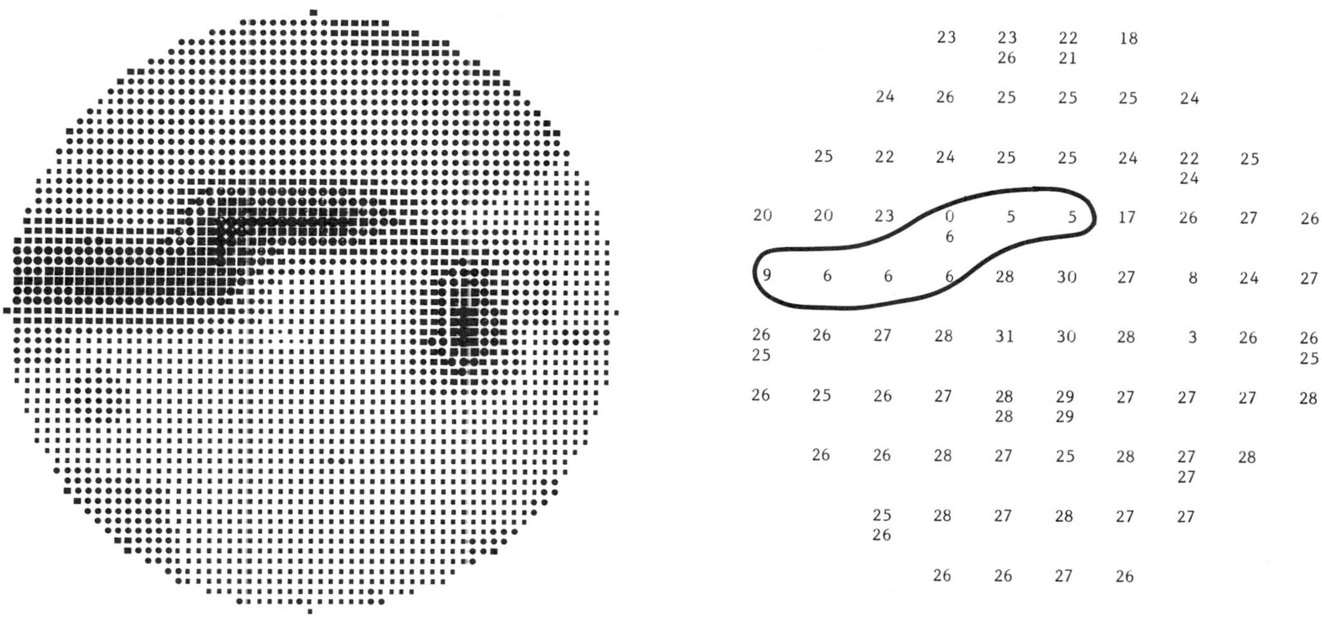
23 23 22 18
26 21
24 26 25 25 25 24
25 22 24 25 25 24 22 25
24
20 20 23 0 5 5 17 26 27 26
6
9 6 6 6 28 30 27 8 24 27
26 26 27 28 31 30 28 3 26 26
25 25
26 25 26 27 28 29 27 27 27 28
28 29
26 26 28 27 25 28 27 28
27
25 28 27 28 27 27
26
26 26 27 26

FIG. 6-5

QUANTIFYING SCOTOMAS

In characterizing a particular scotoma, it is usually not enough to describe the location, size, and shape. The depth and the slope of its boundary should also be described.

FIG. 6-6. Depth of a scotoma.
A, There is a distinction between the approach used to detect and that used to quantify.

TO DETECT THE SCOTOMA WITH SUPRATHRESHOLD TESTING, a spot where the test object is *not* visible must be found. Indeed, the main feature of a scotoma is that a certain test stimulus is not visible that should be visible.

TO QUANTIFY THE DEPTH OF A SCOTOMA, the reverse question is asked: What *is* visible? Or, stated differently, to determine the depth of a scotoma, you ask what the visual threshold within the scotoma is.

B, If the stimulus must be made only slightly more intense or larger to be seen, the scotoma is termed *shallow*. If the stimulus must be made much more intense to be seen, the scotoma is termed *deep*. If the strongest available stimulus on a certain visual field apparatus is not seen, the scotoma is termed a *maximum luminosity* scotoma. If no conceivable stimulus is visible, the scotoma is "absolute." Hence, we can qualitatively speak of the depth of a scotoma as shallow, deep, maximal (for this instrument), or absolute. The physiologic blind spot is an absolute scotoma.

NOTE: It is not possible to quantify visual threshold at a location by determining that a stimulus is *not* seen, any more than it is possible to quantify visual acuity by determining that the 20/20 letters are not seen. The fact that a stimulus is not seen where it should be seen simply uncovers the presence of an abnormality and the next step is to determine what *is* seen.

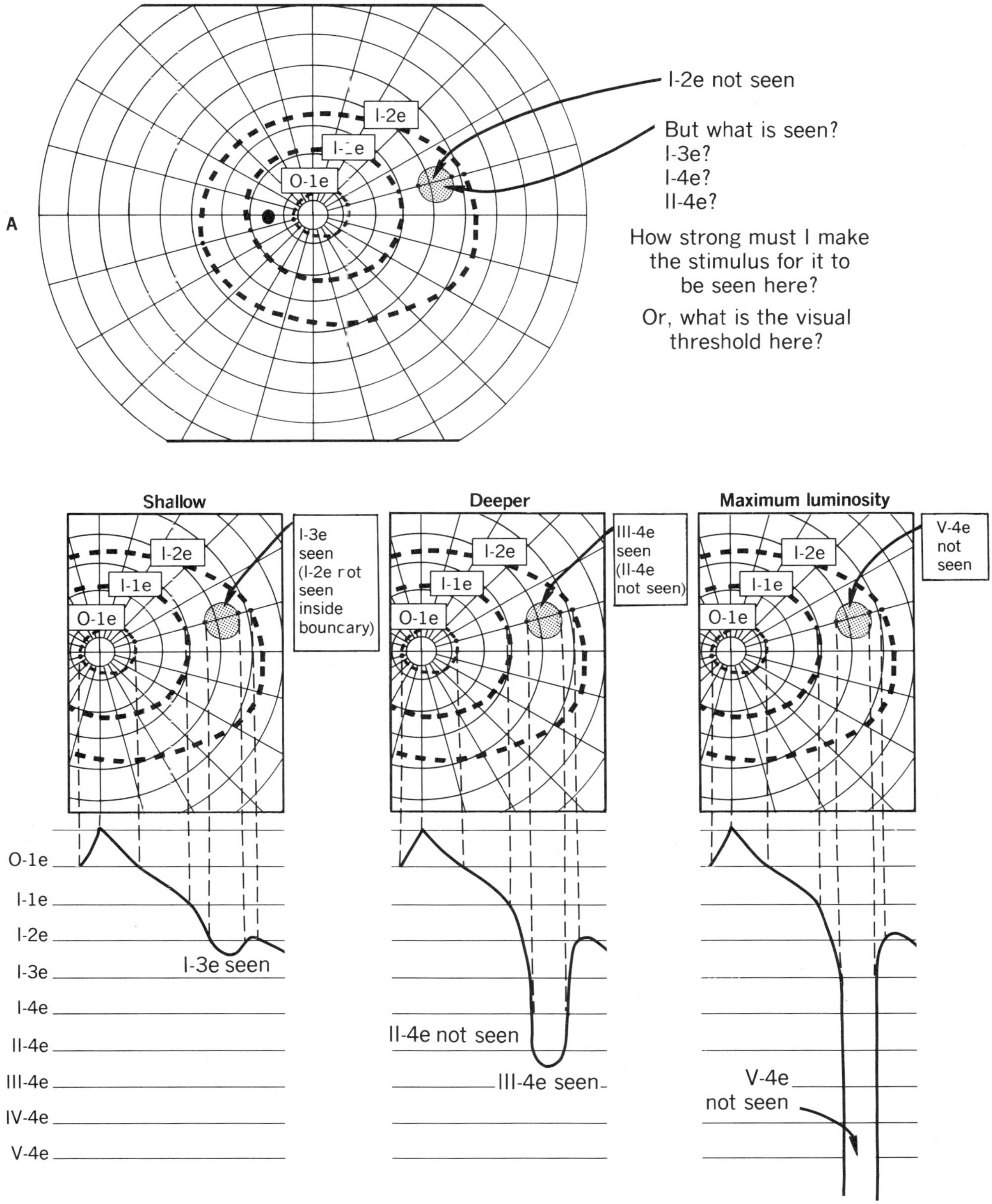
A
I-2e
I-1e
O-1e
I-2e not seen
But what is seen?
I-3e?
I-4e?
II-4e?
How strong must I make the stimulus for it to be seen here?
Or, what is the visual threshold here?
B
Shallow
Deeper
Maximum luminosity
I-3e seen (I-2e not seen inside boundary)
III-4e seen (II-4e not seen)
V-4e not seen
O-1e
I-1e
I-2e
I-3e
I-4e
II-4e
III-4e
IV-4e
V-4e
I-3e seen
II-4e not seen
III-4e seen
V-4e not seen

FIG. 6-6

FIG. 6-7. Slope of the boundary. The depth of the two scotomas illustrated is the same, *II-4e* being the threshold stimulus for both.
A, With a sloping margin the visual threshold changes gradually between the boundary and the deepest part of the center.
B, With a steep margin the visual threshold is very different just inside the boundary as compared to just outside the boundary (right).

The meaning of the terms *sloping* and *steep* is apparent from the profile plots of the two scotomas with the same depth but differing margins.

In the plot of a scotoma the boundary line for each stimulus encloses the region where that stimulus is *not* seen. Of course, the boundary lines for stronger stimuli enclose smaller regions than the boundary lines for weaker stimuli (the opposite of the usual isopters, which enclose regions where the stimulus *is* seen).

Just as with usual isopters (see Fig. 5-3), a sloping contour of the profile is represented by isopters separated one from another whereas a steeper contour is represented by isopters crowded together.

Not all scotomas are as simple as the ones shown. An arcuate (Bjerrum) scotoma, for example, may be of different depth in various places within the scotoma. Moreover, one side may have a steep margin whereas the opposite side may have a sloping margin.

The technique for quantifying scotomas by manual perimetry is covered in Chapter 19.

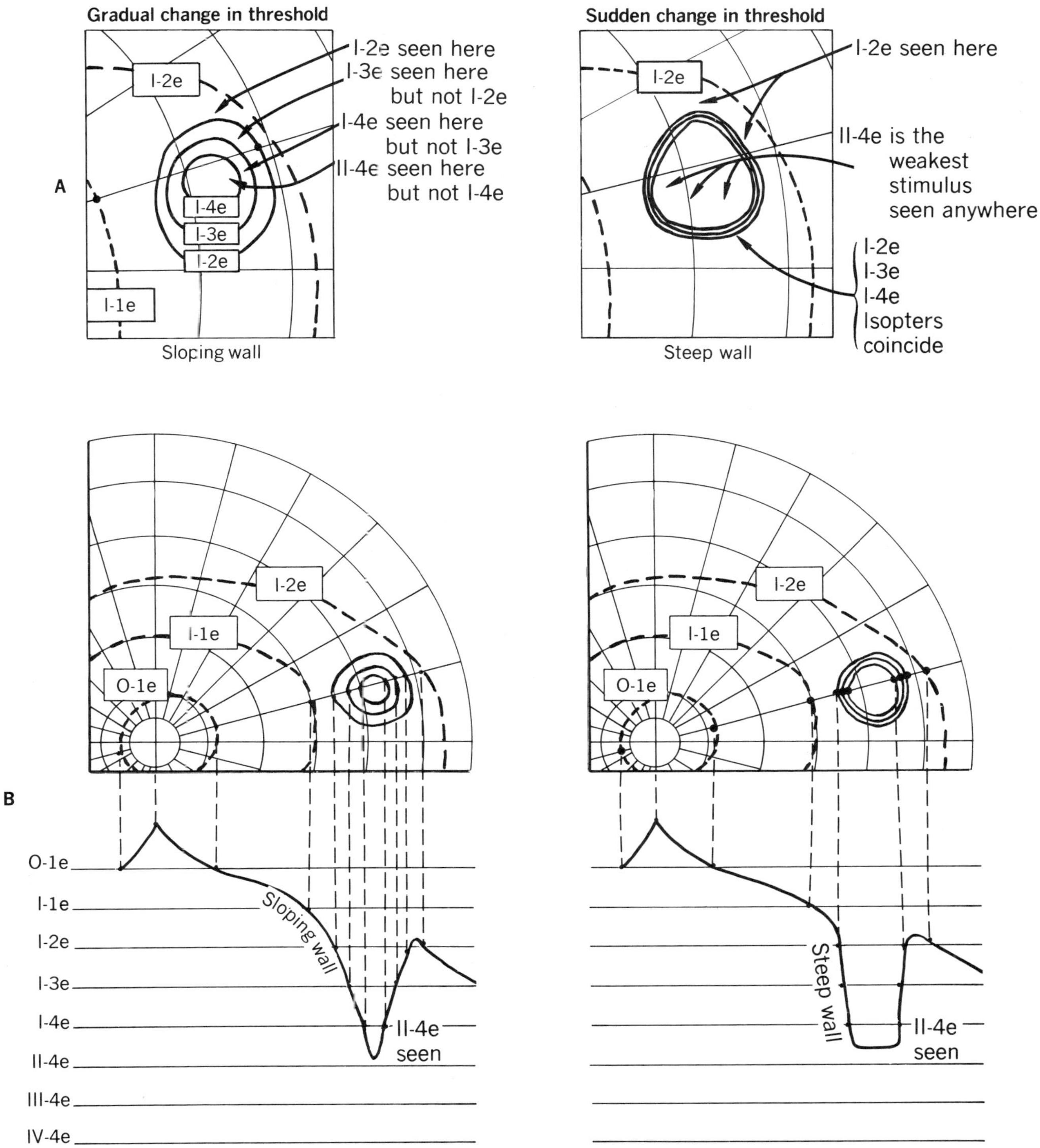

A
Gradual change in threshold
I-2e
I-2e seen here
I-3e seen here but not I-2e
I-4e seen here but not I-3e
II-4e seen here but not I-4e
I-4e
I-3e
I-2e
I-1e
Sloping wall
Sudden change in threshold
I-2e
I-2e seen here
II-4e is the weakest stimulus seen anywhere
I-2e
I-3e
I-4e
Isopters coincide
Steep wall
B
I-2e
I-1e
O-1e
O-1e
I-1e
I-2e
I-3e
I-4e
II-4e
III-4e
IV-4e
Sloping wall
II-4e seen
Steep wall
II-4e seen

FIG. 6-7

When a scotoma has been uncovered by automated suprathreshold testing, the clinical circumstance (Chapter 11) will dictate whether or not the defect needs to be either semiquantified or fully quantified. If it is known in advance that classification of defects is desired, a suprathreshold program can be selected in which the defects are automatically classified (semiquantified) as relative or absolute.

FIG. 6-8. Suprathreshold testing with semiquantitation. In the lower nasal quadrant there is an absolute defect (strongest stimulus not seen) at three adjacent points. Three additional neighboring points are relatively defective (test stimulus not seen, but strongest stimulus is seen).

A semiquantitative classification of defects may suffice for diagnostic purposes, but usually it is not sufficient to follow a chronic condition for possible progression. In such cases the defect (and indeed the entire field, including the normal points) needs to be quantified with static threshold perimetry as a baseline for future comparison.

With automated static threshold perimetry the depth of the scotoma is judged by comparing the sensitivity within the defect to the sensitivity at surrounding locations. Alternatively, the sensitivity at defective points is compared to normal values.

FIG. 6-9. Comparison printout (Octopus) of the scotoma in Fig. 6-5. In the left-hand box the actual threshold values are given and a scotoma is recognized with a sensitivity of only 3 to 9 dB compared to 20 to 30 dB for the surrounding points. In the center box the difference of threshold from the normal value is shown, indicating that the defective points are 15 to 23 dB less sensitive than normal. Note how the deep well-delineated scotoma is highlighted in this type of data presentation. The right-hand box gives the normal threshold values for a person of this age.

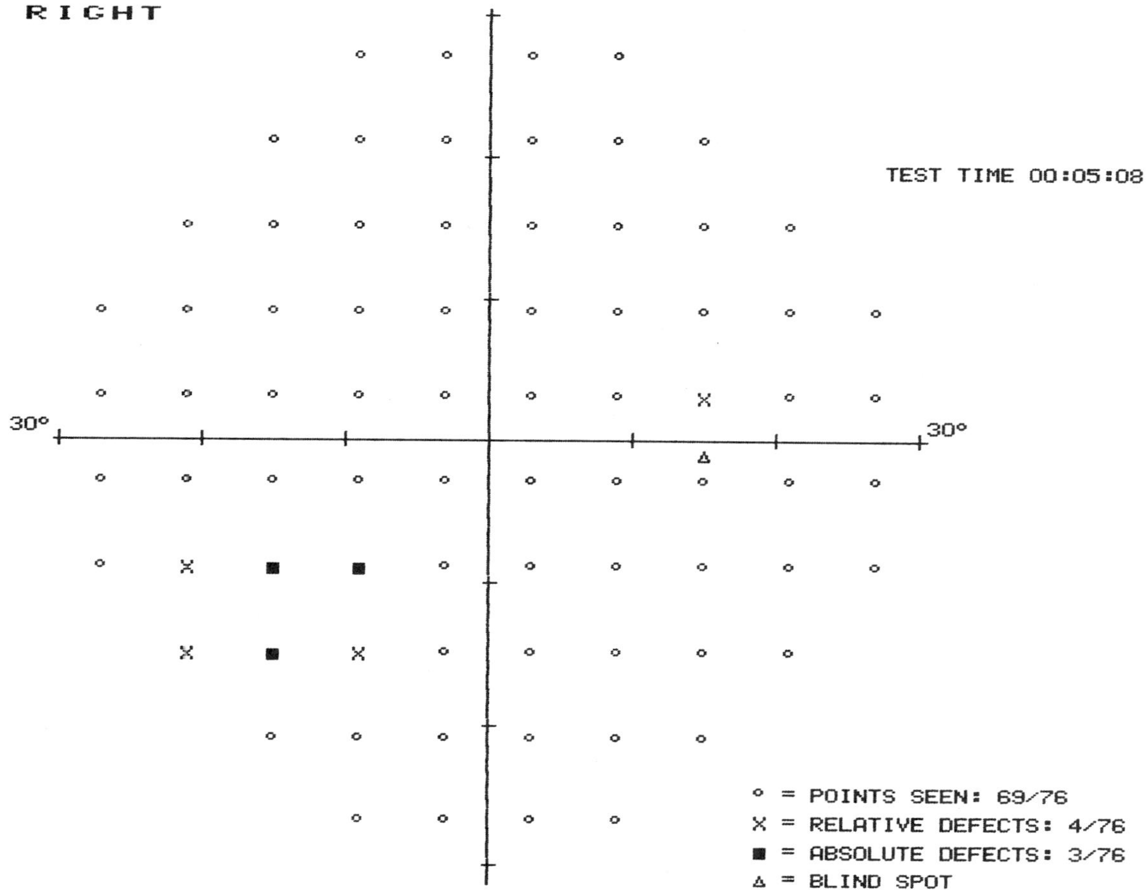
RIGHT
TEST TIME 00:05:08
30°
30°
° = POINTS SEEN: 69/76
X = RELATIVE DEFECTS: 4/76
■ = ABSOLUTE DEFECTS: 3/76
Δ = BLIND SPOT

FIG. 6-8

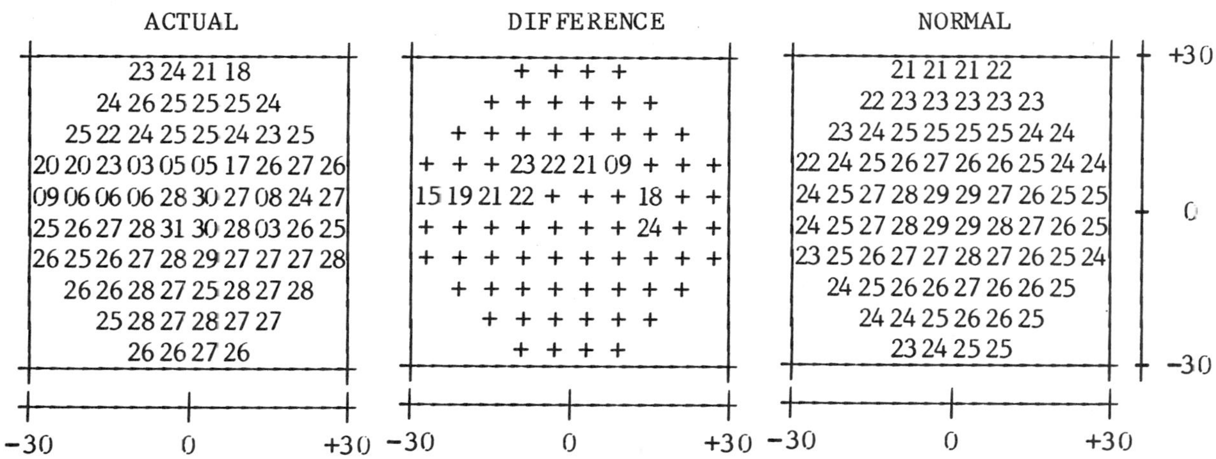
ACTUAL
23 24 21 18
24 26 25 25 25 24
25 22 24 25 25 24 23 25
20 20 23 03 05 05 17 26 27 26
09 06 06 06 28 30 27 08 24 27
25 26 27 28 31 30 28 03 26 25
26 25 26 27 28 29 27 27 27 28
26 26 28 27 25 28 27 28
25 28 27 28 27 27
26 26 27 26
-30 0 +30
DIFFERENCE
+ + + +
+ + + + + +
+ + + + + + + +
+ + + 23 22 21 09 + + +
15 19 21 22 + + + 18 + +
+ + + + + + + 24 + +
+ + + + + + + + + +
+ + + + + + + +
+ + + + + +
+ + + +
-30 0 +30
NORMAL
21 21 21 22
22 23 23 23 23 23
23 24 25 25 25 25 24 24
22 24 25 26 27 26 26 25 24 24
24 25 27 28 29 29 27 26 25 25
24 25 27 28 29 29 28 27 26 25
23 25 26 27 27 28 27 26 25 24
24 25 26 26 27 26 26 25
24 24 25 26 26 25
23 24 25 25
-30 0 +30
+30
0
-30

FIG. 6-9

If the size or slope of the scotoma is not shown in sufficient detail on the standard static threshold test (say, with a 6-degree resolution), there are several ways to quantify the defect in more detail.

FIG. 6-10. Exploration of a scotoma.

A, Discovered by static threshold perimetry with 6-degree resolution (Octopus program 32). The abnormal point represents the end of an arcuate paracentral scotoma, which is drawn in. The physiologic blind spot is also represented.

B, Retesting of the field by a second threshold test with 6-degree resolution but offset 3 degrees from the first both vertically and horizontally (Octopus program 31). The diagram shows the bridge connecting the blind spot and the scotoma. None of the test points includes the physiologic blind spot (see Fig. 13-1).

C, Combined printout, providing a 3-degree resolution of the entire field. The arcuate nature of the scotoma is shown.

D, Static cut along the 0- to 180-degree meridian showing the depth of the scotoma (arrows) on each side of fixation.

In addition, a scotoma can be quantified by a closer grid of points with triple determination (see Fig. 14-1).

The examining physician may use any of these methods whenever he feels uncertain as to the presence of a scotoma in a particular location. For example, there may be two adjacent points in the standard 6-degree program that had a suspicious sensitivity value depressed 5 dB from the normal (see Chapter 13).

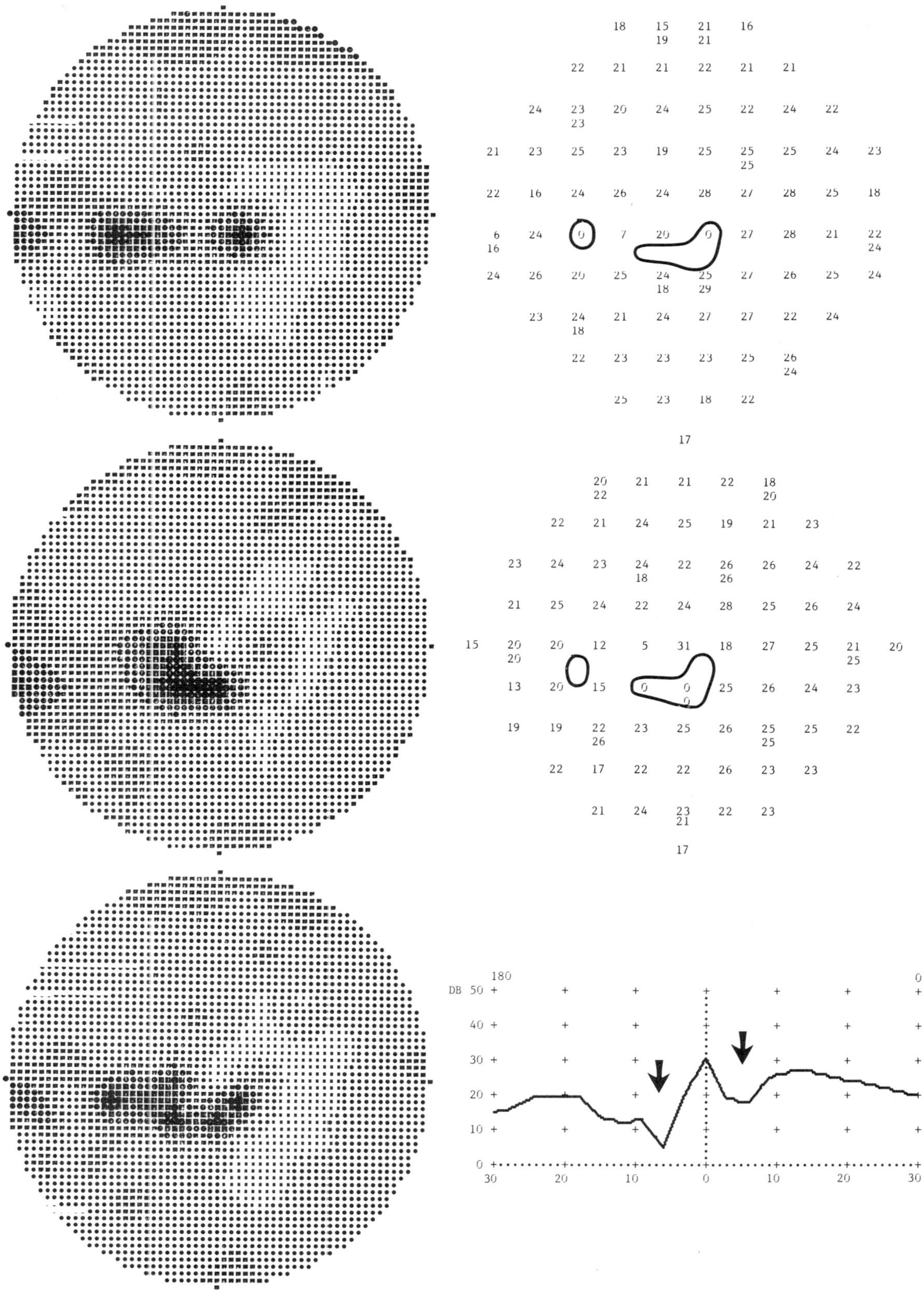
18 15 21 16
19 21
22 21 21 22 21 21
24 23 20 24 25 22 24 22
23
21 23 25 23 19 25 25 25 24 23
25
22 16 24 26 24 28 27 28 25 18
6 24 0 7 20 0 27 28 21 22
16 24
24 26 20 25 24 25 27 26 25 24
18 29
23 24 21 24 27 27 22 24
18
22 23 23 23 25 26
24
25 23 18 22
17
20 21 21 22 18
22 20
22 21 24 25 19 21 23
23 24 23 24 22 26 26 24 22
18 26
21 25 24 22 24 28 25 26 24
15 20 20 12 5 31 18 27 25 21 20
20 25
13 20 15 0 0 25 26 24 23
0
19 19 22 23 25 26 25 25 22
26 25
22 17 22 22 26 23 23
21 24 23 22 23
21
17
180
0
DB 50
40
30
20
10
0
30 20 10 0 10 20 30

FIG. 6-10

CHAPTER 7

Localized depressions

CHARACTERISTICS OF A LOCALIZED DEPRESSION

Visual sensitivity may be reduced in a localized region of the visual field without producing scotomas. Such an area of reduced visual sensitivity is a localized depression.

FIG. 7-1. Isopter plot for a localized depression, A, compared to that for a scotoma, B.
Note that *K* is in a region of reduced visual sensation but is not surrounded *on all sides* by a zone with better sensitivity. The isopter for *I-2e* should continue in a smooth contour enclosing *K,* in which case *I-2e* would be visible at *K*. Instead, the isopter dips inward so *K* is outside the isopter, which means that *I-2e* is not visible at *K* and visual sensation is reduced. *I-2e* should be seen but is not. The *I-2e* is not visible more peripherally than the depressed region—in contrast to the situation existing with a scotoma.

Thus, in a depression the isopter is displaced inward and visual sensation is abnormal; but the abnormality is not a scotoma. The essential difference between a depression and a scotoma is that a scotoma is surrounded *on all sides* by a region of better sensation than within the defect but a depression is not.

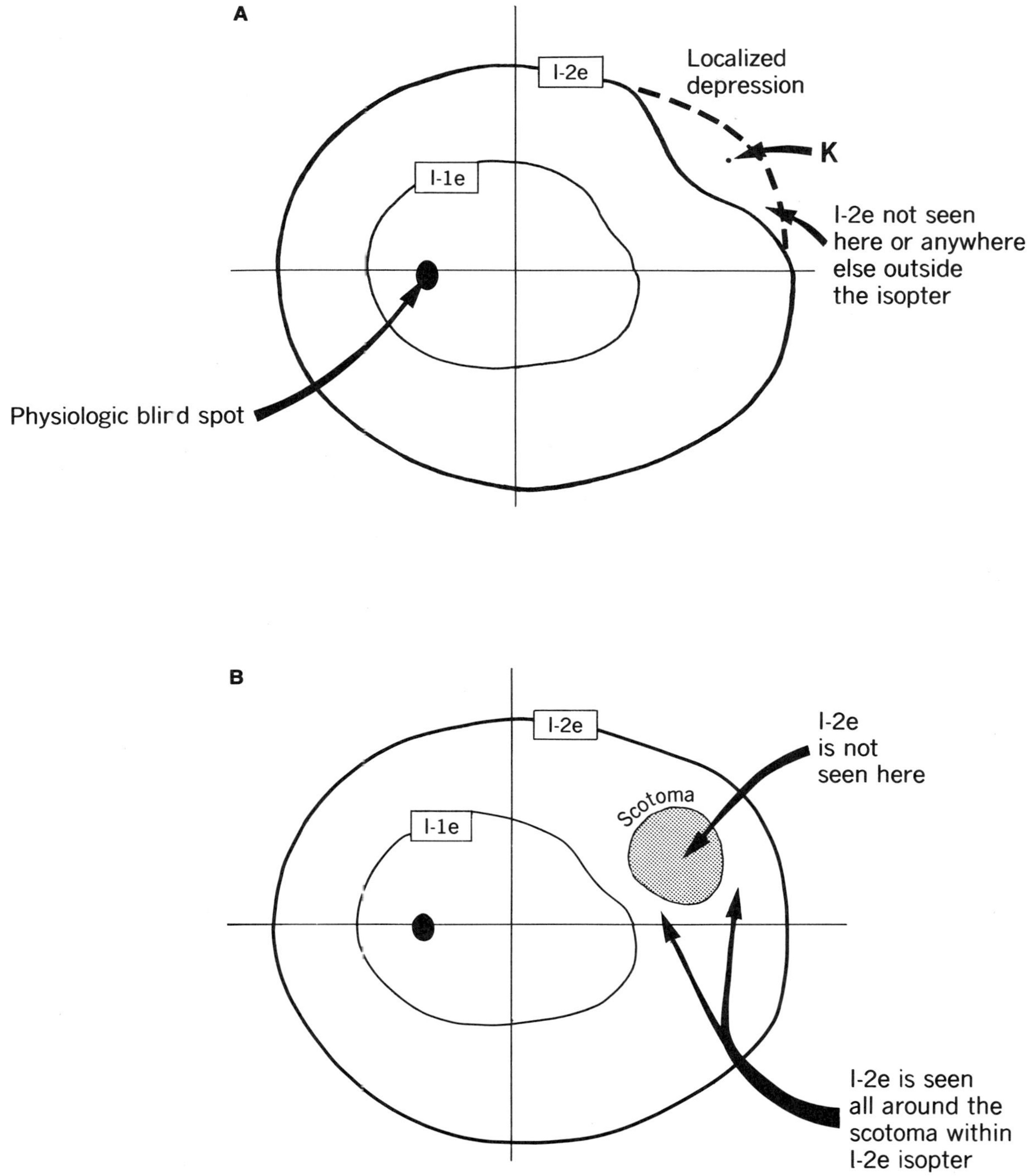
A
I-2e
Localized
depression
K
I-1e
I-2e not seen
here or anywhere
else outside
the isopter
Physiologic blird spot
B
I-2e
I-2e
is not
seen here
Scotoma
I-1e
I-2e is seen
all around the
scotoma within
I-2e isopter

FIG. 7-1

FIG. 7-2. Difference between a pure well-established scotoma (right) and a similarly pure depression (left) in various representations. From top to bottom are shown a three-dimensional sketch of the hill of vision, a meridional profile, an isoper plot, and a greyscale.

The distinction between localized depressions and scotomas has been made because they are differently represented on the field chart. Moreover, they are approached differently for detection and quantitation during manual kinetic perimetry. However, they do have the same underlying basis (reduced visual sensation) and thus they are closely related. The distinction is less important for interpretation in automated perimetry.

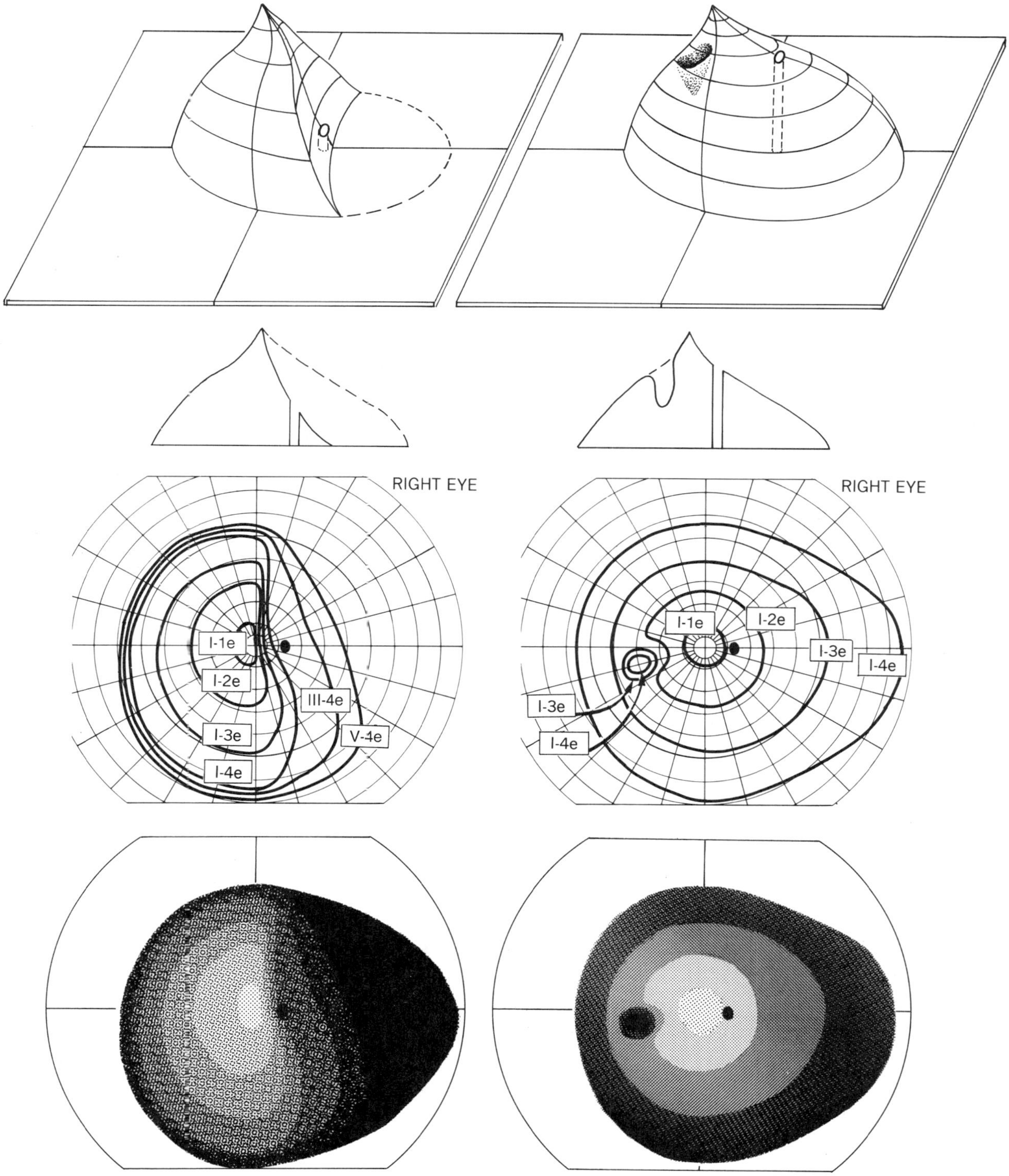
RIGHT EYE
I-1e
I-2e
III-4e
I-3e
V-4e
I-4e
RIGHT EYE
I-1e
I-2e
I-3e
I-4e
I-3e
I-4e

FIG. 7-2

FIG. 7-3. Relationship of localized depressions and scotomas. A scotoma may become a depression if the zone between it and the isopter becomes abnormal. When this occurs, the scotoma is sometimes said to have "broken through to the periphery." The abnormal area, at one time surrounded by a zone of sensitivity, is no longer surrounded by such a zone and hence is no longer a scotoma. Visual sensation in the area that was formerly a scotoma is not charged at all; however, it is no longer a scotoma—not because the scotoma has changed but because an *adjacent area* has changed.

FIG. 7-4. Deviation of an isopter around a scotoma. A region that seems to be a depression because an isopter is deviated inward locally may actually be a scotoma with the isopter (by necessity) simply skirting around it. In this example, if the *I-2c* isopter alone has been plotted, the inward deviation would seem to represent a depression; but in fact it results from a scotoma. Indeed, every scotoma can be made to have an isopter deviate around it if the perimetrist merely plots the isopter that would normally pass through the center of the scotoma. Obviously, if the *I-2e* test object is not seen in the area of the scotoma, a weaker stimulus (*I-2c,* with its isopter closer to fixation than the strong object, *I-2e*) will not be seen either and, hence, the scotoma must lie outside the isopter for *I-2c*.

Diagnostically it is usually the local nature of the reduction of visual sensation and the location or shape of the defect that are important—not whether the defect is a depression or a scotoma.

In automated static threshold perimetry the defectiveness of an area is represented by the threshold values. These are obtained using the same technique in both depressions and scotomas. The defective area may be described as a localized depression or a scotoma; but the interpretation (clinical significance) of the defect depends on its size, shape, and location, as well as on the degree of depressed visual sensitivity (depth of the defect), not on whether it is a scotoma or a localized depression.

Scotoma becoming a depression

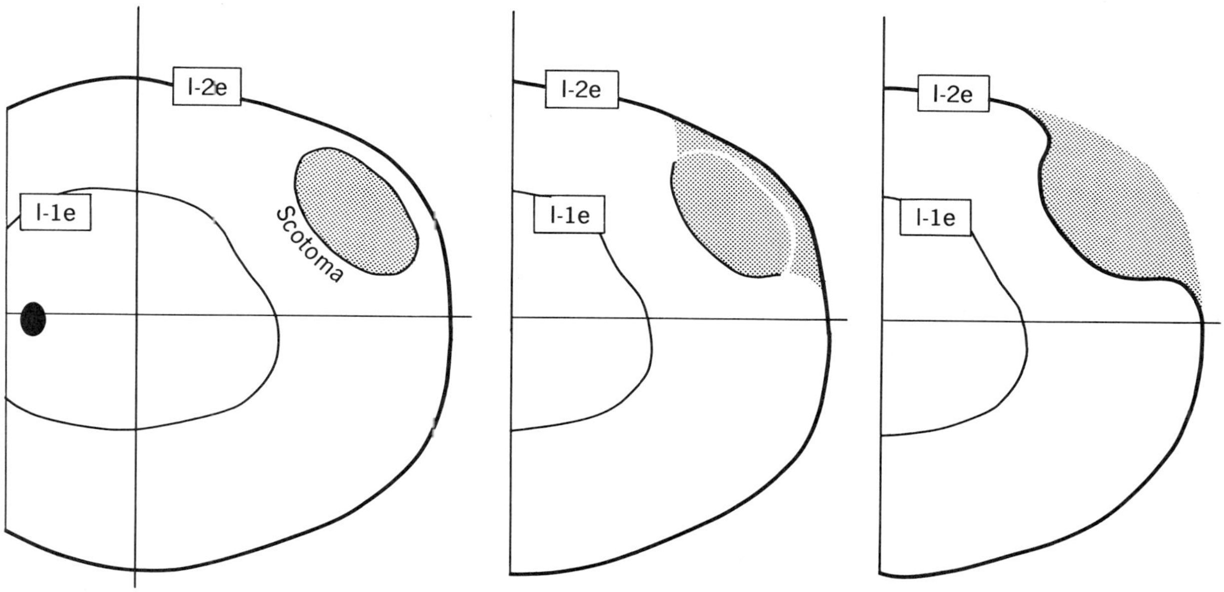

FIG. 7-3

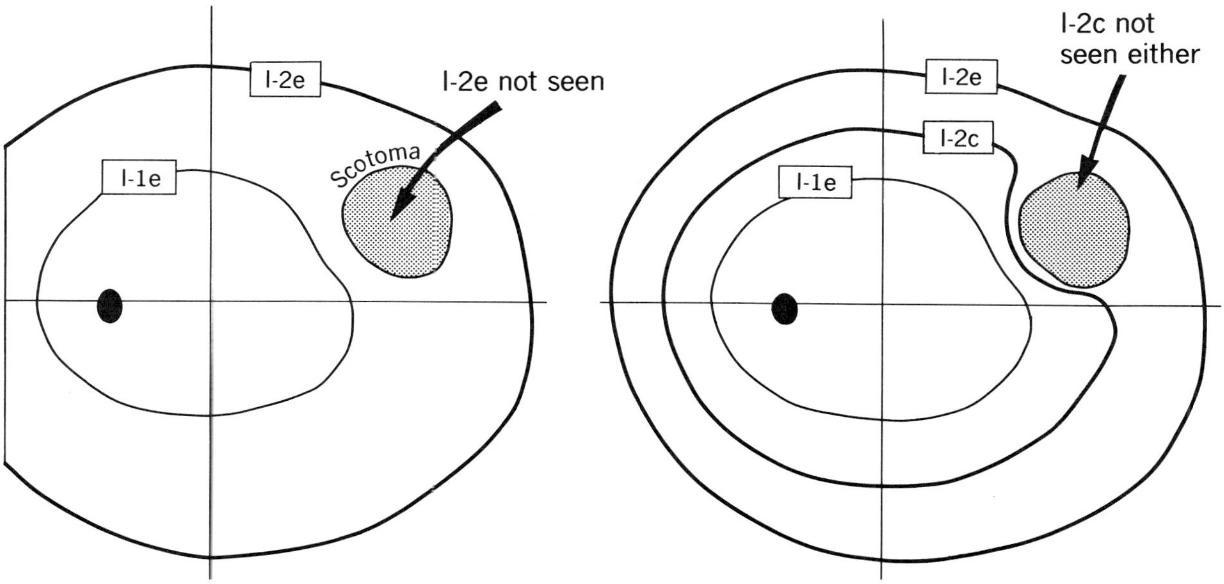

FIG. 7-4

BOUNDARY OF A LOCALIZED DEPRESSION

By automated static threshold perimetry the boundary of an affected region is usually obvious as a darkened region in the greyscale printout or numerical printout of difference-from-anticipated sensitivities.

FIG. 7-5. Static threshold representation of a wedge-shaped defect extending temporally (arrow) from the blind spot. The field is plotted out to 60 degrees. The darkened area nasally (to the left) and superiorly represents the normal edge of the visual field.

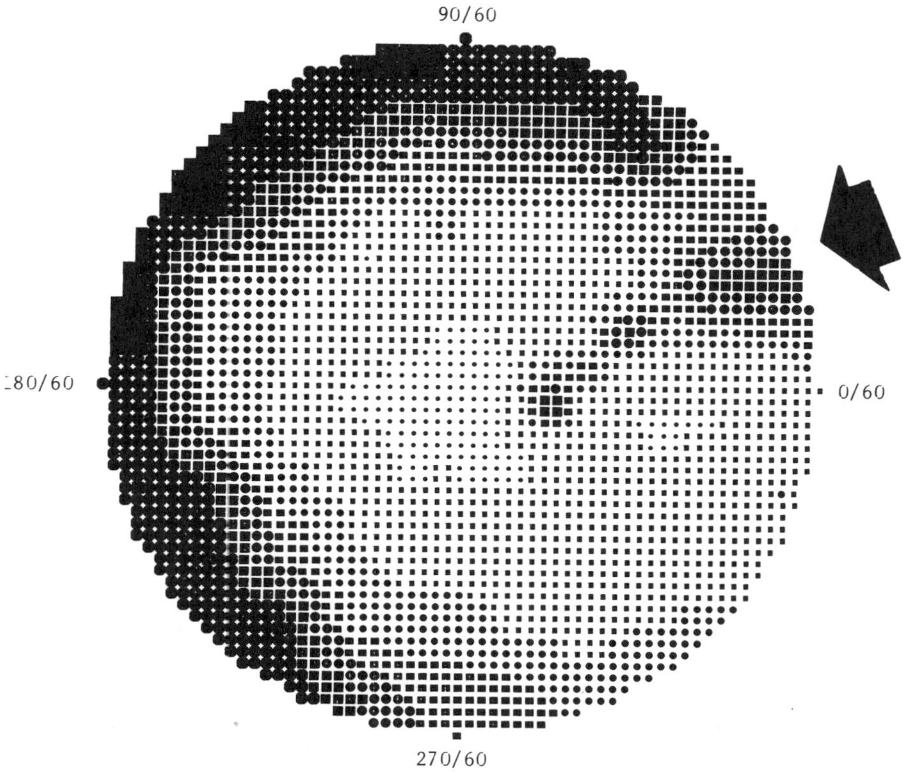

Symb.									
dB	51–36	35–31	30–26	25–21	20–16	15–11	10–6	5–1	0
asb	0,008–0,25	0,31–0,8	1–2,5	3,1–8	10–25	31–80	100–250	315–800	1000

1 asb = 0,318 cd/m²

OCTOPUS®

FIG. 7-5

In an isopter plot the examiner must be careful when trying to recognize the extent of the depression, that is, the extent of the region affected by reduced visual sensation. Visual sensation is reduced in every place where the isopter is deviated inward.

FIG. 7-6. Extent of a localized depression. Visual field charts are never actually marked to show the boundary of a depression, but the extent of the depressed region (emphasized in this illustration) is simply visualized mentally. With attention to all the locally deviated isopters, it is easy to recognize the extent of the area within which there is reduced visual sensation.

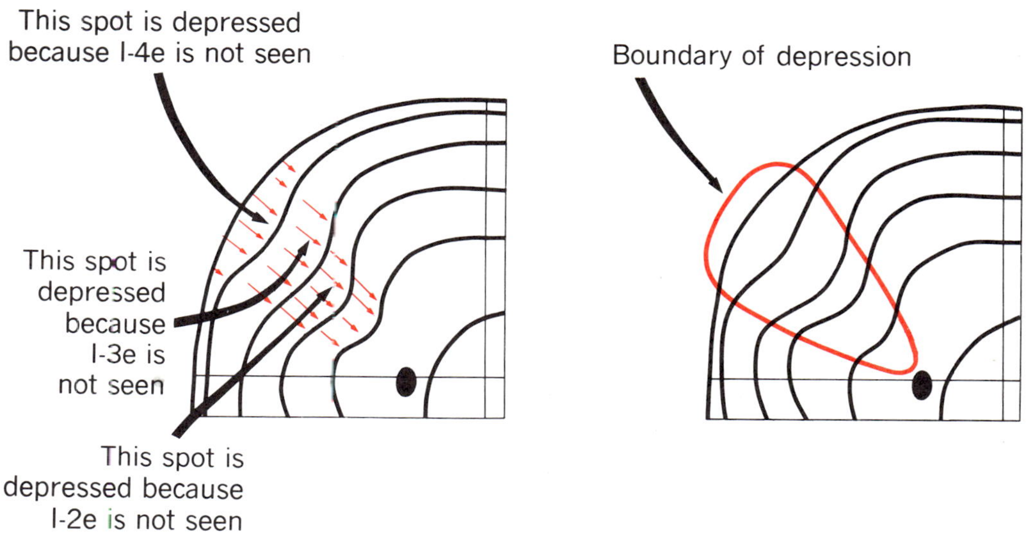
This spot is depressed
because I-4e is not seen
This spot is
depressed
because
I-3e is
not seen
This spot is
depressed because
I-2e is not seen
Boundary of depression

FIG. 7-6

Now the essential distinction between a depression and a scotoma becomes apparent: The boundary of the scotoma is marked by a kinetically plotted isopter separating the region where a particular stimulus is not seen from the region where it is seen; the boundary of the depression cannot be plotted kinetically as an isopter.

FIG. 7-7. Examples of localized depression contrasted with a scotoma. The abnormal region is shaded in red. A depression can contain a scotoma, with the extent of the depression being greater than the boundary of the scotoma. This differs from a pure scotoma, which may show isopters deviating around it but will not show depressed visual sensation outside its boundary.

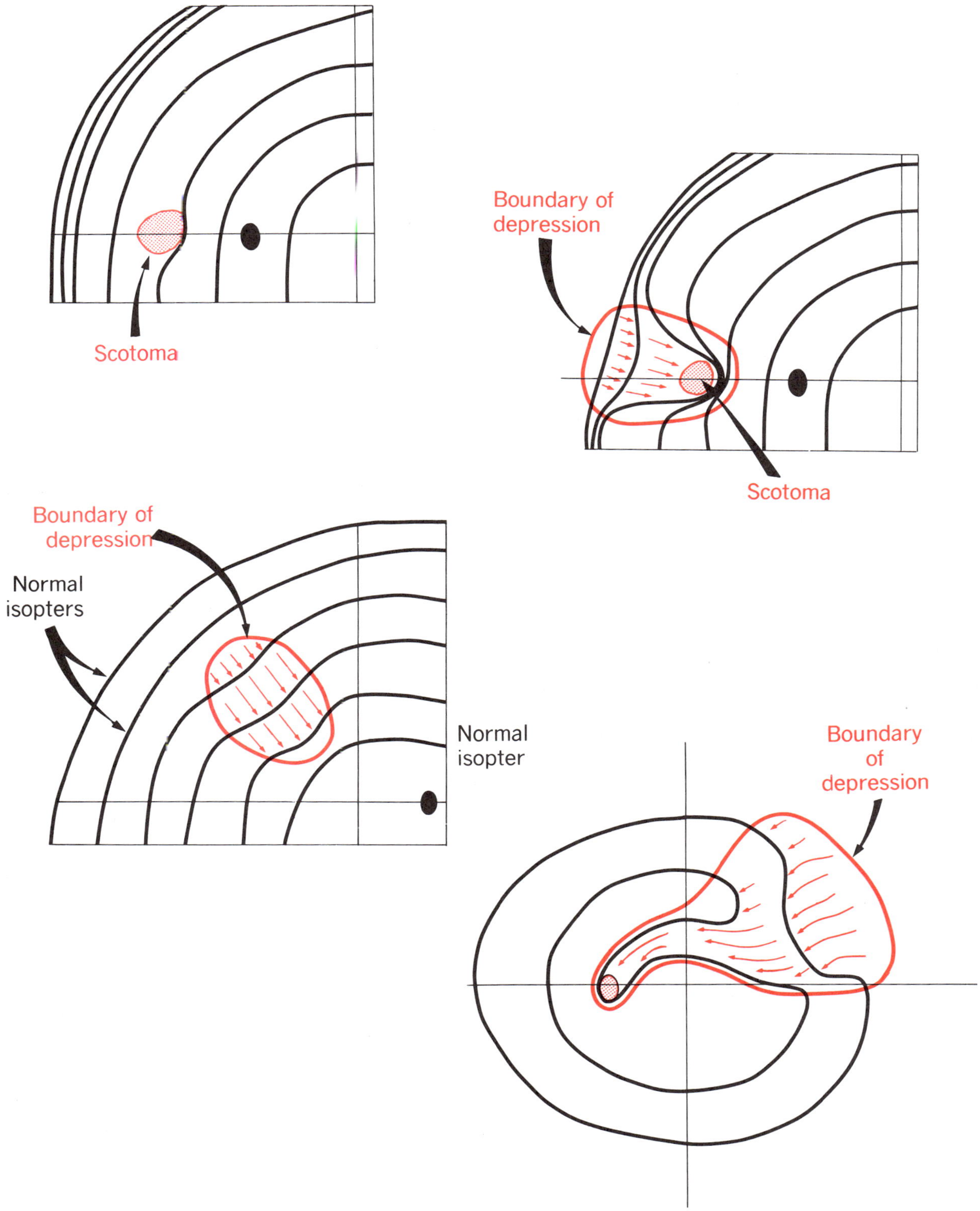
Scotoma
Boundary of depression
Scotoma
Boundary of depression
Normal isopters
Normal isopter
Boundary of depression

FIG. 7-7

FIG. 7-8. Shallow depression. In the isopter plot of the depression the isopters are locally displaced inward only slightly compared to the normal field. At every point within the depression, visual sensation is reduced. For example, at point *R* in the normal field *I-2e* would be seen but at point *R* in the depression *I-3e* would be the weakest stimulus that could be seen. This represents a 0.5 log-unit (5 dB) reduction in visual sensitivity.

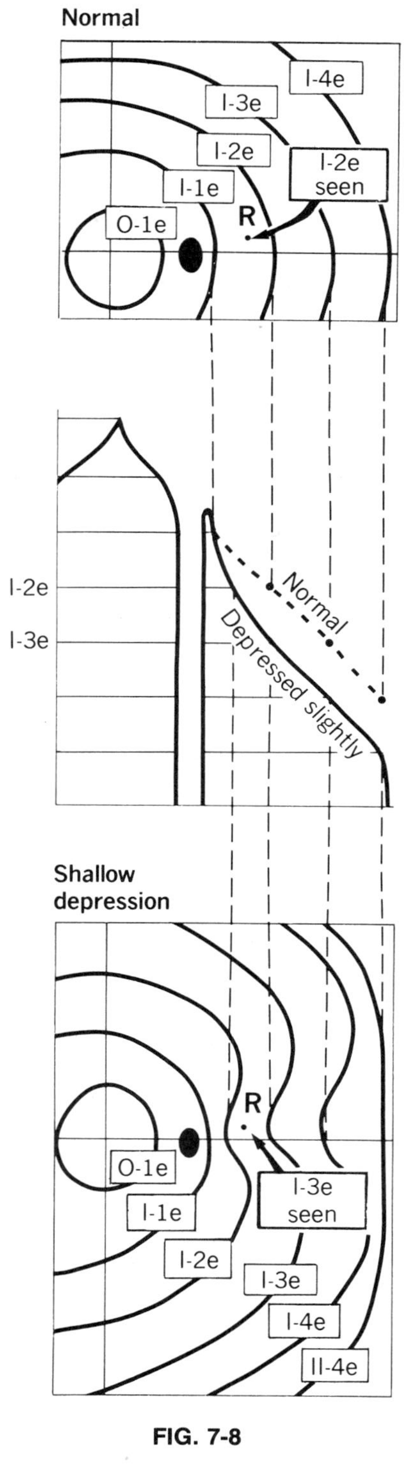
Normal
I-4e
I-3e
I-2e
I-2e seen
I-1e
O-1e
R
I-2e
I-3e
Normal
Depressed slightly
Shallow depression
R
O-1e
I-3e seen
I-1e
I-2e
I-3e
I-4e
II-4e

FIG. 7-8

DEPTH OF A DEPRESSION

Like a scotoma, a depression has depth—the amount of reduction in sensitivity from the expected threshold value.

With automated static threshold perimetry the degree of abnormality is instantly obvious from the numeric printout of the difference-from-expected values. The fact that the boundary of the affected region and the degree of abnormality are both readily apparent is one of the advantages of the static threshold method.

The same threshold information is contained in the isopter plot resulting from properly performed (Chapter 20) kinetic perimetry. However, the abnormality is represented by isopter position rather than by a numerical value. Because of this, the examiner must consciously consider the normal position of the various isopters plotted and calculate the number of log-units of visual change that the isopter displacement represents. The procedure is analogous to digital conversion (i.e., equivalent to the conversion of hand positions on a traditional clock to the numeric readout of hours and minutes on a digital clock).

FIG. 7-9. Examples of localized depression, one with a scotoma, to show how visual threshold at points within the depression can be represented. In the three depressions illustrated any location on the isopter plot may be selected (e.g., point *R*) and the visual threshold known (i.e., the weakest test stimulus visible at that location).

Top, At point *R* in the normal field, *I-2e* is seen.

Bottom left, In a shallow (0.5 log-unit) depression, *I-3e* is the weakest stimulus seen.

Bottom center, In a deeper (1.5 log-unit) depression, *II-4e* is the visual threshold.*

Bottom right, In a depression containing a scotoma, *III-4e* is the threshold.

---

*Of course, the *II-4e* stimulus is larger than *I-4e,* rather than brighter. However, for the present purpose, we can consider the changing from size I to size II as roughly equivalent to an intensity increase of 0.5 log-unit.

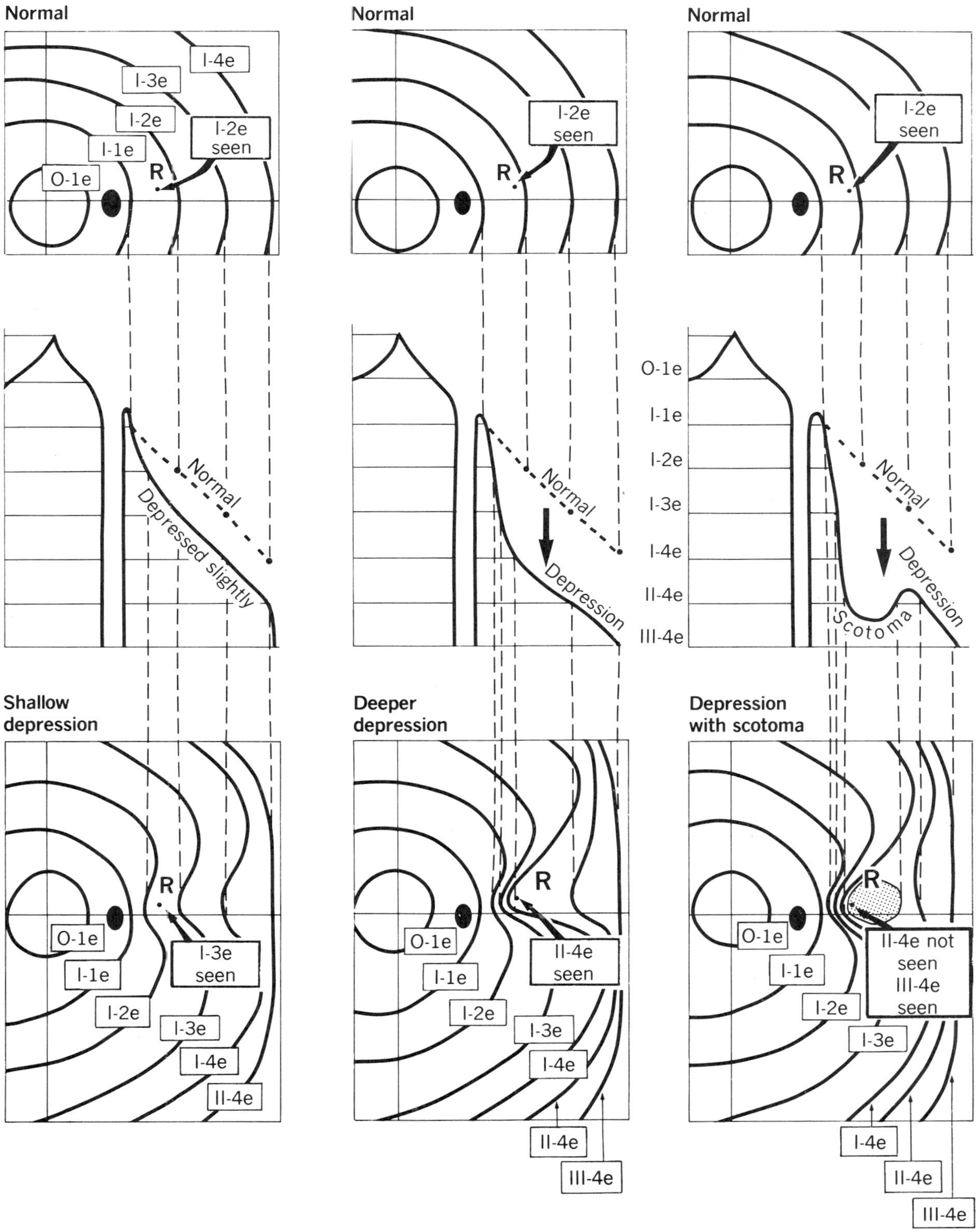

Normal
I-4e
I-3e
I-2e
I-1e
O-1e
I-2e seen
R
Normal
Depressed slightly
Shallow depression
O-1e
I-1e
I-2e
I-3e seen
I-3e
I-4e
II-4e
Normal
I-2e seen
R
Normal
Depression
Deeper depression
O-1e
I-1e
I-2e
II-4e seen
I-3e
I-4e
II-4e
III-4e
Normal
I-2e seen
R
O-1e
I-1e
I-2e
I-3e
I-4e
II-4e
III-4e
Normal
Depression
Scotoma
Depression with scotoma
O-1e
I-1e
I-2e
II-4e not seen III-4e seen
I-3e
I-4e
II-4e
III-4e

FIG. 7-9

CHAPTER 8

Generalized depressions

CHARACTERISTICS OF A GENERALIZED DEPRESSION

There is a generalized depression of the visual field when a depressed (or reduced) sensitivity to light exists *everywhere* in the field. When light sensitivity is less than usual throughout, all test stimuli are generally less visible and the visual threshold becomes abnormal at every spot in the field. This can result from preretinal factors (Chapter 4), such as opacities in the ocular media, or from diffuse involvement of the retina, optic nerve, or some other locus in the visual pathway.

FIG. 8-1. Generalized depression. The normal visual field of a myope is shown in **A,** obtained with the appropriate lens correction. In **B** a generalized depression is simulated by failing to use lens correction and placing a 0.6 log-unit neutral density filter in front of the eye. Throughout the greyscale is darker. In the difference-from-normal printout the sensitivity is reduced everywhere without being strikingly more abnormal in any particular location. (Size III stimulus, Octopus.)

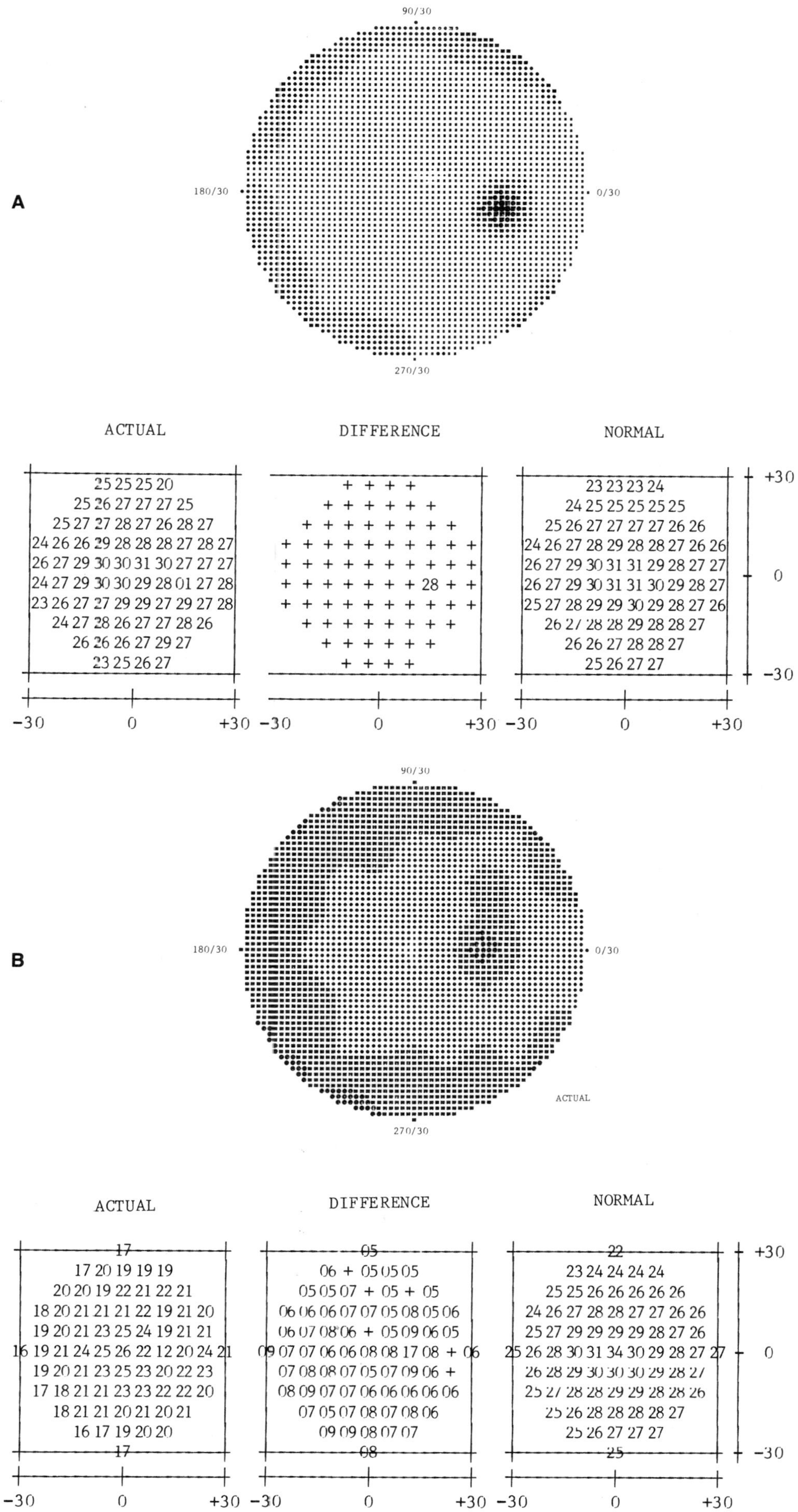
A
90/30
180/30
0/30
270/30
ACTUAL
25 25 25 20
25 26 27 27 27 25
25 27 27 28 27 26 28 27
24 26 26 29 28 28 28 27 28 27
26 27 29 30 30 31 30 27 27 27
24 27 29 30 30 29 28 01 27 28
23 26 27 27 29 29 27 29 27 28
24 27 28 26 27 27 28 26
26 26 26 27 29 27
23 25 26 27
DIFFERENCE
+ + + +
+ + + + + +
+ + + + + + + +
+ + + + + + + + + +
+ + + + + + + + + +
+ + + + + + + 28 + +
+ + + + + + + + + +
+ + + + + + + +
+ + + + + +
+ + + +
NORMAL
23 23 23 24
24 25 25 25 25 25
25 26 27 27 27 27 26 26
24 26 27 28 29 28 28 27 26 26
26 27 29 30 31 31 29 28 27 27
26 27 29 30 31 31 30 29 28 27
25 27 28 29 29 30 29 28 27 26
26 27 28 28 29 28 28 27
26 26 27 28 28 27
25 26 27 27
+30
0
-30
-30 0 +30 -30 0 +30 -30 0 +30
B
90/30
180/30
0/30
ACTUAL
270/30
ACTUAL
17
17 20 19 19 19
20 20 19 22 21 22 21
18 20 21 21 21 22 19 21 20
19 20 21 23 25 24 19 21 21
16 19 21 24 25 26 22 12 20 24 21
19 20 21 23 25 23 20 22 23
17 18 21 21 23 23 22 22 20
18 21 21 20 21 20 21
16 17 19 20 20
17
DIFFERENCE
05
06 + 05 05 05
05 05 07 + 05 + 05
06 06 06 07 07 05 08 05 06
06 07 08 06 + 05 09 06 05
09 07 07 06 06 08 08 17 08 + 06
07 08 08 07 05 07 09 06 +
08 09 07 07 06 06 06 06 06
07 05 07 08 07 08 06
09 09 08 07 07
08
NORMAL
22
23 24 24 24 24
25 25 26 26 26 26 26
24 26 27 28 28 27 27 26 26
25 27 29 29 29 29 28 27 26
25 26 28 30 31 34 30 29 28 27 27
26 28 29 30 30 30 29 28 27
25 27 28 28 29 29 28 28 26
25 26 28 28 28 28 27
25 26 27 27 27
25
+30
0
-30
-30 0 +30 -30 0 +30 -30 0 +30

FIG. 8-1

In manual perimetry, recognizing a generalized depression from an isopter plot requires more conscious effort by the examiner, because the results are presented as isopter positions rather than as numeric values. The *shape* of each isopter may be more or less normal; and to recognize an abnormality, the examiner must consider the *position* of the isopters.

FIG. 8-2. Isopter plot for a generalized depression compared to that for a normal eye. *I-3e* is visible at location *N* inside the *I-3e* isopter of the normal field (above) but in the depressed field (below) *I-3e* is not visible at *N*. On an isopter plot, this means that the *I-3e* isopter has moved inward so it no longer encloses location *N*.

Indeed, since visual sensation is reduced everywhere, all isopters move inward from all sides. Each isopter encloses a smaller area than before; this signifies that each stimulus is visible in a smaller region than before.

Location *N* is still within the *I-4e* isopter, which means that *I-4e* has remained visible at *N*, even though *I-3e* is not visible. Now the threshold at *N* is between *I-3e* and *I-4e* whereas before it was between *I-2e* and *I-3e*.

In a localized depression (Chapter 7) the isopters move inward, but only within a localized region. In a generalized depression the same inward movement occurs but the entire field is involved, so each isopter is moved inward along its entire length. In addition, the diagnostic implications are very different.

At the center of the normal field in Fig. 8-2, *I-1e* and *0-1e* are visible and there are isopters enclosing the regions within which these stimuli can be seen. With a generalized depression, however, these stimuli are no longer visible at all. Therefore, in the plot of the depressed field, the isopters for *I-1e* and *0-1e* are no longer present because there is no region where these stimuli can be seen.

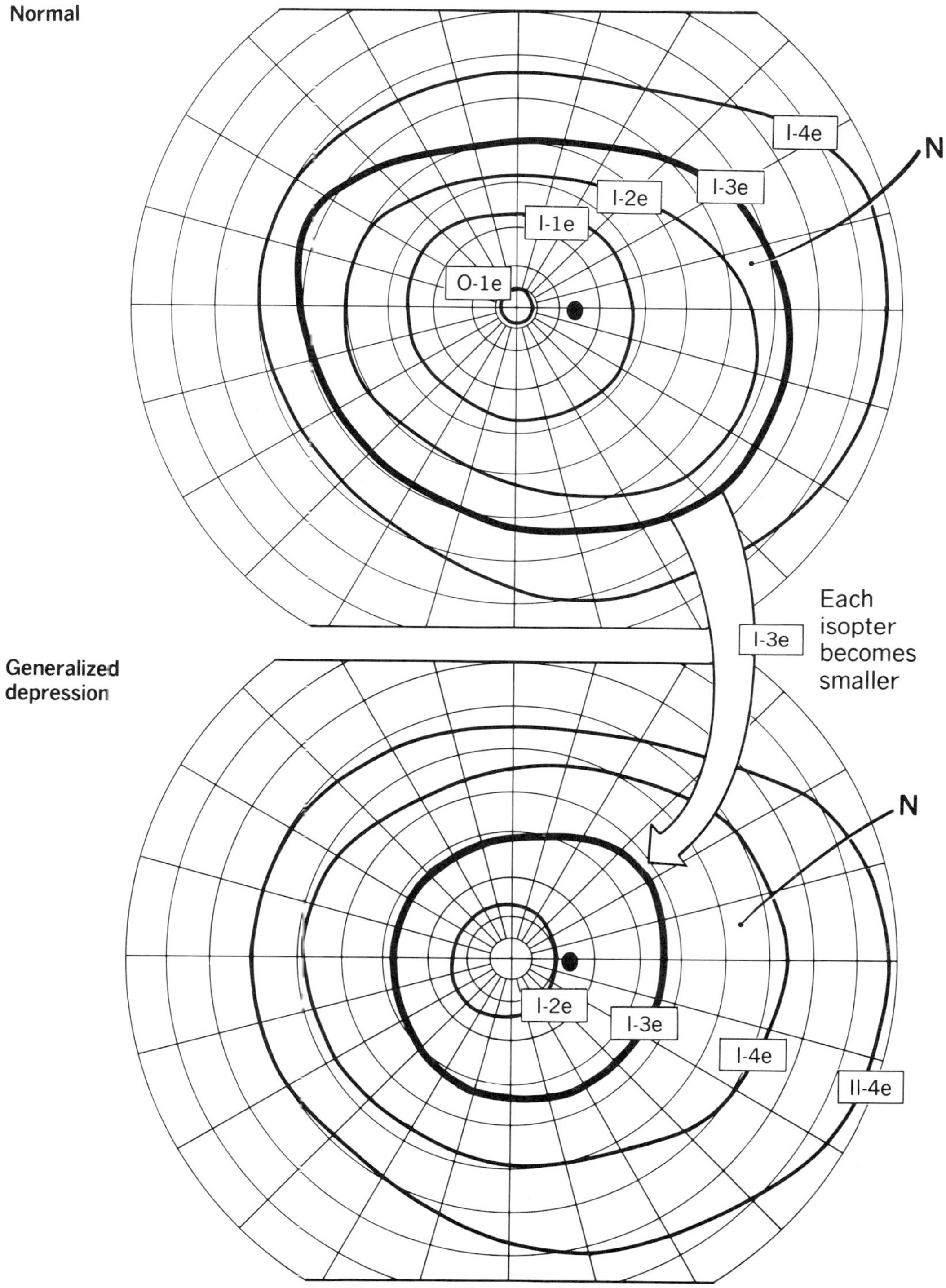
Normal
I-4e
N
I-3e
I-2e
I-1e
O-1e
I-3e
Each isopter becomes smaller
Generalized depression
N
I-2e
I-3e
I-4e
II-4e

FIG. 8-2

FIG. 8-3. Plot for a normal field compared to that for a depressed field.
A, In a normal field of vision, if *I-4e* forms an isopter at the extreme border of the field, then all stronger stimuli will also form isopters at the same place when plotted kinetically; i.e., those stronger stimuli, when brought in from the periphery, will first become visible at the extreme boundary and their isopters will be superimposed on one another. The "isopters" so plotted do not really represent the visual threshold because they are not the *weakest* stimulus visible at the boundary. However, they do enclose the area within which the stimulus is visible. Several isopters superimposed on one another represent a very steep cliff at the extreme border of the hill of vision.
B, When the visual field becomes generally depressed, visual sensation will become reduced at all locations, including *M* (near the periphery), where neither *I-4e* nor *II-4e* is visible any longer but the stronger test stimuli may still be visible. Thus the *I-4e* and *II-4e* isopters move inward and separate from one another so *M* is no longer enclosed by the *I-4e* and *II-4e* isopters. However, isopters of *III-4e* and stronger stimuli remain at the extreme boundary and do enclose *M*.

With a generalized depression the extreme periphery of the visual field does not move inward. This has two practical implications:

1. If the outer limit of the field is routinely plotted only with very strong suprathreshold stimuli, such as II-4e or even V-4e, the extreme boundary will be determined but a depression of the field will not be detected. A depression will be detected only if the isopter for the weakest stimulus that should be at the periphery (I-4e) is plotted and it is discovered that the isopter has moved inward. This principle will be applied when looking for localized depressions in glaucoma (Chapter 21).
2. In the presence of a generalized depression it should be possible to increase the stimulus to a sufficient strength that it becomes visible in the periphery of the visual field. For example, if the I-4e isopter is plotted and found to be constricted, suggesting a depression, it should nonetheless be possible to plot the isopter for a stronger stimulus that will enclose the peripheral field—unless the field is so depressed that it would require a stimulus stronger than the strongest available on the perimeter.

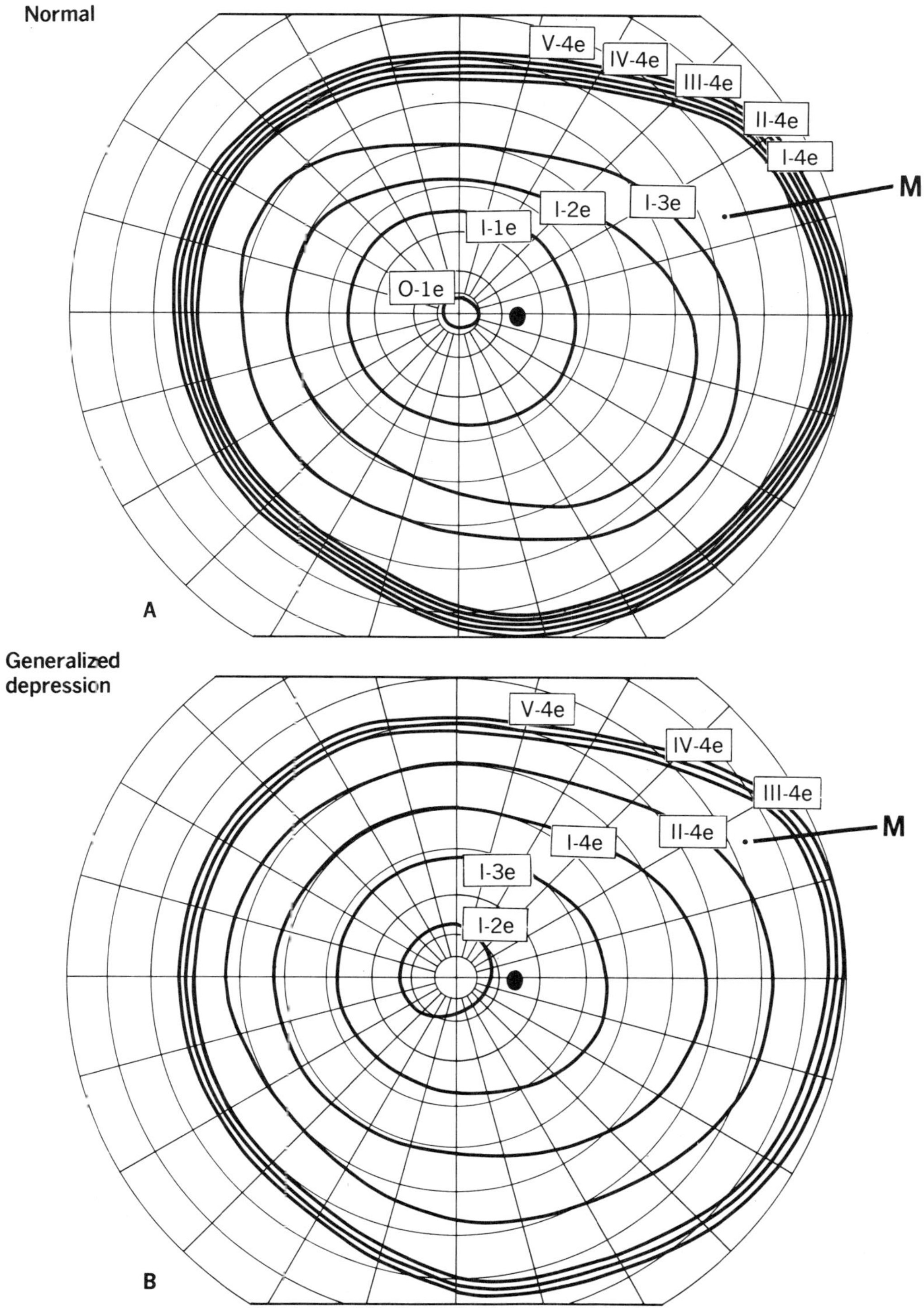
Normal
V-4e
IV-4e
III-4e
II-4e
I-4e
M
I-3e
I-2e
I-1e
O-1e
A
Generalized depression
V-4e
IV-4e
III-4e
M
II-4e
I-4e
I-3e
I-2e
B

FIG. 8-3

FIG. 8-4. Comparison of isopter plots for a normal field and a generalized depression to profile plots. Visual sensation in the depressed field is reduced by 0.5 log-unit* at every point. Thus, where *I-2e* is threshold in the normal field (i.e., at the *I-2e* isopter), the threshold becomes *I-3e*. In other words, the *I-3e* isopter in the depressed field is at the same location that the *I-2e* isopter is normally. Moreover, in the profile plot the hill of vision has the same shape but is moved downward 0.5 log-unit.

In a region where the profile of the field of vision is steep, the isopter will move only slightly with a half log-unit of depression; but in a relatively flat region of the field the isopter will move more. Thus, with the same amount of visual depression everywhere (0.5 log-unit) the isopter moves inward a greater distance in a flat region of the field than in a steeper region. The *I-2e* isopter moved more than 20 degrees inward while the *I-3e* isopter moved in only 10 degrees, having traversed a steeper part of the field. Because the slopes of the visual field on the nasal side and temporal side are not exactly the same, isopters may move to slightly differing degrees on the two sides with a specific amount of depression.

---

*The difference between *I-4e* and *I-3e* is 0.5 log-unit intensity, as is that between *I-3e* and *I-2e* and between *I-2e* and *I-1e*. Also *I-3c* is 0.5 log-unit more intense than *I-2c* (see pp. 32 to 39).

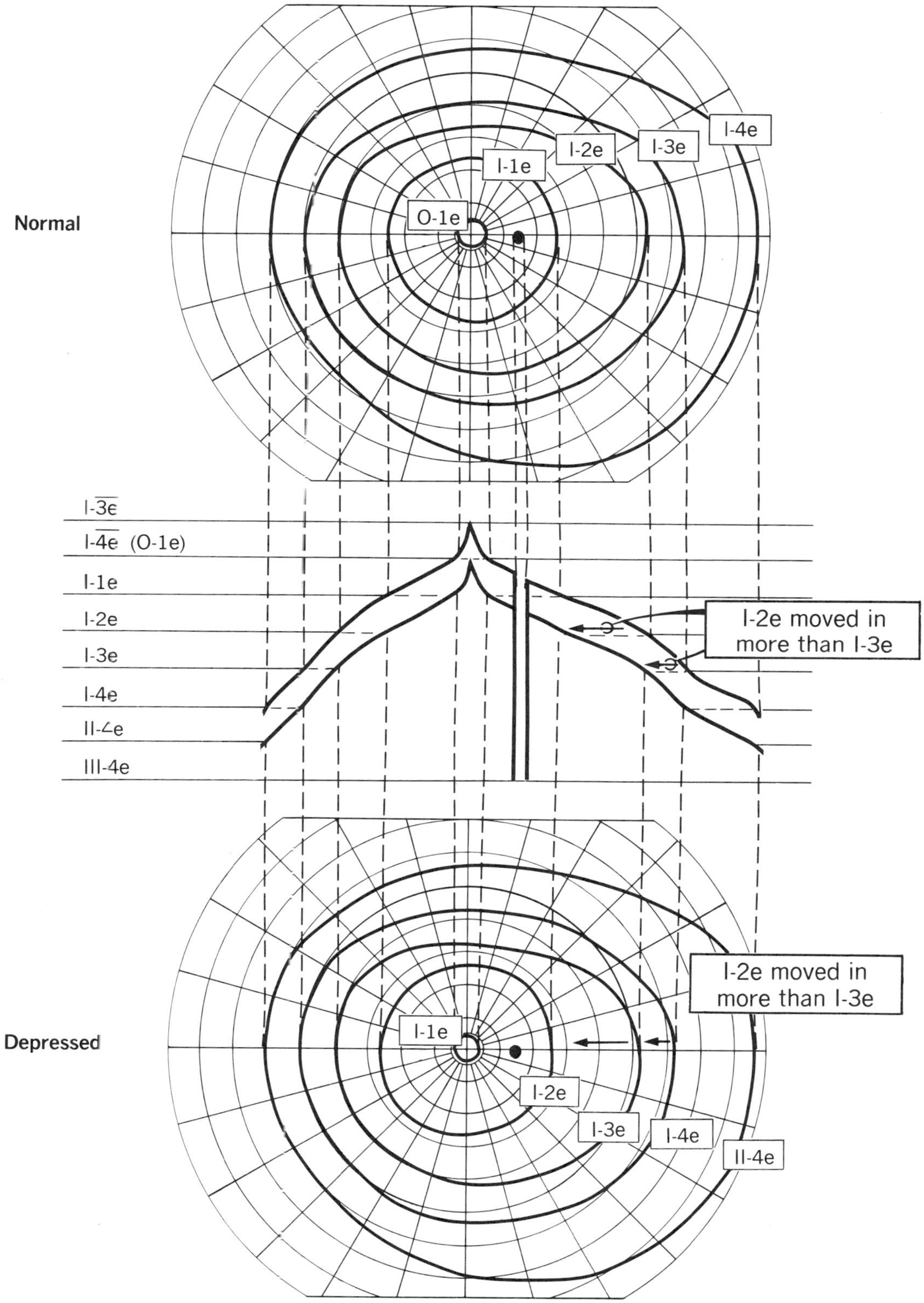
Normal
I-4e
I-3e
I-2e
I-1e
O-1e
I-3̅e̅
I-4̅e̅ (O-1e)
I-1e
I-2e
I-3e
I-4e
II-4e
III-4e
I-2e moved in more than I-3e
Depressed
I-2e moved in more than I-3e
I-1e
I-2e
I-3e
I-4e
II-4e

FIG. 8-4

UNEQUAL GENERALIZED DEPRESSION

The amount of depression is not always the same everywhere in the visual field. For example, with the development of cataract the defocused image may have more effect on the central visual field than on the periphery.

FIG. 8-5. Unequal generalized depression.
A, Static threshold profile of a normal myopic eye. During testing, a −1.75 sphere combined with a +1.00 cylinder axis (108 degrees) was used. This represented a +3.00 add on the patient's distance correction.
B, The field test on this patient with no correction. Because of the blurred retinal image, the foveal peak is flattened and the entire field slightly depressed.
C, Static profile for this patient. The retinal image is blurred because a plus spherical lens was used instead of a minus spherical lens. The field is even more depressed and flattened in profile. This example illustrates the type of depressed field that can occur from a blurred retinal image, which may be caused by disease (e.g., cataract) or can be the result of an artifact due to technical error. (Size I stimulus, Humphrey perimeter.)

A

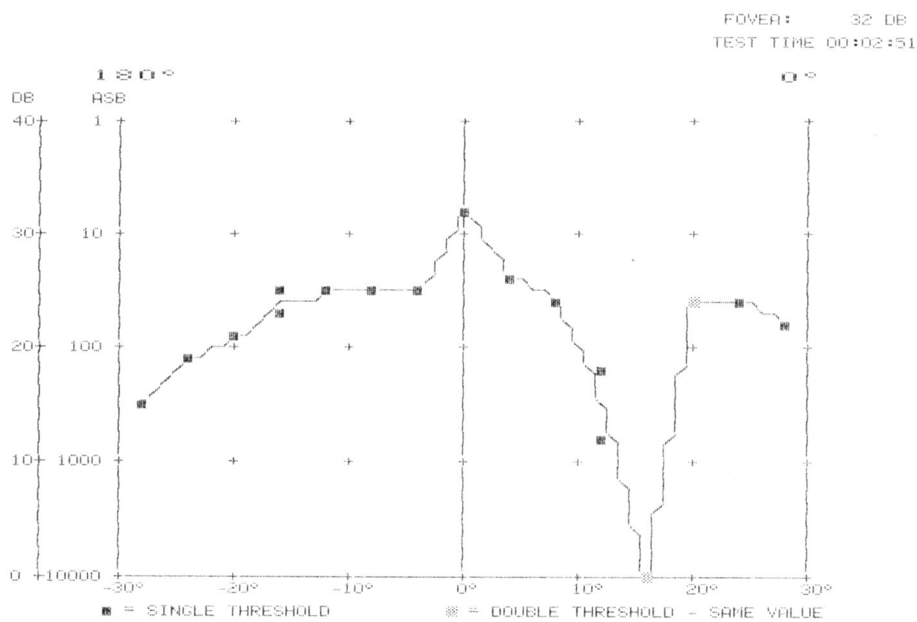

FIG. 8-5

B

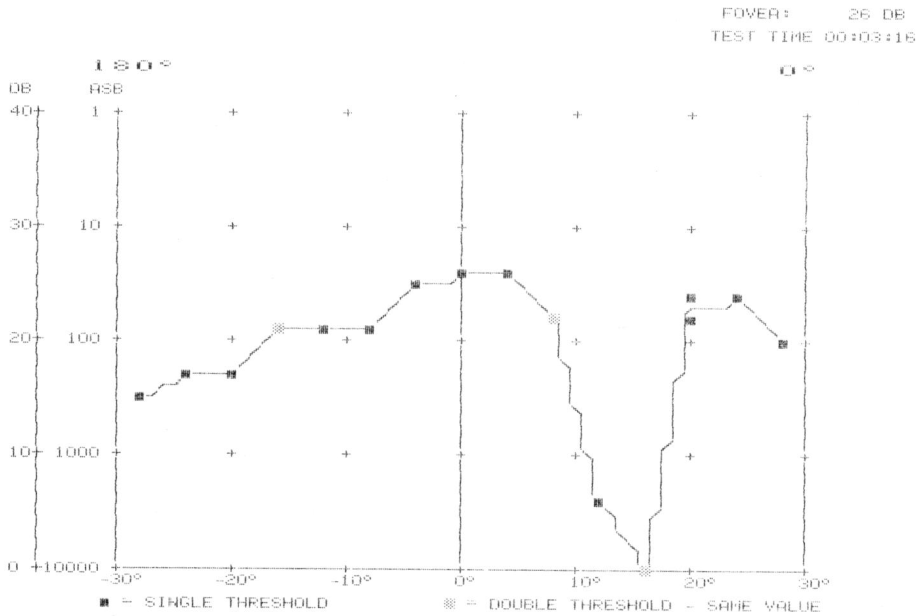

C

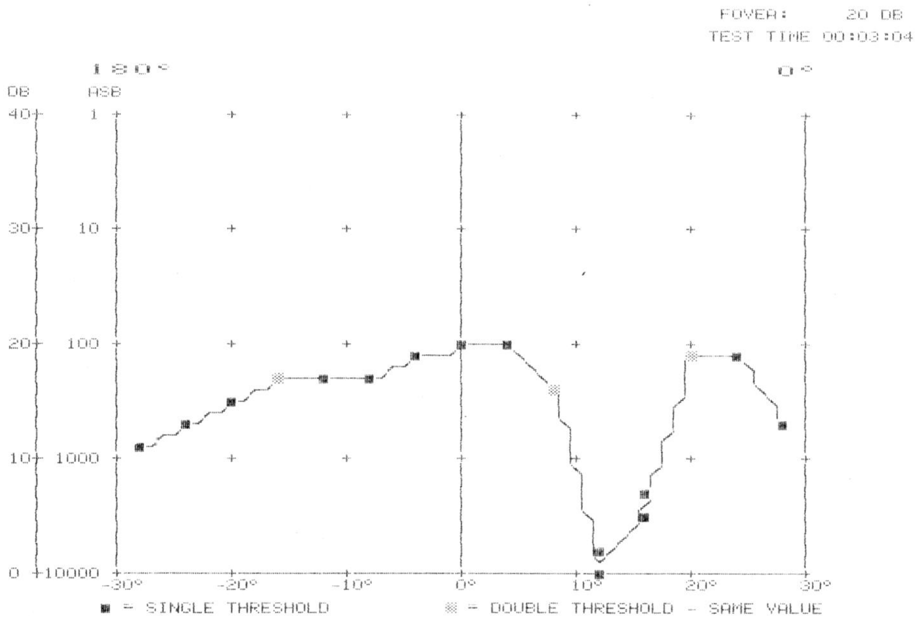

FIG. 8-5, cont'd

The nature of unequal generalized depression is revealed in plots of the hill of vision by manual perimetry. Note in the profile plot that with this type of depression the contour of the hill of vision becomes flatter. This flattening of the field is manifested in the isopter plot by a wider separation between isopters.

FIG. 8-6. Unequal generalized depression. Visual sensation is reduced by 0.5 log-unit in the periphery and by 1 log-unit in the center; however, this is still a *generalized* depression, which means that visual sensation is reduced everywhere, even though not to an equal degree in all places. The slope of the hill of vision has become flatter.

Location *R* in the normal field is within the *I-1e* isopter but in the depressed field is no longer enclosed by either the *I-1e* or the *I-2e*. Thus two isopters, each representing 0.5 log-unit of intensity, no longer enclose point *R* and this represents 1 log-unit of depression. By contrast, point *S* was in the normal field enclosed by the *I-4e* isopter. In the depressed field *S* is no longer enclosed by *I-4e* but is within the next stronger isopter, *II-4e,** and therefore has only 0.5 log-unit of depression.

We will see later how important it is to understand thoroughly generalized depression, and especially the relationship between isopter movement and threshold change.

SIGNIFICANCE OF A GENERALIZED DEPRESSION

There is a certain variability of visual sensation from one person to another—and thus the location of isopters is variable. For example, the I-2e isopter may be at 30 degrees in one person but at 15 degrees in another. Because of this, if the I-2e is at 15 degrees in one individual, it is difficult to say whether this is normal or whether the individual used to have the I-2e isopter at 30 degrees and now has a depressed field. Moreover, the visual field normally undergoes a slow generalized depression with increasing age and thus a relatively inward position of isopters must be considered normal for older people without necessarily signifying the presence of ocular disease (see Fig. 13-25).

However, superimposed on individual variability and age-related changes are abnormal depressions. For example, cataracts or corneal opacities typically cause a generalized depression along with a reduction of visual acuity. In fact, if a patient with reduced visual acuity does not have a generalized depression of the field, you are presented with an important diagnostic clue suggesting that (1) a central scotoma is present to account for the reduced visual acuity and (2) the reduced acuity is not due to a media (cornea, lens, vitreous) opacity.

---

*Of course, the *II-4e* stimulus is larger than *I-4e,* rather than brighter. However, for the present purpose, we can consider the changing from size I to size II as roughly equivalent to an intensity increase of 0.5 log-unit.

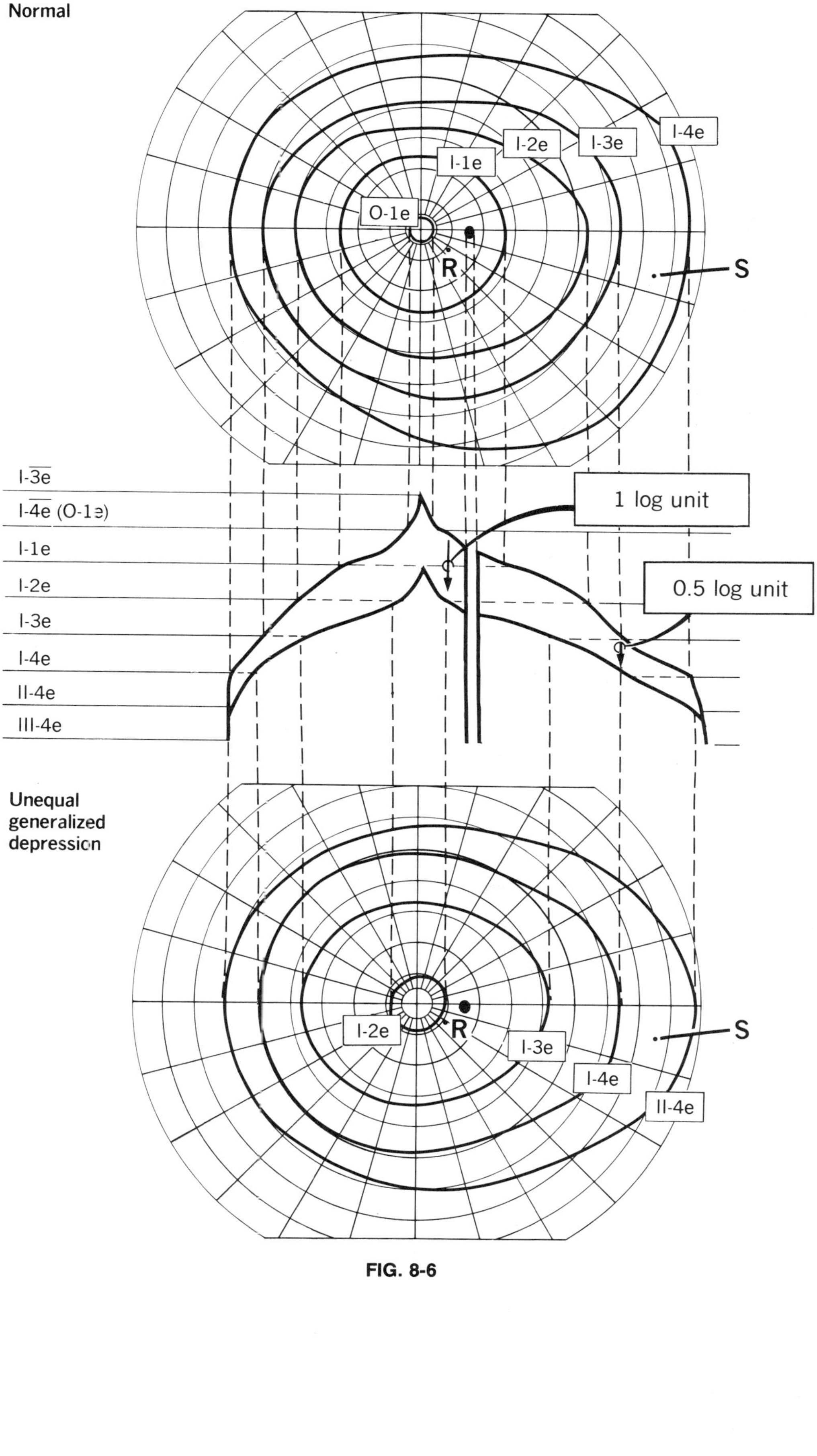
Normal
I-4e
I-3e
I-2e
I-1e
O-1e
R
S
I-3e
I-4e (O-1e)
I-1e
I-2e
I-3e
I-4e
II-4e
III-4e
1 log unit
0.5 log unit
Unequal
generalized
depression
I-2e
R
I-3e
I-4e
II-4e
S

FIG. 8-6

CONTRACTION OF THE VISUAL FIELD

We noted previously (Fig. 8-3) that the extreme boundary of the field does not move inward with an ordinary generalized depression. This contrasts with a contraction of the field in which the extreme boundary does move in.

FIG. 8-7. Comparison of contraction and severe depression.
A, If visual sensation in the periphery of the field is reduced to the point that no stimulus is visible, it is said that the field is contracted. The uninvolved area of the field may have normal visual sensitivity with *I-1e* and *0-1e* isopters in their normal location and all other isopters crowded together at the boundary of the contracted field. The isopter for the strongest stimulus, *V-4e,* is at 25 degrees. Thus, in this example of a contracted field, visual sensation is severely reduced outside 25 degrees but inside 25 degrees it is normal.
B, With a severe generalized depression, visual sensation is reduced everywhere; thus the seeing part of the field has reduced sensation. In this example the *V-4e* isopter is at 25 degrees, the *IV-4e* is at 7 degrees, and the *II-4e* is not visible at all. This situation represents severe depression of the entire field, not just the periphery. The isopters are not crowded together at the limit of the field, and if there were such a thing as a *VI-4e* stimulus we would expect its isopter to be at approximately 40 degrees. Even stronger stimuli would be visible out to the usual extreme boundary of a normal field. By confrontation, in a severe depression (with a restricted field to the strongest test object) there may still be a wide field to hand movements or to light perception with projection. With contraction (an absolute defect) there is no detection of hand movements or light in the periphery (p. 68).

Just like a depression, contraction can be localized (in one area of the field) or generalized. The endstage of glaucoma (Fig. 10-5, *D*) is a contraction of the nasal field. Often a contraction simply results from a severe depression that becomes an absolute defect (as a shallow scotoma can become absolute). At times, however, the distinction between a depression and a contraction is important to the diagnosis because certain diseases produce absolute defects without accompanying or surrounding depression. One clue in such cases can be whether or not there is a generalized depression within the seeing area of a contracted field. Hence, if plotting a restricted field, it is never adequate simply to plot the outer boundary of a contracted field; rather it must be determined what can or cannot be seen in the seeing zone. In other words, visual threshold must be determined in all the seeing area. This is important not only in establishing the diagnosis but also in being able to follow the progress of chronic conditions such as glaucoma.

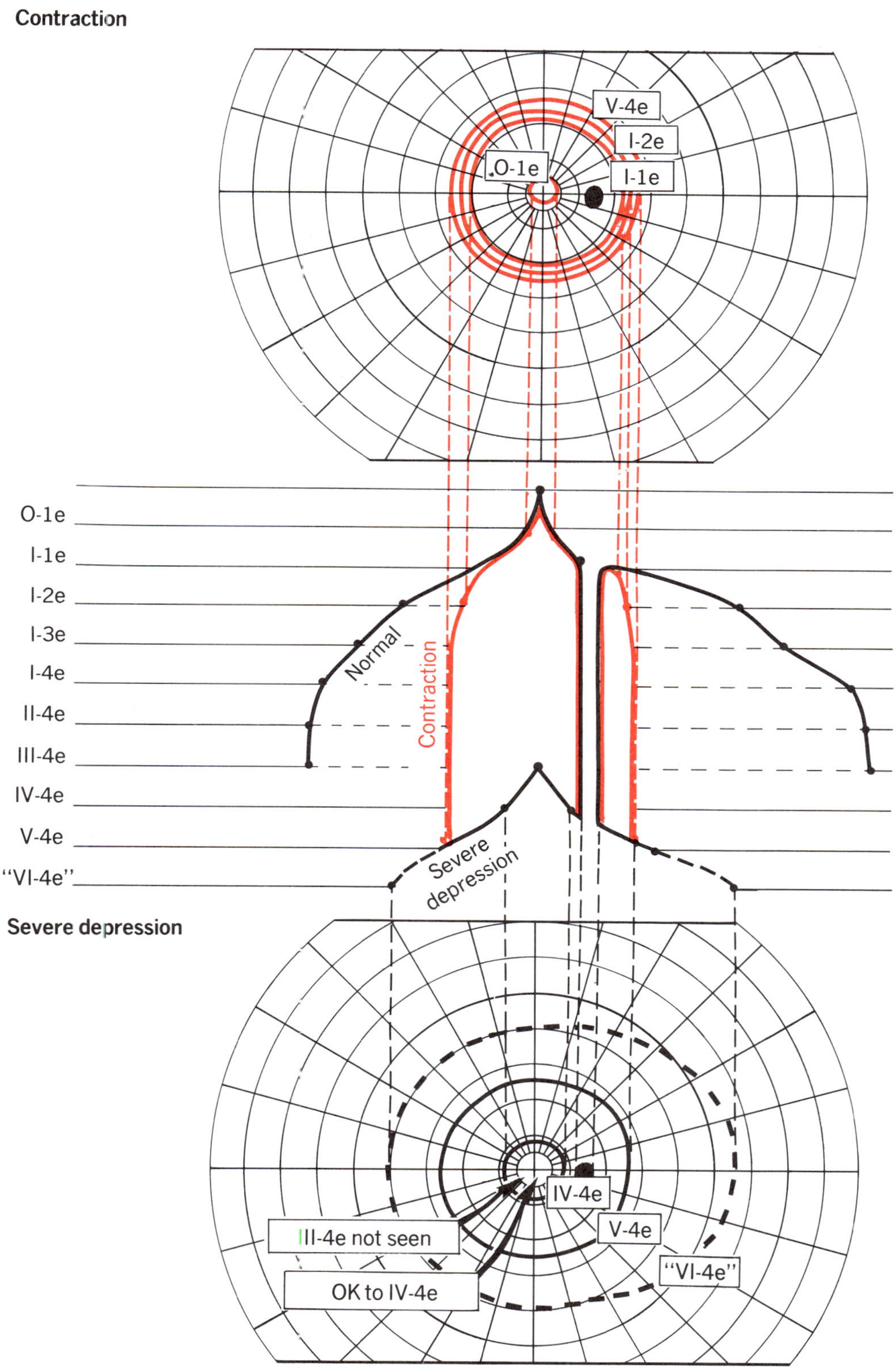

Contraction
V-4e
I-2e
O-1e
I-1e
O-1e
I-1e
I-2e
I-3e
I-4e
II-4e
III-4e
IV-4e
V-4e
"VI-4e"
Normal
Contraction
Severe depression
Severe depression
IV-4e
V-4e
III-4e not seen
"VI-4e"
OK to IV-4e

FIG. 8-7

CHAPTER 9

Topographic classification of visual field defects

ANATOMIC BASIS

All field defects can be classified topographically as prechiasmal, chiasmal, or postchiasmal depending on the anatomic location of the disease that produced the visual abnormality.

FIG. 9-1. Anatomic basis of topographic classification. The optics of the eye (cornea and lens, Fig. 4-1) focus an image on the retina. The retina converts the light to nervous impulses that are processed and conducted ultimately to the occipital (or visual) cortex.

Some of the nerve fibers from each eye cross at the optic chiasm to the opposite side of the brain in such a manner that impulses derived from objects to the right side of the field of vision are received by the left visual cortex and objects to the left are received by the right visual cortex. Thus a stimulus in the right (temporal) visual field of the right eye is seen by the nasal retina of the right eye and nerves carrying these impulses cross at the chiasm to the left side of the brain. However, objects to the left of fixation seen by the right eye in its nasal visual field stimulate points in the temporal retina of the right eye and nerves carrying these impulses from the temporal retina (pathway in red in Fig. 9-1) do not cross the chiasm but remain on the right side of the brain. The point dividing the nasal and temporal halves of the retina is the fovea (represented by fixation), not the optic nerve head (represented by the physiologic blind spot).

In this chapter the characteristics of field defects are discussed in relation to the location of the lesion in the visual pathway. The techniques to use in looking for different types of defects are discussed in later chapters.

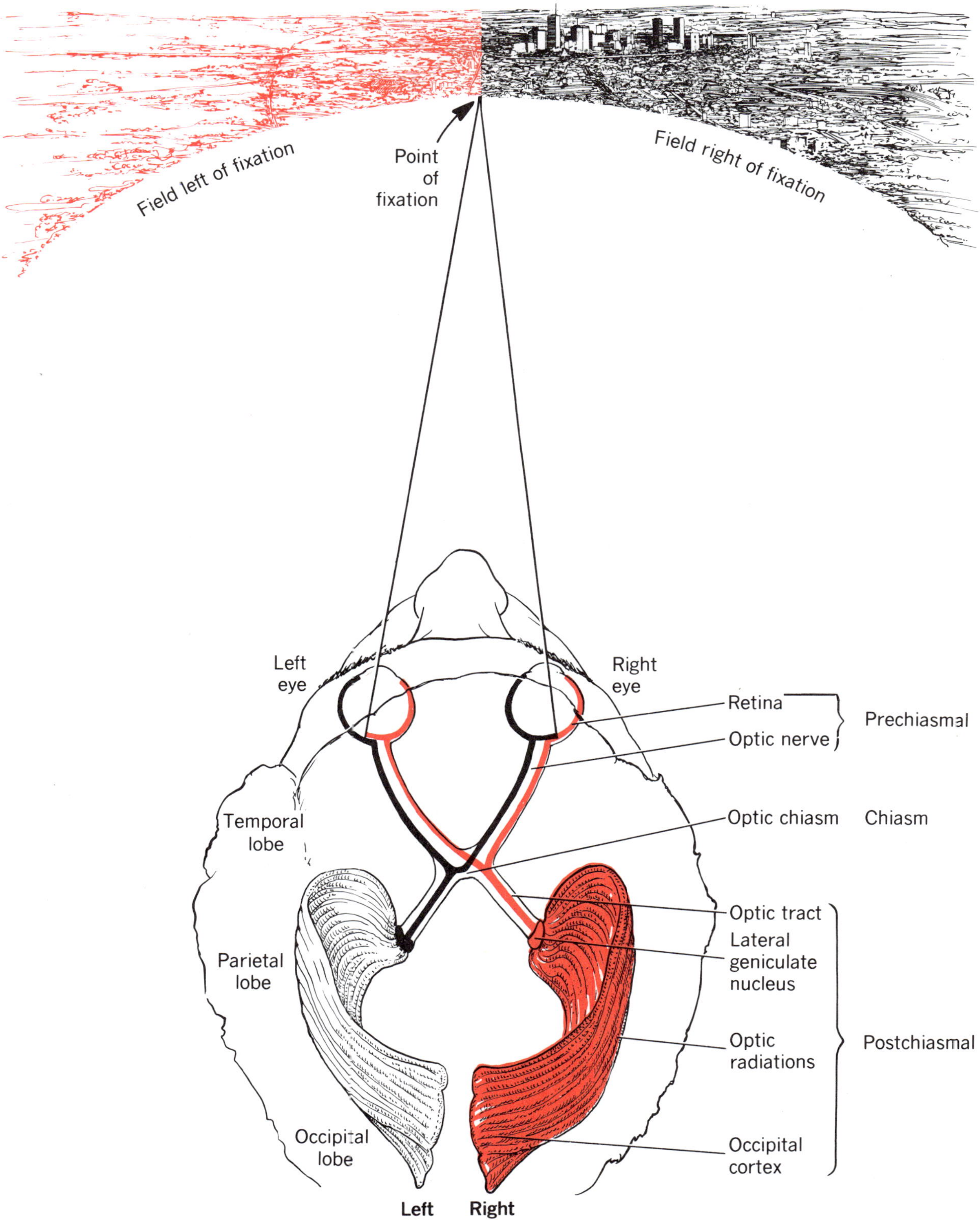
Field left of fixation
Point
of
fixation
Field right of fixation
Left
eye
Right
eye
Retina
Optic nerve
Prechiasmal
Temporal
lobe
Optic chiasm
Chiasm
Optic tract
Lateral
geniculate
nucleus
Parietal
lobe
Optic
radiations
Postchiasmal
Occipital
lobe
Occipital
cortex
Left
Right

FIG. 9-1

PRECHIASMAL DEFECTS

Prechiasmal lesions include abnormalities in the refractive properties and transparent ocular media of the eye (cornea, lens, vitreous) as well as a variety of diseases affecting the retina and optic nerve. Glaucoma, a disease characterized by intraocular pressure damaging the optic nerve, is one example of a prechiasmal lesion.

Prechiasmal lesions produce visual field defects with the following characteristics:

1. The defect is in one eye only—unless the disease affects both retinas or optic nerves, in which case both eyes may have visual field defects. If there is a visual field defect in one eye only and the other eye has no defect at all, the lesion must be prechiasmal. Moreover, if there is no preretinal or retinal lesion (almost any of which would be visible on examination of the eye) to explain the defect, it must be an optic nerve lesion.
2. The defect may extend uninterrupted across the vertical meridian. The diagnostic importance of this fact is that a defect resulting from a postchiasmal lesion does *not* cross the vertical meridian. Therefore, if a defect crosses the vertical midline uninterrupted, the lesion is not postchiasmal but prechiasmal (or combined chiasmal and prechiasmal).
3. If the defect in the nasal visual field results from a lesion of the optic nerve (or the retinal nerve fiber layer), it *may* end abruptly with a straight horizontal border nasal to fixation (i.e., a nasal step or a scotoma with a flat horizontal edge). However, if it results from a lesion in the temporal retina or choroid, it may extend across the horizontal meridian uninterrupted. If it has a sharp horizontal border nasally, it is undoubtedly due to a prechiasmal lesion. If it does not have a horizontal nasal border, it may or may not be due to a prechiasmal lesion.
4. There are quite a variety of scotomas and depressions produced by prechiasmal lesions. Selected typical examples are shown on the opposite page.
5. A prechiasmal visual field defect may be associated with any of the following:
   a. Reduced visual acuity (e.g., a generalized depression resulting from media opacities or a central scotoma resulting from macular or optic nerve disease)
   b. Abnormal pupil reaction (afferent pupillary defect)
   c. Abnormality evident by ophthalmoscopy
   d. Abnormal color vision

FIG. 9-2. Prechiasmal field defects.

A, Generalized depression with flattening of the hill of vision. This typically results from opacity of the ocular media. Some diffuse diseases of the retina or optic nerve may also produce generalized depression or constriction of the visual field. The visual acuity is reduced.

B, Centrocecal scotoma. These and central scotomas may be due to lesions of the macula or the optic nerve, particularly the posterior optic nerve, and are associated with a reduced visual acuity.

C, Arcuate and wedge-shaped defects that point toward the blind spot. These are characteristic of lesions that destroy bundles of nerve fibers in the retinal nerve fiber layers or the anterior optic nerve. Glaucoma is an example. Note that the defect may cross the vertical meridian uninterrupted and may have a sharp horizontal border nasally. The visual acuity may remain normal.

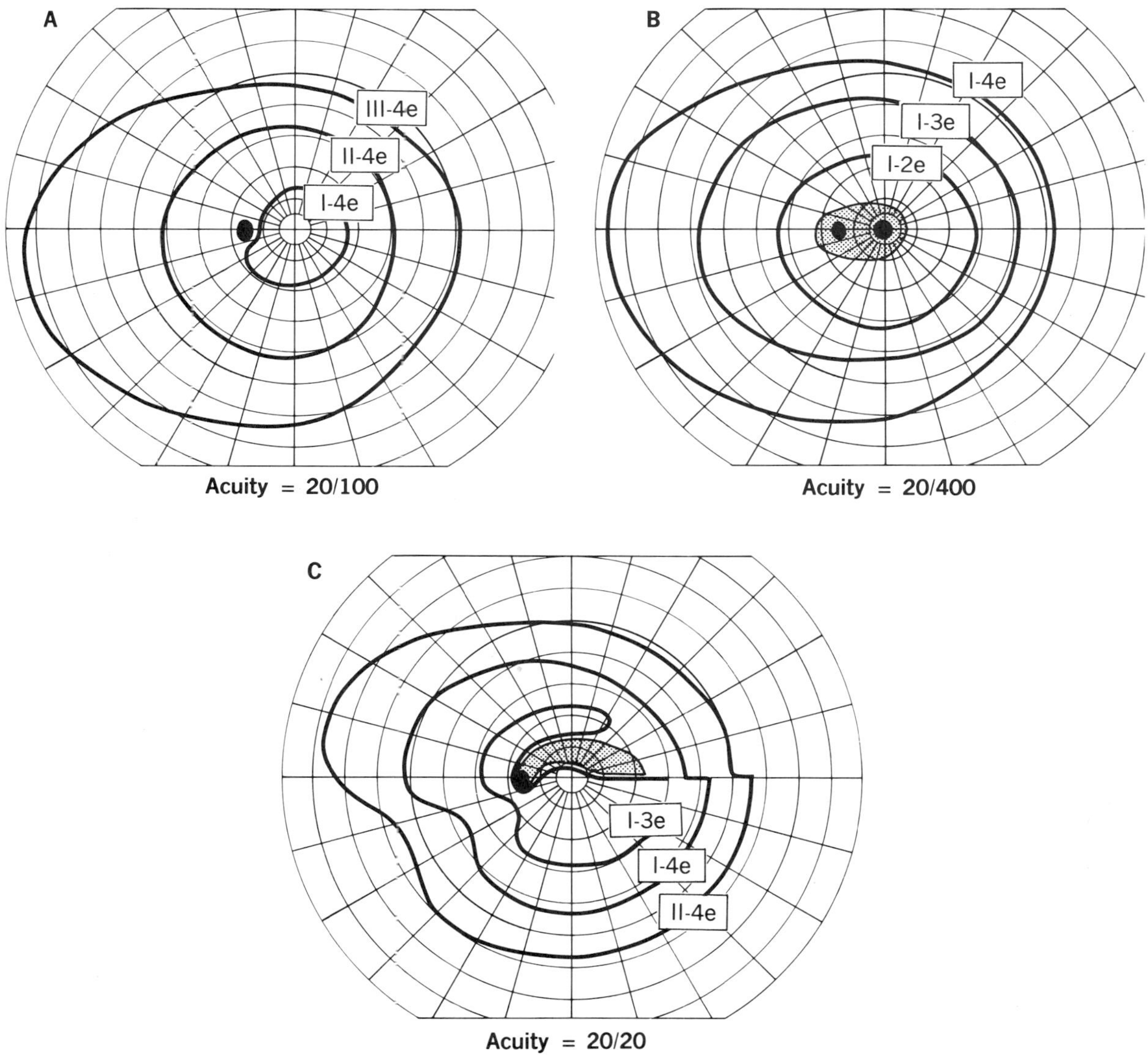

FIG. 9-2

The prechiasmal causes for field defects can conveniently be subdivided into three "territories":

1. PRERETINAL FACTORS (Chapter 4). Abnormalities in the optical pathways may produce a defocused image, scattered light, or blockage of light. The result is a generalized visual depression, often with flattening of the slope of the hill of vision. Sometimes a localized opacity in the media will produce a shadow on the retina, resulting in a localized depression but not a scotoma.
2. LESIONS OF THE OUTER RETINA AND CHOROID. This area is called *territory I* of the neural visual pathway by Trobe and Glaser,* and lesions here can produce a variety of defects that may not have any specific or characteristic features. The defects do not respect the vertical or nasal horizontal meridians but correspond to the portions of the retina involved.
3. THE RETINAL NERVE FIBER LAYER AND OPTIC NERVE. Trobe and Glaser call this *territory II* of the neural visual pathway. Typical field defects include central or centrocecal scotomas, paracentral or arcuate defects in the Bjerrum region (as if emanating from the blind spot), scotomas or localized depressions that respect the nasal horizontal meridian, and wedge-shaped defects with the apex pointed at the blind spot (not hemianopic wedges with the apex pointed at fixation).

CHIASMAL DEFECTS

Lesions affecting the chiasm (Trobe and Glaser's *territory III* of the neural visual pathway), e.g., a pituitary adenoma, produce visual field defects in the temporal field of both eyes (bitemporal hemianopia†).

FIG. 9-3. Bitemporal hemianopia. The defective vision is in the temporal field of each eye, ending abruptly at the vertical meridian; but, as is usually the case, it is not of the same extent in the two eyes.

The field defect ends abruptly at the vertical meridian if only the chiasm is affected. Often, one or both optic nerves are affected by the same tumor that presses on the chiasm; thus characteristics of a prechiasmal (optic nerve) lesion may be present in addition to the temporal hemianopia.

FIG. 9-4. Bitemporal hemianopia associated with a central scotoma in the left eye. Such a defect would be caused by a tumor compressing the optic nerve of the left eye in addition to the chiasm.

With chiasmal lesions the visual acuity is normal unless the optic nerve is also involved.

---

*Trobe, J.D., and Glaser, J.S.: The visual fields manual: a practical guide to testing and interpretation, Gainesville, Fla., 1983, Triad Publishing Co., Chapter 3, pp. 26-62.

†*Hemianopia* is defective vision within half of the visual field. *Temporal hemianopia* is defective vision confined to the temporal half of the field. *Bitemporal hemianopia* is temporal hemianopia in both eyes.

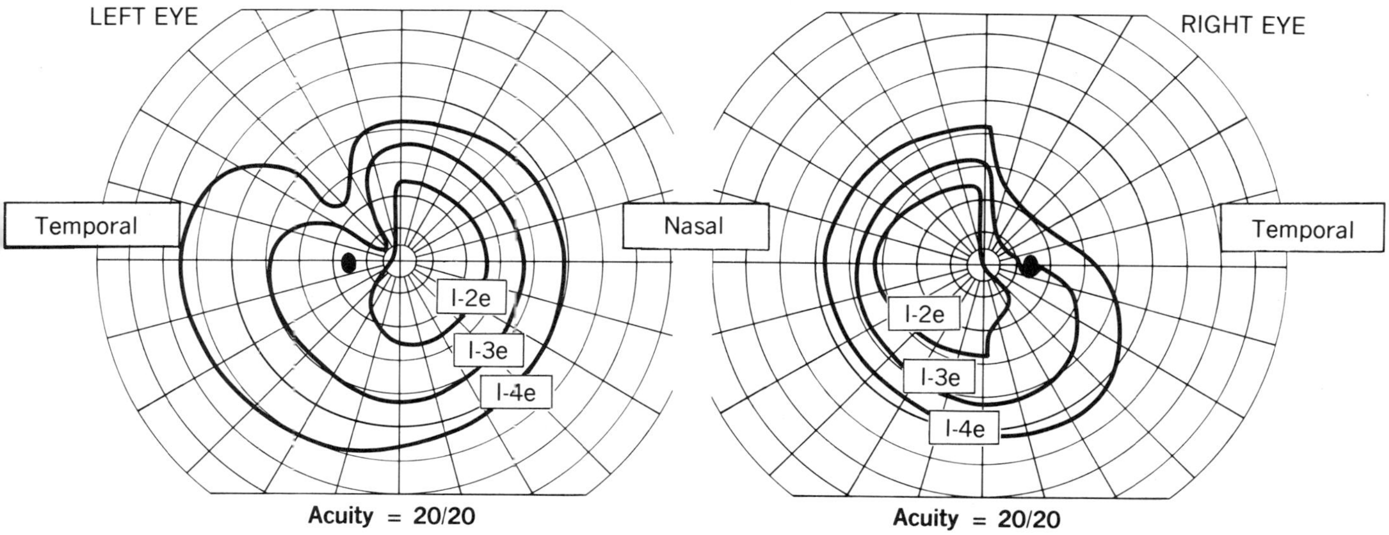
LEFT EYE
RIGHT EYE
Temporal
Nasal
Temporal
I-2e
I-3e
I-4e
I-2e
I-3e
I-4e
Acuity = 20/20
Acuity = 20/20

FIG. 9-3

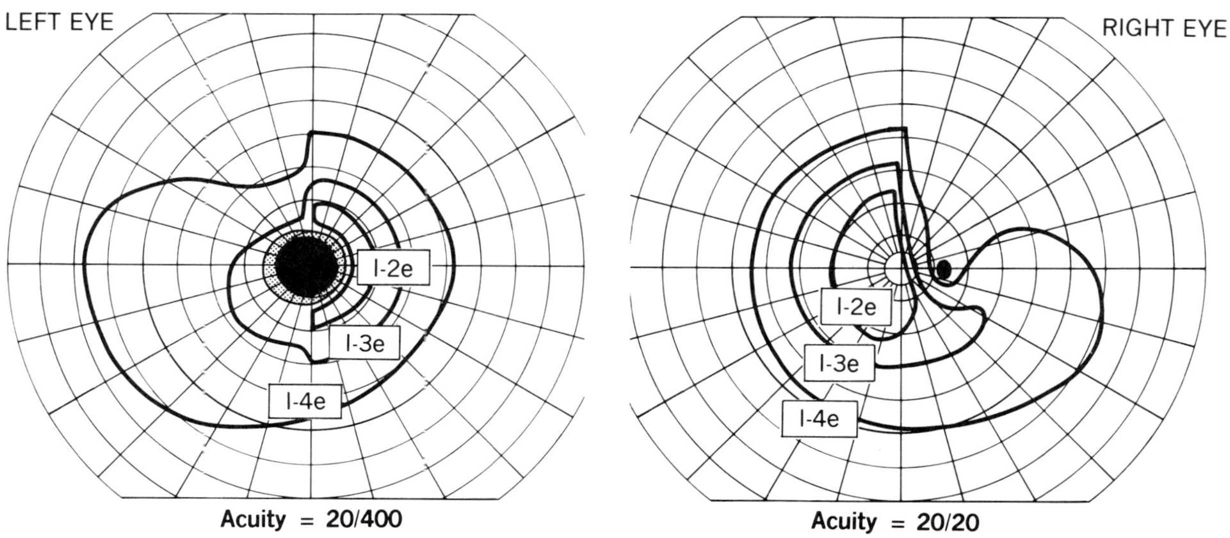
LEFT EYE
RIGHT EYE
I-2e
I-3e
I-4e
I-2e
I-3e
I-4e
Acuity = 20/400
Acuity = 20/20

FIG. 9-4

POSTCHIASMAL DEFECTS

Lesions affecting the postchiasmal visual pathway (*territory IV* of the neural visual pathway in Trobe and Glaser's classification) produce visual field defects in both eyes, but the two eyes may not be affected equally. The field defects are limited to half the field (hemianopia) and end abruptly at the vertical midline.

The hemianopic defects are *homonymous*. In homonymous hemianopia, the defects of the two eyes are both to the right or both to the left. Therefore the defect is nasal in one eye and temporal in the other.

When the lesion is of the occipital cortex (usually vascular), the defects tend to be identical *(congruous);* but lesions in most other locations (e.g., optic tract or temporal lobe), usually tumors, typically produce *incongruous* defects.

Associated findings are sometimes important to a diagnosis when there is homonymous hemianopia:

1. With postchiasmal lesions the visual acuity is almost always normal except when there is postchiasmal involvement on both sides.
2. The pupillary reactions are normal (unlike those with prechiasmal lesions), except that with optic tract lesions there may be a *hemianopic* pupil with a reduced reaction to light on the involved side of the visual field. This should occur only with optic tract lesions and not with lesions behind the lateral geniculate body.
3. Ophthalmoscopy is typically normal, with two exceptions: (a) there may be papilledema associated with a brain tumor and (b) in the rare instance when the hemianopia is caused by an optic tract lesion, the optic disc is pale and ''bow-tie'' shaped in the eye on the opposite side of the lesion while the disc of the eye on the same side shows temporal pallor.
4. Opticokinetic nystagmus may be abnormal toward the involved side with postchiasmal lesions.

FIG. 9-5. Postchiasmal field defects.

A, Incongruous left homonymous hemianopia, as would be produced by a tumor of the right temporal lobe, affecting the left side of the visual field in both eyes. Note that the defect ends abruptly at the vertical midline (making it a hemianopia), that the left half of the field is affected in both eyes (making it homonymous), and that the defect is not of equal severity in the two eyes (making it incongruous).

B, Congruous homonymous hemianopia, typical of occipital lobe lesions, often the result of vascular occlusion.

C, Congruous homonymous scotmatous hemianopia, the result of a small occipital lobe infarction.

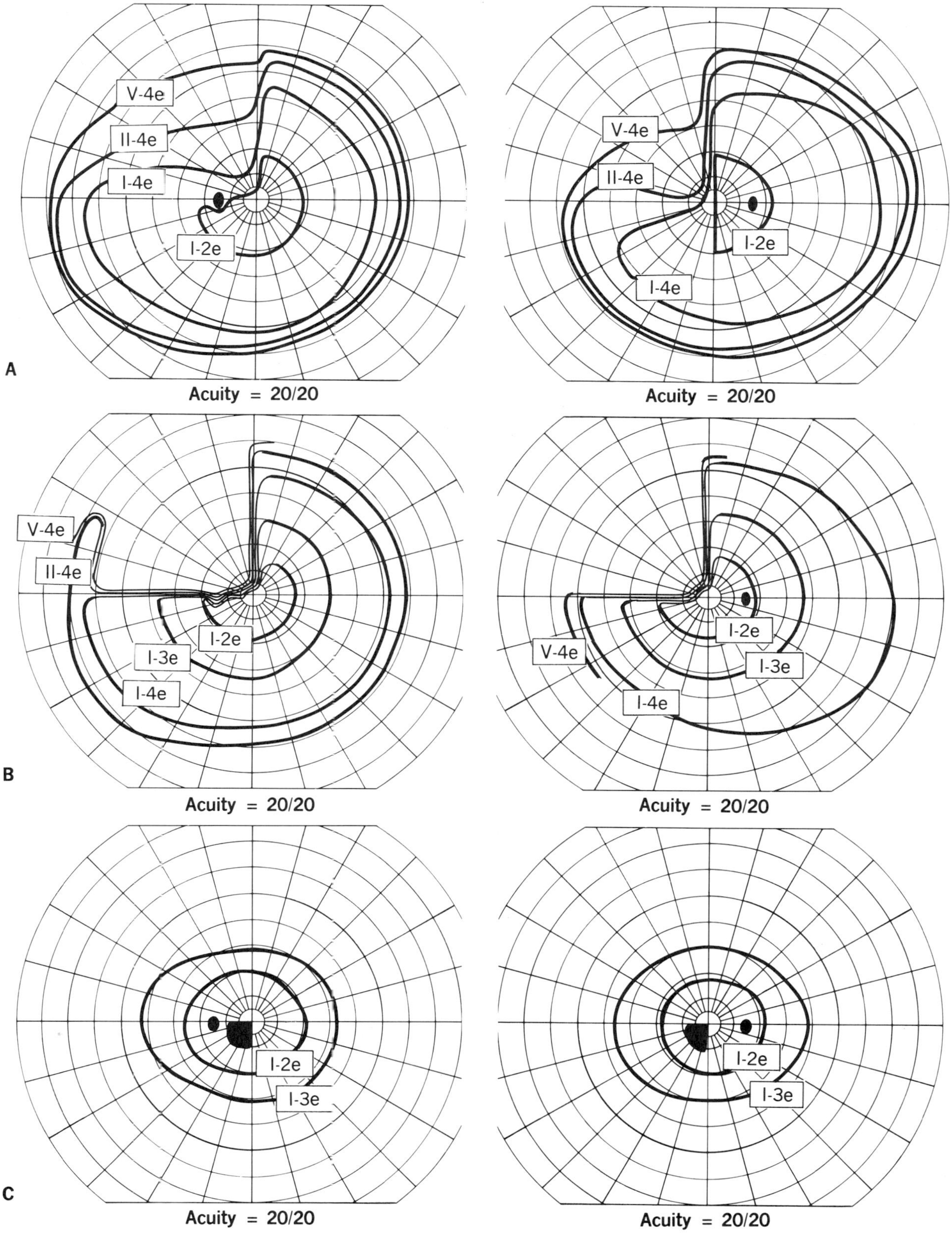
V-4e
II-4e
I-4e
I-2e
A
Acuity = 20/20
V-4e
II-4e
I-2e
I-4e
Acuity = 20/20
V-4e
II-4e
I-2e
I-3e
I-4e
B
Acuity = 20/20
I-2e
V-4e
I-3e
I-4e
Acuity = 20/20
I-2e
I-3e
C
Acuity = 20/20
I-2e
I-3e
Acuity = 20/20

FIG. 9-5

RIDDOCH PHENOMENON

Sometimes within a hemianopic field defect a test stimulus *is* visible if it is moving but is *not* visible if stationary, as if there were a much greater abnormality of visual threshold with static stimuli than with kinetic stimuli. The result is that an isopter for a certain stimulus may be plotted kinetically but in static spot-checking the stimulus will not be visible over a broad area inside the isopter. However, it *is* visible inside the isopter if the stimulus is moving.

This marked difference in visibility between moving and nonmoving stimuli within an abnormal region of the visual field is known as the Riddoch phenomenon, after the British neurologist George Riddoch (1888-1947). When such a region is encountered by an unsuspecting perimetrist, it can be very confusing because it appears, with the usual combined kinetic and static spot-checking technique, as though the patient is being inconsistent. However, once it is realized that the field defect is displaying the Riddoch phenomenon, it is possible to outline a normal seeing area (inside the kinetic isopter), where the stimulus is seen only if moving, and a nonseeing area (outside the kinetic isopter), where the stimulus is not seen whether moving or not.

FIG. 9-6. Hemianopic field defect displaying the Riddoch phenomenon.

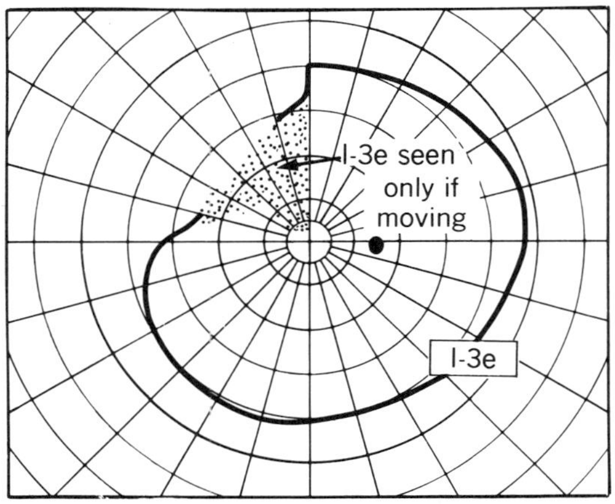

FIG. 9-6

It is sometimes difficult in the presence of the Riddoch phenomenon to outline isopters accurately. Fortunately, when dealing with hemianopias, it is often necessary only to know that there is a definite abnormality; its exact boundary is less important. If quantitation is required, it may best be achieved by static perimetry, which will show a denser abnormality than the kinetic stimulus and will give the most consistent patient responses.

ADDITIONAL READING

For those who wish more details on the topographic approach to visual field diagnosis as relevant especially to neurologic conditions, considerable information can be found in the following:

Duane, T.D., editor: Clinical ophthalmology, vol. 2, New York, 1976, Harper & Row, Publishers.

Ellenberger, C., Jr.: Perimetry: principles, technique, and interpretation, New York, 1980, Raven Press.

Glaser, J.S.: Neuro-ophthalmology, New York, 1978, Harper & Row, Publishers, pp. 47-167. *This is almost the same as the Duane, reprinted with slight modification.*

Harrington, D.O.: The visual fields: a textbook and atlas of clinical perimetry, ed. 5, St. Louis, 1981, The C.V. Mosby Co.

Huber, A.: Eye signs and symptoms in brain tumors, ed. 6, St. Louis, 1976, The C.V. Mosby Co.

Hughes, B.: The visual fields. A study of the applications of quantitative perimetry to the anatomy and pathology of the visual pathways, Springfield, Ill., 1954, Charles C Thomas, Publisher.

Scott, G.: Traquair's clinical perimetry, ed. 7, London, 1957, Henry Kimpton.

Traquair, H.M.: An introduction to clinical perimetry, ed. 6, St. Louis, 1949, The C.V. Mosby Co. *It is hard to beat the valuable information found in this great classic.*

Trobe, J.D., and Glaser, J.S.: The visual fields manual: a practical guide to testing and interpretation, Gainesville, Fla., 1983, Triad Publishing Co.

Walsh, F.B., and Hoyt, W.F.: Clinical neuro-ophthalmology, vol. 1, ed. 3, Baltimore, 1969, The Williams & Wilkins Co., pp. 43-97.

CHAPTER 10

Visual field loss in glaucoma

Glaucoma is an example of a prechiasmal cause of visual field loss. It is the most common reason for performing a visual field test in the usual clinical practice and thus is the subject of a separate chapter.

In glaucoma, axons (nerve fibers) of the optic nerve are damaged and visual function is diminished or lost in the retinal area served by the damaged axons. Sometimes the axon damage is diffuse (scattered at various parts of the optic nerve) so there is a diffuse or generalized decrease of visual sensation throughout the entire retina and visual field. Other times the damage is more localized, affecting bundles of axons that serve a particular portion of the retina, so visual sensitivity is reduced only in some locations. Perhaps most typically there is some degree of diffuse axon damage, but with a greater degree of damage in certain locations, so a localized field defect is superimposed on a generalized depression.

GENERALIZED DEPRESSION

When the axon damage is evenly diffuse, it may be difficult to diagnose glaucomatous generalized depression for two fundamental reasons:

1. If the depression is mild, the visual sensitivity may still be within the normal range (though reduced from the previous visual threshold in that patient). It may require loss of half the axons to produce a 0.5 log-unit (5 dB) reduction in visual sensitivity; thus the damage is far advanced before the static threshold or isopter position is recognizably outside the normal range, especially if one takes into account the variability of results under clinical testing conditions.
2. Patients with such depression may also have preretinal conditions (e.g., small pupil, mild cataract, another dysfunction) that accompany age. Thus, when generalized depression occurs, it cannot automatically be attributed to glaucomatous optic nerve damage, even in the presence of an elevated intraocular pressure. Similarly a generalized depression cannot easily be attributed to damage from high intraocular pressure (IOP) in eyes that are anatomically outside the normal range (small eyes with hyperopia, large eyes with myopia, misshapen eyes with astigmatism), that are frankly anomalous (microphthalmic, nanophthalmic, etc.), or that have diffuse ocular disease (uveitis, diabetic retinopathy, etc.). When such eyes have high intraocular pressure, as they often do, generalized depression may not represent glaucomatous damage.

Despite these limitations, generalized depression can be recognized as a result of glaucomatous optic nerve damage. For example, it may be recognized when static thresholds or isopter positions are being compared to a previous visual field examination in that patient (instead of being compared to the normal range), provided the visual decline is confirmed not to be due to long-term fluctuations (see Chapter 13). It may also be recognized as glaucomatous if the visual sensitivities in the two eyes are recognizably different, especially if the eye with the lower sensitivity also has a higher IOP and larger excavation of the optic nerve (and provided also that the difference is not explained by amblyopia, anisometropia, asymmetric media opacity, or other accompanying difference between the two eyes). A third clue to recognizing pathologic generalized depression (even when the sensitivity remains within the normal range) is that certain localized areas may be more affected than others. When some regions have more sensitivity loss, there is an unevenness in the contour of the hill of vision. With automated static perimetry this unevenness may be recognized by calculating "loss variation" (see Chapter 13) or with manual perimetry may be represented by local regions of variable response. When more pronounced, localized areas that are more affected than others become localized visual field defects and these are even more distinctly recognizable as abnormal.

FIG. 10-1. Generalized depression in glaucoma.
A, Greyscale and difference-from-normal printouts. There is a mild (averaging 7 to 8 dB) reduction of sensitivity throughout the central 30 degrees, with no exaggeration in any location.
B, Greyscale representing static threshold perimetry out to 60 degrees in a more advanced case (left eye). The sensitivity is reduced everywhere, although more in the upper nasal quadrant.

A

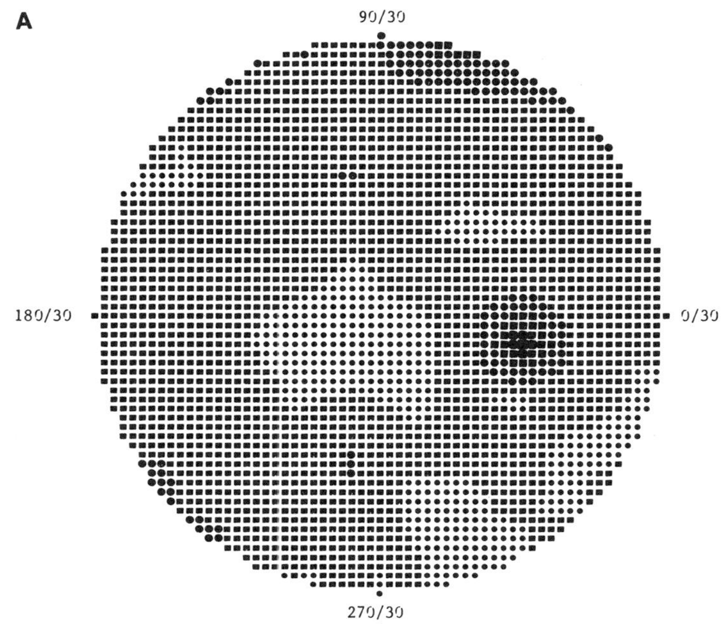

ACTUAL

16 18 14 11
18 18 19 19 20 18
21 20 17 15 19 20 19 20
20 19 19 20 20 20 21 21 20 19
19 20 20 20 21 20 19 17 20 20
19 20 20 22 23 22 19 00 20 20
17 16 18 21 20 21 20 21 18 21
17 19 19 15 20 20 19 22
17 18 16 21 21 20
20 19 20 22

-30 0 +30

DIFFERENCE

06 + 08 12
05 06 05 05 + 06
+ 05 09 11 07 06 06 05
+ 06 07 07 08 07 06 05 05 06
06 06 08 09 09 10 09 10 06 06
06 06 08 07 07 08 10 28 07 06
07 10 09 07 08 08 08 06 08 +
08 07 08 12 08 07 08 +
08 07 10 06 06 06
+ 06 06 +

-30 0 +30

NORMAL

22 22 22 23
23 24 24 24 24 24
24 25 26 26 26 26 25 25
23 25 26 27 28 27 27 26 25 25
25 26 28 29 30 30 28 27 26 26
25 26 28 29 30 30 29 28 27 26
24 26 27 28 28 29 28 27 26 25
25 26 27 27 28 27 27 26
25 25 26 27 27 26
24 25 26 26

-30 0 +30

+30 0 -30

FIG. 10-1

B

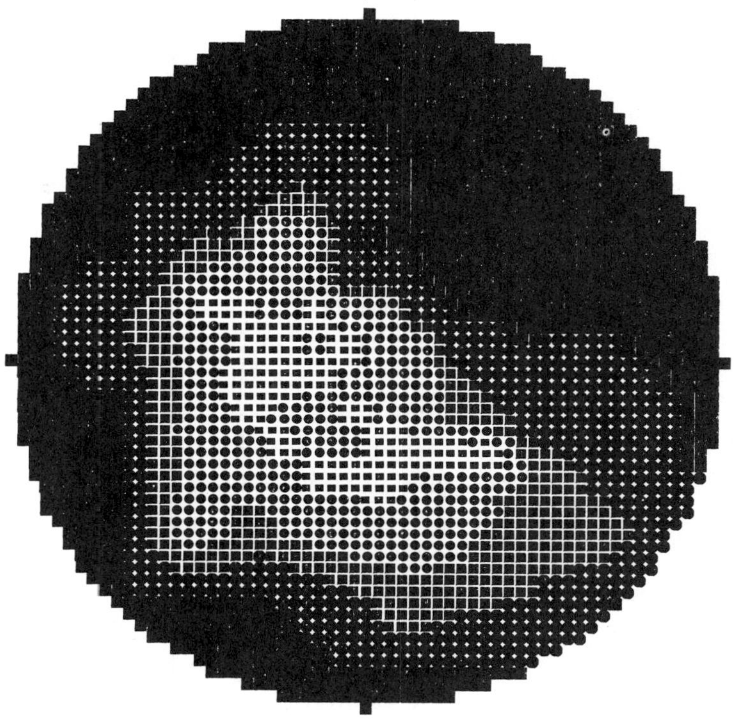

FIG. 10-1, cont'd

LOCALIZED DEFECTS

Although they are often accompanied by generalized depression, typical localized field defects of the nerve fiber bundle type are considered more characteristic of glaucoma than is pure generalized depression. They are indeed common in glaucoma and also more specific, not being mimicked by relatively common preretinal conditions. However, they are mimicked by other causes of nerve fiber bundle defects that are less common than glaucoma.

In contrast to generalized depression, localized defects may be recognized when overall only a small percentage of the nerve fibers are destroyed. A bundle of axons may be completely destroyed and produce an unmistakable dense scotoma but still represent 5% or less of the total number of axons in the optic nerve.

Anatomic basis of localized defects

As discussed in Chapter 4, each location in the retina corresponds to a certain direction in the visual field; for example, a specific location on the inferior retina corresponds to a location in the superior visual field. The nasal retina represents the temporal visual field. The fovea represents the point of fixation and thus separates the nasal from the temporal side.

The optic nerve exits from the nasal side of the fovea. Therefore the physiologic blind spot is in the temporal visual field. Because the visual field diagrams show the field "as the patient sees it," the blind spot is to the right of fixation for the right eye and to the left of fixation for the left eye.

Nerve fibers pass from every point in the retina to the optic nerve head, or optic disc. The pathway of the nerve fibers is important. From the retina nasal to the optic disc, the fibers take a straight course to the disc. Fibers from the nasal side of the fovea also pass rather directly toward the temporal margin of the disc but take an increasingly curved course as they go farther above or below the horizontal meridian. However, the fibers from the retina temporal to the fovea extend in an arcuate pathway around the fovea to pass into the upper and lower poles of the optic disc. The arrangement is quite orderly. Thus, if the retina is divided by an imaginary horizontal line on the temporal side of the fovea, fibers from above the line arc around the fovea superiorly and enter the upper pole of the disc. Similarly, fibers from below the line arc inferiorly around the fovea to enter the inferior pole of the disc.

FIG. 10-2. Relationship of the retina to the visual field.

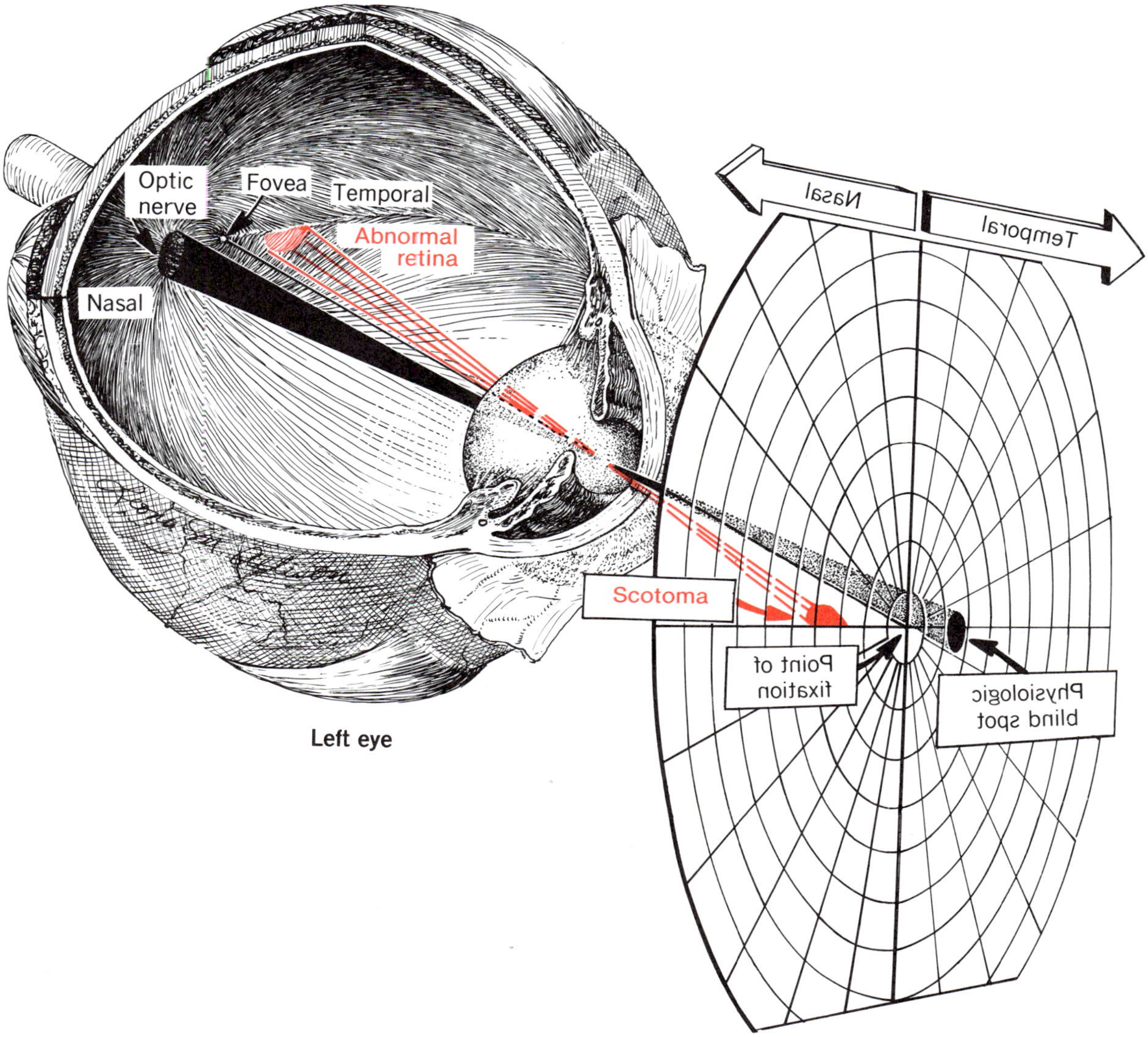
Optic nerve
Fovea
Temporal
Abnormal retina
Nasal
Nasal
Temporal
Scotoma
Point of fixation
Physiologic blind spot
Left eye

FIG. 10-2

In glaucoma, when bundles of nerve fibers are damaged at the optic disc, the visual field supplied by them loses its sensitivity and the result is a scotoma or a localized depression.

Typically the first nerve fibers affected as bundles in glaucoma are those entering the upper or lower pole of the optic disc. Because of this, paracentral scotomas appear within an arcuate region around fixation, the *Bjerrum region,* or there is a depression in the nasal field of vision, or both.

FIG. 10-3. Glaucomatous damage to nerve bundles and resulting visual abnormalities. Damage at the lower pole of the optic disc causes abnormalities in the visual field as shown (left eye).

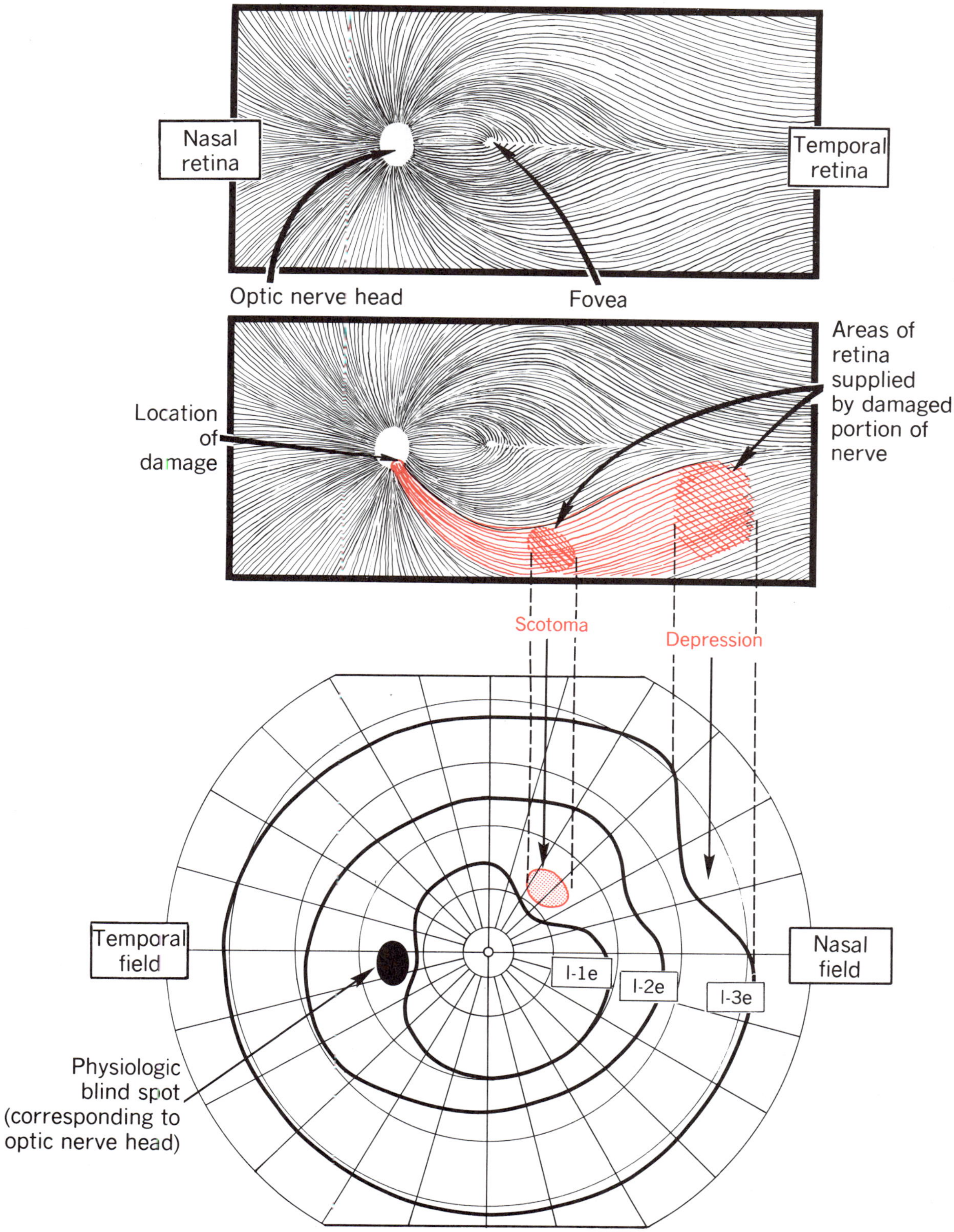
Nasal
retina
Temporal
retina
Optic nerve head
Fovea
Location
of
damage
Areas of
retina
supplied
by damaged
portion of
nerve
Scotoma
Depression
Temporal
field
Nasal
field
I-1e
I-2e
I-3e
Physiologic
blind spot
(corresponding to
optic nerve head)

FIG. 10-3

Nasal steps

The arcuate route of the nerve fibers around the fovea causes the retina to be divided into an upper and a lower portion on the temporal side of the fovea, which is represented nasal to fixation in the visual field. Thus, temporal to the fovea, nerve fibers originating below an imaginary horizontal line enter the bottom of the optic disc whereas those above the line enter the upper pole of the disc.

FIG. 10-4. Basis of the nasal step.
A, When a bundle of nerve fibers that enters the bottom of the optic disc is damaged in glaucoma—or in other diseases affecting the optic nerve head—a scotoma may result in the upper nasal visual field.
B, Such a scotoma may be close to the horizontal meridian on the nasal side of fixation. However, it will not cross the horizontal meridian because the nerve fibers supplying the area just below the horizontal meridian enter the side of the optic disc opposite the location of the damage. The scotoma will have a flat edge along the horizontal meridian, and the isopter that skirts around it will have a "step."
C, This sharp demarcation along the horizontal nasal meridian applies not only to scotomas but also to peripheral depression. If there is upper nasal depression, it will end abruptly at the horizontal meridian, producing a "step" in the isopter.
D, The arcuate (Bjerrum) scotoma typically ends with a steep edge at the horizontal meridian. If there are Bjerrum scotomas both above and below, they will not meet exactly and, thus, they will not likely form a perfect ring-shaped scotoma but will have an abrupt horizontal step on the nasal side.

A nasal step may result either from a scotoma or from a nasal depression. There are two reasons why the nasal step is important in visual field screening and diagnosis of glaucoma.

First, it is easy to look for a nasal step. Threshold values above and below the nasal horizontal meridian can be compared easily, and kinetic techniques are particularly sensitive in detecting nasal steps (with proper technique, Chapters 21 to 23). When there is a nasal step, there is almost always also a scotoma somewhere in the paracentral region that may have escaped detection.

Second, generalized depression may occur as a result of many causes, e.g., age or cataract. Such generalized depression is common and would be difficult to distinguish from the depression of glaucoma if it were not for the fact that age and cataract will *not* produce a nasal step. However, if there is any unevenness in the depression it may show up as a nasal step, revealing that the depression is caused by damage to the optic nerve.

Therefore, in glaucoma visual field testing, particular attention is paid to the horizontal meridian on the nasal side. It is very important to know whether or not the isopters have a nasal step. Although glaucoma is the most common cause of field defects with nasal steps, other less common diseases affecting the optic nerve head can cause an identical field defect.

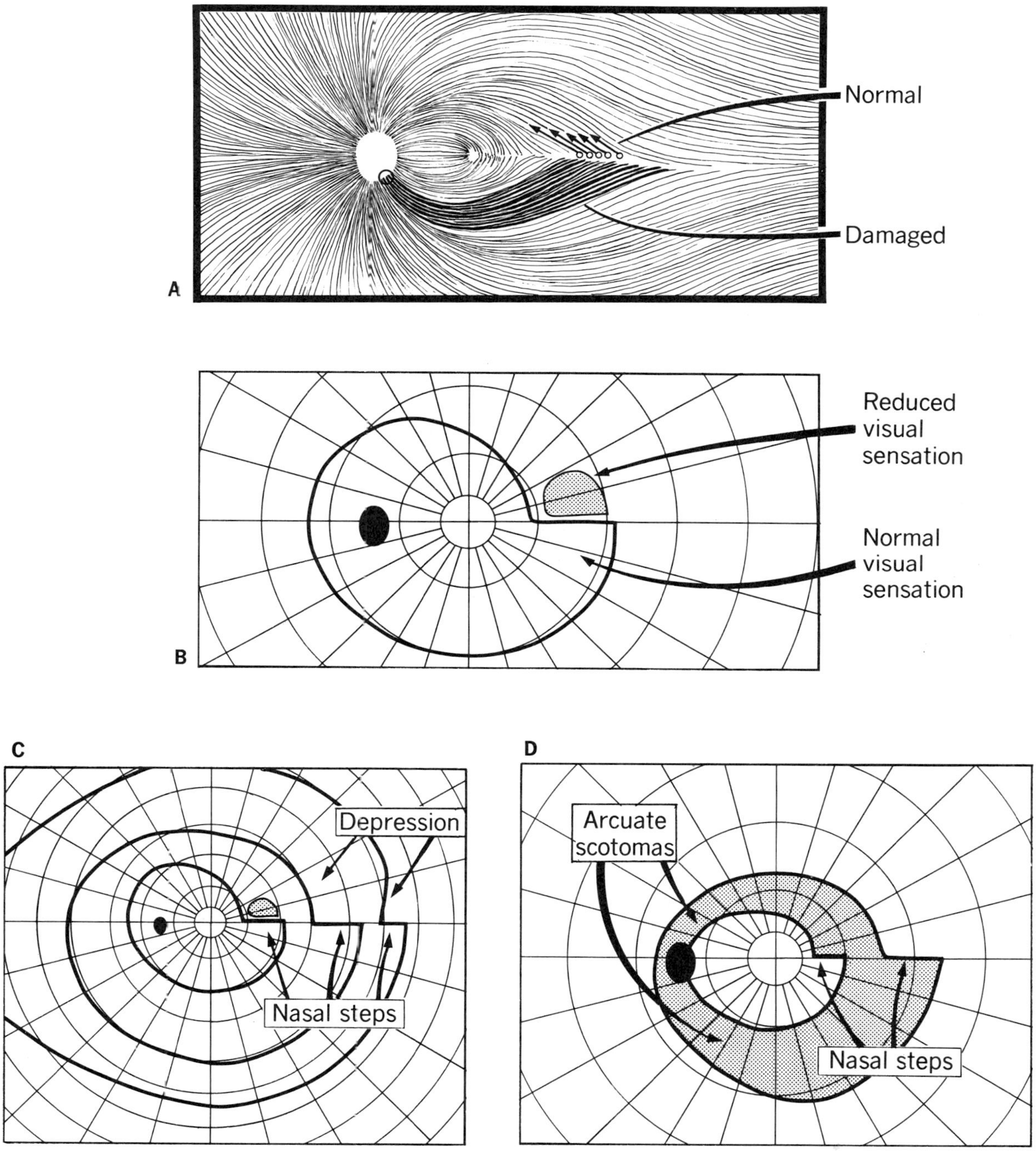
Normal
Damaged
A
Reduced visual sensation
Normal visual sensation
B
C
Depression
Nasal steps
D
Arcuate scotomas
Nasal steps

FIG. 10-4

PROGRESSION OF FIELD LOSS

Typically, either a paracentral scotoma or a peripheral nasal depression is the first localized abnormality to appear. As the disease progresses, additional areas become abnormal and visual sensation becomes worse in the already abnormal areas.

FIG. 10-5. Stages in the progression of glaucomatous visual field loss.
A, An arcuate (Bjerrum) scotoma to *I-3e* superiorly contains two dense nuclei where *V-4e* is not seen. A peripheral nasal depression is also seen.
B, In a more advanced stage of glaucoma the *I-3e* isopter in the depression moves inward to meet and unite with the *I-3e* isopter that formed a boundary of the arcuate Bjerrum scotoma. The scotoma and the depression become one, and it is said that the "scotoma breaks through to the periphery." The two nuclei remain as paracentral scotomas within the arcuate depression. A shallow scotoma to *I-3e* is also in the lower Bjerrum region.
C, At a more advanced stage of glaucoma, visual sensitivity is worse in both the upper and the lower arcuate regions, with a dense arcuate abnormality above and a shallower arcuate defect below.
D, After arcuate scotomas have formed both above and below and have broken through the periphery, there remains a central island of vision and a temporal crescent of vision. At this stage, by imaging a line vertically through fixation, it is possible to see that nearly all the nasal field of vision is gone. However, the temporal half of the field of each eye is present and each compensates for the absent nasal field of the other such that with both eyes open the patient is often unaware of the visual loss. The temporal field of vision of the right eye covers the area to the right of fixation and the temporal field of vision of the left eye covers the area to the left of fixation.

Ultimately both the central island and the temporal crescent become smaller, and then one or the other is lost completely. When both are lost, the patient is blind in that eye.

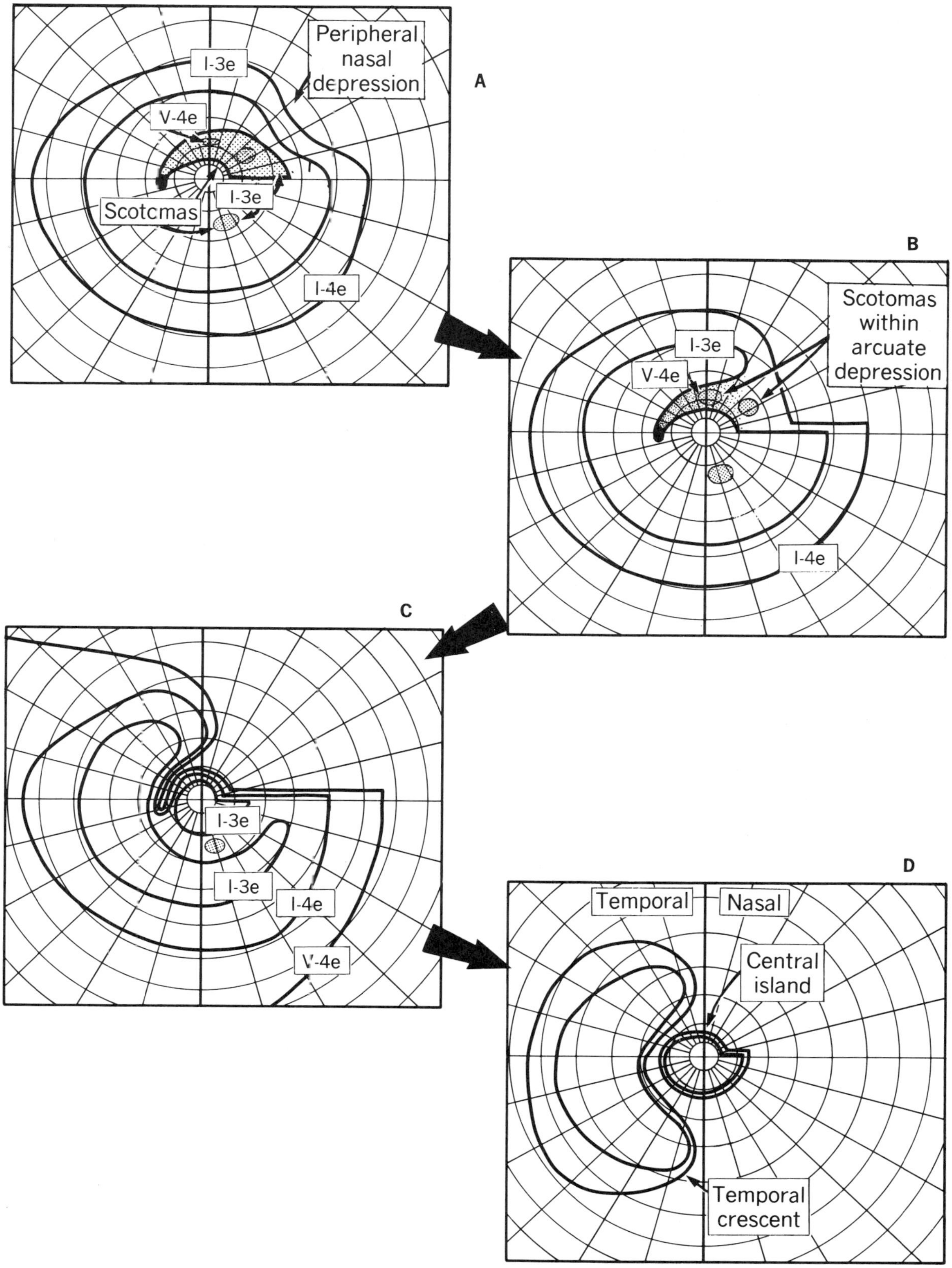
A
Peripheral nasal depression
I-3e
V-4e
Scotcmas
I-3e
I-4e
B
Scotomas within arcuate depression
I-3e
V-4e
I-4e
C
I-3e
I-3e
I-4e
V-4e
D
Temporal
Nasal
Central island
Temporal crescent

FIG. 10-5

POINT OF FIXATION

Although a central island of vision is typically preserved until late in the course of glaucomatous optic nerve damage, visual function at the point of fixation may be affected by diffuse loss of axons (generalized depression of the field) or by a localized field defect impinging on the point of fixation. In such cases tests of central acuity, color vision, and contrast sensitivity may be detectably abnormal. Mild abnormality at or around fixation is common, but it is atypical for a scotoma affecting fixation to predominate. Cases in which the point of fixation and its immediate surround are more densely affected than the rest of the visual field are perhaps more common in myopic eyes. However, central scotomas are infrequent in glaucoma. The examiner must always be on guard, because a person with elevated IOP may also have a compressive lesion of the optic nerve producing a progressive central scotoma.

OTHER DEFECTS

There are several less common but typical visual field defects in glaucoma. One example is a localized depression consisting of a wedge on the temporal side with its apex pointed at the blind spot (see Fig. 7-5). Another is a scotoma on the nasal side outside 30 degrees. A third is reduced visual sensation in the arcuate region that may be represented by depressed isopters instead of by a scotoma.

FIG. 10-6. Less common defects. Wedge-shaped temporal depression pointing at the blind spot and a midperipheral nasal scotoma with a nasal step in one isopter.

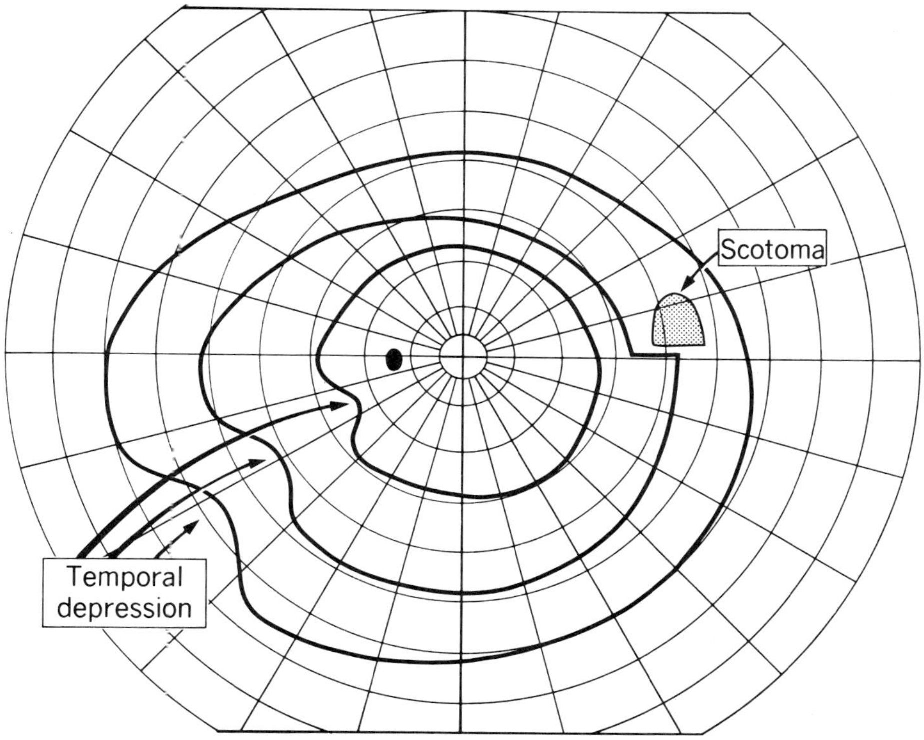

FIG. 10-6

SUMMARY

In addition to generalized depression, the visual field loss in glaucoma typically consists of paracentral scotomas that may enlarge and join together to become an arcuate or Bjerrum scotoma. Depression on the nasal side may merge with the reduced visual sensation of the arcuate scotoma. Nasal steps are produced because the depression and the scotomas are of unequal severity above and below the horizontal meridian.

FIG. 10-7. Typical localized glaucomatous defects. This composite of visual field defects might occur in moderately advanced glaucoma.

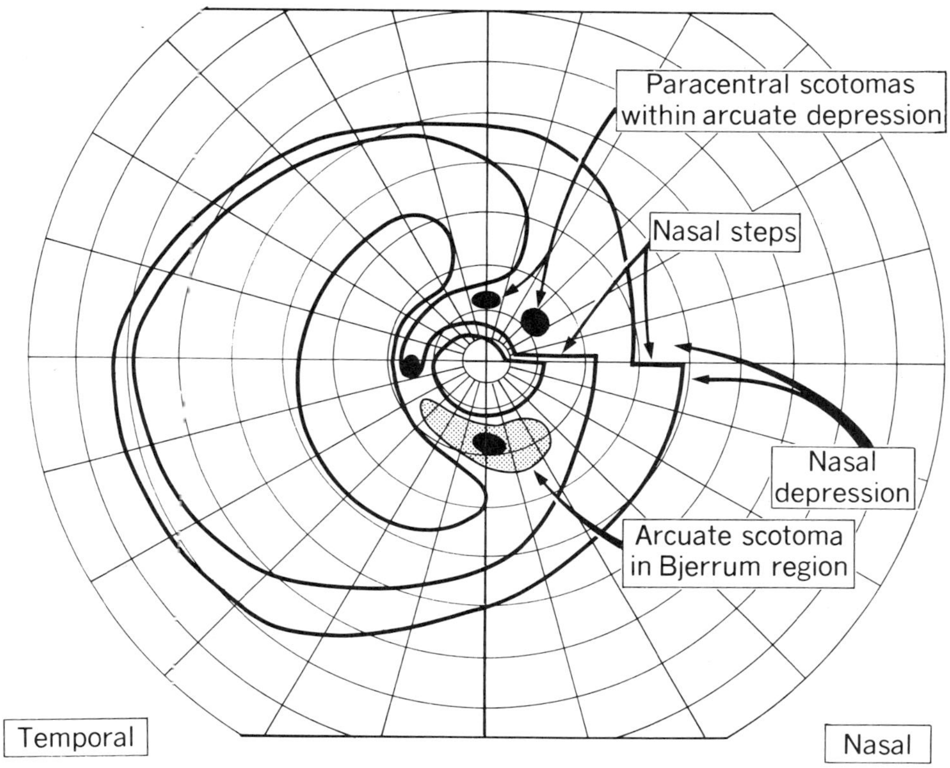
Paracentral scotomas within arcuate depression
Nasal steps
Nasal depression
Arcuate scotoma in Bjerrum region
Temporal
Nasal

FIG. 10-7

FIG. 10-8. Combined localized and generalized loss
A, Generalized loss with low sensitivity everywhere. The loss is greatest as a superimposed localized defect in the inferior arcuate region and lower nasal quadrant. The actual threshold values are shown in the center panel. The difference-from-expected printout, which highlights the localized loss (see Fig. 2-8 for an explanation) but hides the presence of generalized depression, is at the bottom.
B, Scotoma in the upper arcuate region near the blind spot. The greyscale shows the scotoma and draws attention to the abnormal threshold value (circled) in the center panel. The difference-from-normal printout (bottom) shows that there is a generalized depression (nearly all locations are affected), but it does not call attention to the scotoma.

These examples show that glaucoma often includes both localized and generalized loss. They also illustrate that generalized loss is judged by a comparison to normal values but localized loss is judged by comparison to other locations that may be normal or at least less abnormal.

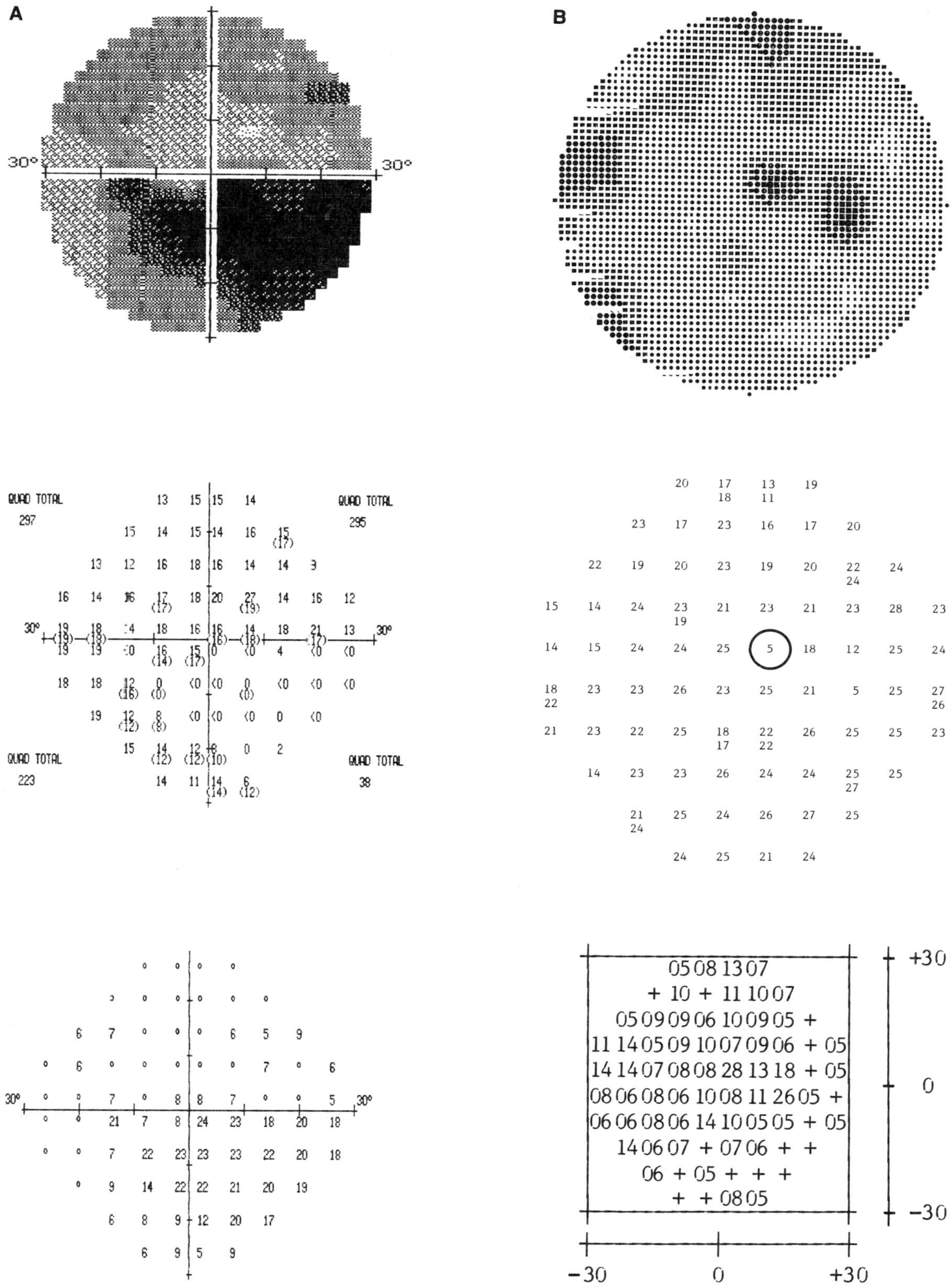
A
B
30°
30°
QUAD TOTAL
297
QUAD TOTAL
295
QUAD TOTAL
223
QUAD TOTAL
38
+30
0
−30
−30
0
+30

FIG. 10-8

CHAPTER 11

Purposeful examination of the field

TYPES OF EXAMINATION

There is no such thing as a standard visual field examination, because there are many different reasons for performing the test. A manual technique or automated program must be chosen according to the purpose at hand. There should always be a specific clinical question in mind to be answered. Four general types of examination are as follows:

1. *General screening examinations*. These are performed on large groups of people (e.g., all patients seen in the office, all individuals renewing their driver's license, or all individuals entering the U.S. Air Force) to detect any kind of field defect.

   The process includes screening of nonsuspects, and it must be distinguished from the screening for visual field defects of individuals who have some clinical sign or symptom that makes them suspect for a disease. Applicable techniques may range from simple finger-counting confrontation fields, to the kinetic plotting of an isopter or two with static spot-checking centrally, to simple supraliminal static spot-checking without plotting an isopter. The choice depends on the sensitivity desired, the types of defects that are most important to detect in the group being tested (e.g., asymptomatic conditions for which early treatment is beneficial, or defects that would be a hazard for automobile driving or aircraft piloting), and the time and energy that the examiner can devote to the detection (cost-effectiveness).
2. *Screening examinations for a particular defect*. These are directed at deciding whether or not a particular type of visual field defect is present and may be performed on a person with a symptom or clinical sign that makes him suspect for a particular disease.

   For example, in the case of an individual with poor visual acuity, the question might be whether or not a central scotoma is present. In another individual with medical evidence of endocrine abnormality suggesting a possible pituitary tumor, the question might be whether or not a bitemporal hemianopia is present. Field testing could be done on an individual taking chloroquine because he was at risk of developing maculopathy. In a person with elevated intraocular pressure, there might be a question of whether or not glaucomatous optic nerve damage had occurred. Specific glaucoma screening examinations could also be directed toward people who were not individually suspect but were in a high-risk group, such as those living in a retirement center.

The exact nature of the screening examination will depend on the type of defect for which the examiner is looking: the screening examination performed to look for a hemianopia will not be the same as one performed to look for a glaucomatous defect.

3. *Diagnostic examinations.* These are performed to establish or help establish a diagnosis.

   At times there is not much distinction between a screening examination and a diagnostic examination. For example, if a pituitary tumor is suspected because the patient has endocrine abnormalities and a field examination shows a bitemporal hemianopia, the presence of a pituitary tumor is both detected (screening) and established (diagnosis). Another way in which screening and diagnosis are performed at the same time is when a screening strategy is used until the abnormality is found and the perimetrist or a computerized program proceeds immediately to define in detail the nature and extent of the defect that has been detected.

   In some settings, however, detection and diagnosis are kept separate. It may be more efficient to use a relatively rapid general screening technique (perhaps with a fair number of false-positive results) to look for glaucoma in a large general population in which only a few people will have glaucoma. Only those who seem to have a defect by the screening technique will then, at another time and place, undergo a more time-consuming, but also more accurate, examination for diagnosis. The purpose of the second examination is to separate individuals who have false-positive results by the first test from those who truly have defective vision. The distinction between screening and diagnosis in these cases is that a rapid screening examination detects the *possible* (or *probable*) presence of an abnormality while the diagnostic examination establishes the presence of a defect and defines its nature with sufficient certainty to enable a diagnosis to be made (and perhaps indicate the need for treatment).

   Occasionally a diagnostic examination takes the form of distinguishing between two types of defects. For example, in the case of reduced visual acuity it may be necessary to know whether the visual reduction is due to a generalized depression or to a central scotoma. Such a diagnostic test consists of looking for both suspected defects, expecting only one to be found.

4. *Following progressive conditions*. Detailed quantitative definition of a defect may not be necessary for detection and diagnosis. However, it is important if a patient has a condition that may worsen or improve and the progress of the condition must be followed so therapeutic decisions can be made. Glaucoma, a prominent example used throughout much of this book, is such a condition. Another is recurrence of a brain tumor after irradiation.

Some instrumentation and test strategy may apply to one circumstance but not to another. There is no point in going through a fully quantitative visual field examination for half an hour when the question at hand is simply whether or not the patient has a hemianopia or a central scotoma, questions that can be answered rather quickly with less elaborate techniques. In fact, a highly quantitative field examination covering the entire area may be less accurate for this: The examiner may do a fairly extensive quantitative visual field test and still miss a small central scotoma that was accounting for the patient's 20/60 vision unless it is kept in mind that the goal of performing the field test in this patient was to look for a central scotoma and therefore make a concentrated effort at the central 2 or 3 degrees of the field.

Both for manual techniques and for the selection of automated programs, the examiner needs to consider the context in which the examination is being performed—the type of defect possible (e.g., a central or paracentral scotoma, a hemianopia) according to the disease suspected, the features of the field defect that will help distinguish one diagnosis from another (e.g., a quadrantic defect with its apex at fixation as opposed to the blind spot, the presence or absence of a strict limit of the defect at the vertical meridian), and whether or not any defect found should immediately be quantified (either to help with the diagnosis or because the progress of the chronic condition will subsequently need to be followed).

Routine office visits

A complete eye examination should probably include a rapid determination by confrontation that the patient is able to count fingers 3 or 4 feet away and 45 degrees from fixation in each of the four quadrants, along with an examination of the pupils, an alternate cover test, and other components of a complete routine eye examination. Such a quick confrontation examination is routine in our institution and may pick up such things as glaucomatous visual field defects in the upper nasal quadrant, an unsuspected hemianopia, or a field defect that results from an unsuspected retinal detachment (although the existence of these conditions might also be detected in the course of the remainder of the eye examination).

Although formal field testing with perimetric equipment is not routinely part of a complete eye examination in most offices and clinics, with the increasing availability of automated perimetry it is tempting to incorporate a visual field screening routinely into every complete eye examination. This would most logically be an automated suprathreshold test of the central 30 degrees, perhaps supplemented by a suprathreshold test of the peripheral field with a stronger stimulus. It remains to be seen, however, whether this would be cost effective and how often it would detect the existence of a condition that might not have become apparent in the course of the remainder of the eye examination, including confrontation field testing and ophthalmoscopy. Cost consciousness should dictate that such screening tests not be overutilized and the charge for them not be out of line (e.g., not the same as for lengthier quantitative programs used in following the progress of glaucoma).

General screening of a population

The screening visual field examination—e.g., with an automatic perimeter that uses a suprathreshold spot-checking strategy—may be useful, along with determination of visual acuity, to look for visual abnormalities in members of large groups. The main consideration in judging such screening projects is whether or not a sufficient number of visual field defects are detected to be worth the effort and expense. This depends on how many defects exist in the population (prevalence), how serious the existing defects are, if there is benefit to finding the disease or visual deficit earlier than might otherwise happen, and how effectively the testing time can be kept brief without losing sensitivity in detecting the people who have abnormalities.

An important consideration in planning a screening program is the rate of false-positive results (the percentage of people with normal vision who seem to have a field defect but, in fact, do not) compared to the prevalence of true visual field defects. It is discouraging if most of the positive results uncovered during a screening project are false alarms. This will happen if the rate of false-positives (e.g., 5%) exceeds the prevalence of true defects (0.5%) in a population. Moreover, the additional time it takes to do more definitive examinations on the false-positives to distinguish them from true-positives must be taken into account when judging the cost and time expended in detecting the people with true defects. (This is not as great a problem when vision screening is being done in an office setting, however. The patient is undergoing a complete eye examination anyway, and the rest of the clinical examination will assist in interpreting the meaning of borderline visual field findings.)

The ratio between false-positive and true-positive results can be made more favorable by increasing the true-positive rate or by decreasing the false-positive rate. The former can be accomplished by conducting the screening examination on a selected group (e.g., elderly persons) with a high prevalence of true visual defects. The latter can be accomplished by selection of the test strategy. For example, to reduce the rate of false-positive results in a suprathreshold test, the examiner can use a somewhat stronger stimulus than might be used in another setting. Also, the criteria for normalcy may be kept lax so that indefinite findings are not considered evidence of abnormality. (These measures will, however, also reduce the sensitivity of the test in detecting mild cases of true abnormality—see p. 164.)

A threshold-related stimulus selection can be used if there is a high priority on detection of localized defects and if mild generalized depression is to be ignored. However, if attention is going to be paid to all defects, including mild generalized depression, then it might be wise to forego the use of a threshold-related strategy for stimulus selection and thereby save time. To reduce time expenditure (cost), it is also important to keep the number of test locations small.

Taken together, these considerations suggest that the best strategy in mass screening might be to test between 75 and 100 points with an eccentricity-compensated stimulus that ought to be suprathreshold at all points in virtually all normal people. Missed points would be retested and any missed a second time would be considered an abnormality. Whenever it becomes obvious during a test that the field is abnormal, time can be saved by stopping the test, because it has already been determined that a more definitive test will be necessary.

Small or shallow defects may not be detected when a stronger stimulus is used to lessen the rate of false-positive results and the number of tested locations is limited to keep the time within acceptable limits. In a screening program this reduced sensitivity in detecting abnormalities is accepted with the realization that the defects missed will be small or shallow and will be the less important or even inconsequential ones. However, it is hoped that all the more important defects exceeding a certain size and depth will be discovered. Of course, sensitivity should not be compromised needlessly: Eccentricity-compensated stimuli should be used, because the test takes no more time than one-level screening.

There may be advantage to using a semiquantitative program—i.e., one that classifies abnormal points into relative and absolute defects. With appropriate criteria of what constitutes an abnormal screening field (see Chapter 13), a lower rate of false-positive results may be obtained without losing much sensitivity. At first glance, it would seem that a semiquantitative program would take longer; but this is not true. The time needed for an entirely normal field will be the same. An abnormal field will not take longer if the test is stopped as soon as it is certain that the criteria for an abnormal screening test have been fulfilled.

Glaucoma screening projects

In the past many glaucoma screening projects in the general population have consisted simply of measuring the intraocular pressure. Unfortunately, many individuals with glaucoma are not detected by a single pressure reading, especially if the cutoff point of abnormality is raised to reduce the number of false-positive results. To supplement the pressure readings, examinations of the optic disc or screening visual field examinations would improve the detection rate. However, disc examination is a feasible method only if there are available personnel skilled in recognizing glaucomatous cupping by ophthalmoscopy. Most practitioners interested in a screening project can easily be trained to perform a simple screening examination with the Goldmann perimeter (a suitable protocol might be to spot-check the central 25 degrees with the I-3e stimulus or a stimulus that was threshold at 30 degrees), and instruments that simplify or automate the use of a threshold static spot-checking strategy can be operated by personnel with even less training. It becomes still more feasible to incorporate field testing into a standard glaucoma detection project, although for the sake of time-(cost-)effectiveness, the test will be usually done only on the central 30 degrees. Nonetheless, an efficient eccentricity-compensated automated program might profitably also test a few points in the peripheral field without much additional effort.

The visual field component of the glaucoma screening program differs from the general visual field screening program in that it is aimed specifically at glaucomatous visual field defects. However, many of the same considerations apply: It is important to aim the program primarily at persons in whom there is a particular risk of glaucoma (the elderly, those with a family history of glaucoma, etc.). It is also important to use a screening technique with criteria for abnormality that will yield a low false-positive rate lest it become too time consuming to perform on all who seem to have a defect (most of whom will turn out to be normal). The use of semiquantitation may make true abnormalities more obvious and permit the use of stricter criteria for abnormality, thereby reducing the false-positive rate. In the attempt to achieve a quick simple screening test without too many false diagnoses, some early field defects will escape detection, but these can be minimized by using stimuli that are eccentricity compensated. If it is decided to concentrate on localized defects and ignore mild generalized depression that might be due to a nonglaucomatous cause, a threshold-related strategy for stimulus selection can be used.

Perhaps the only difference from a general screening project is that, for glaucoma detection, it would be more sensible specifically to use a test pattern that highlights points above and below the horizontal meridian nasally, points in the arcuate region, and points near fixation.

Glaucoma detection and diagnosis in the clinical office

In an ophthalmologist's office a combination of pressure measurement and careful examination of the optic disc constitutes an efficient method for glaucoma detection in patients who come for a complete eye examination. Visual field screening for glaucomatous visual field defects can be performed on individuals who have a particular sign of glaucoma, perhaps an elevated pressure (whether or not the disc appears to be damaged) or an excavated disc (whether or not the pressure is elevated) or for some other reason (e.g., a strong family history of glaucoma).

The examination method used in this setting should be more sensitive than that used for screening the general population. The presence or absence of a field abnormality is a prime consideration in the decision to initiate therapy. Because of this, there has been considerable emphasis on high sensitivity in detecting the earliest field abnormality. Of course, the false-positive rate must be kept acceptably low; but for the sake of gaining sensitivity, the false-positive rate can be allowed to go somewhat higher than in population screening programs. Among glaucoma suspects the proportion of true-positives is higher than in the general population. Therefore, even with a somewhat higher false-positive rate, the ratio between true- and false-positives will remain acceptable.

For **manual perimetry** this means that the static suprathreshold spot-checking must be done with a marginally suprathreshold stimulus by using individualized stimulus selection (p. 398). In addition, some degree of eccentricity compensation is needed so a weaker stimulus can be used for the central 10 to 15 degrees than for the region from 15 to 30 degrees (p. 404). All defects detected must be quantified to establish them as real and to set a baseline for judging future progression. Once a field is known to be abnormal, all regions—not just those that are usually screened—should be searched for abnormalities and quantified as a baseline.

With **automated perimetry,** the best approach for all glaucoma suspects is to use a fully quantitated static threshold program. Threshold determination provides better information than suprathreshold tests can about the presence or absence of a visual field defect. Furthermore, with the development of calculated indices to judge the presence of an abnormality, this type of program may become even more sensitive. Additionally, the fully quantitated threshold test gives a baseline that allows future judgment about the presence of a defect to be made by comparing the field to the patient's own previous baseline rather than to a broader range of normal values. For ease in recognizing defects that represent the nasal horizontal meridian, a pattern of points that straddle the horizontal meridian should be selected rather than one whose tested points fall along the horizontal meridian (e.g., program 32 of the Octopus or 30-2 of the Humphrey perimeter rather than program 31 or 30-1 respectively). It is sometimes helpful to include the point of fixation and a cluster of points surrounding fixation in the pattern, such as program G1 of the Octopus perimeter, or to select the option of including the fovea with program 30-2 of the Humphrey instrument.

An alternative, eccentricity-compensated, threshold-related, supraliminal strategy may also be used, similar to the one used in community glaucoma screening. Then, to interpret the presence of a generalized depression, attention is paid to the stimulus level selected by the threshold-related program. The criteria for what constitutes an abnormality may be such that with a relative defect more attention is given to just a few spots because the rate of false-positives is not so big a problem as it is in a community screening program. Whenever the field is determined to be abnormal, a fully quantitated field (with a manual perimeter or with a static threshold automated program) must be performed to act as a baseline for detecting future progression.

An even less sensitive alternative is an eccentricity-compensated supraliminal program that is not threshold related but uses standard stimuli for age. This will reveal localized defects in the presence of a generalized depression if the thresholds of abnormal points are determined (programs 33 and 34 of the Octopus perimeter) but will not reveal shallow defects in an individual who happens to have an overall supernormal hill of vision.

There is a difference of opinion about the value of testing the peripheral field in addition to the central field by automated perimetry. Cases exist in which defects are detected only in the periphery, and it makes sense that the addition of a peripheral field examination should achieve the goal of detecting the earliest field defects in as many individuals as possible. However, when sensitive methods are used in the central field, isolated peripheral defects are even less frequent. Additionally, such isolated peripheral defects do not represent an imminent threat to practical visual function. Some authors may even argue that if additional time is available it would be better spent doing double determinations of threshold in the central field, or doubling the number of points tested in the central field, rather than exploring the peripheral part of the field. At present, most clinicians test only the central field, simply because the test becomes too lengthy if peripheral threshold testing is included. A compromise is to test the central field with a fully quantitated program but the periphery with a suprathreshold program followed by depth classification of any defective points (program G1 of the Octopus, a combination of 32 and 07 of the Octopus, combinations of 30-2 and nasal step programs of the Humphrey, etc.).

Following potentially progressive glaucoma or neurologic disease

Suprathreshold static spot-checking or quick plotting of one or two isopters may reveal some cases of progression in which there is considerable enlargement of the visual field defect. However, these methods will not reveal deepening of defects or milder degrees of progression.

A fully quantitated manual field examination with multiple kinetic isopters and quantitation of the depth of all defects is an excellent traditional mainstay in watching for progression. The manual techniques are described in detail in Part II of this book.

A fully quantitated automated field has become a popular alternative (static threshold perimetry). As with screening, some clinicians regularly test the peripheral field in addition to the central field; however, others save time by testing only the central field, trusting that significant progression in the periphery will be infrequent without simultaneous detectable progression in the central 30 degrees. A program with a pattern of test points straddling the horizonal meridian (e.g., 32 of the Octopus or 30-2 of the Humphrey) is of advantage. Determining threshold at the point of fixation, likewise, may be advantageous to supplement visual acuity determinations and monitor foveal vision.

After a set of baseline quantitated field tests is on record, a time-saving program is one that tests each point in the field by supraliminal static spot-checking with a stimulus intensity that is a fixed small amount greater than the mean of the preceding baseline values. If the stimulus is seen, it can be safely assumed that the point has not deteriorated a detectable amount. Any defective points, of course, must be quantified; and if sufficiently numerous points have changed, a new quantitated baseline may be needed for judging further progression.

Although many program options are available (patterns of stimulus location, stimulus size, background intensity, etc.), it is probably wise to use a standard program with standard parameters in the absence of compelling reasons to do otherwise. This will make for ease in comparing the visual fields from one time to another, especially as a patient may later go to another office for examination.

However, the availability of nonstandard options is of great advantage in certain special cases when a closer grid of points or more detailed testing of particular regions is required. Sparingly the examiner may substitute or supplement with a special pattern, may use a different stimulus size, or may even adjust the background for specific clinical or research purposes.

For example, if there are field defects near fixation, if fixation is split, or if only an island of vision around fixation remains, it becomes important to quantify the central 5 or 10 degrees with extreme care. A program can be chosen to determine static threshold values at points in a close grid surrounding fixation (e.g., 61 of the Octopus or a "macula program"). Alternatively, a static cut with 1-degree resolution may be chosen. The equivalent is accomplished in manual perimetry by plotting precisely the position of any isopters in the region, including especially the weakest stimuli visible in the area, and the boundaries of defects with the strongest stimuli that are invisible (see Chapter 23).

As another example, if there are many points in the field where the maximum intensity stimulus is not visible with the standard size, it may be advantageous to use a larger *nonstandard* size. Progression cannot be recognized at points where the maximum intensity stimulus (0 dB) of standard size is not seen: If the threshold value is already 0, it cannot become less than that. However, if a particular submaximum stimulus becomes visible with a larger size, then a measurable threshold exists and can be followed for deterioration. If a considerable portion of the field remains blind to the larger stimulus size, a program must be used that allows a closer density of points to be followed within the area of the field that does remain.

FIG. 11-1. Three ways to follow a small amount of remaining vision.
A, The Goldmann field shows a small central island and a temporal crescent. Isopters to the weakest visible stimulus must be plotted (p. 394).
B, The standard 30-degree field has only five seeing points with a measurable threshold to the size 3 test stimulus; however, a measurable threshold exists nearly everywhere to the size 5 stimulus, which is roughly equivalent to a 10 dB increase in intensity compared to the size 3.
C, Pattern of points with high spatial resolution (test locations 2 degrees apart) with triple determination of threshold at each location. (See Fig. 13-54 for an example of progression followed in this manner.)

The same principles used in following the progression of glaucoma apply to monitoring other chronic conditions—such as retinitis pigmentosa, hemianopic lesions (to look for recurrences after neurosurgery), progressive optic nerve involvement from thyroid exophthalmos, changes in macular threshold values in individuals taking chloroquine. It is necessary to quantify with multiple isopters or static threshold the areas of the visual field relevant to the problem at hand.

A

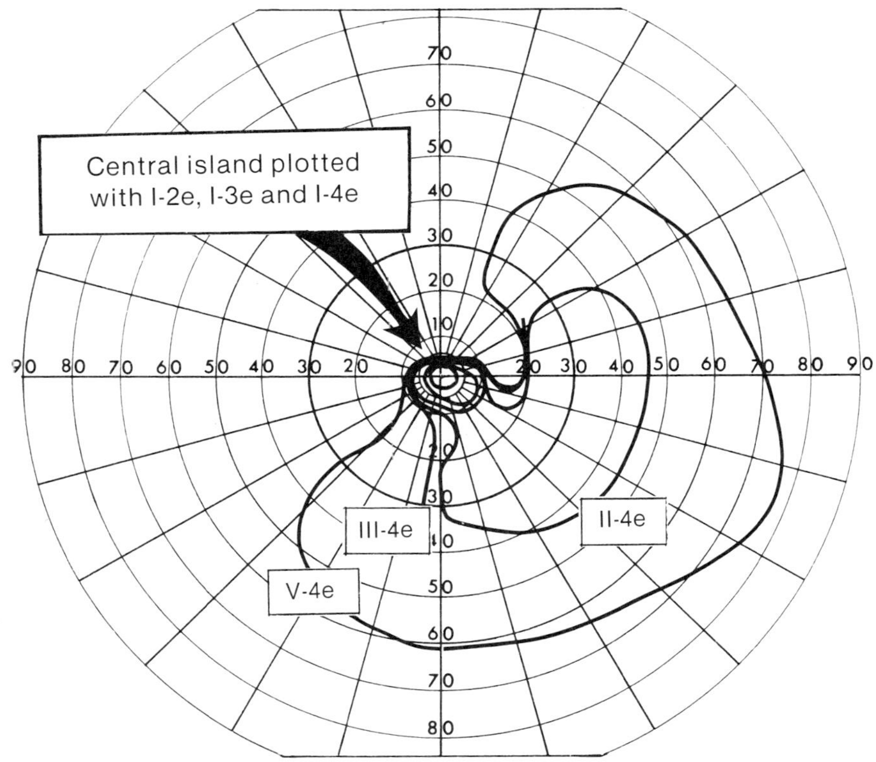

FIG. 11-1

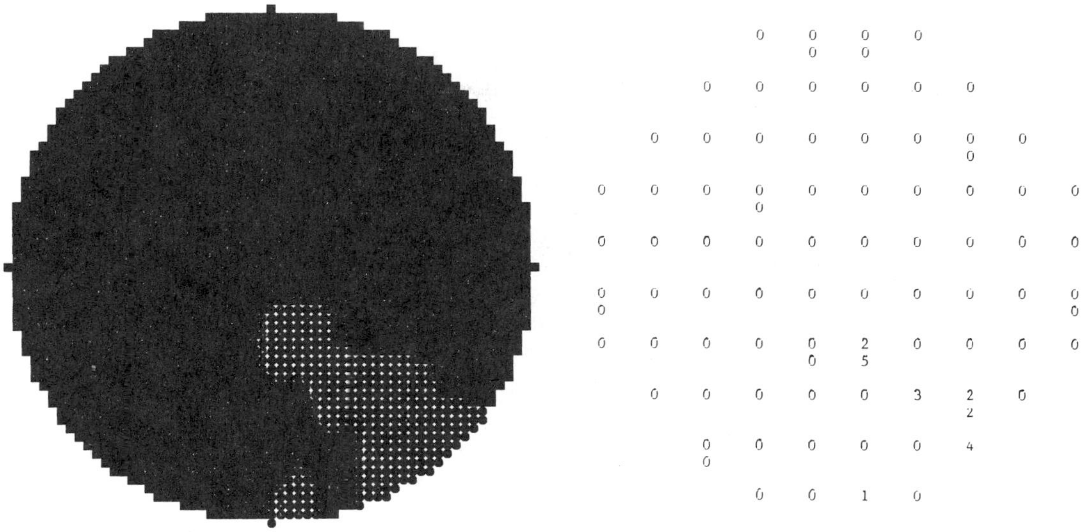

B

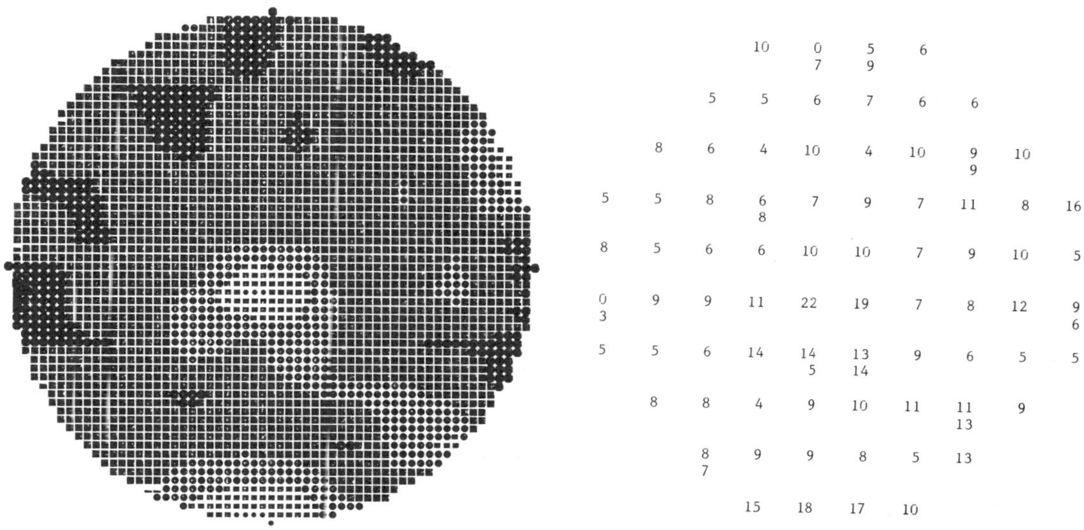

C

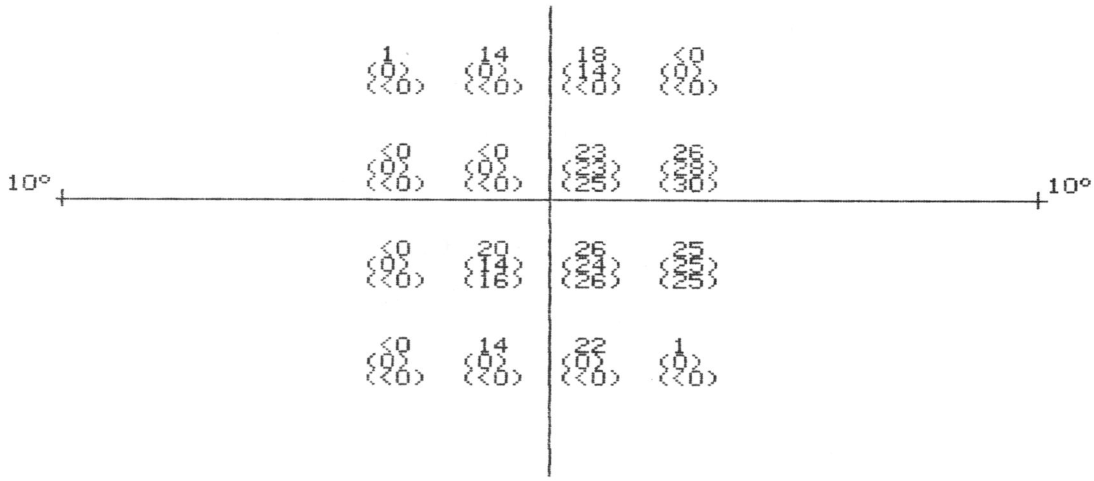

FIG. 11-1, cont'd

REDUCED VISUAL FUNCTION

Perimetry is sometimes performed to assist in the diagnosis of an unexplained visual symptom or unexplained loss of visual acuity.

If a patient has unexplained visual symptoms but his acuity is correctable to 20/20, then the search is for either a broad defect such as a hemianopia or a small scotoma near but not actually affecting the point of fixation. The former may be suggested by a complaint of deficient peripheral vision, the latter by a complaint of difficulty in reading or doing tasks that require detailed vision.

If the acuity is abnormal, there should be an abnormal visual threshold at fixation. It is diagnostically helpful to determine whether reduced foveal threshold is associated with a generalized depression of the field or with a central scotoma, or both.

Broad defect

To look for a broad localized defect (altitudinal defect, hemianopia, etc.) or a generalized depression, the examiner must test with an adequate sampling of points within the central 30 degrees. Only infrequently will testing of the peripheral field add to the diagnostic information obtained from testing the central field. Isolated peripheral visual field defects are not likely to be symptomatic, and then the cause for such symptoms of reduced acuity should be reflected in the central field. Suprathreshold static spot checking with standard stimuli for age is a rapid means to rule out the presence of a broad field defect or to establish its presence, and may be all that is required. If no defect is found but one is strongly suspected, the test can be repeated with somewhat weaker stimuli.

Some clinicians always use a fully quantitative technique to look for broad defects. They avoid thereby the need ever to have to repeat the suprathreshold test. Moreover, if a field defect is present, a quantitative method (static threshold determination or plotting of multiple isopters) may often be required anyway to establish the diagnostic nature of the defect or to quantify its severity.

If the clinical history is such that the presence of a broad field defect is reasonably likely, it may be more efficient in automated perimetry to go directly to a quantitated technique. An appropriate selection would be static threshold determination over the central 30 degrees (program 32 of the Octopus or 30-2 of the Humphrey), perhaps supplemented with suprathreshold testing in the peripheral field (07 of the Octopus or a full field screen of the Humphrey). In manual perimetry the central field is explored in the same manner as for glaucoma, with immediate quantitation of any defects discovered. Do not make the mistake of plotting only a large isopter (e.g., V-4e) just because the visual acuity is poor. Determine whether the isopters for moderate stimuli (I-2e, I-3e) are in their normal location or moved inward or if perhaps the stimuli cannot be seen at all.

Central scotoma

Although the search for broad or generalized defects is essentially the same as for glaucomatous defects, the search for small defects at or immediately around the point of fixation requires a more concentrated effort within the central 5 or 10 degrees. For example, in a standard automated program the points tested are 6 degrees apart but a defect of much smaller diameter may be visually important if it is at or near the point of fixation. With automated perimeters static threshold determination by a close grid of points is the appropriate choice to look for scotomas near or at fixation. Of course, fixation itself needs to be included in the points tested.

With manual perimetry on the Goldmann perimeter, the inner 2 degrees of the field is occupied by the fixation target and the telescope port and cannot be tested without a special attachment. Central scotomas extending more than 2 degrees from fixation can be detected, but smaller scotomas require a special eccentric fixation device for the perimeter (not readily available) or another method must be used. Fortunately, the Amsler grid often gives sufficient diagnostic information.

The Amsler grid and a confrontation test with a red object (p. 74) are quick and useful in detecting scotomas at or near fixation. In the presence of very poor vision, a central scotoma can be determined even when there is also a severe generalized depression by asking the patient to compare the brightness of a penlight at fixation to the brightness at other locations in the field. Such a confrontation test may help determine whether or not the person with cataract also has macular disease, glaucomatous involvement of the fixation point, or optic atrophy that would prevent a good visual return after cataract extraction.

If a central scotoma is present, especially when unilateral and unexplained, it is not sufficient to test the area around fixation with an Amsler grid or a macular program in automated perimetry. A broader visual field test must also be performed to look for temporal hemianopia, especially superiorly. Both eyes must be tested, not just the eye with poor acuity, because chiasmal lesions may involve the optic nerve, producing a central scotoma in one eye, and be associated with a temporal field defect in the opposite eye as well as the eye with a central scotoma.

Other tests

There are additional visual tests that may be used to analyze the cause of reduced acuity:

1. Look for abnormal pupil reactions, especially with the swinging light test. Central scotomas resulting from optic nerve disease will typically have an afferent pupillary defect or Marcus Gunn pupillary sign. Central scotomas resulting from macular disease will typically not have an abnormal pupil reaction, nor will generalized depression resulting from a cataract or other opacity of the normally transparent ocular media.
2. When checking central vision with the Amsler grid, ask if the central region is blurred or absent and whether it is distorted with wavy lines. Distortion of the image, called "metamorphopsia," suggests the presence of macular disease as the cause for poor central vision.
3. If the visual acuity is reduced but still better than 20/80, a photo stress test can be performed by having the patient look at a bright penlight for 10 seconds and then having him look at a visual acuity chart to determine how long it takes for the visual acuity to return to the level he had before staring at the light. If macular disease is present, recovery may take longer than 30 to 50 seconds, or the recovery time in one eye may be more than 20 seconds longer than in the other. However, patients with central scotomas as a result of optic nerve disease, like those with normal eyes, will recover to their usual acuity sooner.
4. If there is reduced acuity but no scotoma under the usual monocular testing circumstances, there may be amblyopia, perhaps as a result of a monofixational phoria, which can be discovered by stereopsis testing. Another way to determine whether or not a reduced acuity is the result of amblyopia is with a 2.0–log-unit filter. Such a filter placed before a normal eye will reduce the acuity two lines (20/20 to 20/40). When it is placed before an amblyopic eye, the vision is affected less than two lines and may even improve; however, when placed in front of an eye with vision reduced organically (retinal or optic nerve disease), the visual acuity will be worsened by at least two lines and sometimes dramatically more.
5. Tests of contrast sensitivity, color vision, and glare will help document the basis of a visual symptom when the cause has not been apparent in the rest of the clinical examination.

Especially if it is reduced, the visual acuity should always be recorded on the visual field chart.

MISCELLANEOUS PRECHIASMAL LESIONS

An optic nerve lesion (*territory II,* Chapter 9) may produce a central scotoma and poor visual acuity (p. 134) or nerve fiber bundle defects that are similar to glaucomatous defects. Nerve fiber bundle defects can be examined by the technique used for glaucoma.

Retinal and chorioretinal lesions (*territory I,* Chapter 9) may produce many different defects. In selecting the appropriate strategy for visual field examination, the clinician must consider the purpose at hand (detection of the defect, differential diagnosis of the defect, quantitation of the severity of the defect) as well as the nature of the disease(s) present or suspected to be present. If the disease is known to be confined to a particular location in the retina, it makes sense to concentrate the visual field exploration in the appropriate sector.

For example, if the purpose is to detect beginning retinopathy in a patient taking chloroquine, careful static threshold determinations (with white, red, or blue test stimuli) in the central 10 degrees may be appropriate along with Amsler grid screening. If it is desired to quantify the rate of progression of retinitis pigmentosa, quantitation with static threshold perimetry or plotting of many isopters in the central and peripheral regions may be appropriate. If the purpose is to document growth of a choroidal mass, the field examination may concentrate on the involved area of the field, plotting the defect with multiple isopters, with a grid of static threshold determinations, or with static cuts, depending on the instrumentation available.

If serial examinations are being performed to look for progression of a disease, some of the same principles used to look for glaucoma will apply. A case in point would be that when stability of the condition has been established over three quantitated visual field examinations deterioration can be detected by suprathreshold perimetry with stimuli based on the average previous threshold at each location.

THE NEUROLOGIC FIELD

A visual field examination may be performed when there are clinical signs, symptoms, or laboratory evidence of a condition that might affect the neural visual pathway from the eye to the occipital cortex. There is quite a variety of clinical circumstances, each requiring a slightly different approach to testing. At times a general screen is required. For a patient complaining of headaches the clinician may obtain an erythrocyte sedimentation rate and a visual field test, expecting the findings to be normal but occasionally finding evidence of a tumor or vascular malformation. Sometimes the purpose is more specifically to look for evidence of a pituitary adenoma in a patient with abnormalities of endocrine function. In another patient it may be desired to quantify a known defect to look for a recurrence of tumor after irradiation.

In general, the simplest test that will accomplish the purpose at hand should be selected. Particularly when the patient is neurologically impaired or otherwise enfeebled, the simplest examination may sometimes provide more diagnostic information than a quantitated visual field (which can be hard for the patient to tolerate).

The approach to *prechiasmal* lesions, especially those affecting visual acuity, has been described. The search for nerve fiber bundle defects is done as for glaucoma, one of the main prechiasmal lesions. Usually this means a full threshold test of the central 30 degrees.

Four different techniques can also be used to demonstrate the presence of *chiasmal* and *postchiasmal* lesions.

Comparison techniques. In searching for evidence of a hemianopia, and particularly a bitemporal hemianopia, the strategy of asking the patient to compare the two sides of the vertical meridian by confrontation is helpful (p. 72).

The patient may be asked to compare the quality of vision with respect to two hands held to the right and left of the vertical meridian or to compare the color of a sizable red object to the right and left of that meridian. When he reports having dimmer vision on one side than on the other, it is important that the object be moved across the vertical meridian from one side to the other and that he report when the change occurs. If the change occurs gradually, the presence of a hemianopia is not convincingly demonstrated; but a hemianopia is demonstrated if he reports a sudden change in visibility precisely when the vertical meridian is crossed (p. 74).

Comparison tests are good because they are quite sensitive in detecting hemianopias: If an alert patient is certain that there is no difference in visibility on the two sides of the vertical meridian, it is unlikely that a hemianopia is present. On the other hand, a convincing difference of visibility across the vertical meridian is rather specific evidence that a hemianopia is indeed present.

Because important neurosurgical diagnostic decisions may be based in part on the field examination, it is well to have corroborating evidence of the hemianopia by one of the other methods given below, especially if the patient responded with uncertainty when tested by confrontation comparison methods. Nonetheless, the color comparison by confrontation is so accurate, despite its simplicity, that it may be used routinely both to detect a hemianopia and to double-check the findings with other perimetric methods.

Isopter plotting. A second method for demonstrating hemianopia is to plot isopters, paying particular attention as the isopters cross the vertical meridian. Dr. J. Lawton Smith performs this kinetic examination on the tangent screen; but instead of using regular test objects, he uses a projected spot of light from a focused flashlight, controlling its intensity by partially covering the end of the flashlight with his hands.* In essence, he dims the stimulus on the tangent screen until it is of appropriate intensity to form an isopter somewhere between 15 and 30 degrees from fixation and uses this projected stimulus to plot the isopter kinetically.

The advantage of Smith's method is its simplicity. Nothing more elegant is required if the examiner wants to determine whether or not a hemianopia is present. The technique can be performed in a classroom against a chalkboard or in almost any hospital room on a blank wall. It is not necessary to move a debilitated patient to a room with special perimetry equipment. Of course, if the patient happens to be in a clinical examining room equipped for visual field testing, the ordinary tangent screen, Auto-Plot, or Goldmann perimeter can be used, provided the test is convenient and comfortable.

With the perimeter it is possible to plot several isopters, particularly across the vertical meridian, similar to testing the horizontal meridian in glaucoma. Not only is the presence of a hemianopia demonstrated by plotting isopters across the vertical meridian, but the extent and depth of any defect, as well as the congruence of the defect between the two eyes, can be delineated by plotting the full circumference of the isopters. Comparison testing can be done, in addition, by asking the patient to judge the intensity of a stimulus to the right and to the left of the vertical meridian, as in confrontation fields, but this should not be to the exclusion of plotting isopters.

Static spot-checking. The third basic method of finding a hemianopia is suprathreshold static spot-checking. The Friedmann Visual Field Analyser or an automated perimeter that uses static spot-checking strategies will uncover a hemianopia, provided the stimulus is appropriately chosen to be suprathreshold on one side of the vertical meridian but infrathreshold on the other. A pattern of test points with the loci concentrated just to the right and left of the vertical meridian is most appropriate. The method is rapid and efficient as well as accurate. Some authors recommend testing the full field (threshold related, with or without eccentricity compensation) with semiquantitation for chiasmal and postchiasmal lesions.

---

*Smith, J.L.: The optic nerve. Neuro-ophthalmology Tapes (9820 S.W. 62 Court, Miami, Fla., 33156) pp. 55-57, 1957.

Suprathreshold spot-checking can also be performed on the Goldmann perimeter, typically in conjunction with the plotting of isopters. The technique is similar to that used for glaucoma, with the modification that the isopters are plotted especially carefully as they cross the vertical meridian and the examiner looks for a vertical step in the same way that he looks for a nasal step in glaucoma.

Static threshold determination. The presence of a hemianopic field defect may be nicely documented by static threshold perimetry, provided the pattern of test locations is such that a comparison can be made of points to the right and to the left of the vertical meridian. You can also get an indication of the extent and depth of the visual field defect, indicating the severity of an underlying lesion. A static cut may help define the hemianopic boundary (Fig. 13-44). In some clinical contexts it may not be necessary to quantify the defect in such detail and a less tedious visual field test will suffice. In other contexts (e.g., when later looking for recurrent tumor growth) a fully quantitated field may be necessary.

DETERMINATION OF VISUAL DISABILITY

Legal (statutory) blindness and visual disability are determined by visual acuity and by the extent of the intact field.

The visual field component for determining statutory blindness or the percent of visual efficiency has traditionally been determined with a kinetic 0.5-degree stimulus (a 3/330 test stimulus) under an illumination of 7 footcandles or a III-4e test stimulus on the Goldmann perimeter. In an aphakic patient without a lens implant and without a contact lens, a 6/330 test stimulus or the IV-4e Goldmann stimulus is used. The position of the isopters is determined along eight standard meridians without spectacle or trial lenses in front of the eye. According to the Social Security definition,* legal blindness is present if the field is contracted to 10 degrees or less in the better eye or if the widest diameter in the better eye is 20 degrees or less. To determine percent visual field efficiency according to the AMA standards,† add the distance of the isopter from fixation in degrees along the eight principal meridians. If scotomas are present along any of these meridians, subtract the width of the scotoma. However, this is not done for central scotomas, because visual acuity is separately taken into account when net visual efficiency is being calculated. If a principal meridian forms a boundary of the visual defect (as in a hemianopia), that meridian is given a value of half its normal

---

*As defined in Social Security Regulations, Nos. 4 and 16, Listing of impairments, the adult listings, special senses and speech, Ophthalmology (20 CF 404.1525 and 416.925, Appendix One, Part A, para. 2.00A). Every federal, state, or local agency has its own definition, revised from time to time, and the definition may be different for each legal purpose (e.g. Internal Revenue Service, or various welfare agencies).

†Guides to the evaluation of permanent impairment, ed. 2, Copyright 1984, The American Medical Association, the visual system portion of which is reprinted in *PDR: The Physician's Desk Reference for Ophthalmology*.

Table 11-1. Minimal normal extent of visual field from point of fixation

	Degrees
Temporally	85
Down temporally	85
Down	65
Down nasally	50
Nasally	60
Up nasally	55
Up	45
Up temporally	55
TOTAL	500

extent according to Table 11-1. Because the total in a normal field is 500, the result is divided by 5 to determine the percentage of field retained.

More recently visual sensation in each region of the field is determined and a score, which gives greater weight to the regions around fixation, is determined as a measure of visual function compared to a normal standard. To use this method, one must have an appropriate Esterman grid. At the tangent screen a 2/1000 white stimulus is used, and a 25 degree isopter gives a score of 100. For a perimeter the 0.5 degree stimulus (3/330 or III-4e) is used. Grids have also been devised for automated suprathreshold screening tests and for binocular evaluation of the field.

The percent loss of visual field is combined with loss of acuity and ocular motility to determine the net impairment of the visual system, and this may be combined with other physical impairments to calculate the impairment of the whole person. To accomplish these calculations in the standard way, one must consult the AMA Guide.

SUMMARY OF EXAMPLES OF FIELD TEST STRATEGY SELECTION

Routine office visits

Use *confrontation finger counting* routinely. An effective alternative (if cost can be kept low) may be a fast automated *suprathreshold screen* (eccentricity-compensated) with criteria to yield a low false-positive rate.

General screening in the community

Use an *automated fast suprathreshold screen* with a pattern of points selected to detect the types of defects that would be meaningful in the group screened—provided the defects detected will be important enough to warrant the effort (cost-effectiveness). Criteria for abnormality must be chosen to keep the false-positive rate low. Use a *threshold-related stimulus selection* to reduce the number of patients with mild generalized depression who are called abnormal; however, this takes longer. *Semiquantitation* may help identify true abnormalities with more certainty. *Eccentricity compensation* should be routine.

Glaucoma screening in the community

Use an *automated eccentricity-compensated suprathreshold screen* of the central 30 degrees with a standard stimulus (or threshold-related stimulus). Some authors advocate suprathreshold testing of the peripheral field. Aim the program at high-risk groups (e.g., the elderly or those with a family history of glaucoma). Criteria for abnormality must favor a low false-positive rate. *Threshold-related stimulus selection* may improve the detection of localized defects, as well as the specificity. *Semiquantitation of abnormal points* may also help identify true defects.

With manual perimetry the *Armaly-Drance single-level spot-checking* technique with minimal isopter plotting (Chapter 22) may be used if technical expertise is available.

Screening and diagnosis of glaucoma suspects in the clinical office

Sensitivity in detecting mild defects takes on more importance, and the goal of lowering the false-positive rate takes on less importance, in individuals with signs of glaucoma (high pressure, disc cupping, etc.). A lengthier test can be used than in community screening programs without losing cost-effectiveness.

With automated perimetry, use a *static threshold examination* of the central 30 degrees straddling the horizontal meridian, with or without suprathreshold testing of the peripheral field (program 32 of the Octopus and 30-2 of the Humphrey instrument). This method is preferred not only to enhance detection but also to provide a baseline for future judgments of abnormality in these glaucoma suspects. An alternative is *eccentricity-compensated threshold-related suprathreshold testing* of the central (or central and peripheral) field—with semiquantitation or quantitation of abnormal points, or with a follow-up static pattern of all fields in which abnormalities are detected.

With manual perimetry (Chapters 21 to 23), *spot-check* inside 15 degrees with a weaker stimulus than is used for the region between 15 and 30 degrees (p. 404).

Following progressive disease

With automated perimetry, use a *static threshold program* covering the relevant portion(s) of the field. In glaucoma it may be sufficient to follow the central 30 degrees, but some authors advise threshold testing of the peripheral field as well. If the field remains stable after several examinations, you can subsequently evaluate it using a *suprathreshold strategy* that tests each point with a stimulus slightly brighter than the average of the preceding threshold values at that point.

If large regions of the field are blind to size 3 stimuli of maximum intensity (0 dB), it may be possible to follow the region with *size 5 stimuli*. To follow small defects, especially those close to fixation, defects that split fixation, or where there is a small central island remaining, a *close grid of points* or static cuts of 1-degree resolution may be used.

With manual perimetry, use *kinetic quantitation* of both normal and abnormal regions of the field (as described in Chapters 21 to 23).

Diagnosing reduced visual function and unexplained visual symptoms

In these patients, look for both small scotomatous defects affecting the point of fixation and broad depressions affecting a large region including the point of fixation.

For small defects near fixation the *Amsler grid* is of prime importance in evaluating vision around the fovea. A static threshold determination on a grid of close points, or a macular program, will also evaluate this region. If a central scotoma is found, be sure to look for a temporal hemianopia in the other eye.

For broad defects a *suprathreshold screen* with a standard stimulus that tests the central field (similar to the programs used for glaucoma) is appropriate. Alternatively, a more time-consuming *static threshold test* can be used.

With manual perimetry the same basic technique used for glaucoma will pick up broad defects of many causes; but pay special attention to the vertical meridian, to find a temporal hemianopia in the opposite eye, and special attention also to the region surrounding the point of fixation.

Defining retinal and optic nerve lesions

For central scotomas and nerve fiber bundle defects (territory II), use the *methods for reduced acuity and for glaucoma* respectively. For retinal lesions (territory I) the choice of test depends on the clinical circumstance. Pay special attention to the region of the field where a defect is expected based on the location of the retinal lesion. *Suprathreshold testing* in the appropriate location may be done if detection of an abnormality is desired, but *quantitation with static threshold methods* or *kinetic perimetry* may be needed if the degree of abnormality is important in the diagnosis or management of the condition.

Diagnosing neurologic fields

Confrontation comparison methods are excellent for detecting hemianopias, which may also be documented by isopter plotting, by automated suprathreshold testing of the full field with semiquantitation, or by a static threshold program of the central field. Expert clinicians differ in their preferences, and selection may vary according to the neurologic defect under consideration. For example, it may be necessary to establish whether or not a hemianopia is congruous.

CHAPTER 12

Administering the visual field test

TEACHING THE NATURE OF THE TEST

Only the patient knows what he can or cannot see. Success in quantifying the visual field depends on the perimetrist's ability to get the patient to report accurately what he can see. This is just as important as knowing how to manipulate the switches on the instrument.

The patient needs to understand that the nature of the test is for him to report what he sees peripherally while maintaining visual fixation on a specific location. Sometimes all that is needed is an explicit instruction to look straight ahead at the fixation target and push the button when a light is seen anywhere within the field of view. Especially for a patient who has not experienced field testing before, it is helpful to begin with a confrontation test, in which the patient practices reporting what he sees in his peripheral vision. At the same time the examiner gets a clue about any major field defect that might be present. This information is helpful in deciding which eye to test first at the perimeter, in anticipating the defect that will be found by manual kinetic perimetry, or in selecting appropriate programs to use on an automated perimeter.

FIG. 12-1. Educating the patient by confrontation testing. Initially it does not matter whether he has one eye covered or not. The patient can be asked to look at your nose. Holding up your arms 1 foot to each side of the line of sight, you can instruct him to tell you which hand is wiggling. He cannot look at both hands while waiting to see which one moves, and it becomes obvious that he can look at only one point of fixation (your nose) and he must tell you something about what is happening to the sides without actually looking. You can then have him cover one eye if he has not already done so and ask him to count your fingers in the four quadrants (see Chapter 3, p. 66) until he seems able to hold fixation and report what he sees, and until you have an estimate of how severe any existing field defect may be.

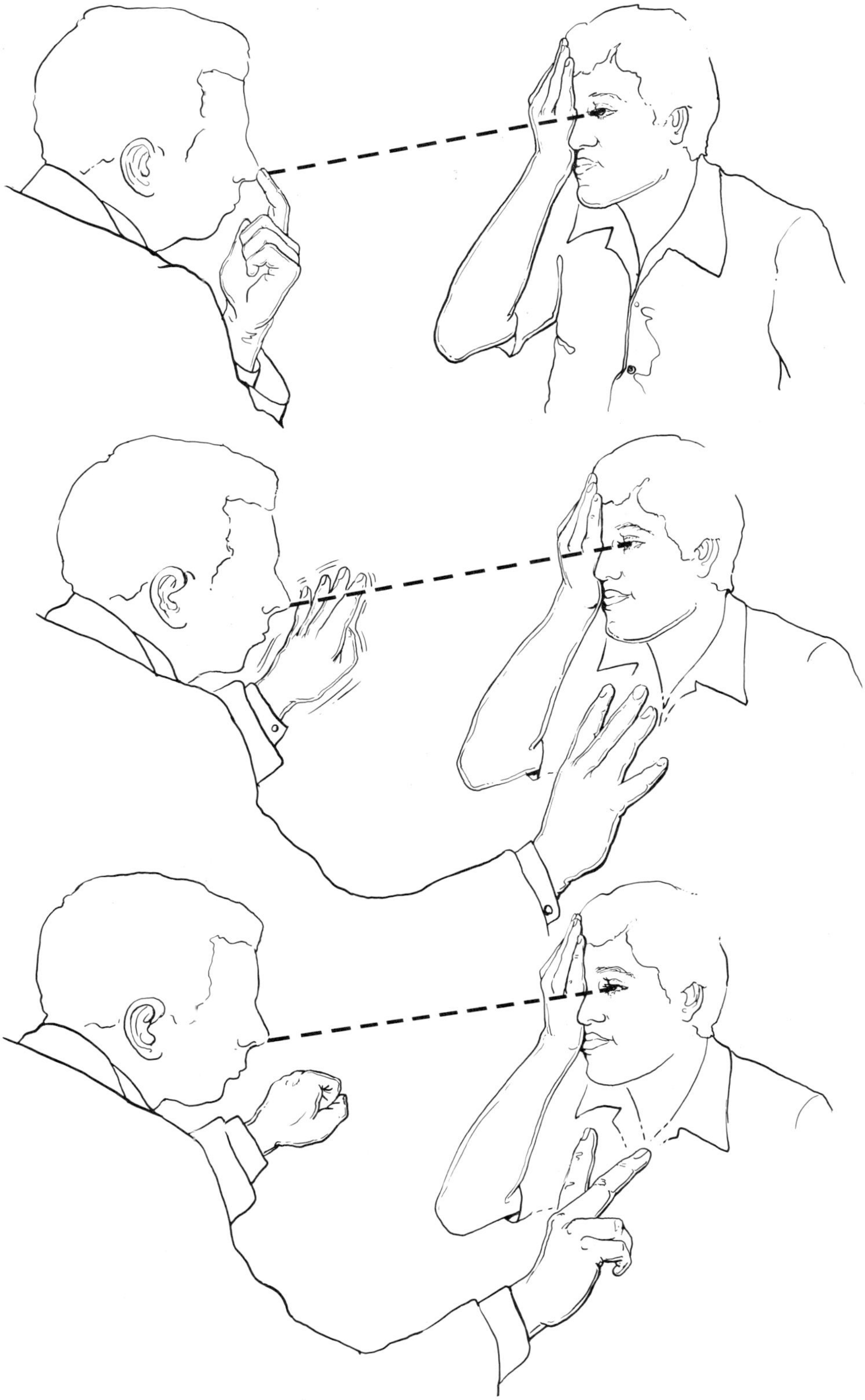

FIG. 12-1

In manual kinetic perimetry, after the demonstration by confrontation, additional instruction can be brief because the patient learns the nature of the test at the perimeter (Fig. 12-5). As the test proceeds, he learns that a light will appear repeatedly, that after he responds it will disappear, and that he should wait for another (pp. 370, 378, and 380).

Special instructions are needed for automated perimetry, especially if the patient has undergone manual perimetry previously. In automated perimetry he needs to be told that the light will be a brief flash and following it there will be an interval during which the machine waits for a response. Unlike manual kinetic perimetry, in automated perimetry the light does not stay on until the patient responds. He needs to know that it is all right to respond after the light goes off. He should not feel frustrated or inadequate when he discovers that it is impossible to respond while the light is still on, as he did with kinetic perimetry. He should answer quickly (before the time is up) but not so quickly as to respond in error.

He should also be told that some of the stimulus presentations will be very dim. In kinetic perimetry the stimulus is dim when first perceptible, but it gets subjectively brighter (as it moves inward) until the patient is sure he sees it and then responds. In static perimetry the patient finds himself responding to dim stimuli that are not reaffirmed by becoming a bit brighter before he must make up his mind whether he saw it or not (pp. 334-336). He should be told to expect dim stimuli and to respond when he sees them, but to respond only when he is sure because there will be times when the machine will pretend to present stimuli (catch trials, p. 226).

POSITIONING THE PATIENT AT THE PERIMETER

Especially if the patient has never undergone perimetry before, it is best to test the better seeing eye first. You can learn from the patient's history, by testing his visual acuity, or from the confrontation field test which eye is better. Otherwise, it would be traditional to test the right eye first.

The eye not being tested is covered. For comfort and to avoid pressure, the patch should form a slightly concave cup over the eye and allow the eye to be open beneath it. An eye pad taped over the closed eye or a patch that puts pressure on it should not be used. The patch should fit the face snugly to prevent the covered eye from seeing stimuli in the peripheral field.

Goldmann advocated the use of a white translucent cover that would maintain light adaptation of the covered eye, but it seems to make little actual difference in the test results if a black patch is used because the eye light-adapts quickly when uncovered. The translucent patch gives a background glare that subjectively seems to rival the test stimulus in the uncovered eye; however, the threshold measurements seem to be the same whether the untested eye is covered with a white or a black patch.

The eye to be tested is centered squarely in front of the fixation target. The face may be turned slightly to the left when testing the right eye, and slightly to the right when testing the left eye, so the nose does not obstruct the nasal periphery of the field.

FIG. 12-2. Face turn during perimetry. The turn should be very slight. A straight ahead position is usually quite acceptable. The main reason for a slight turn away from the eye being tested is to ensure that the face is not turned wrong if the head drifts a bit during the test. Remember: The patient may be uncomfortable if you overposition the head.

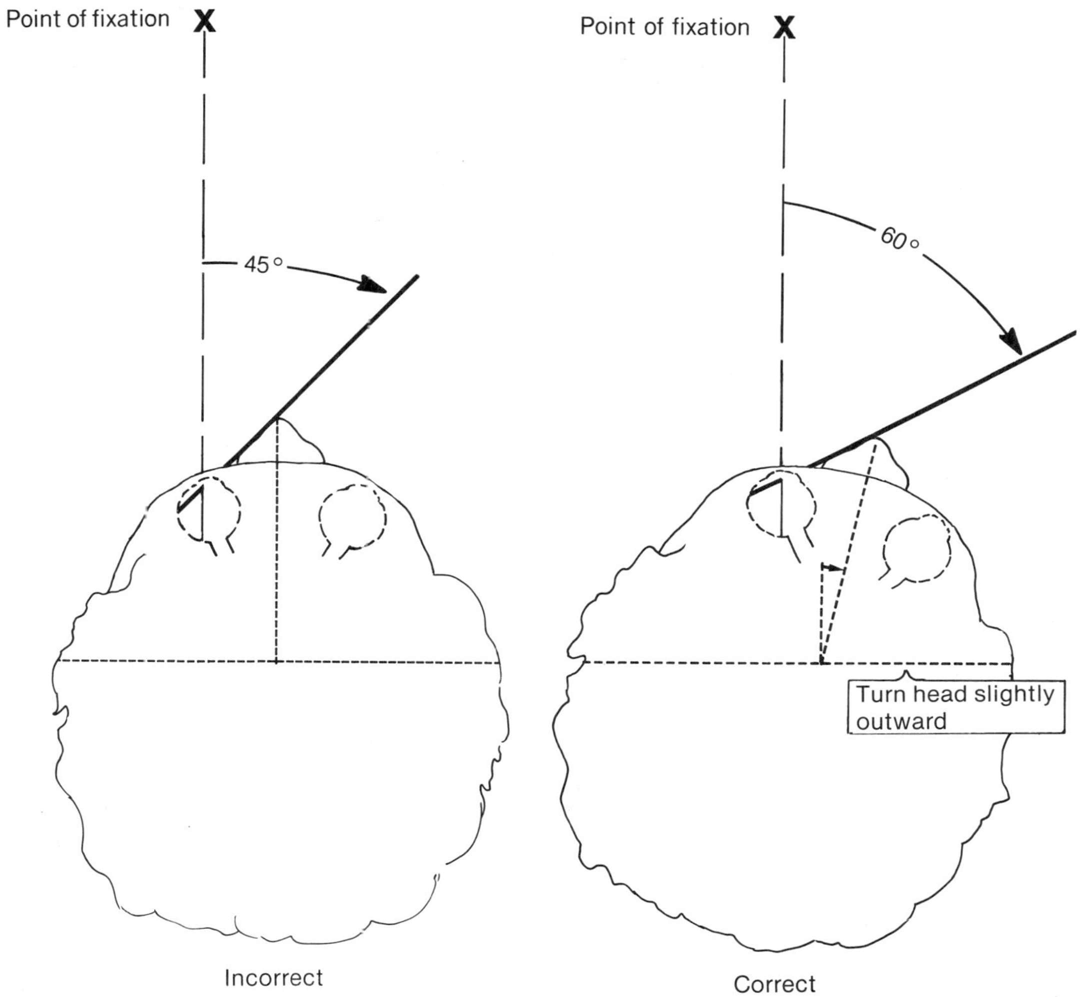

FIG. 12-2

Likewise, the chin should be positioned such that the plane of the face is directed forward or ever so slightly upward (thus putting the eye in slight down gaze to see the fixation target) to reduce the interference of the eyebrows and upper eyelids. The side turn and upward tilt of the face should be neither exaggerated nor uncomfortable. A slight downward and temporal gaze position is preferred only to ensure that the eye is not in a nasal or up gaze position, which would cause facial structures to shade the peripheral field.

FIG. 12-3. Effect of tilting the face. If the patient's face is tilted forward (the forehead against the forehead rest but the chin not fully forward), his eye will be in slight upgaze when looking at the point of fixation. His eyelid and eyebrow may interfere with the upper portion of the visual field. However, with his face straight, or perhaps slightly tilted backward (the chin forward), interference by eyelid and eyebrow is reduced. These greyscales are of an automated static threshold test done on the author with his head in the illustrated correct and incorrect positions. There is no ptosis of the eyelid—only an incorrect head position.

An additional problem is that with improper forward tilt of the head, the correcting lens cannot be positioned close to the eye (p. 200). The upper edge may be touching the eyebrow, but the lower edge will be distant from the cheek and block some of the inferior visual field. In this situation the upper edge of the field will be shaded by the eyebrow and the lower edge by the correcting lens (and the lens holder).

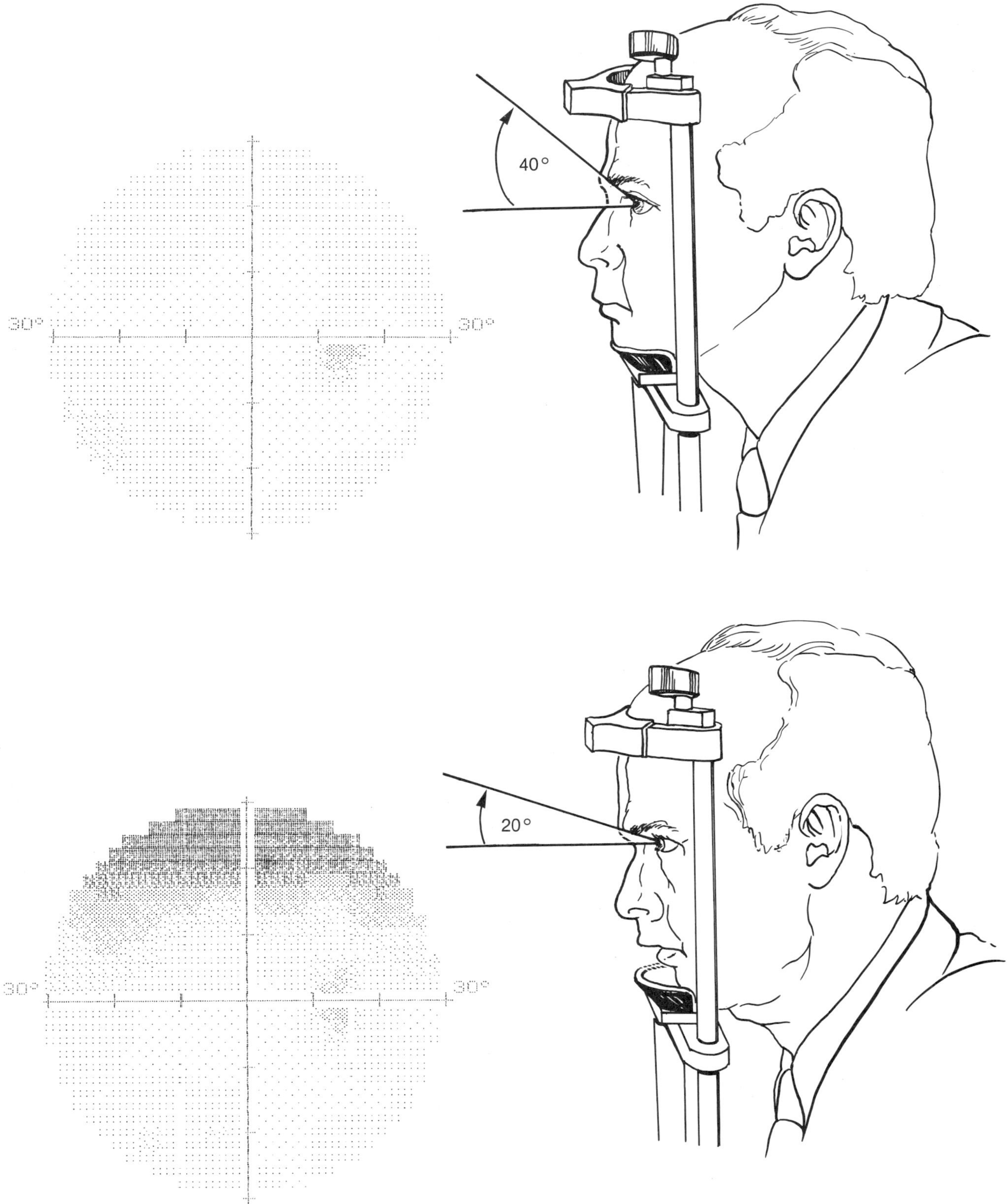

FIG. 12-3

The height of the instrument must be such that the patient is comfortable and able to concentrate on the task of responding to the visual stimuli. He should not have to bend over or stretch up to reach the chin rest.

Besides the considerations of comfort, if the patient must stretch to reach the chin rest (instrument too high or chin too low) then as he relaxes during the test his forehead will drift backward and his eye be too far behind the correcting lens (see p. 200). A lens rim artifact will result when points near the edge of the 30-degree central field are being tested. Also, if the instrument is too low (or the chair too high) the patient's neck may be flexed and his chin a bit backward when the forehead touches the forehead bar. This will make it difficult to position his face so the eyebrows and eyelids do not impinge on the upper part of the field.

The distance of the chair from the instrument should be coordinated with the height of the instrument so the patient leans slightly forward (Fig. 12-4, *A*).

If the chair is too far away or the perimeter too low, the patient will be bent uncomfortably forward during the test. His face may be tilted forward and, once again, his eyelids and eyebrows in a position where they interfere with testing of the upper visual field (Fig. 12-4, *B* and *C*). If the patient is heavyset, he may have to lean forward more than is optimal so his head will reach beyond the anterior protuberance of his body (Fig. 12-4, *D*). In such cases the examiner must be particularly careful to set the chin forward in the chin rest, even though hyperextension of the neck may be uncomfortable and difficult to maintain.

If the chair is too close or the perimeter too high (Fig. 12-4, *E* and *F*) the patient may be off balance and continually straining to maintain his position at the perimeter. The instrument may be too close if he feels the need to prop himself up with his arms back or hold onto the instrument to keep from falling backward *(E)*.

FIG. 12-4. Influence of chair and instrument positions on the patient's comfort and face position.

A, Correct position, leaning slightly forward.

B, Instrument too low, which not only makes the patient uncomfortably hunched but also causes his face to tilt forward so his chin moves backward in the chin rest.

C, The patient is leaning uncomfortably forward too far.

D, The heavyset patient may have to lean forward so his face will reach the instrument.

E, Instrument too close. The patient must sit perfectly straight instead of comfortably leaning slightly forward.

F, Instrument too high, causing the forehead to drift back from the forehead rest (and the eye back from any correcting lens in place). This position is also uncomfortable because the patient must stretch upward in a vain effort to keep his forehead in place.

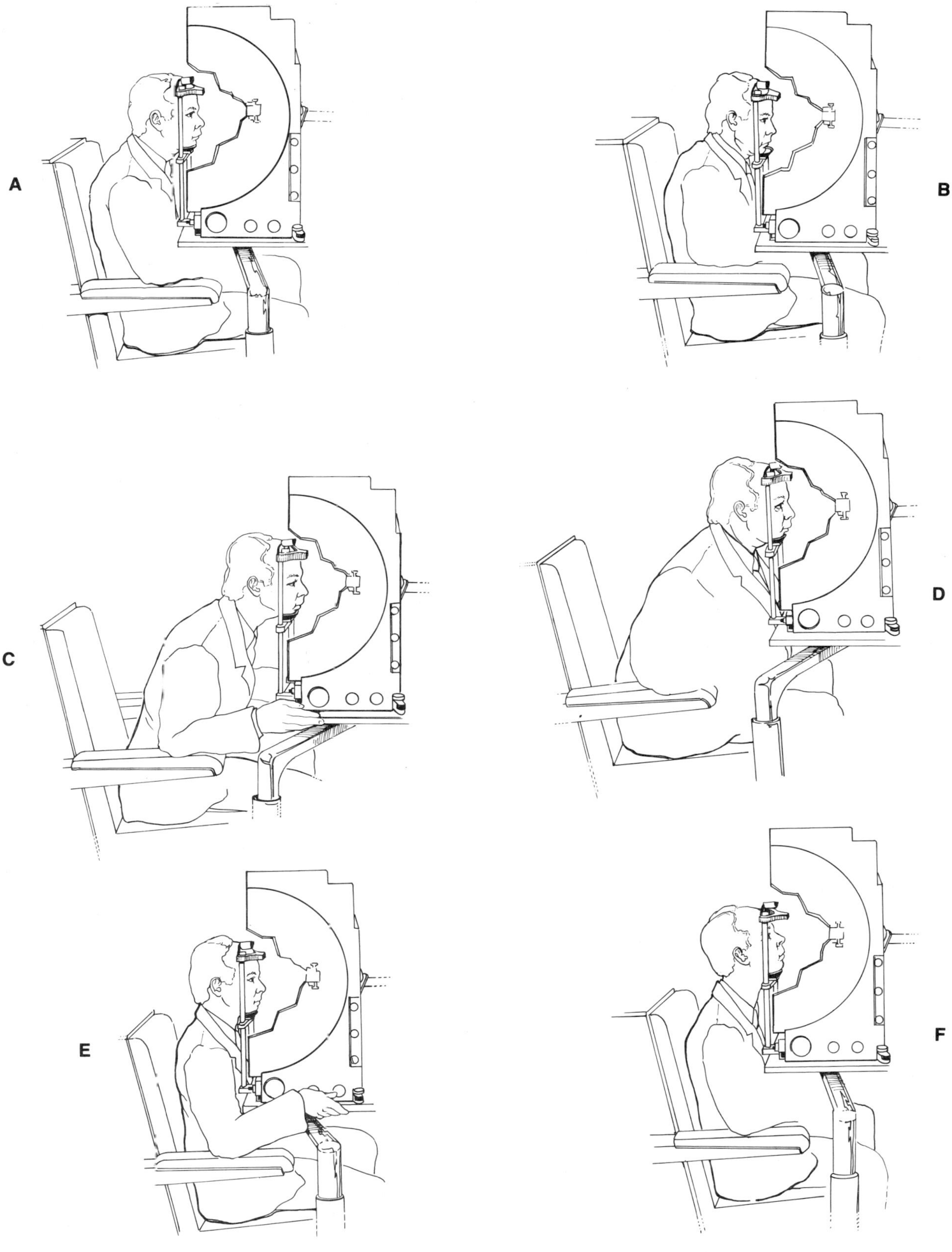

FIG. 12-4

EDUCATION AT THE PERIMETER

A practice run is important when someone is undergoing testing for the first time. Its omission may cause the first field test to be inaccurate.

Automated perimeters often have a program that gives a brief sequence of stimulus presentations (whose responses are not recorded) to be used for practice before the real test begins.

Training is also important with *manual* perimeters and can be accomplished quickly and easily.

FIG. 12-5. Educational sequence at the Goldmann perimeter. With the eye not to be tested covered, the patient is instructed to look at the fixation target.

1. The largest and brightest test object *(V-4e)* is then flashed for ½ second at about 5 degrees from fixation and the patient is asked if he saw it. He is then given a button to sound the buzzer when he next sees a flash of light, or some other signal (e.g., tapping a coin on the table) is established; but he should not speak because this moves the eye away from its centered position.
2. Then a large bright object can be placed further from fixation. If the patient shifts his fixation to look at the projected spot, warn him not to do so, explaining that you want to test what he can see without looking directly at it. If necessary, repeat the presentation of a large object until the patient responds without shifting fixation.
3. Next, a small bright object *(I-4e)* is placed near fixation.
4. Next, a small dim light *(I-2e)* is placed near fixation. During this process it becomes obvious to the patient that the objects may vary in size and in location. Also, he learns that as soon as he responds the stimulus disappears, and he then awaits another.
5. Having proceeded this far, you can now begin to use some weaker stimuli further from fixation in four or five random locations to get an approximate idea of what the patient can or cannot see in various locations (e.g., 15, 25, and 35 degrees from fixation). This should include being sure that the patient can see the *I-4e* at 25 to 30 degrees.
6. Finally, the physiologic blind spot is plotted with the most intense but smallest test object *(I-4e)* as proof that you are ready to proceed. Something is suboptimal if a known absolute scotoma (the blind spot) cannot be detected and plotted. If you cannot plot the physiologic blind spot, there may be some problems that need solving before you proceed. Have you covered the other eye? Is the patient holding fixation? Are you using stimulus size I, or is the object too big? Is the stimulus shutter switch set correctly so the stimulus is on when the shutter switch is depressed? Is there a pathologic field defect that prevents plotting of the physiologic blind spot?

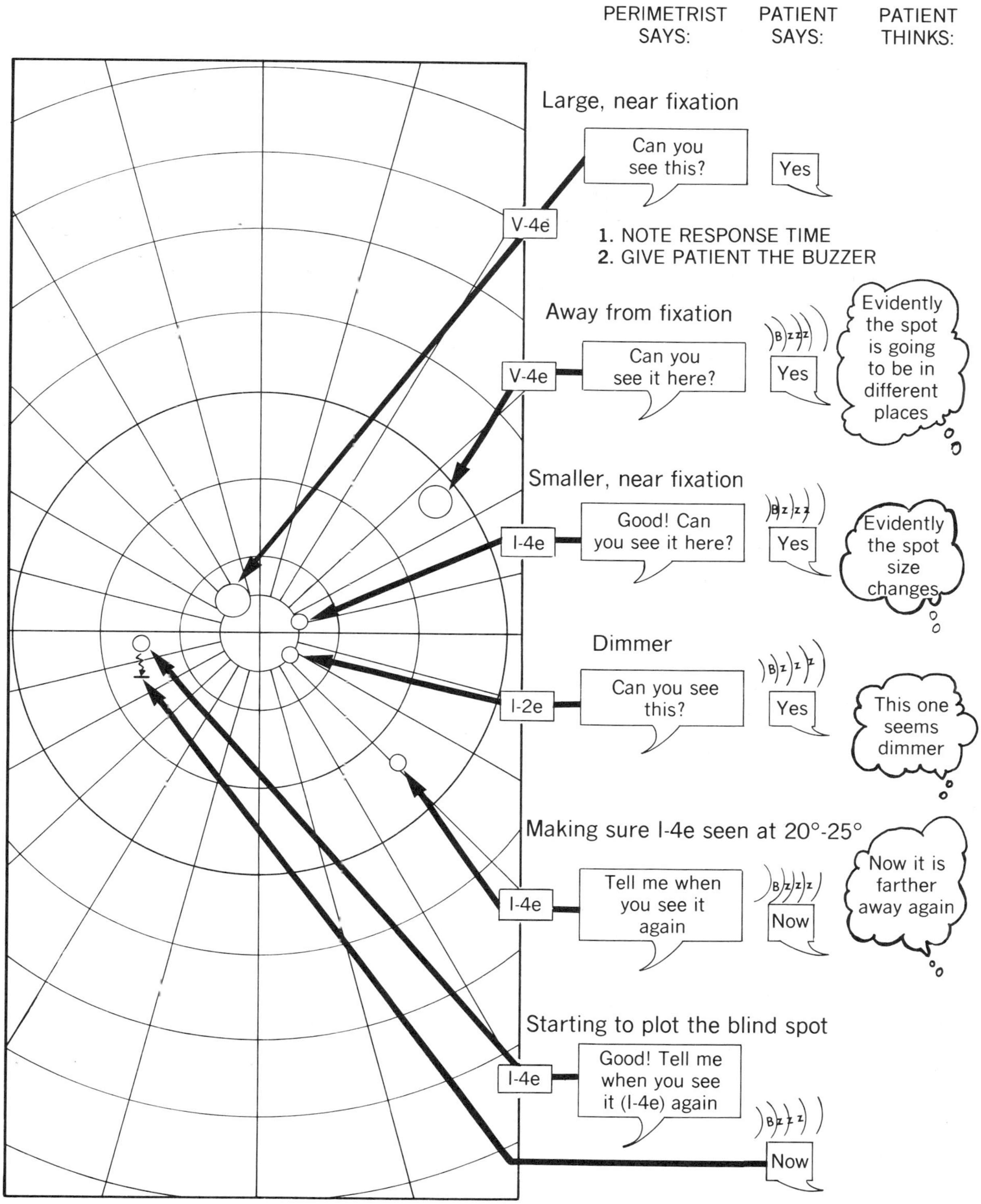
PERIMETRIST SAYS:
PATIENT SAYS:
PATIENT THINKS:
Large, near fixation
V-4e
Can you see this?
Yes
1. NOTE RESPONSE TIME
2. GIVE PATIENT THE BUZZER
Away from fixation
V-4e
Can you see it here?
Yes
Evidently the spot is going to be in different places
Smaller, near fixation
I-4e
Good! Can you see it here?
Yes
Evidently the spot size changes
Dimmer
I-2e
Can you see this?
Yes
This one seems dimmer
Making sure I-4e seen at 20°-25°
I-4e
Tell me when you see it again
Now
Now it is farther away again
Starting to plot the blind spot
I-4e
Good! Tell me when you see it (I-4e) again
Now

FIG. 12-5

EDUCATION AT THE TANGENT SCREEN

FIG. 12-6. The same basic method used at the tangent screen. A good-sized object (5 mm) is placed on the side (not the end) of the wand covered with black felt. The wand is placed with its end near fixation but with the object hidden from view. It is rotated, exposing the object, and the patient is asked if he saw the white bead. Then he is instructed to respond when he sees it again. The wand is held in the same position and again rotated to get the patient's response. Immediately it is obvious to him that he is supposed to respond when he sees the white bead and not when he simply sees the end of the wand.

Several wands with different-sized objects can be held in one hand while the other hand holds the wand at the tangent screen (see Fig. 2-1). Wands are interchanged and held in different positions until the patient realizes that the test objects may be of different sizes and in different locations. Finally, the blind spot is plotted, and the next step is to proceed with plotting the appropriate isopters.

The same principle can be applied with any technique for visual field examination. An obvious advantage of the projection method, e.g., the Auto-Plot, is that the patient has no prior clues as to where the test object will be projected and there may thus be less incentive to lose fixation. With the wand, the patient knows where the object will appear and he is more apt to glance at the wand while looking for the test object.

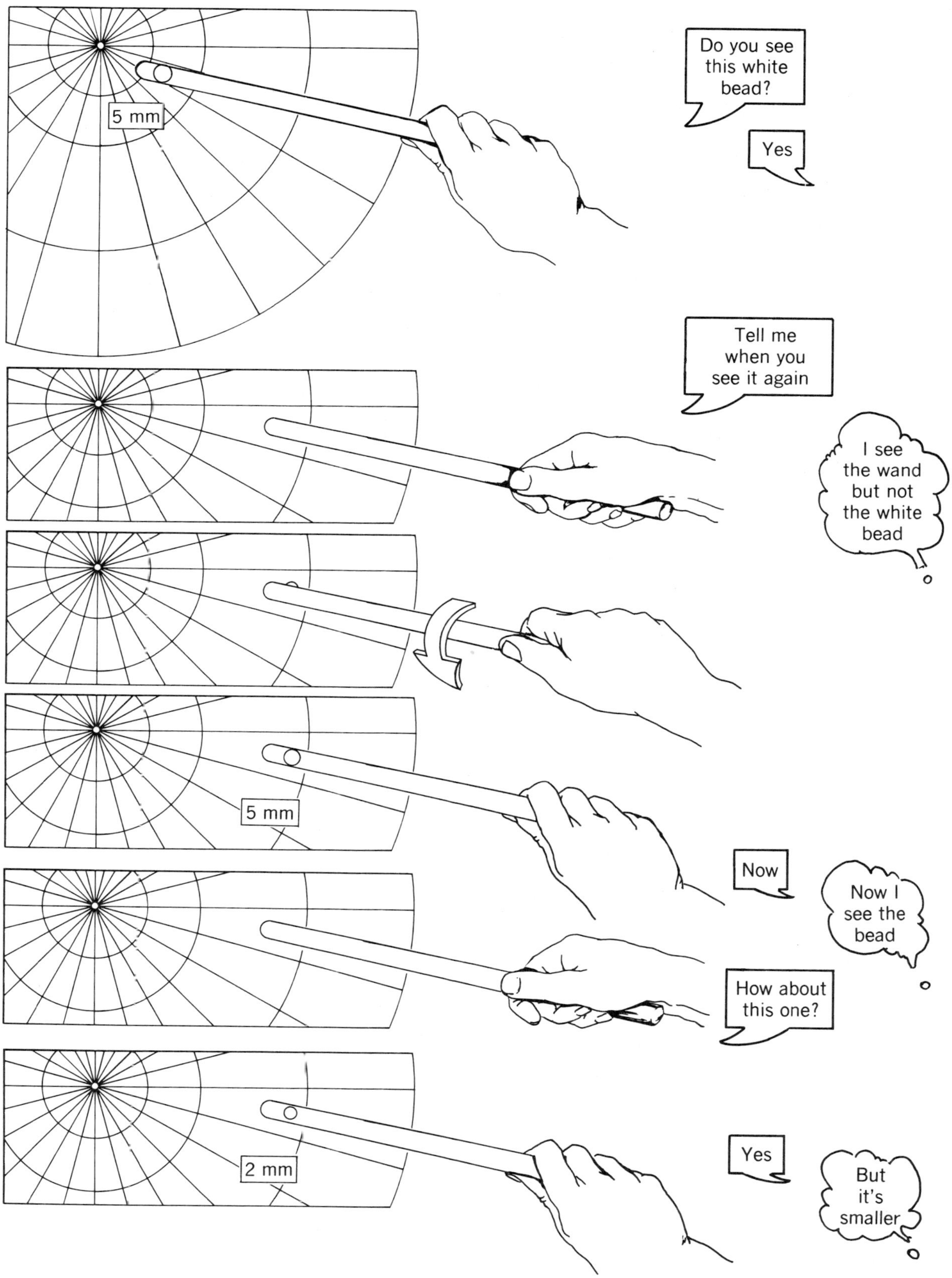
5 mm
Do you see this white bead?
Yes
Tell me when you see it again
I see the wand but not the white bead
5 mm
Now
Now I see the bead
How about this one?
2 mm
Yes
But it's smaller

FIG. 12-6

CORRECTIVE LENSES

General principles

For optimum visualization of test stimuli, they must be in focus on the retina. Therefore, the patient may need corrective lenses to obtain an optimum visual field examination with consistent responses. Optical correction for the entire visual field would be ideal; however, as a practical matter, the rim of the lens gets in the way and therefore a lens cannot be used outside 30 degrees. Fortunately, there is less need for a sharply focused retinal image in the peripheral field than in the central field.

To determine the appropriate lenses, the examiner must consider (1) the refractive error of the patient at distance; (2) an added adjustment (provided by accommodation or by a lens) so the patient can see the test stimuli, which are 30 cm away in the case of the Goldmann perimeter; and (3) the amount of near add that can be provided comfortably by the patient's accommodative ability, which reduces the amount needed from the lenses. The patient's accommodative ability is determined by his age but is 0, no matter what the age, if the eye is aphakic or under the influence of a cycloplegic drug.

Choosing the appropriate lens power

The first step is to determine the **best distance correction** for the patient. This can be done by means of a complete refraction, but more often you do it by establishing the power of the patient's present distance glasses and determining the visual acuity at distance. If the visual acuity is 20/20, or if it is less but cannot be improved with a pinhole, the present glasses probably represent the best distance correction. If a pinhole improves the vision, plus or minus spheres can be placed over the present glasses to see if the vision is improved to a satisfactory level. If so, the combination of the spheres and the present glasses is considered the best distance correction. As a general rule, +0.50 and −0.50 D spheres should be tried over the glasses if the vision is in the range of 20/50. Similarly, +1.00 and −1.00 D spheres should be tried if the vision is 20/100.

If a cylinder correction is included in the "best distance correction," it should simply be ignored if it is a 0.25 D cylinder or less. If the power of the cylinder is 0.50 to 0.75 D, no cylindric correction is used for the visual field test but the distance sphere is adjusted by 0.25 D to maintain spheric equivalence. However, if the power of the cylinder is 1.00 D or more, the cylindric lens is used for the visual field test. Be sure that the lens is placed in the lens holder at the correct axis.

The **spheric lens used for visual field testing** is the "best distance sphere correction" combined with an add according to the patient's age. Table 12-1 gives the add recommended by Goldmann for his perimeter and the equivalent adds for other perimeters. These are generous adds so the patient uses some of his accommodation but is not fatigued by having to use most of it. Note that the selection of the add for perimetry is not determined by the patient's own reading glasses. The full add used for patients with no ability to accommodate is +3.25 D on the Goldmann perimeter, which is quite close to the +3.33 D sphere add corresponding to the 30 cm testing distance. The full +3.25 D add used for those over 60 years old is also used at any age in aphakia, after cycloplegia, and in patients who are more than 3.25 D myopic.

The reason for not choosing the full add on all persons but requiring them to use some of their own accommodation is that the prismatic and other effects of the lenses are minimized with the weakest lens possible. The principle is to use the weakest lens possible but to provide a generous enough add that the patient is comfortable without having to use all his accommodative reserve. However, more add than the table recommends may be used if the increased power would result in the need for a weaker minus lens—provided the maximum add (recommended for that instrument for patients over 60 years of age) is not exceeded.

In summary, the lenses used for perimetry are (1) the *cylindric,* as required by the patient for distance if it is 1.00 D or more, and (2) the *spheric*. The power of the spheric lens is the patient's own distance correction adjusted by +0.25 D if it includes a +0.50 or +0.75 D cylinder that is not being used for perimetry and adjusted further according to the patient's accommodative ability—i.e., age and other factors.

Table 12-1. Add (to the best distance correction) for perimetry

	Bowl radius			
Age (yr)	**30 cm (Goldmann, Perimat, Fieldmaster 101)**	**33 cm (Humphrey, Digilab 750, Dicon)**	**42.5 cm (Octopus 2000, 500)**	**50 cm (Octopus 201, Squid)**
30 to 40	+1.00	+1.00	+0.50	—
40 to 45	+1.50	+1.50	+1.00	+0.50
45 to 50	+2.00	+2.00	+1.50	+1.00
50 to 55	+2.50	+2.50	+2.00	+1.50
55 to 60	+3.00	+3.00	+2.50	+2.00
Over 60	+3.25	+3.00	+2.50	+2.00

Positioning the cylinder axis

It is easy to place cylindric lenses incorrectly. The standard notation for the axis of the cylinder is in keeping with standard mathematical coordinates as the examiner looks at the patient's face. Thus 45 degrees is toward either the upper nasal quadrant of the right eye or the upper temporal quadrant of the left eye.

FIG. 12-7 Axis of the cylindric lenses used for astigmatism.

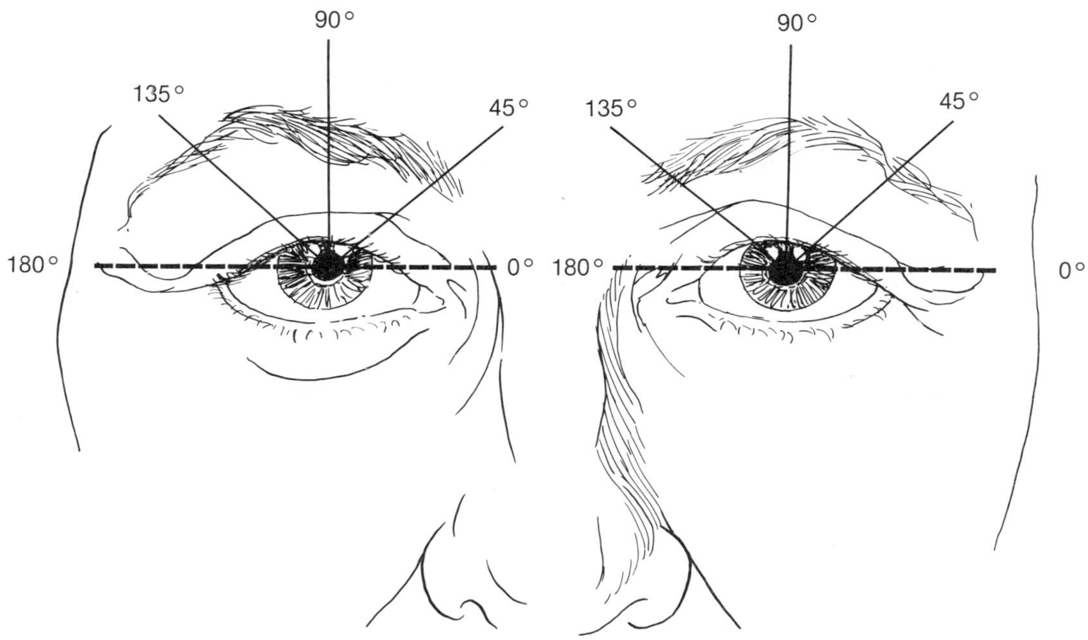

FIG. 12-7

There is an important difference between perimeters, however, that must be observed when placing lenses in the lens holder. With some the perimetrist inserts the lens while looking at the lens holder from the side that will be toward the perimetric bowl. With others he inserts the lens while looking at the side that will be against the patient's face. It is important to pay attention to this difference when placing lenses.

FIG. 12-8. Angle of cylindric axis for lens holders viewed from the bowl side when placing a lens (Goldmann, Octopus 201).

FIG. 12-9. Angle for cylindric lens placement in a lens holder viewed from the patient side when placing a lens (Humphrey, Dicon).

Three other important considerations pertain:

1. When placing a lens in the lens holder, be sure that the spheric lens goes in the slot that will be nearest the patient's face and the cylindric lens goes in front toward the bowl. If two spheric lenses are used (to achieve the total add required), the stronger one goes closer to the eye.
2. Use a full-aperture lens with a narrow metal rim around the glass, not a lens with a broad rim around a smaller glass.
3. Keep straight in your mind whether the patient's correction is expressed in plus or minus cylinders and use the appropriate type. They are not the same.

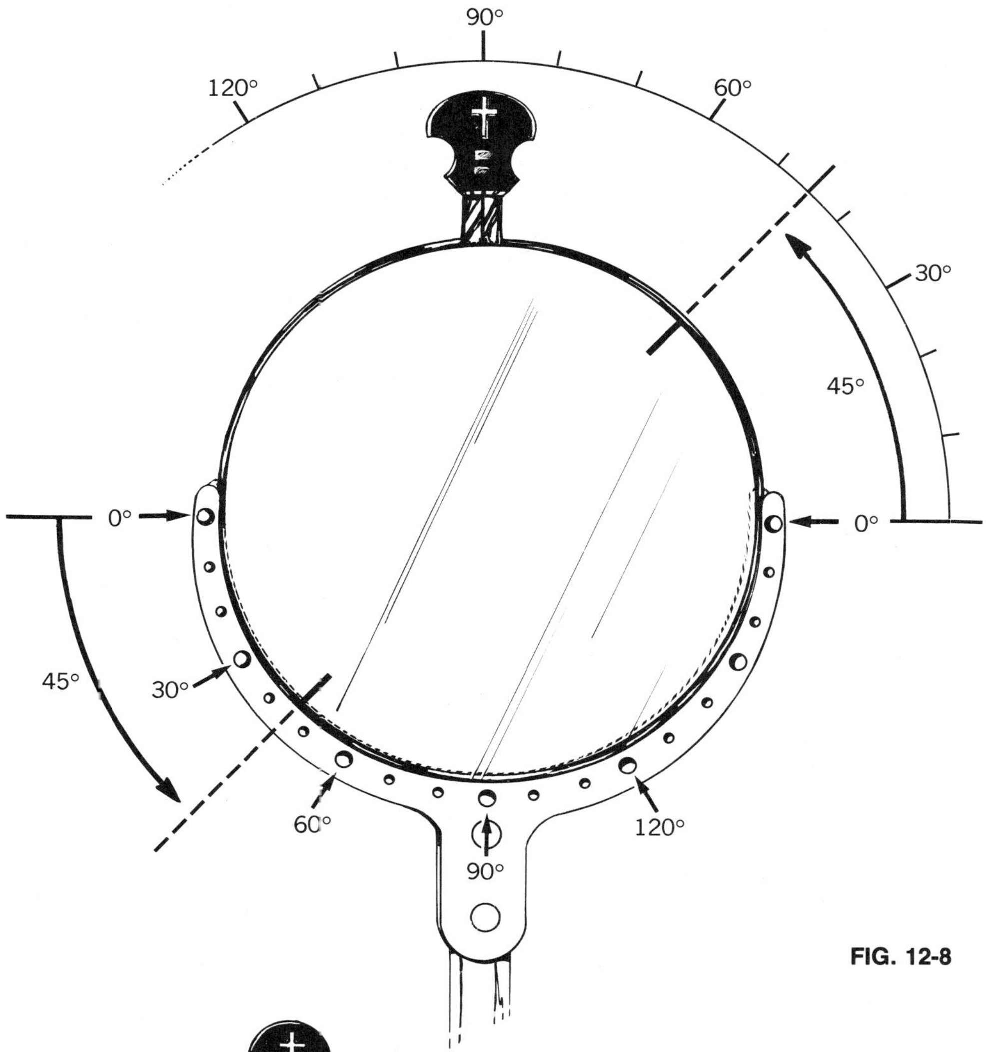

FIG. 12-8

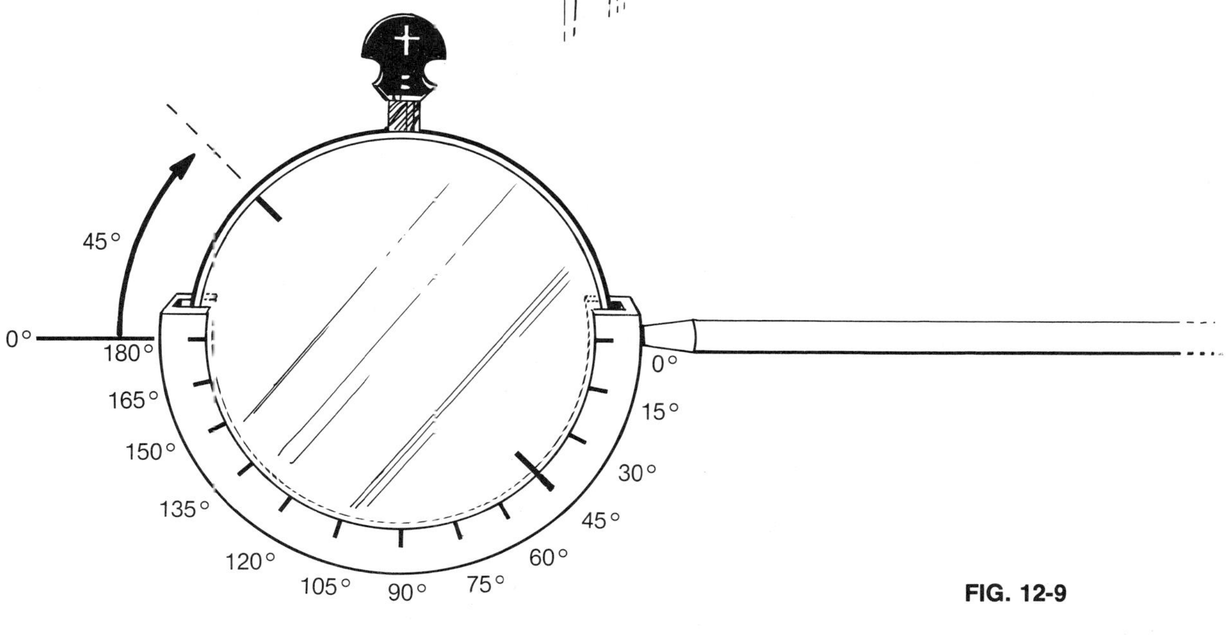

FIG. 12-9

Assuring the proper corrective lens position

It is important that the corrective lens be close to the face, almost touching the eyelashes. Otherwise, its edge will impinge on the edge of the 30-degree field to be tested.

FIG. 12-10. Effect of lens distance on the limits of field that can be tested. See Fig. 13-32 for an example of the artifact that can result.

Also the eye must be centered with respect to the corrective lens. For the lens to be centered over the pupil, it must be positioned snugly against the bridge of the nose. It is easy for the patient's head to drift away from the correct position, so the lens position relative to the eye must be monitored continually lest the patient's head drift during the course of the test. This must be done in addition to monitoring fixation (p. 206).

FIG. 12-11. Correctly centered lens (left) and incorrectly centered lens (right). In the incorrect position the upper nasal portion of the field is blocked by the lens rim. Stimuli presented in that quadrant may not be seen, simulating visual field loss. Note that even the slight misalignment shown here can cause a false field defect, examples of which appear in Figs. 13-59 and 13-62.

Also, be aware that an improper head tilt (p. 186) will cause the lower edge of the lens to be far from the eye (blocking the lower part of the field), even if the upper part of the lens is as close as possible to the eyebrow.

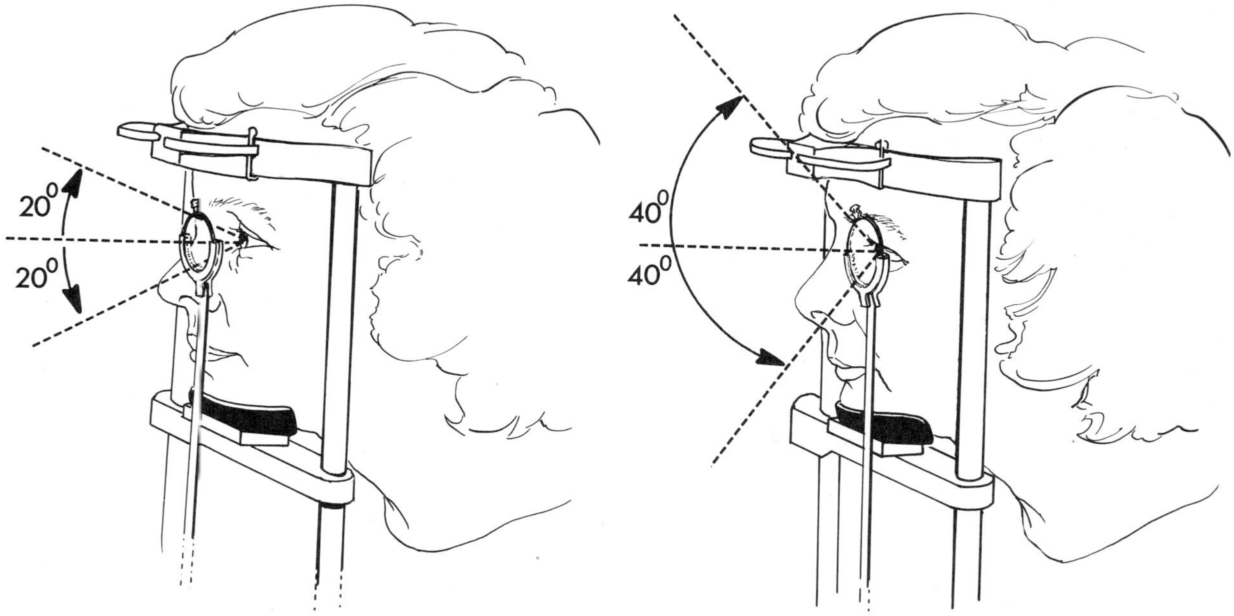

FIG. 12-10

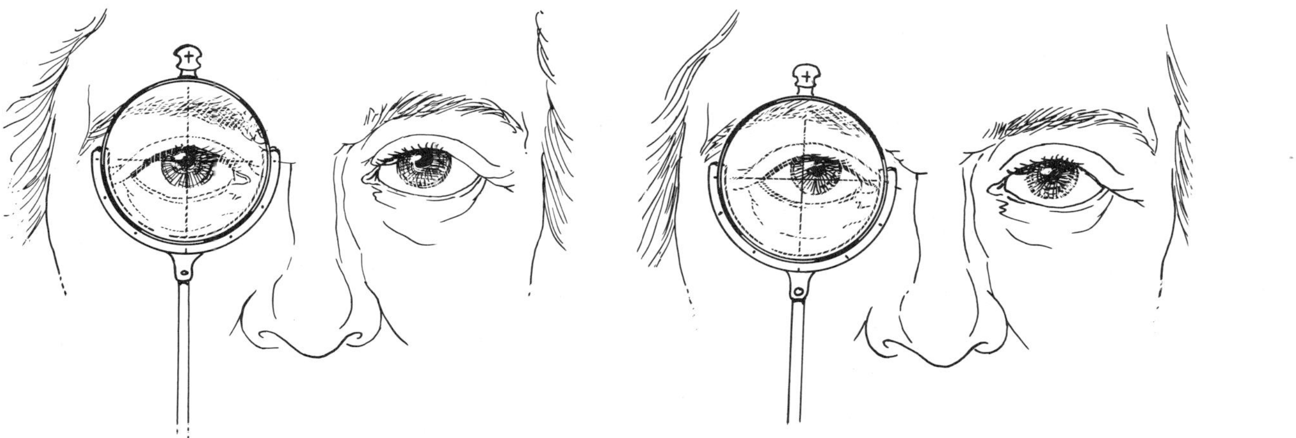

FIG. 12-11

Cycloplegia

If a patient has been given cycloplegic drops to dilate the pupil or for a refraction, the full add in Table 12-1 is required for any age because the cycloplegic drug will have eliminated all accommodative ability.

Contact lenses

If the patient wears contact lenses representing his proper distance correction, the contact lenses are left in for the entire field examination (both central and peripheral fields). The contact lens alone is used for the peripheral field; but when testing the central 30 degrees of the field, the required add for perimetry is provided by using a loose trial lens along with the contact lens. In essence, the patient who wears only distance contact lenses is considered to have no refractive error at distance, requiring an add just for perimetry in the central 30 degrees according to his accommodative ability. If he wears glasses over the contact lenses for distance, the spectacle correction is considered the distance refractive error to be used as the starting point in determining the near correction for perimetry.

Aphakia

After cataract extraction a patient no longer has accommodation and will require a full add regardless of his age. If he wears contact lenses, a +3.25 D add combined with a *distance* overcorrection in the spectacles will be needed in addition to his own contact lens for the central 30 degrees. The contact lens alone will be adequate for the peripheral field outside 30 degrees. If he does not wear contact lenses, the distance spectacle correction plus the full add for perimetry (Table 12-1) will be needed.

However, there are problems with such strong lenses. First, their prismatic effects cause the central field to be miniaturized on the field diagram—the blind spot migrating toward fixation and the apparent limit of the field produced by the lens edge moving inside 30 degrees. Second, the vertex distance (from the lens to the cornea) is critical with strong lenses and it is difficult to maintain the proper vertex distance during the entire field examination, especially for elderly patients.

To overcome these problems, it is good to use contact lenses for the visual field examination in patients with aphakia, even if they do not usually wear contact lenses. Contact lenses that provide both the distance correction and the full add for perimetry are used for both the central and the peripheral field examinations. Using contact lenses for testing the peripheral field provides the additional theoretical advantage of allowing stimuli to be adequately focused on the retina, which seems to improve the peripheral field examination when there is a strong refractive error (as in aphakia) even though corrective lenses are not extremely important for testing the peripheral field in the presence of the usual refractive error.

A hard contact lens of 10 mm diameter and a steep base curve (7.60 mm) is used to reduce lens movement, which would be disturbing to a patient not accustomed to wearing contact lenses. A steep immobile lens is tolerated by the cornea for the duration of the examination, even though it would not be suitable for regular wear. Additional comfort is provided by instilling topical anesthetic before putting the lens in place.

A selection of four lenses is kept for use in perimetry (+13.00, +16.50, +19.00, and +21.00 D). To select the proper lens, the examiner determines the spectacle correction, adding together the sphere and the cylinder expressed in plus form (the minus cylinder is ignored), and makes +3.25 D add for perimetry. The vertex distance of the spectacle is calculated and the total required correction (sphere, +cylinder, and +3.25 D add) is converted to a vertex distance of 0. Then the strength closest to this result is selected from among the four standard lenses. Often this will be the +16.50 D lens.

Of course, because the corneal curvature was not considered, the correction of the refractive error will rarely be perfect. Plus and minus spheres can be used over the contact lens, and the patient then asked which superimposed trial lens brings the fixation spot into best focus. Any additional lenses required can be used along with the contact lens for the central 30 degrees, but the contact lens alone is used for the peripheral field.

It is not always practical to spend the time needed to achieve a perfect correction. Most of the time a +16.50 D contact lens will do an adequate job. When a little extra care is needed, calculation of the lens strength from the spectacle correction and vertex distance may be warranted. For patients in whom it is expected that visual field examinations will be required often, e.g., a patient who has glaucoma, it may be worth the effort to perform an overrefraction with spheres over the contact lenses selected to determine which contact lenses and which loose trial lenses will be required. The same lenses can be used for all subsequent field examinations without having to go through the effort of determining the best lens each time.

Refinements

Ideally lens thickness should be minimized to avoid distortions and prismatic effects. For this purpose, as already noted, it is not necessary routinely to use the full add on all patients. Nonetheless, to reduce even further the need to use unnecessarily strong lenses, two additional principles can be applied:

REDUCE THE STRENGTH OF MINUS SPHERES as long as the patient is using any accommodation. There is the double advantage of reducing the strength of the minus sphere while simultaneously reducing the need for the patient to accommodate.

AVOID USING A CYLINDER WHOSE SIGN IS OPPOSITE that of the sphere. When the sphere and cylinder are of like sign, the cylinder augments one meridian of the sphere and the strength of the spheric lens is less than it would be with the opposite cylindric form. When the sphere and cylinder are of opposite sign, the cylinder weakens one meridian of the sphere.

To implement these principles, start with the distance spectacle refraction of the patient expressed in the plus cylinder form and apply the following rules:

1. If the sphere component is a plus lens, use the spherocylinder combination calculated by providing the usual add for age from Table 12-1.
2. If the sphere component is between −3.25 D and plano for the Goldmann perimeter,* use the age correction to calculate the required near correction for perimetry. If the calculated required sphere is plus, use it and any plus cylinder that is needed. If the calculated sphere is minus, then use no sphere but only the plus cylinder that is needed.
3. If the sphere component of the distance correction represents more myopia than the full add of the perimeter being used, calculate the near correction for perimetry by using the full add. Convert the result to the minus cylinder form and use it. EXCEPTION: Do not convert to the minus cylinder form if the plus cylinder power happens to be more than twice the minus sphere in the spherocylinder lens needed for perimetry. Use the lenses in the plus cylinder form.

Tangent screen

The distance to the tangent screen is 1 m, and the +1.00 D add can usually be ignored. Therefore the patient's own glasses may be used. This is especially helpful for patients with aphakia because there need be no concern about the vertex distance if properly fitting lenses are used. However, one must beware of the reading segment of bifocals, which can interfere with testing the inferior arcuate region. To test the inferior portion of the field, it may be necessary to have the patient tilt his head down while looking straight ahead, thereby moving the reading segment downward and out of the way.

---

*Between −3.00 and plano for instruments with a bowl radius of 33 cm, between −2.50 and plano for instruments with a bowl radius of 42.5 cm, and between −2.00 and plano for instruments with a bowl radius of 50 cm.

CAUSES OF UNSTEADY FIXATION

There are three reasons why the patient may look away from the fixation target:

First, an inborn reflex exists in everyone that whenever something flashes or moves in the peripheral field we quickly glance at it (for example, to see whether it is a harmless rabbit or a man-eating tiger). Most of us can consciously overcome this reflex during field testing, but there remains an urge to look at the test stimulus, especially if it is quite dim and we are not certain that it is really there. The patient naturally wants to look to verify that the light is on before pushing the button.

Second, in a testing situation most people want to do a good job. If the patient knows or thinks that the next stimulus will be in a certain direction from fixation, he not only concentrates his attention in that direction, he may even look quickly that way from time to time searching for the stimulus. If the location of the next stimulus cannot be anticipated, he may search in all directions.

Third, the patient may not be able to see the fixation target because of his visual loss.

The first motive is not a major problem during field testing. A patient cannot look at the test stimulus (to verify that it is really there) unless in fact he did see it in the first place, at least dimly. Thus the accuracy of the test is not much affected, although the test may be slowed by his continuous eye movements followed by the perimetrist's urging that he hold his eye still. If this type of unstable fixation is recognized (by virtue of the fact that the loss of fixation always occurs in response to a seen stimulus) and urging the patient not to look at the stimulus fails, the test can still be done. With manual perimetry the next stimulus is not presented until the patient has again taken up fixation. In automated perimetry it simply must be assumed that fixation has been reestablished by the time the next stimulus is presented. Fixation can be monitored, and if necessary the rate of stimulus presentation slowed, to ensure that fixation has been regained by the time the next stimulus is presented.

The second motive is more of a problem in that it causes the patient to look away from the fixation target *before* the stimulus is presented. With such anticipation, if the eye is not centrally fixated, the stimulus is presented to some part of the retina other than that intended and the response or lack of response indicates the visual status of some unknown position in the visual field.

The problem of looking in a specific direction for the next stimulus is reduced if the stimulus presentations are in an unpredictable sequence of locations. Many (but not all) automated programs are like this, and most patients have steady fixation when the direction of the next stimulus is unpredictable. In manual perimetry the perimetrist monitors fixation and continually reminds the patient, and in most cases fixation is adequately stable. For those patients who cannot resist looking when an isopter is plotted in sequential meridians, the perimetrist may present the stimulus in an irregular sequence of meridians (45 degrees, then 150 degrees, then 130 degrees, then 280 degrees, then 80 degrees, and so on). Some perimetry teachers have advocated always using a random sequence to stabilize the patient's fixation. Others teach that an orderly sequence be used for the majority of patients in whom fixation is quite adequate. An orderly sequence is a bit quicker, but the real reason for advocating a regular sequence is that the reproducibility of the responses is greater when the patient can direct his attention to a specific area (provided he does not also shift his gaze in that direction).

There remain a number of patients who will be constantly searching everywhere for the stimulus. Some of these simply cannot resist looking around (unconsciously); others will be unable to see the fixation target. A large random element exists in these responses—the patient may happen to be looking at a spot near the place of stimulus presentation or may happen to be looking somewhere else. In such cases the printout of an automated field has an irregular checkerboard or Swiss cheese pattern (see Fig. 13-41) and the report indicates that there were many fixation losses, many false-positive responses, and perhaps many false-negative responses. Such patients are better tested by manual perimetry with an understanding and experienced perimetrist who constantly monitors fixation and accepts only those responses occurring in the intervals while the patient is centrally fixating.

MONITORING FIXATION

Manual perimeters have a telescope through which the perimetrist observes the eye position continually (p. 354). Most automated perimeters are similarly equipped with a telescope, peephole, or television screen for this purpose. The intent is to encourage and remind the patient if he falters in maintaining fixation, to pause for readjustment of his position if his face drifts to the right or left or backward, and to help him stay awake and alert to the task if his eyelids begin to droop.

With manual perimeters, if a stimulus is presented at an instant when the eye is deviated, the response is ignored; but with current automated instruments it is not possible to signal that a given response is invalid. Automated perimeters may have a device that observes the eye and sounds a warning buzzer if the eye position changes. However, these devices only act as a supplement and are not a substitute for an attentive perimetrist. In addition, they may be affected by a change in head position, even when the eye is still centrally fixating; and if their sensitivity is adjusted to eliminate false alarms, they may not adequately detect fixation losses. In any event, most patients are more responsive to the gentle reminder of a perimetrist to maintain fixation than they are to the warning buzzer of a machine.

Some automated programs monitor fixation by the Heijl-Krakau method of occasionally presenting stimuli in the center of the previously mapped physiologic blind spot. If the patient is centrally fixating, the stimulus will not be seen. At a minimum, the printouts report the percentage of time that the stimulus is seen in the blind spot, which is one measure of the accuracy of the field test on this occasion. The instrument may also sound a reminding buzzer if the stimulus is seen. In addition, the machine may be programmed to assume that the most recent responses are inaccurate and to repeat all the stimulus presentations since the last time that fixation was tested. This programmed assumption, however, is often false. If the patient is alternately fixating and searching, then whether or not he was fixating when a stimulus was presented in the blind spot may not indicate that he was fixating during each of the preceding 10 stimulus presentations; and repetition of the stimulus presentation does lengthen the test considerably.

All told, the present methods of automated fixation monitoring are not optimal. The perimetrist still must watch the patient's eye position. Moreover, he must remain alert to whether the eye is centered behind the corrective lens, is close to the lens, and has not drifted backward so the rim of the lens produces an artifactual defect in the visual field.

KEEPING THE PATIENT AT HIS BEST

The task of concentrating on a fixed spot for the better part of an hour and responding quickly to a rapid sequence of visual stimuli is not easy. Some patients will be tense in a testing situation, or they may be anxious about the threat to their vision. Others may be bored. The constant brightness in the perimetric bowl may seem to fade in and out, and there may appear to be dim flashes of light when actually none exist. While staring into an empty white space with monotonous flashes of light and rhythmic repetition of sounds, the patient may drift in and out of sleepiness. If motivated, he may fight to stay awake and may tire easily. An awkward position can be difficult to maintain.

Perimetrists need to appreciate the nature of the experience. Perhaps every clinician and perimetrist should undergo field testing annually. It could help them understand and empathize with their patients, to be understanding about patient inconsistencies, and to realize the importance of encouragement.

The test should be made as easy as possible for the patient, because only the patient can know if he does or does not see the stimulus. It is up to the examiner to set the patient at ease, to help him achieve to the fullest his part of the test, and to obtain the greatest amount of diagnostic information possible within the limits of his ability. Even with automated instruments, the perimetrist can make a difference in how well the patient is able to do the task.

During the test there should be occasional voice contact with the patient. Especially with automated perimetry it is helpful to the patient to know that a person is sharing the experience with him. It is not just he and the machine. This contact is accomplished in part by the occasional need to remind the patient to look at the fixation target. (This should always be done in an encouraging and friendly tone, never with implied criticism that could add to the patient's tenseness.) An occasional "you're doing great" or "we're about halfway through now" will keep the perimetrist and patient in touch. The comments should be brief and not require an answer, especially with automated perimetry. After all, the patient is busy concentrating and the machine does not pause for the patient to listen while you speak. How often you utter an encouraging word and what you say are judgments that you make and will depend on the individual patient. Be sure also not to have a solicitous, condescending, or impersonal air.

A patient may wish to pause for a few seconds. During manual perimetry this can be done by merely inviting him to close his eyes and relax for a few seconds (for example, while you are drawing an isopter). During automated perimetry when there is a pause between phases of the programming, you may ask "How are you getting along?" or "Ready to go again?" The patient should be told that by simply holding the response button depressed he can stop the automated test any time he wants to pause and rest.

The perimetrist should have, and show, a genuine interest in the patient's comfort and the quality of the test result. There should never be an expression of dissatisfaction with performance, an impatient remark, or some other indication of being in a hurry. Because performing the test repeatedly can become routine for you, always guard against becoming automatic in your responses or uncaring in your attitude.

When patients with large dense field defects are tested, there may be a long series of presentations that they do not see. This can be very disconcerting to a patient, who may worry about his visual loss or may wonder whether the test is still proceeding or has been concluded. In manual perimetry, if three or four stimuli are not seen a visible stimulus should be presented in a known seeing area to maintain the patient's attention and reassure the perimetrist that the patient is still attending to the task. Automated perimeters do not do this, and whenever the patient has not responded to a series of presentations the perimetrist should reassure him that everything is going well, that the machine is testing the limits of his vision with some stimuli too dim for him to see, that he need not worry but should wait for a stimulus that he can see. It is reassuring to know that someone is there and paying attention, that the test has not been terminated, and that it is all right for a series of stimuli not to be seen.

Some patients may be concerned if they make a false response that they know is ill timed or mistaken—one that they wish they could retract. They should be reassured that the computer program allows for a number of these and will not be affected by a few erroneous answers.

The perimetrist should pay attention to the patient's posture. If his forehead tends to wander backward, perhaps he is having to stretch to reach the chin rest. On the other hand, he may be squirming because of back pain from leaning forward too much or some other discomfort. These are important. Artifactual field defects will result when an eye moves away from the lens. Apart from the fact that the patient should not suffer unnecessarily, an uncomfortable patient cannot concentrate.

Finally, it is important that nothing distract the patient. The perimetrist should refrain from making or receiving phone calls or conversing with others while administering the test. The waiting room should be adequately sound proofed so crying babies or conversations are not audible to the patient.

AFTER THE TEST

The record of the field test must include the patient's name (as well as his date of birth), the date of the test (including the year), any corrective lenses used, the size of the pupil, and which eye was tested. In automated perimetry any information not printed out must be added by hand. It is sometimes customary to record the visual acuity and intraocular pressure on the field diagram, for this information may help in the interpretation. Any comments on the reliability of the test or other factors that may affect the interpretation should also be recorded.

HOW MUCH THE TECHNICIAN SHOULD KNOW ABOUT DIAGNOSIS

The responsibility of the technician varies from one office or clinic setting to another. It depends on the personality of the clinician and how much responsibility he wants to delegate, whether or not the perimetry is manual or automated, and the skill and experience of the technician currently holding the position.

To be done adequately, manual perimetry demands some familiarity with the types of field defects, information about what is under exploration in the particular patient, an ability to choose the exact technique for the purpose at hand, and skill at modifying the details of the method to define a defect better when one becomes apparent as the test is conducted. Part II of this book is for technicians who will be doing manual perimetry.

With automated perimetry the technician need not at first be quite so familiar with all the types of field defects and how fields are interpreted. Typically someone else (the "boss") will decide which program is to be done. The technician's responsibility is to administer the test. However, the attentive technician who becomes familiar with the reasons for selecting different tests under differing conditions and who has the opportunity to see how the tests are interpreted may come to know when a certain program should be used instead of, or in addition to, the usual one. He may realize that when the acuity is abnormal the point of fixation must be tested if it is not already included in the selected program. After looking at the printout, he may understand what circumstances prompted the clinician to request another program to explore the situation further, may recognize eyelid and lens rim artifacts that require the test to be repeated, or may be able to discern that a particular result is equivocal with respect to the diagnosis in question. In this last case he may know that a specific region requires a closer grid of points or perhaps that a threshold test is needed to follow up on an equivocal suprathreshold test, that a 30-to-60-degree program is needed to evaluate a seeming abnormality near the periphery of the 30-degree test, or maybe that the test should be done with a dilated pupil if there seems to be progression compared to a previous examination, and so on. Even if not given the responsibility for making such decisions, the technician can recognize when the clinician should be asked about the possible need for an additional test while the patient is still seated at the perimeter.

The technician will certainly not be in a position to make a diagnosis, which after all depends on correlating the field results with the symptoms and other clinical findings that the patient shows; and, besides, he does not have the formal schooling required. However, he can (and should) pay attention to the clinical circumstances that required the field test and he may learn how the results are interpreted for use in making diagnostic and therapeutic decisions. After learning this through months and years of experience, he may be able to contribute significantly to the quality of patient care by augmenting the visual field test appropriately to establish the diagnosis. At least he should add to the efficiency of patient care by reducing the need for repeated tests because the first test did not achieve the diagnostic goal intended.

CHAPTER 13

Interpretation

THE APPROACH

Interpretation is an art that improves with experience. Even when testing of the field is automated, interpretation is not.

Interpretation is not easy at first, and clinicians who receive the plotted results of manual or automated field examinations yearn for a simple set of rules that will yield an interpretation of the field. If simple accurate criteria existed, the computer could handle the interpretation of automated visual field tests. This will never happen. Any criteria meant to include 95% of normals will sometimes (in fact, 5% of the time) label a normal field as abnormal. On the other hand, when field loss first starts, the mildly deficient visual sensation will for a while remain within normal limits.

Similarly, any criteria for progression will be exceeded by the natural fluctuations of visual sensation in a certain small percent of normal people, yielding a false-positive result. At the same time the criteria may fail to recognize a slight but genuine progressive visual deterioration, especially if they are made lenient to avoid false-positives.

Therefore visual field information often cannot be definitively interpreted without taking into account other clinical findings. Two or three points that seem abnormal at the lower nasal edge of a central 30-degree field test may be judged an early field defect if there is elevated intraocular pressure (IOP) and some cupping of the disc. The same visual field finding may be judged a normal variant in another patient who has no sign of ocular disease, or perhaps an artifact caused by the rim of a correcting lens may be suspected. Even in the presence of an elevated IOP, the abnormality may be considered related to cataract or retinal abnormalities rather than to glaucoma if the clinical examination reveals that these other conditions are present and there is no cupping of the optic disc.

In the same way, worsening of the field may be accepted as genuine glaucomatous progression in the presence of marginally controlled IOP or equivocal enlargement of a disc excavation. In the presence of well-controlled pressure the significance of the same field change may be questioned, necessitating that the examination be repeated or the ocular media and fundus be examined more carefully to look for other explanations for the changes in visual threshold.

As another example, the topographic nature of a defect or visual field change may be out of line with that of the known or suspected disease, leading the clinician to feel that a reexamination is necessary to find the presence of another condition not previously recognized.

Finally, both the visual field and the other clinical findings may be so equivocal that final diagnostic interpretation must be deferred until a later time, when suspected mild disease may or may not have developed more definitive manifestations.

In some sense this approach to visual field examination is not ''objective'' but is biased by the other available clinical information. The subjectivity of interpretation is quite appropriate to most clinical settings in which any subjectivity is called ''clinical judgment'' and is, hopefully, astute. There are, however, two settings in which the visual field information may need to be interpreted without the aid of other clinical findings: *visual field screening* and *certain research projects*.

In visual field screening programs it may be impractical to obtain all the necessary clinical information for definitive diagnosis. Clearly defined criteria are needed to reach the decision to refer an individual for more definitive evaluation—which can include both a more thorough field test and a more comprehensive clinical examination to look for corroborative evidence of the suspected disease. It may be tricky to establish criteria that will minimize the number of people with mild disease who are missed (and not referred for definitive examination) and at the same time minimize the number of people with no disease who are unnecessarily subjected to the cost of a definitive examination only to have it found out that the screening exam had given a false-positive result.

In certain scientific studies it may similarly be necessary to establish objective criteria so a group of individuals can be classified as normal or abnormal without any knowledge of their clinical status. Even if some of the "positive results" are artifacts (caused by a lens rim or by disease other than the one under study), the artifactual result will appear equally in the two groups being compared and thus not affect the determination that there is a difference between the two groups. Strictly objective criteria are needed in this setting lest, for example, the scientific investigator induce a bias by labeling a lower nasal defect as real in one group he thinks to be under less effective treatment but excuse the same defect as artifactual in another that he thinks is under more effective treatment. In a scientific study, maintaining unbiased data takes priority over achieving absolute accuracy, provided the frequency of inaccuracies is limited. To cite a case in point, if two groups in a study are found to differ by having (in one) 80% abnormality and (in the other) 40%, it makes little difference if there has been a 10% error so that in reality a 70% abnormality exists in the first group and 30% in the second. The conclusion remains: group A has a substantially higher rate of abnormality, and the investigator was successful in determining that group B is better off. In some study designs judgment may be permitted as long as the interpreter is kept from knowing to which group the individual subject belongs.

In clinical practice, interpretation isolated from other clinical findings is undesirable. The examiner is interested primarily in the individual, not in the average of a group. It makes perfect sense that if the IOP has been running a bit high and the excavation of the disc seems a bit larger than before then a new abnormality in the field is likely real. On the other hand, if the same defect appears as a surprise on routine follow-up in a patient who seems stable, it is sensible to suspect an artifact or some other cause and to at least repeat the field test before accepting it as real.

If the reader wishes to be analytical about this assertion, the viewpoint can be taken that any isolated clinical finding is not to be believed until it is confirmed by some other clinical finding or by a repeat of the abnormal test. In one case an apparent mild change in the excavation and the apparent change in the visual field serve to confirm each other. In a second case the repeat field, if abnormal, confirms the first field test.

Another way of looking at it is that a particular visual field finding does not have a fixed probability of being abnormal but rather simply increases the probability of abnormality that existed *before* the test was done. Suppose a patient is judged 40% likely to have ocular damage on the basis of high pressure and the appearance of the disc. This may not be enough to reach a decision to alter management yet it will be enough to decide to look for more evidence. When there is a particular finding on the field test, the probability may be increased to 80%, enough for the clinician to decide that a change in management is warranted. Now, consider another patient who is judged very likely normal or stable on the basis of the clinical findings before the field test is done, perhaps with only a 5% chance that there has been progressive damage. This 5% chance is enough to do a routine or follow-up field as a matter of course. If the suspicious finding appears on the field test in this patient (which has a 95% unexpectedness), it may be judged that the probability of abnormality in this patient has risen from 5% to 20%. This is enough to explore the situation further by repeating the visual field examination or having another look at the optic disc, but it is not enough to reach the decision to change the management.

The risk of abnormality *before* the test is done also affects how an abnormal test on a screening examination is to be interpreted. Consider, for example, that 5% of normal individuals may have one or two abnormal points on a screening field examination and that 1% of people in a certain age bracket have glaucoma. If 100 such people in a condominium are screened, 6 abnormal results may turn up—5 who are normal but have false-positive results, plus 1 who really does have previously undetected glaucoma. Of those with a positive result on field examination, only one of the six actually has glaucoma. Beforehand, everyone who was screened entered the field examination with a 1% chance of having glaucoma. In those with a positive test, that probability rose to 17% (one out of six), high enough to warrant exploring the situation further but not high enough to allow a diagnosis to be certain without the performance of a more extensive examination.

Suppose the same test is made on an office patient with an elevated IOP and questionable cupping. Maybe a third of such patients will have a true field defect. When 100 such patients are examined, 36 positive results may be obtained—33 true defects, and 3 false-positives (5% of the remaining 66 patients with undamaged optic nerves). For those with a positive test the probability of having real glaucomatous damage rose from 33% to 92% (thirty-three out of thirty-six).

The point is that the circumstances and the other clinical findings must be taken into account when interpreting the field test result. Clinicians who want to study further the mathematical reasoning that makes this approach valid should consult a statistics book that describes how the predictability of a test result (with a certain sensitivity and specificity) is influenced by the prevalence of abnormality in the population subjected to the test, or by the a priori probability that the individual has a defect.

These principles apply not only to screening tests but also to the more definitive diagnostic tests. If the individual is already a suspect because of other clinical findings or because of a specific screening test, the examiner may choose a test with greater sensitivity (but a higher false-positive rate) without losing predictability. In other words, he can pay more attention to equivocal findings.

The same analysis holds when testing for progression of field defects, if the test is considered a means of detecting (or screening for) progression. Again, there is a greater likelihood that apparent progression is real in those with high pressure or suspicious disc changes than in those who lack these corroborating clinical findings.

Although a certain subjectivity is essential for interpretation, the judgment exercised must be astute and careful. It is possible to use *poor* clinical judgment. In the clinic the examiner must be "scientific" enough to demand good evidence to confirm a suspicious finding. Test results must be in keeping with other clinical findings or must be confirmed by a repeat of the test. If the result is uncertain or contradicts other clinical findings, he is permitted to repeat the test or may defer judgment to observe the clinical course further. Sometimes he will be forced to make a decision about management in the face of uncertainty. Factors other than the disease status may come into play—e.g., an anxious patient who wishes more aggressive treatment and who reaps peace of mind therefrom even when the therapeutic benefits are uncertain. Another patient might easily want to wait a few months to see how things progress before making a commitment to a more aggressive management with its attendant risks or side effects. If this person's level of anxiety were already low, he would not reap a gain from immediate action.

The preceding introductory essay should make it obvious that there are no plain rules. We cannot say, for example, "If X number of points deviate from the expected value by Y amount or more, then condition Z is present (or progression has occurred, or whatever)." To be sure, some sensible guidelines can be formulated; but every field test and every clinical circumstance are a little different, and there is always an element of judgment.

DEFECT DETECTION WITH SUPRATHRESHOLD TESTING

The negative result

It is always necessary to judge the reliability of each test individually. When the test stimuli are seen at all points tested, it is important to consider whether the test performed was adequate to have detected a defect of interest. Specifically one must look at

- Stimulus intensity. Was it too great? How deep a defect might have been present and still escaped detection? (If the stimulus intensity was not eccentricity compensated, a defect near fixation would have had to be deeper than another minimally detectable one at the edge of the tested region.)
- Number of points tested. Were there enough? How large a defect might have been present and still fit between the tested points? (For example, a defect the size of the physiologic blind spot [5 degrees wide] would not have been detected if it was positioned appropriately in a grid of points 6 degrees apart—a typical pattern for many automated perimeters.)

FIG. 13-1. The physiologic blind spot and a scotoma the same size can each fit between points 6 degrees apart.

- Pattern of test points (location). Was it appropriate for the lesion suspected? (Consider, for example, a central scotoma or one impinging on fixation. It may be small and yet visually significant. If such a defect is suspected but not discovered, the interpreter should consider whether or not the point of fixation was tested and whether a sufficient number of points near fixation were included in the pattern. A frequent mistake in manual perimetry is not to test the area around fixation carefully enough. Likewise, in automated perimetry an evenly spaced grid of points 6 degrees apart screens the central field for moderate-sized defects but may leave the region just around fixation inadequately tested for small, though visually significant, defects.)

FIG. 13-2. Central scotoma not detected by a grid of points 6 degrees apart straddling (but not including) the point of fixation.

(In a similar way the interpreter should consider whether the pattern of points was appropriate to discover any other suspected defect, be it a hemianopia, a nasal step, or a peripheral defect caused by a chorioretinal lesion.)

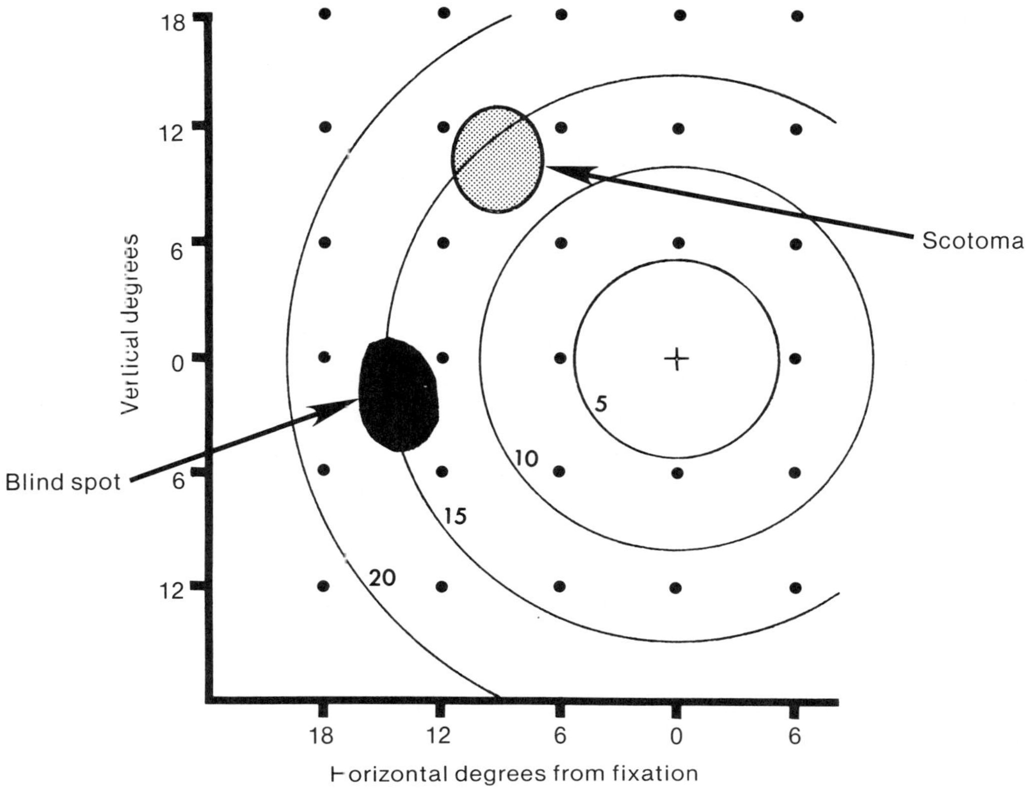

FIG. 13-1

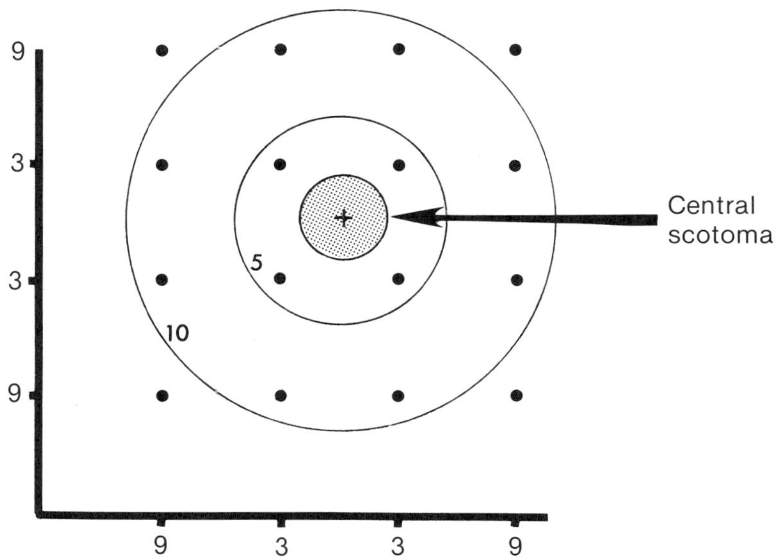

FIG. 13-2

- Possible presence of generalized depression. Suprathreshold spot-checking strategies are designed particularly to uncover localized defects, especially if the stimuli are selected by determining threshold at some location(s) prior to beginning the spot-checking. (In manual perimetry the interpreter can recognize that a generalized depression may be present [without a localized defect being detected] if the perimetrist, by virtue of static or kinetic threshold determination temporal to the blind spot, selects a stronger-than-normal stimulus for spot-checking. Similarly, the interpreter must know the strategy used in automated perimety and must specifically note whether the perimeter found an abnormal threshold anywhere in selecting a stimulus intensity for suprathreshold screening.)

Remember also that the circumstances surrounding the test can influence the interpretation of a negative result.

In a population screening program in which the prevalence of visual field abnormalities is low, the negative test is not surprising. Even if the test strategy is selected to have a low-false positive rate (high specificity) at the cost of a lower intensity for early defects, the chances are still quite high that a person with a negative outcome will in fact have a normal visual field.

By contrast, if a person has an elevated IOP and what appears to be glaucomatous optic nerve damage or if he has reduced acuity with an afferent pupillary defect, this may force the examiner to conclude that a visual field defect is present but is too small or too shallow for the test to uncover.

Between these two extremes is the person with less compelling but suspicious clinical findings (e.g., elevated IOP with uncertain enlargement of the optic nerve cup) in whom the negative field test must be viewed with uncertainty.

• • •

To summarize, the interpretation of a negative test must include the consideration that either there is no defect or else a defect is present that is smaller or shallower than the test was able to detect. In the case of a population screen, the likelihood is that the field is indeed normal. In the case of rather certain evidence of damage to the visual system, the likelihood is that a field defect is present but undiscovered. In an intermediate clinical situation, either possibility has a reasonable likelihood and the clinician must decide whether or not to use another test to look for a defect of lesser magnitude than could be detected by the one already performed.

Equivocal and positive results

Everyone is entitled occasionally to fail to respond to a stimulus (say, because of a blink or lapse of attention). Even when all missed responses are rechecked, it is common for several points to be registered as "not seen." There are no absolute criteria by which to decide whether a given field with one or several missed responses is normal or abnormal, but in general

- A cluster of two or more adjacent misses is far more significant than individual misses at several nonadjacent points. Whatever proportion of points a person is missing at random, it is unlikely that they will be clustered together as a chance event in a normal visual field (Figs. 13-4 and 13-5).
- Points are more likely to be truly abnormal if stronger stimuli presented at that location are also not seen (suprathreshold testing with semiquantitation or quantitation of defective points) (see Fig. 6-4).
- Defects detected by manual perimetry with spot-checking are likely real if their boundaries can be plotted kinetically, especially if a denser nucleus can be found and plotted.
- Missed points in a typical location for the disease under suspicion (Figs. 13-5 and 13-6) deserve more attention than points atypically located (Fig. 13-8).
- Points at the edge of the tested area (e.g., at 30 degrees) are more likely to be missed than are points in other locations in a normal field. The variability of response is greater in the periphery than near the center when the stimulus intensity is not adjusted for eccentricity. Therefore points are more likely to be missed at the edge because the stimulus may be near threshold whereas centrally it is much stronger than threshold. Edge points may be missed also because of interference by the edge of a correcting lens (Figs. 12-10 and 12-11). Finally, points may be missed in the upper position of the field both because of the eyelid and/or eyebrow (Fig. 12-3) and because of the slight physiologic depression of the field superiorly (pp. 84-87).
- If a patient misses a handful of stimulus presentations at random, a different set of points will be missed if the test is repeated (Fig. 13-7). When the same set of points is missed on repeat testing, the abnormality is likely real.
- The clinical circumstances will dictate how much attention should be paid to a certain pattern of missed points.

FIG. 13-3. A single missed point may be ignored if the examiner is expecting the field to be normal. Even when a spot is missed with more intense stimuli and the defect is reproducible on repeat testing, it may just be that the spot happens to have fallen on a retinal vessel or small retinal scar. There may not be an abnormality produced by the disease under consideration. Yet if such a reproducible defect occurs in an eye with an elevated IOP and suspicious cupping, the clinician should justifiably be suspicious enough to test the area with a finer grid of points or some other, more definitive, test. After all, every advanced defect was once a minimally detectable abnormality.

FIG. 13-4. Several scattered missed points, even a dozen or more, may be entirely normal. If these are isolated (separated by points where the stimulus is seen), the examiner's first impulse may be to discount their significance. In the setting of a population screen they would certainly have to be ignored. On the other hand, they may be more significant if the right eye shows no missed points while the left eye has a higher pressure and a larger excavation of the disc. After all, the latter could indeed represent the beginnings of reduced visual sensation in the region typically affected by glaucoma. Therefore, taken alone, this finding is equivocal; but if the clinical circumstances raise enough suspicion to repeat the visual field examination, the abnormality is likely real when the same points are again missed with the stimulus remaining visible everywhere else in the field. The missed points also deserve more attention if the reduced visibility is confirmed by stronger stimuli (presented during semiquantitation or quantitation).

FIG. 13-5. An almost certain abnormality. A few points clustered together in a typical location are very unlikely to be abnormal. Nonetheless, the examiner must still confirm by clinical examination that such a defect corresponds to the region of the disc that is excavated and that there is no other cause (e.g., branch retinal artery occlusion or artifact of testing) to account for its presence.

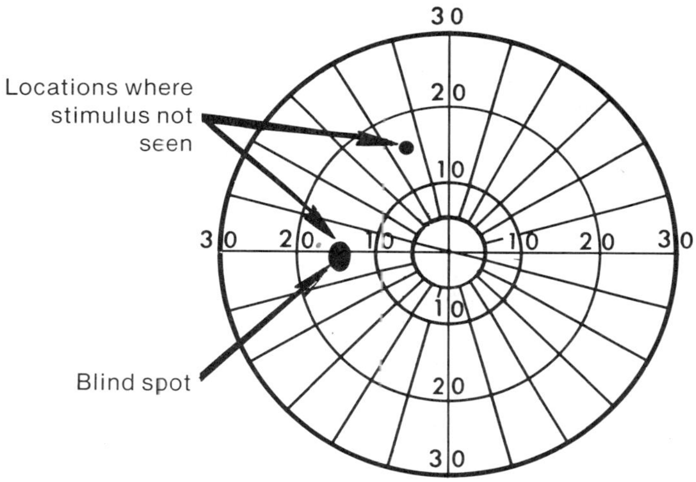

FIG. 13-3

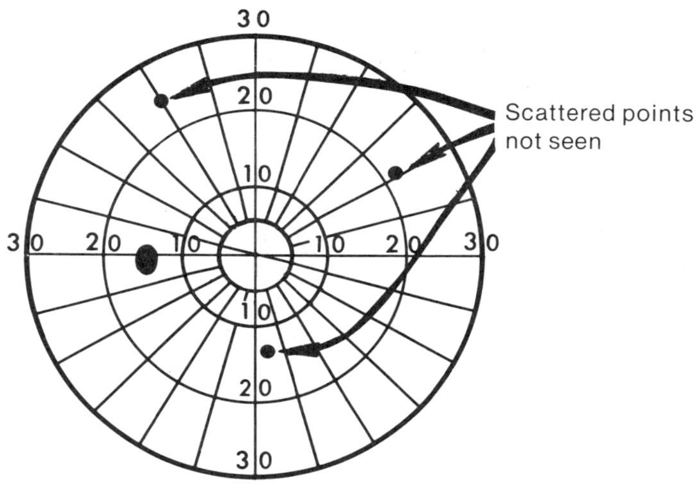

FIG. 13-4

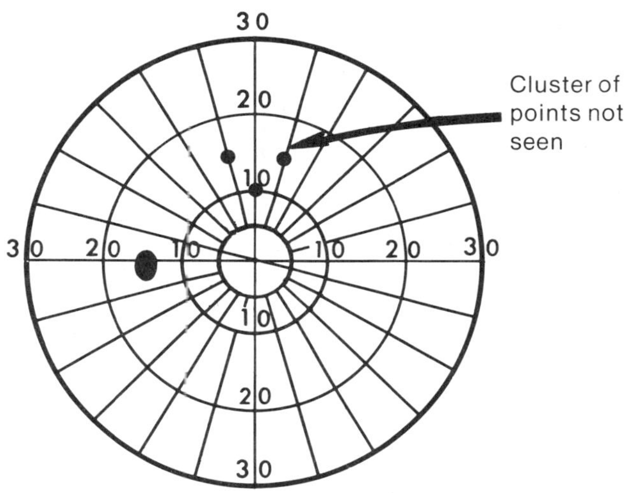

FIG. 13-5

Several exceptional circumstances need to be described:

Sometimes there is a confined region of inconsistent responses where several points may be missed in a confined region but they are not adjacent. On retesting, several points in the same region are again missed but not necessarily the exact same ones. Such a region is consistently inconsistent, so to speak, and must be considered likely abnormal if the stimuli are reliably seen in the remainder of the field.

FIG. 13-6. Field with an inconsistent zone. On retesting, another set of points are missed but in the same region.

A generalized depression may be represented by random intermixing of seen and not seen stimuli. If the stimulus level is close to the generally depressed sensitivity level of the region, repeat testing may even show a different selection of points missed and seen. This circumstance is like the consistently inconsistent region representing a shallow scotoma, except that the entire field is affected; it is an exception to the rule that requires an individual point to be not seen on retesting if it is to be counted as a true defect. In the case of a mild generalized depression most locations would be classed as ''seen'' if the missed stimuli were tested with stronger stimuli. If the test were repeated with a stimulus level 0.5 log-unit more intense, the abnormality would disappear.

FIG. 13-7. Mild generalized depression with scattered missed points throughout the field. A different set of points are missed on retesting.

An isolated missed spot or a string of adjacent missed points at the edge of a 30-degree region tested are often found in normal fields. There are several causes. Sometimes the eyelid or eyebrow accounts for it in the superior field, or the eye may be decentered or too far back from a correcting lens (or empty lens holder). Edge points may be missed, even in the absence of these artifacts, because there is a broader range of normal threshold values (so the sensitivity may be less in one normal individual than in another) and a greater variability in responsiveness at points further from fixation. When the stimulus is not compensated for eccentricity, points at the edge may be missed for the additional reason that they are near the isopter of the stimulus used and therefore the stimulus is very near the threshold at that location.

FIG. 13-8. Edge points missed. A cluster of missed edge points is an equivocal finding that might be due to an artifact or to a true defect. The location of the points on the temporal edge of the field is not typical of a glaucomatous field defect, so a lens rim artifact would be suspected in this example. See Fig. 13-32 for a similar artifact on threshold testing.

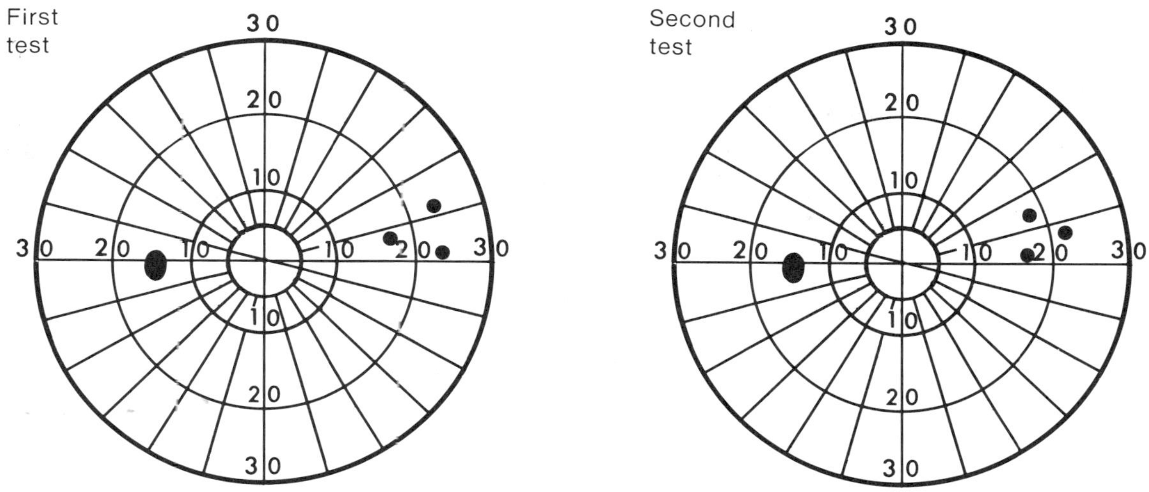

FIG. 13-6

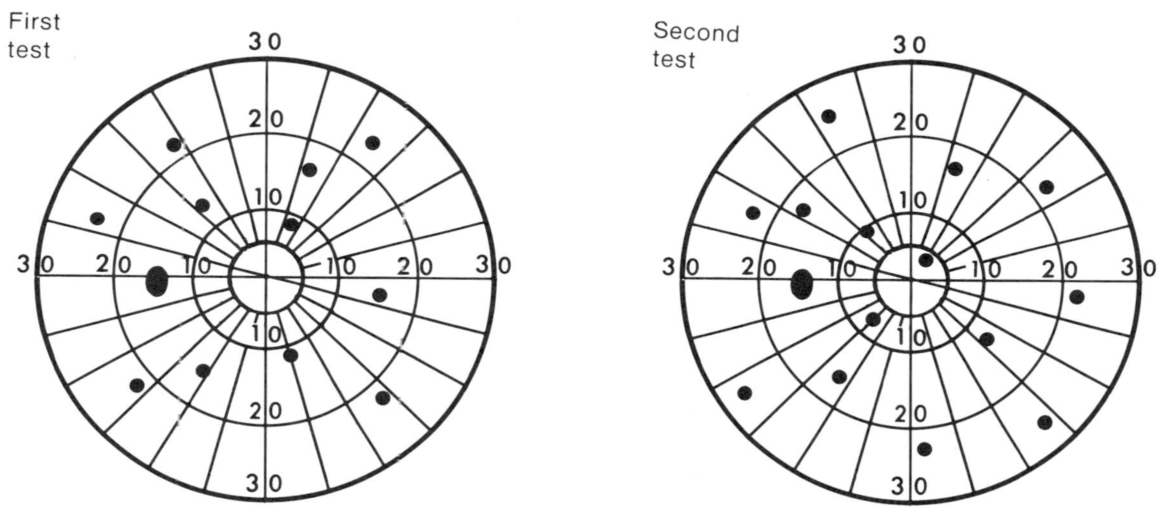

FIG. 13-7

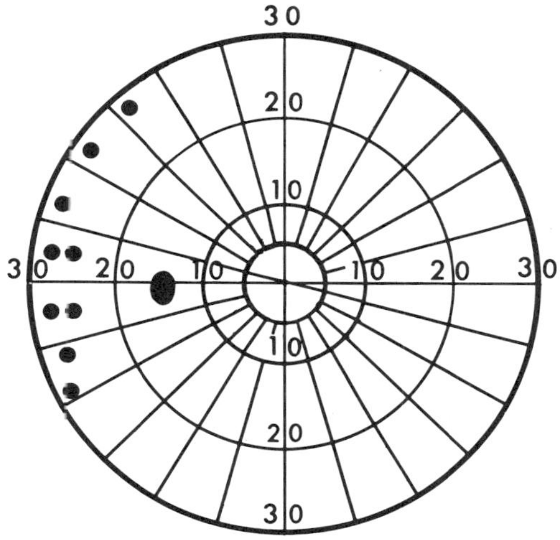

FIG. 13-8

The central points may be missed (and the rest seen) when there is a central scotoma. It may also happen that the central points are not seen and the remainder are seen whenever eccentricity compensation is used and the hill of vision is flatter than normal. This may occur as a normal variant, but it may also happen when cataract or other preretinal factors produce a blurred image, because the central points are the most affected by a blurred image. Be careful therefore not to interpret this finding as necessarily representing a central scotoma.

FIG. 13-9. Pseudocentral scotoma. The central points are missed with eccentricity-compensation strategy when the very center of the field is more depressed than elsewhere.

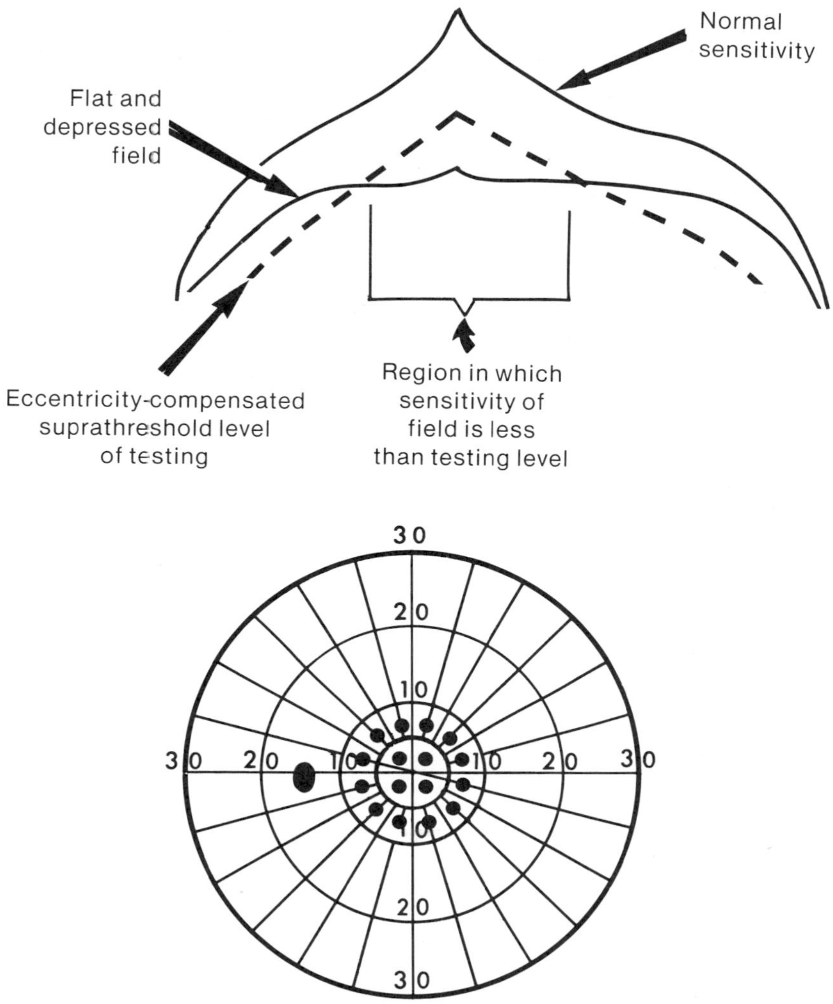
Normal
sensitivity
Flat and
depressed
field
Eccentricity-compensated
suprathreshold level
of testing
Region in which
sensitivity of
field is less
than testing level
30
20
10

FIG. 13-9

RECOGNIZING ABNORMALITIES WITH AUTOMATED STATIC THRESHOLD PERIMETRY

Quality of the test

As always, interpretation begins with considering the reliability of the individual test.

Catch trials. One aspect of the quality of the test session is patient responsiveness. Automated perimeters can utilize three strategies to measure the quality of the test:

1. PRETEND STIMULUS PRESENTATIONS. From time to time the perimeter will imitate presentation of a light stimulus, perhaps even clicking the shutter, to record how often the patient responds when in fact no light stimulus was presented. The results are tabulated as the proportion of false-positive responses (e.g., 1 out of 7).
2. SUPRATHRESHOLD PRESENTATIONS. From time to time the patient will be presented with a stimulus well above threshold in a known seeing region of the field. If you have the test performed on yourself, for example, you can recognize these catch trials because the stimulus will appear much brighter than stimuli presented for threshold determinations. The results are tabulated as the proportion of false-negative responses (i.e., when the patient failed to respond to a known suprathreshold stimulus).

3. FIXATION LOSSES. Some automated strategies monitor fixation by presenting an easily visible stimulus in the location of the physiologic blind spot from time to time. The proportion of times that the patient responds to the stimulus presumably indicates how often he was not maintaining straight-ahead fixation. Along with the other two types of catch trials, this gives some measure of the overall reliability of the patient's responses.

There are two circumstances that may lead to a reported high rate of fixation loss when the patient in fact had maintained fixation well. First, there may be a high rate of false-positive responses, with the patient responding even when he does not see the stimulus (see Fig. 13-42). Second, the location of the blind spot may have been inaccurately determined at the beginning of the test so the stimulus is being presented in a seeing location instead of in the blind spot of that individual.

Frequency-of-seeing curve, zone of uncertainty, short-term fluctuations, and root mean square. If threshold is determined several times, there will be some variability in the values obtained due possibly to patient unreliability and/or inconsistency. However, even for patients who are perfectly alert and attentive, who maintain perfect fixation, and who never blink at the moment of stimulus presentation, there is likely to be a certain minimum variability of responsiveness to stimuli near the boundary between visible and invisible stimuli. This zone, several decibels wide, is represented by the *frequency-of-seeing curve*.

FIG. 13-10. Frequency of seeing curve. There is a range of stimulus intensities in which the stimulus is seen only sometimes, and this range represents a zone of "uncertainty."

Thus, at a given point, a certain stimulus intensity may be clearly infrathreshold (never seen); a stimulus 1 dB more intense may be seen 30% of the time and when picked out be barely perceptible or maybe ambiguous; a stimulus 1 dB more intense may be seen 60% of the time and often with a greater degree of certainty; and, finally, a stimulus 1 dB even more intense may be seen more than 99% of the time or virtually always. An accurate determination of threshold in these circumstances would require repeated presentations of stimuli at each of the intensities in this zone of uncertainty, with threshold defined as the intensity that was seen *50% of the time*.

In clinical testing, repeated presentations for each threshold determination are usually not practical. Instead, threshold is estimated with a certain crudeness based on presenting a series of stimuli 4 dB apart, perhaps with a refinement to the closest 2 dB. As it is being determined, the last several presentations will be within the zone of uncertainty and have a certain likelihood of not being seen. The value reported as "threshold" depends on whether or not the patient happens to respond to each of these last several stimuli. If the same sequence of stimuli were to be presented immediately again, the patient might respond to a stimulus intensity to which he previously had not, or vice versa. The threshold value determined and reported on the printout would be a bit different. Both determinations are estimates.

The intratest variability that would occur in the reported threshold values if tested several times (which would result from both the psychophysiologic "frequency of seeing curve" and the algorithm or strategy used by a given computer program to estimate threshold) has been called *short-term fluctuation*. It is the variability of repeated threshold determinations that occurs within a given testing session. Short-term fluctuations (intratest variability) are typically in the range of 2 to 3 dB. Some authors have found this magnitude of variability throughout the field, but others have found it somewhat larger in locations away from fixation (e.g., 5 to 6 dB near 30 degrees).

FIG. 13-11. Static cut "true" threshold values as a smooth curve. Surrounding this is a zone of uncertainty with physiologically inconsistent responses. Actual threshold values as might be determined during static threshold perimetry are indicated in red, with the error bar showing short-term fluctuations.

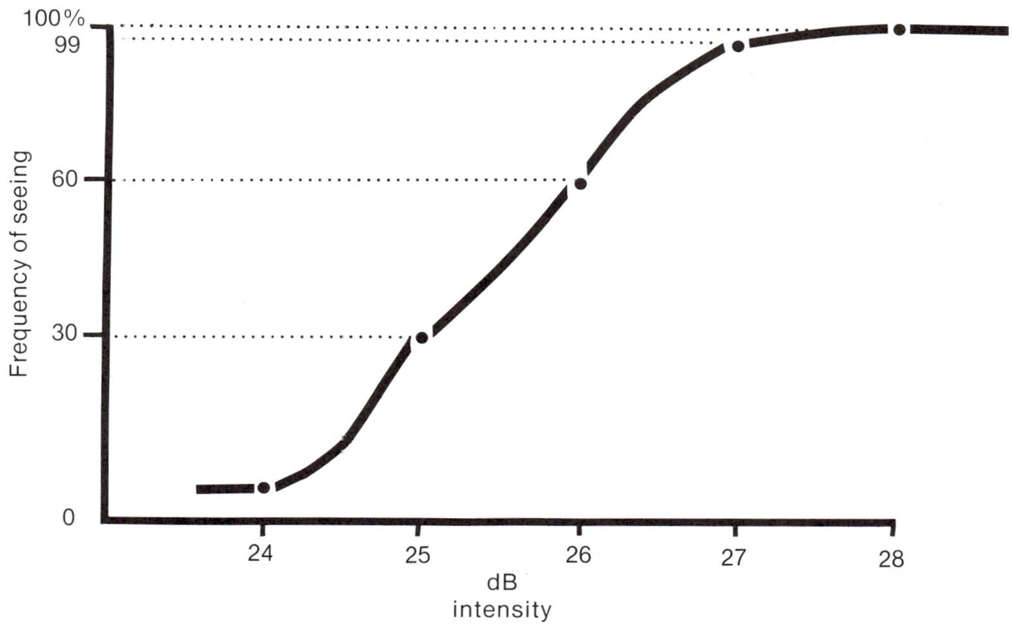

FIG. 13-10

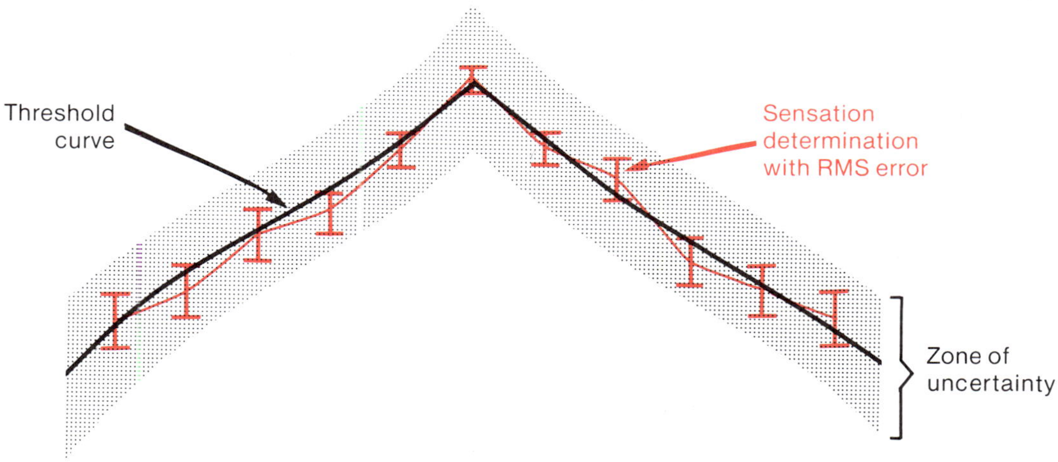

FIG. 13-11

To calculate the intratest variability in a given patient (eye) on a given occasion, many automated programs perform duplicate (or multiple) determinations of threshold at selected locations or even at all locations. The variability is essentially equivalent to the standard deviation of the repeat measurements and is reported as the *root mean square* (RMS) or fluctuation. It constitutes an estimate of the accuracy of the threshold determinations on this occasion in this patient and can be taken to mean that, for 68% of the points tested, the reported value is within 1 RMS of the "true" threshold value and that 96% of the reported values will be within 2 RMS of the true threshold.

The intratest variability score has a certain minimum obtainable value, which is the short-term fluctuation determined by the frequency-of-seeing curve and the test strategy. However, the fluctuation score can be made larger by imperfect patient attentiveness or inconsistent responsiveness, which is the reason for actually measuring the variability in a given patient on a given occasion. Thus a fluctuation score of 2 to 3 dB would be considered usual under the best of circumstances whereas one of 5 or 6 dB (or even larger) would reflect inconsistent patient responsiveness, which would have to be taken into account when interpreting the results.

FIG. 13-12. Numeric printout of static threshold tests on two patients. The reliability of the field test is judged by the false-positive rate, the false-negative rate, the frequency of fixation loss, and the fluctuation.
A, The numeric value of *21* dB (circled) is an estimate, and with a fluctuation score of *1.6* dB a 64% likelihood exists that the actual threshold is in the range of 21 ± 1.6 dB (19.4 to 22.6 dB). There is also a 96% likelihood that the sensitivity is in the range of 21 ± 3.2 dB (17.8 to 24.2 dB). Thus there is a 4% chance that the error is more than 3.2 dB and that it may occur at 2 to 4 points in a field where 76 points are being tested. The number of questions asked was *436* and indicates how many stimulus presentations were made, which reflects the length of time the test took.
B, The fluctuation value in this example is *2.32* dB. The number of questions asked *(513)* is indicated as well as the actual time of the test (*16* min, *57* sec).

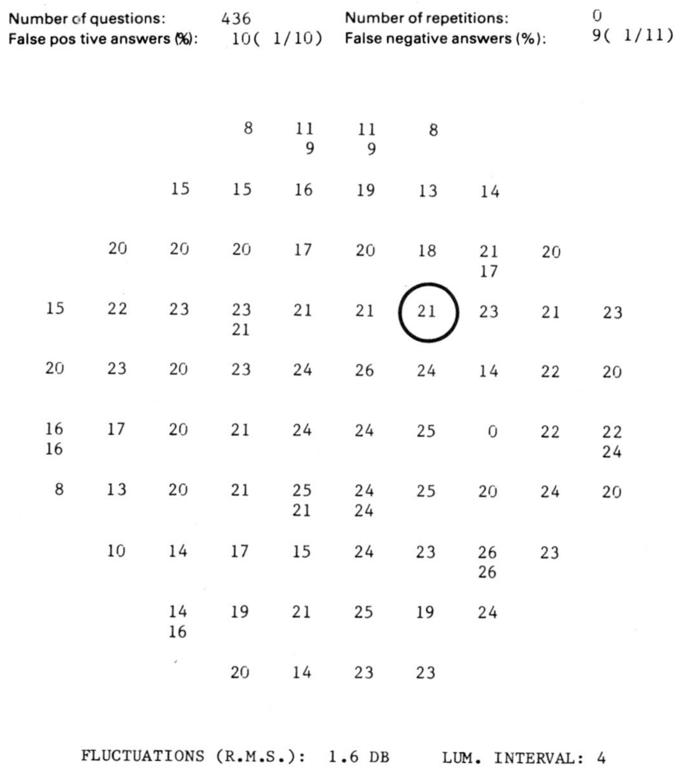
Number of questions: 436
Number of repetitions: 0
False pos tive answers (%): 10(1/10)
False negative answers (%): 9(1/11)
FLUCTUATIONS (R.M.S.): 1.6 DB
LUM. INTERVAL: 4

A

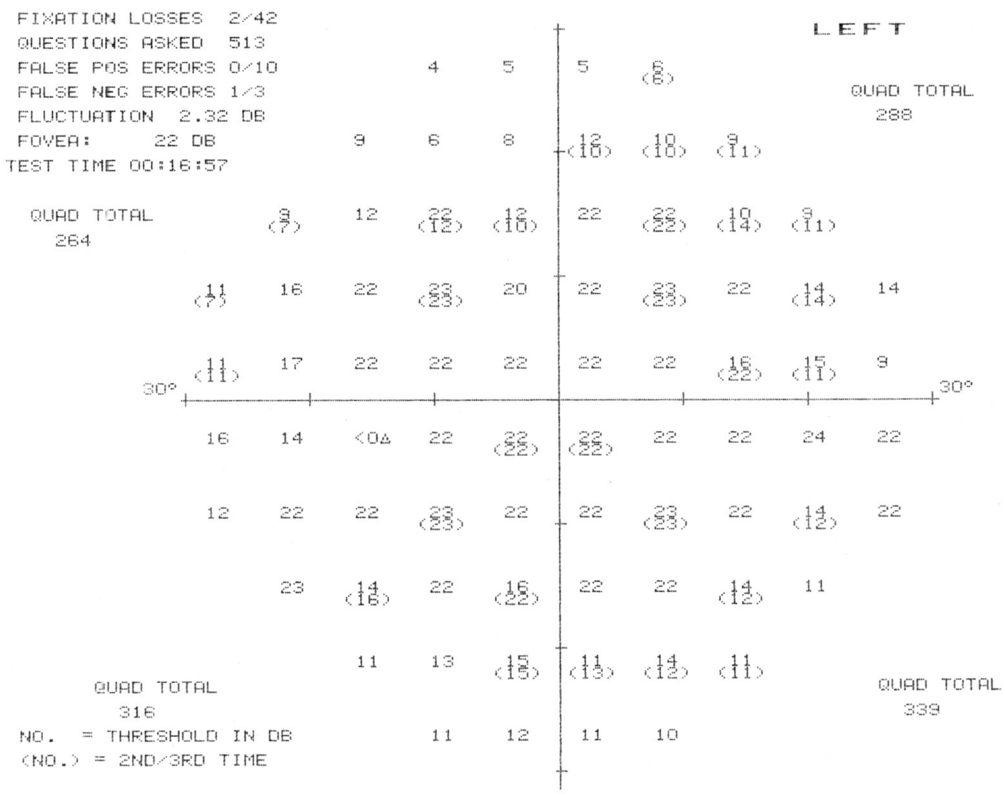
FIXATION LOSSES 2/42
QUESTIONS ASKED 513
FALSE POS ERRORS 0/10
FALSE NEG ERRORS 1/3
FLUCTUATION 2.32 DB
FOVEA: 22 DB
TEST TIME 00:16:57
LEFT
QUAD TOTAL
288
QUAD TOTAL
264
QUAD TOTAL
316
QUAD TOTAL
339
30°
30°
NO. = THRESHOLD IN DB
(NO.) = 2ND/3RD TIME

B

FIG. 13-12

The sensitivity values reported in Fig. 13-12 are estimates of threshold, and their variability is a gauge of the likely amount of error in the estimate. The examiner may wish not merely to estimate the error but also to reduce it when it is critical. The error of a threshold estimation can be reduced by determining sensitivity several times and taking the average. In some automated programs, if a limited number of points are tested, threshold is determined two or three times at each point. In other programs threshold is routinely redetermined at points where the first value was out of keeping with the expected based on the threshold of adjacent points. The reasoning is that if adjacent points have similar sensitivity values the values are mutually confirmatory and the errors are probably small. However, when a point has a deviant sensitivity value, it may be either an erroneous determination or a defective location in the field. A repeated test of such a point will help make the distinction.

Incidentally, the intratest variability is greater at points with reduced sensitivity (see Figs. 13-14 and 14-1) and a high variability of threshold determination is expected in abnormal regions of the field. A high variability in threshold values at such points does not indicate that the patient is unreliable in his responses. When judging the meaning of high fluctuations in score, the examiner must know whether the particular program used only normal points or both normal and abnormal to calculate the variability score.

See Figs. 14-2 and 23-7 for implications of the zone of uncertainty in kinetic perimetry.

Localized defects

A localized defect is present if there is some region in the field where visual sensitivity is reduced while other areas are unaffected or are affected to a lesser degree. A localized defect can be recognized and evaluated in several types of data presentations:

1. NUMERIC PRINTOUT. The display of actual sensitivity values gives the most complete information. Localized defects are recognized by comparison of all the data points with (a) surrounding points and (b) equivalent points in a mirror-image location (e.g., points to the right and to the left of the vertical meridian, or above and below the nasal meridian). Often the examiner may have to consider other printouts first to get an initial clue concerning localized defects before looking at the numeric printout.
2. GREYSCALES. Many localized defects can be instantly appreciated by examination of a greyscale. Especially when the greyscale suggests a small or shallow defect, the clinician should examine the numeric printout of actual threshold or sensitivity values to be able to judge the depth of a reduced sensitivity before reaching a conclusion as to the presence of a localized defect.

3. DIFFERENCE-FROM-NORMAL PRINTOUT (CO or Total Deviation printout). This indicates the amount of depressed visual sensation from the normal sensitivity for age. As a rule of thumb, the following may be useful: the minimum defect to which attention can be paid is a single point depressed more than 10 dB from normal, two points depressed at least 8 or 9 dB from the mean normal, or three or more points in a typical location depressed 5 or 6 dB from normal.

   It should be noted that this printout gives a comparison with the normal value at each point; however, the criterion for a localized defect is a depressed sensitivity compared to surrounding points, not compared to normal values. Therefore, when only a few points are mildly abnormal, the printout of actual threshold values must be consulted. For example, all the points in the visual field may be 3 or 4 dB less sensitive than the average normal value but are still within the normal range. Because of short-term fluctuation, there may be several points whose reported sensitivity is an additional 2 or 3 dB less, in total bringing these points 5 dB lower than the average sensitivity for a person of that age. Yet these points may not be actually depressed (as a localized defect) compared to surrounding points.

   The contrary situation may also exist: In a given normal person all the points in the visual fields may be 3 or 4 dB more sensitive than the average normal value, and within the field there may be a cluster of points distinctly depressed 7 to 9 dB below the surrounding points and thus representing a scotoma; however, because the sensitivity values remain within the "normal" range, even for these points, there is no indication of the scotoma on the difference-from-normal printout.

   Therefore, although the greyscales and the difference-from-normal printouts may assist by calling attention to certain regions that need careful attention, it is always necessary to look at the numeric printout of actual sensitivity values.

4. DIFFERENCE-FROM-EXPECTED PRINTOUT (Pattern Deviation printout). This highlights localized defects by compensating for slight variances in the height of the hill of vision. It utilizes threshold information from a few selected points to calculate an anticipated value for all the tested points, based on the assumption of a certain normal slope to the hill of vision. It indicates the difference between measured threshold and expected threshold.

5. PROBABILITY-OF-ABNORMALITY PRINTOUT. The probability that a given point is deviant from the average normal value (i.e., outside the normal range for that point) can be calculated from not only the average normal value but also the range or variability of normal values; the variability may be greater for points away from fixation than for those near fixation.

To decide if a localized defect is absent or present, the clinician must apply some of the same principles used for suprathreshold testing (see p. 219 and Figs. 13-1 to 13-9). Two, three, or four points of slightly depressed sensitivity and clustered together in a typical location are not likely to be an accident of testing. A single such point or several in scattered locations might be the result of lapses in attention or a chance occurrence from short-term fluctuation. Nonetheless, a single point may be worthy of attention if its sensitivity is extremely reduced, representing a small but very deep scotoma.

FIG. 13-13. Well-developed localized defect. The defective points superiorly have a reduced sensitivity compared to surrounding points and compared to equivalent points in the inferior field. They are also indentified on the difference-from-expected printout and the greyscale. See Fig. 6-5 for another example.

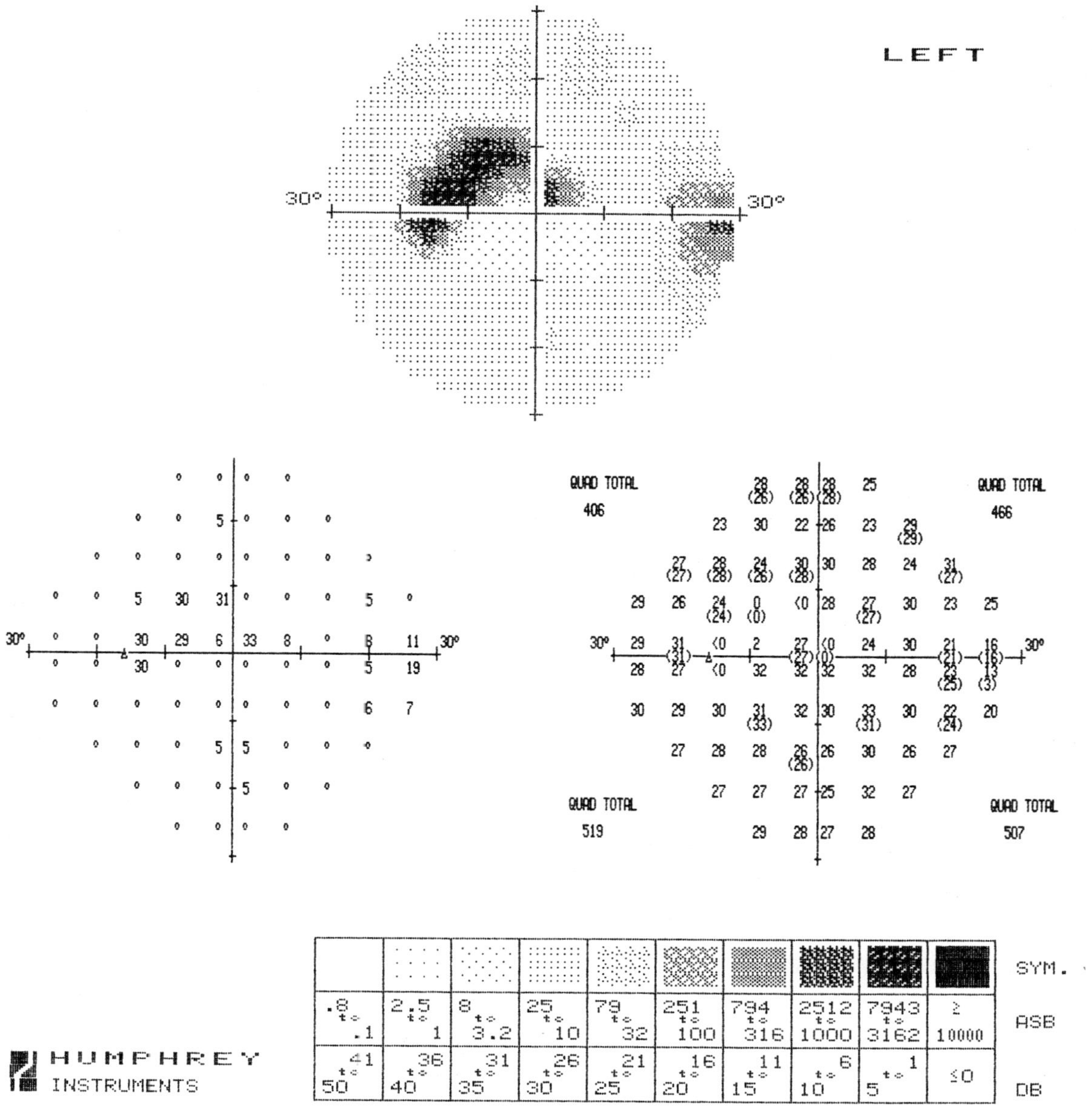
LEFT
30°
30°
QUAD TOTAL
406
QUAD TOTAL
466
QUAD TOTAL
519
QUAD TOTAL
507
HUMPHREY
INSTRUMENTS
SYM.
ASB
DB

FIG. 13-13

FIG. 13-14. Visual field with a small scotoma affecting one test point. This abnormality was confirmed in three subsequent tests and corresponded to the clinical observation of a splinter hemorrhage at the lower temporal margin of the disc with an early glaucomatous cup.

Of note is that the root mean square (RMS) is quite low, indicating a reliable field and low variability of response at the normal points. The abnormal point, however, has a much larger variability than the normal points (sensitivity of 0, 1, 8, and 15 dB on the four occasions). Although the variability of the sensitivity noted over several different test sessions includes both long-term fluctuation (to be discussed later) and short-term fluctuation, a large short-term fluctuation here was confirmed in this patient (see Fig. 14-1).

Exam #1

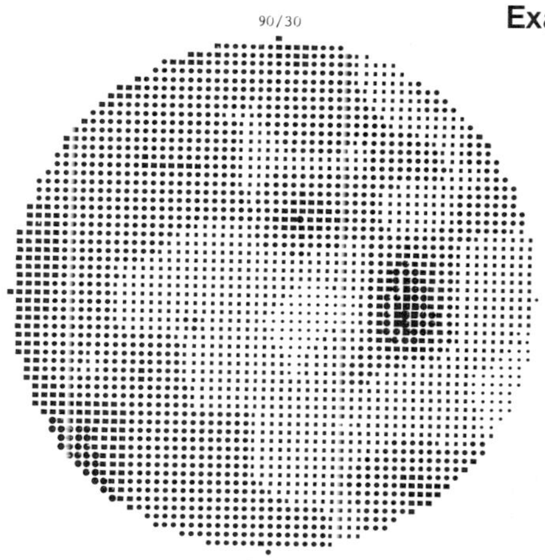

FLUCTUATIONS (R.M.S.): 1.5 DB   LUM. INTERVAL: 4

			20	23 23	21 19	26			
		23	25	26	23	25	26		
	24	20	20	27	26	26	23 25	26	
19	22	23	27 23	25	(15)	23	29	25	25
18	25	26	29	28	30	30	12	26	28
20 20	23	28	25	30	32	31	3	26	30 28
20	27	20	27	29 27	30 32	23	30	30	32
	16	22	25	25	28	31	28 26	29	
		24 22	25	25	29	25	20		
			22	22	23	27			

Y
FLUCTUATIONS (R.M.S.): 1.5 DB   LUM. INTERVAL: 4

Exam #2

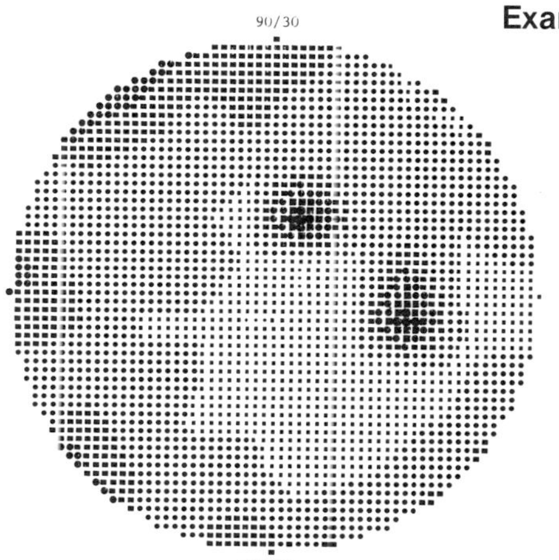

FLUCTUATIONS (R.M.S.): 1.3 DB   LUM. INTERVAL: 2

			17	20 18	18 20	23			
		17	23	19	23	22	25		
	20	23	23	25	22	24	23 24	25	
22	23	24	24 26	27	(0)	22	25	25	22
16	23	22	21	27	31	28	15	27	26
17 18	21	26	26	31	30	27	1	25	28 28
23	23	25	25	29 27	30 28	28	29	26	24
	19	23	26	26	27	26	25 27	25	
		20 23	24	24	28	26	25		
			21	19	23	22			

Y
FLUCTUATIONS (R.M.S.): 1.3 DB   LUM. INTERVAL: 2

Exam #3

			18	21 20	20 20	21			
		19	22	21	23	23	24		
	20	22	22	25	19	21	24 23	22	
9	23	23	26 24	25	(8)	21	26	24	24
17	16	25	24	26	28	26	20	26	27
16 19	18	28	28	28	30	30	0	26	27 27
19	23	22	23	27 26	29 29	26	28	25	28
	20	21	24	27	28	26	27 25	25	
		18 21	25	27	28	24	23		
			20	21	23	23			

Y
FLUCTUATIONS (R.M.S.): 1.2 DB   LUM. INTERVAL: 2

Exam #4

			19	20 19	18 20	17			
		21	18	22	24	24	24		
	24	20	22	24	20	22	24 25	24	
17	23	24	22 24	24	(1)	21	25	22	25
17	20	22	24	27	30	26	21	26	27
22 21	21	25	27	29	28	30	0	24	26 28
20	22	24	25	28 28	29 27	26	29	27	26
	21	23	22	26	28	26	25 25	27	
		17 20	25	26	29	27	25		
			19	20	22	23			

Y
FLUCTUATIONS (R.M.S.): 1.2 DB   LUM. INTERVAL: 2

FIG. 13-14

In addition to looking for points with sensitivities that are depressed from normal values (or depressed compared to points in the immediate surround), the clinician should compare the value of an average representative cluster of points with that of an equivalent cluster in the opposite hemifield. For example, when looking for a hemianopia, he can compare points to the right and to left of the vertical meridian. Similarly the points above and below the nasal horizontal meridian can be compared when looking for a glaucomatous visual field defect. Also, equivalent regions in the upper and lower arcuate regions can be compared. Of course, it must be taken into account that superiorly the visual field normally has a slightly depressed sensitivity compared to the inferior field (pp. 86-87).

FIG. 13-15. Comparison of the upper arcuate region (sensitivity, about 20 dB) with the lower arcuate region (sensitivity, about 28 dB). This may be more than the physiologic degree of depression of the upper field as compared to the lower field and is suspicious. Its significance can be judged only from the clinical examination. (Is there cupping of the disc toward the inferior rim? Is there ptosis of the upper eyelid?)

FIG. 13-16. More definite abnormality of the superior field. Either a lens rim artifact or an upper nasal depression from glaucoma can produce the severely reduced threshold value at the upper nasal edge of the field. Glaucomatous abnormality is more likely because blocks of points in the upper field, but not at the edge, are depressed compared to equivalent points in the lower field.

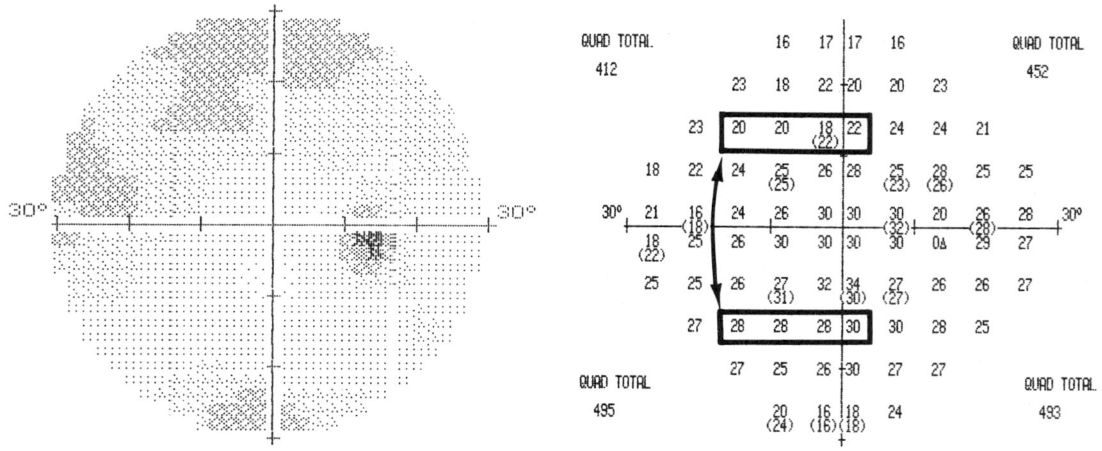

FIG. 13-15

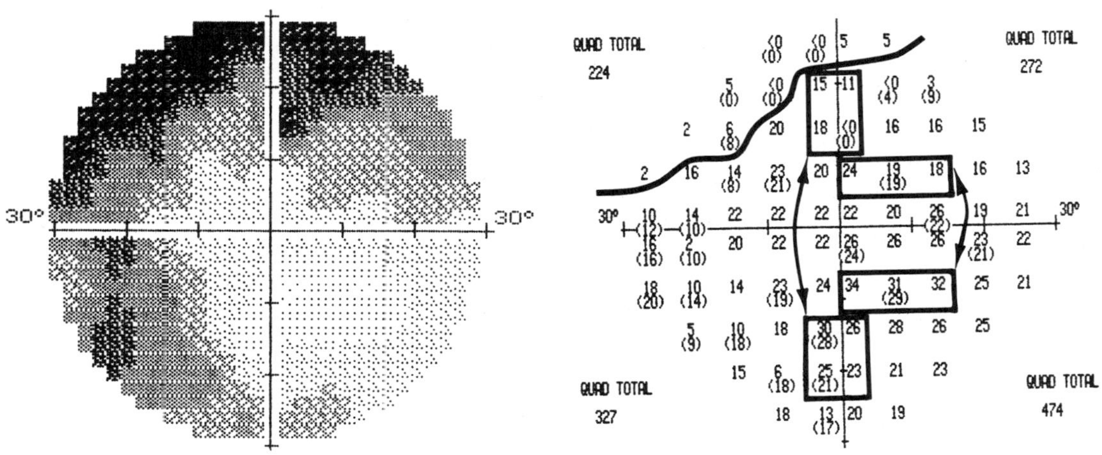

FIG. 13-16

FIG. 13-17. Irregular localized defects. In both the upper and the lower arcuate regions certain points (circled) are depressed compared to surrounding points (i.e., they denote scotomas). Additionally, a block of four points in the lower nasal quadrant is depressed compared to equivalent points in the upper nasal quadrant. There is, furthermore, an overall depression of sensitivity in the left compared to the right eye (note the four points around fixation in each eye). The mean sensitivities in this patient were 18.8 dB for the left and 24.0 dB for the right eye. Fig. 13-28 shows the manual kinetic field of this patient.

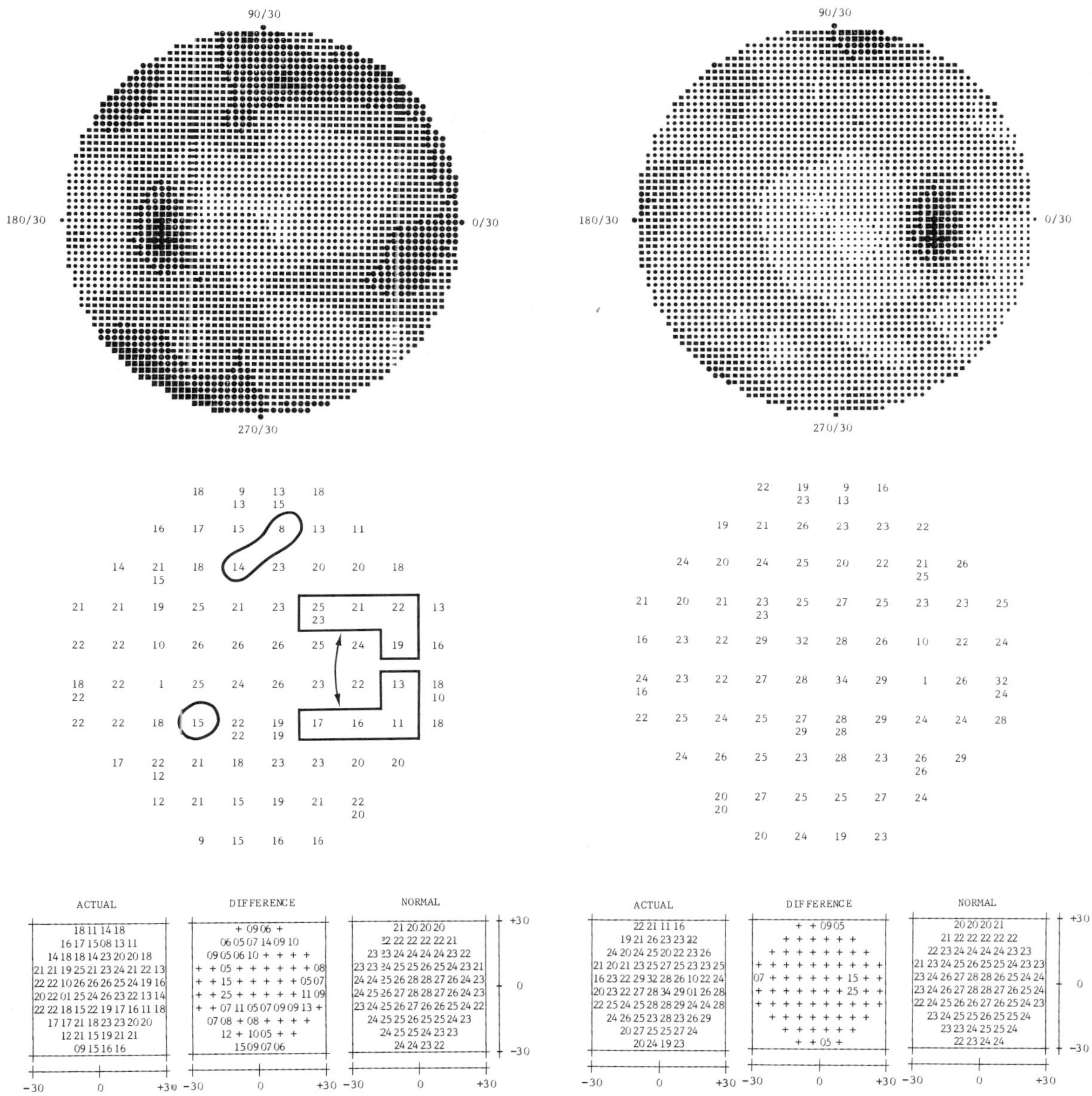

FIG. 13-17

Finally, the clinician can look at the shape of isopters (i.e., the lines that enclose all points with sensitivity greater than 25 dB, greater than 20 dB, greater than 15 dB, etc.). He then may draw lines on the numeric printout to indicate these boundaries or, equivalently, may look at a greyscale printout, which separates threshold values into such groupings. An abnormality may be indicated by a wedge of depressed sensitivity compared to equivalent wedges in other meridians, or by flattening of the normal ovoid shape of the isopter on the nasal side.

FIG. 13-18. Nasal depression of the field. Isopters for 10 and 20 dB are drawn in. Compare with Fig. 13-31, which shows the manual kinetic field of this patient.

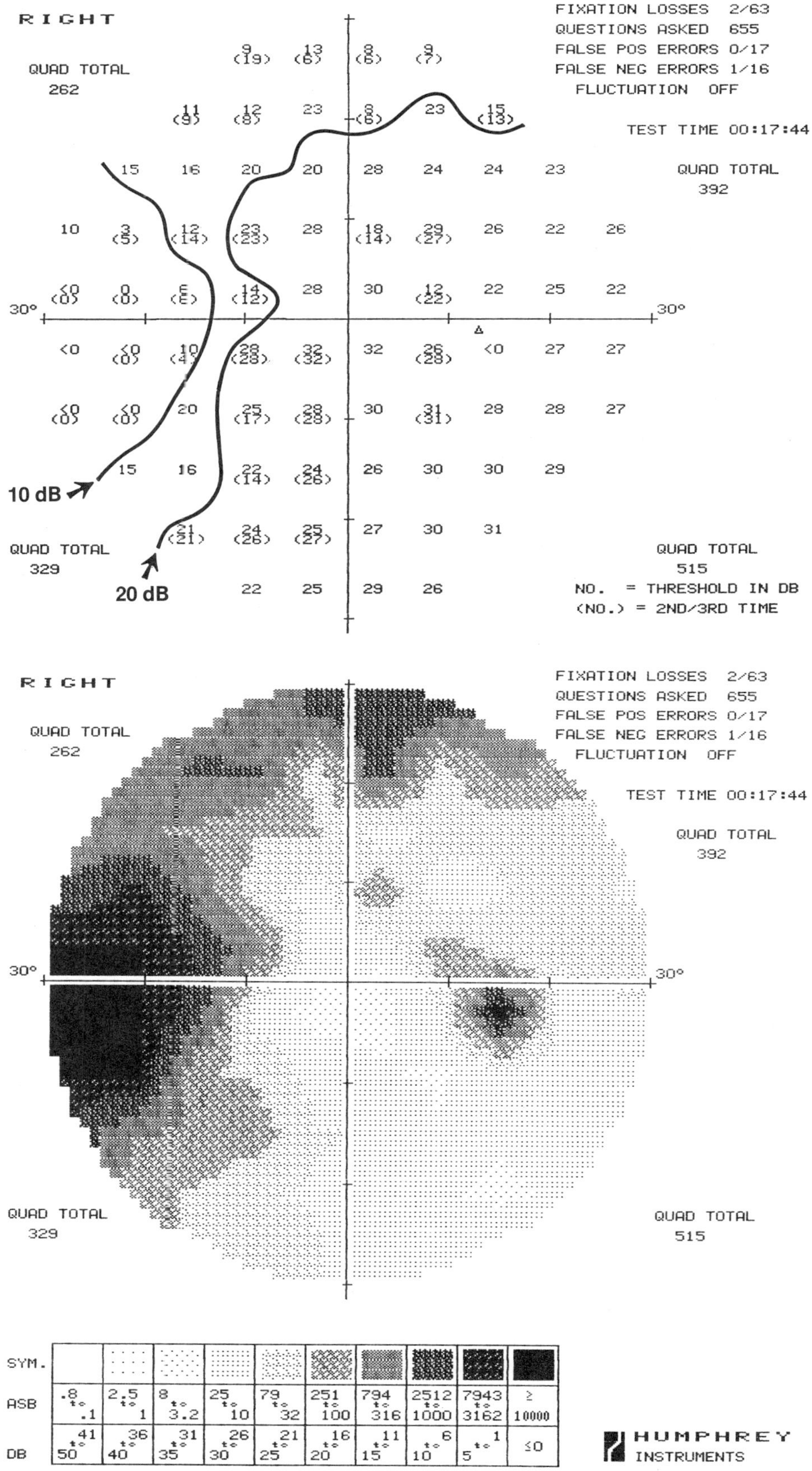
RIGHT
QUAD TOTAL 262
FIXATION LOSSES 2/63
QUESTIONS ASKED 655
FALSE POS ERRORS 0/17
FALSE NEG ERRORS 1/16
FLUCTUATION OFF
TEST TIME 00:17:44
QUAD TOTAL 392
30°
30°
10 dB
20 dB
QUAD TOTAL 329
QUAD TOTAL 515
NO. = THRESHOLD IN DB
(NO.) = 2ND/3RD TIME
RIGHT
QUAD TOTAL 262
FIXATION LOSSES 2/63
QUESTIONS ASKED 655
FALSE POS ERRORS 0/17
FALSE NEG ERRORS 1/16
FLUCTUATION OFF
TEST TIME 00:17:44
QUAD TOTAL 392
30°
30°
QUAD TOTAL 329
QUAD TOTAL 515
SYM.
ASB
.8 to .1
2.5 to 1
8 to 3.2
25 to 10
79 to 32
251 to 100
794 to 316
2512 to 1000
7943 to 3162
≥ 10000
DB
41 to 50
36 to 40
31 to 35
26 to 30
21 to 25
16 to 20
11 to 15
6 to 10
1 to 5
≤0
HUMPHREY
INSTRUMENTS

FIG. 13-18

Generalized depression

Localized defects occur when a disease process affects certain regions in the retina or certain bundles of neurons in the visual pathway while other regions or bundles are unaffected or are affected only to a lesser degree. The shape and location of the visual field defect typify and characterize the location and nature of the disease. They are recognized by comparing visual sensitivity in the affected region to that elsewhere in the visual field.

By contrast, a given disease may produce generalized visual depression either through some preretinal interference in light transmission to the retina or following diffuse involvement of the retina or other neuronal structures. Unlike localized defects, a generalized depression does not provide a topographic feature that will characterize a particular portion of the visual pathway. The presence of defective visual sensation is judged not by comparing a particular location in the field to another location but, instead, by comparing visual sensitivity at each or all locations to one of the following:

1. The range of normal values for age (pp. 245-247)
2. The values in the other eye (pp. 248-250)
3. The previously known values in that patient (p. 250)

The term *generalized depression* can be taken to mean that the sensitivity is reduced diffusely throughout all regions of the field. In the purest example the amount of reduction is about the same everywhere. However, there may be a greater decline near the center (flattening of the hill of vision), as is typical of cataract. In diffuse neuronal disease (which may occur with glaucoma) some nerve fiber bundles are more affected than others and thus the hill of vision develops an irregular contour as it is depressed (see discussion below on the loss variance index). The more affected points may correspond to locations typical of the more diagnostic localized defects. In such cases the defect is arbitrarily considered as either localized with a superimposed generalized loss (Fig. 13-17) or basically generalized with an uneven degree of involvement (Fig. 10-1, *B*). The two descriptions are equivalent.

If generalized depression is present, the clinician should not ignore it as nonspecific. Rather, he should seek to attribute it to a particular cause. If the presence of cataract does not explain the deviation from normal values or the asymmetry between eyes, he should entertain the possibility that another cause of generalized depression might be present (glaucoma, thyroid orbital disease, retinitis pigmentosa, papilledema [pseudotumor cerebri]). Any accompanying localized defects may be helpful in making the diagnosis.

Comparison to normal values. In cases with moderate generalized depression it may be easy to recognize that, on the whole, sensitivity values are 10 dB depressed compared to average normal values. Of course, some points will be 7 or 8 dB depressed compared to average values while others are 12 to 13 dB depressed, the difference representing the effect of intratest variability (short-term fluctuation, root mean square). It is possible also to take an average of all the measured sensitivities and discover that it is 10 dB less than the average of the normal sensitivities at these points.

Recognizing a 2 to 3 dB generalized depression from inspection of the numeric printout is more difficult because the depression may be hidden within the variability of the threshold determinations. Some points will have threshold determinations better than normal, and others worse than normal, and it will take careful analysis to discern that the slightly lower values are more numerous. The effect of this variability on measuring any individual point can be practically eliminated by taking the average (mean) of the sensitivities of all the points measured—points where the inaccuracy provided a falsely high threshold will be offset by an approximately equal number of points where it gave a falsely low value. As a rule of thumb, 95% of the population is included in the value ±3 dB from the mean normal and 99% are within 4 to 5 dB of the normal. Thus it may take 5 dB of depression for the abnormal to be recognizable. However, in the appropriate clinical context a 2.5 to 3 dB depression of the mean value should arouse suspicion.

FIG. 13-19. A 10 dB depression of the field. This can be recognized by comparing the actual threshold values to the normal values.

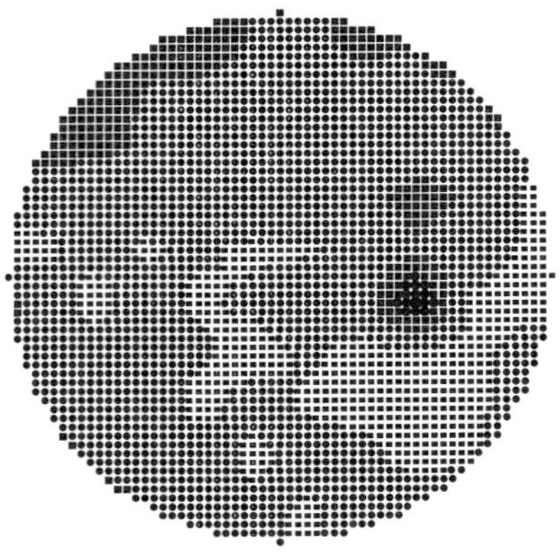

ACTUAL

			07	11	11	10			
		11	12	12	12	11	12		
	09	11	11	13	12	12	13	12	
13	14	13	13	13	12	12	09	11	16
17	14	16	15	16	16	14	11	13	16
12	17	14	16	15	13	13	00	16	17
12	14	15	15	17	15	17	17	17	14
	13	12	17	14	16	17	17	17	
		13	12	17	13	14	17		
			12	13	17	12			

−30 0 +30

DIFFERENCE

			13	09	09	11			
		10	10	10	10	11	10		
	13	12	13	11	12	12	10	11	
08	09	11	12	13	13	13	15	12	07
06	10	10	12	12	12	12	14	11	08
11	07	12	11	13	15	14	26	09	07
10	10	10	11	09	12	09	08	07	09
	10	12	08	11	10	08	08	07	
		10	11	07	12	11	07		
			10	10	07	12			

−30 0 +30

NORMAL

			20	20	20	21			
		21	22	22	22	22	22		
	22	23	24	24	24	24	23	23	
21	23	24	25	26	25	25	24	23	23
23	24	26	27	28	28	26	25	24	24
23	24	26	27	28	28	27	26	25	24
22	24	25	26	26	27	26	25	24	23
	23	24	25	25	26	25	25	24	
		23	23	24	25	25	24		
			22	23	24	24			

−30 0 +30

+30 0 −30

FIG. 13-19

FIG. 13-20. A mild generalized depression. As shown in the difference-from-normal printout, intratest variability causes randomly scattered points to have sensitivity values more than 5 dB depressed from normal. The mean sensitivity is 3 to 4 dB less than the normal value, and this field would be judged suspiciously abnormal in the appropriate clinical context. See Figs. 8-1 and 10-1 for other examples of generalized depression.

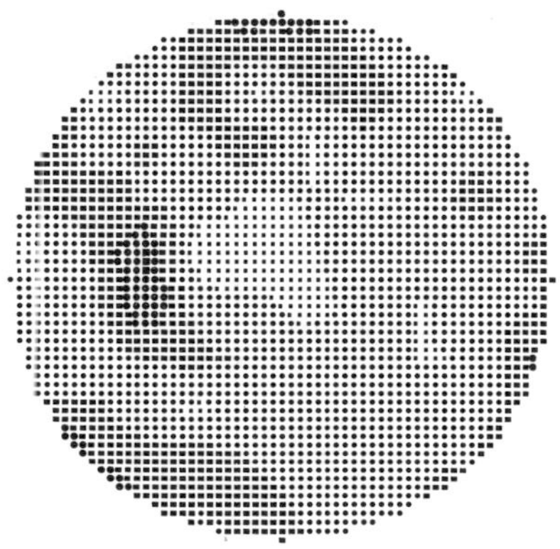

ACTUAL

```
            18 17 16 22
         24 17 27 20 17 23
      22 20 22 16 27 22 24 22
   19 19 21 21 27 25 26 25 18 23
   26 20 10 30 30 26 23 22 25 20
   23 22 11 23 24 28 23 26 23 21
   24 24 20 19 22 22 21 26 25 16
      19 24 27 22 23 25 22 24
         18 17 21 23 23 22
            21 17 22 22
-30             0             +30
```

DIFFERENCE

```
            06 06 07  +
          +  08  +  05 08  +
       +  06 05 11  +  05  +   +
   07 07 06 07  +   +   +   +  08  +
    +  07 18  +   +  05 07 07  +  06
    +  06 18 07 07  +  07  +   +  05
    +   +  08 10 08 07 08  +   +  09
      08  +   +  07 05  +  05  +
         09 11 07  +   +   +
            06 10  +   +
-30             0             +30
```

NORMAL

```
            24 23 23 23
         25 25 25 25 25 24
      26 26 27 27 27 27 26 25
   26 26 27 28 28 29 28 27 26 24
   27 27 28 29 31 31 30 29 27 26
   27 28 29 30 31 31 30 29 27 26
   26 27 28 29 30 29 29 28 27 25
      27 28 28 29 28 28 27 26
         27 28 28 27 26 26
            27 27 26 25
-30             0             +30
```

+30

0

-30

FIG. 13-20

Comparison to the other eye. Although there can be a 5 dB range of normal values among individuals, there is probably much less variation between the two eyes of a given individual. Thus, if no anisometropia or other difference is present between the two eyes, a consistent 1 or 2 dB mean sensitivity difference between the two eyes may represent mild generalized depression acquired from some disease.* (For example, in Fig. 13-17 it was noted that in the left eye even the points with normal sensitivities were depressed compared to equivalent points in the right eye, illustrating that generalized depression can be recognized by comparing the two eyes; and it was noted that both localized and general involvement can occur in the same eye.)

FIG. 13-21. Generalized depression in the right eye, A, compared to the normal left eye, B. The central reference level (arrows) is 32 dB in the left eye but less than 26 dB in the right eye. The central four points are 4 to 8 dB less sensitive in the right eye. Note that the difference-from-expected printout (lower left in **A** and **B**), which is designed to highlight localized defects, does not indicate any localized abnormalities.

---

*Brenton, R.S., et al.: Interocular differences in the visual field in normal subjects, Invest. Ophthalmol. Vis. Sci. **27**:799-805, 1986.

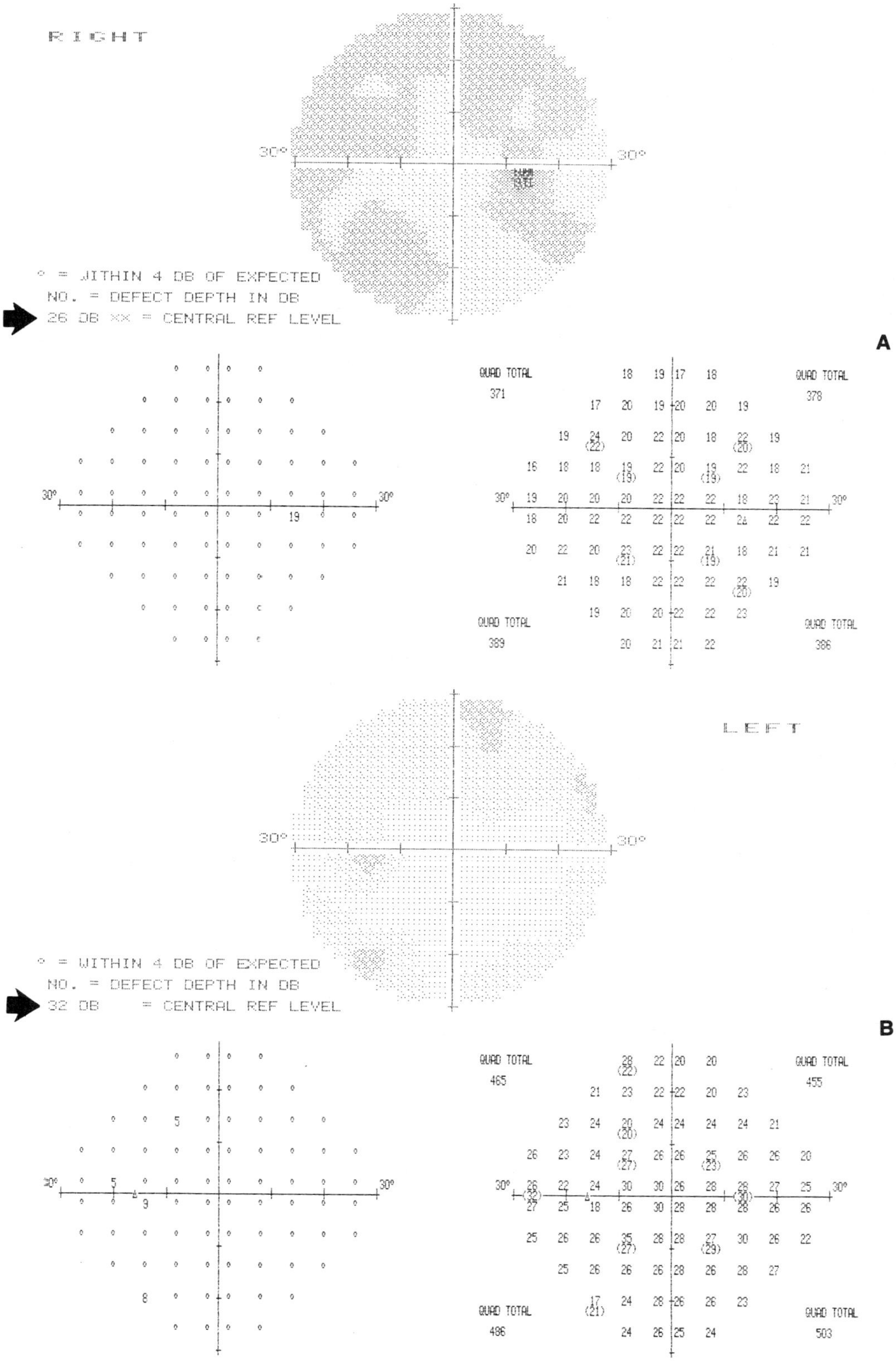
RIGHT
30°
30°
° = WITHIN 4 DB OF EXPECTED
NO. = DEFECT DEPTH IN DB
26 DB xx = CENTRAL REF LEVEL
A
QUAD TOTAL 371
QUAD TOTAL 378
QUAD TOTAL 389
QUAD TOTAL 386
LEFT
° = WITHIN 4 DB OF EXPECTED
NO. = DEFECT DEPTH IN DB
32 DB = CENTRAL REF LEVEL
B
QUAD TOTAL 465
QUAD TOTAL 455
QUAD TOTAL 486
QUAD TOTAL 503

FIG. 13-21

FIG. 13-22. Very slight generalized depression in the right eye compared to the left eye. Except in the lower temporal quadrant, the sensitivities on three consecutive occasions are consistently about 1 dB lower in the right eye than in the left. This can be perceived by looking at the numeric printout and comparing equivalent points in the two eyes (e.g., the four points around fixation). The summary tables at the bottom of the figure show average (mean) sensitivity values on the three dates. The averages of all points together, of points in each quadrant, and of points in three zones of eccentricity are given for each date. The normal mean appears in parentheses; *N: 24.1* denotes that the normal mean value is 24.1 dB.

In this patient the right eye has an elevated IOP, and its optic nerve a somewhat larger excavation, than the left eye. Such depression is recognizable only by comparing the two eyes. That it is a true defect is confirmed by its repeatability and its compatibility with other clinical findings. Note that the threshold and mean sensitivity values are within the normal range, even in the slightly depressed right eye.

Probably the most frequent cause of acquired adult generalized depression is cataract, although diffuse damage to the nerve fibers (e.g., from glaucoma) must always be considered if the clinical context is appropriate. When glaucoma produces diffuse neuronal damage, there is likely also to be some other clinical asymmetry between the two eyes so the eye with the depressed field has a slightly larger cup and higher pressure. A localized defect may not occur unless there is a localized extension of the cup caused by more severe neuronal loss in a particular sector than in other sectors.

Comparison to previous sensitivities. Given the broad range of normal values, a person who begins with a visual sensitivity in the upper part of normal may need more than 5 dB of depression before his sensitivity falls outside the normal range. The sensitivity values of all points may remain within normal limits on the difference-from-normal printout, and the mean sensitivity may be within 3 dB of the normal mean value, even though 6 or 7 dB depressed from that point's previous value.

Thus it is inevitable that there will be some individuals with early disease who will still have mean visual threshold values in the normal range. These can be recognized by comparison with the individual's own previous mean sensitivity value, taking into account long-term fluctuation as discussed on p. 310. In general, a 1 to 2 dB change up or down from one occasion to another is the expected normal long-term fluctuation; however, a greater change or a consistent downward trend signifies the development of generalized depression. The criteria are the same as for judging progression (p. 296).

Left eye

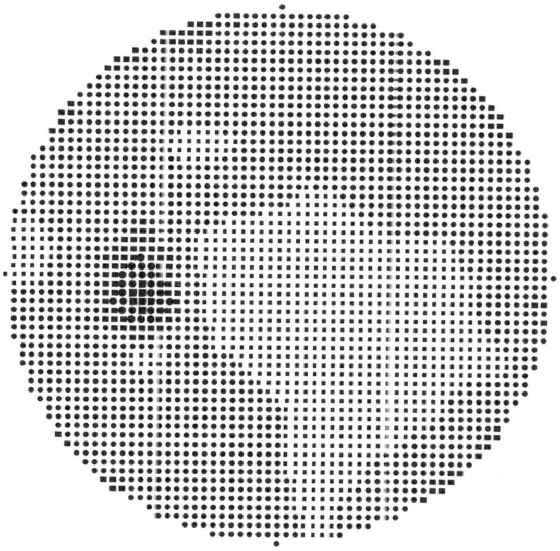

Right eye

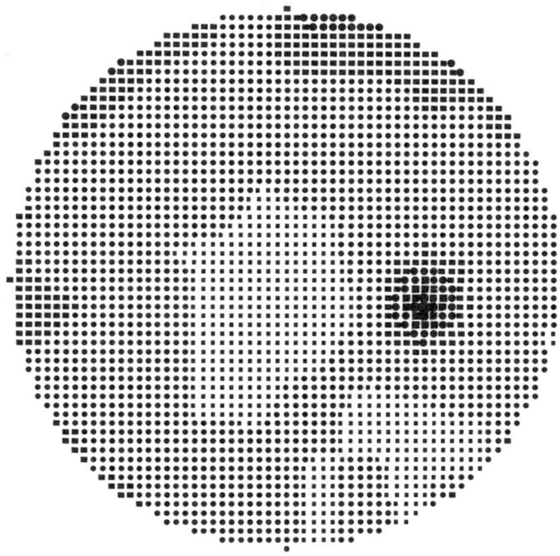

			20	22 22	24 24	24			
		2◂	21	24	24	23	24		
	24	25 25	27	25	23	25	22	23	
24	24	24	24	24	26	26 25	22	25	23
27	23	17	26	28	28	26	27	25	25
25 25	24	5	25	30	28	27	27	26	22 21
25	24	25	25	26 27	27 28	27	27	27	25
	25	25 24	21	25	26	28	27	24	
		24	24	25	26	26	25 24		
			23	23	26	25			

			20	22 22	16 17	16			
		21	22	21	22	22	20		
	21	22	23	24	25	23	22 21	22	
21	23	24	25 24	26	25	25	22	22	22
22	24	25	26	26	27	24	20	22	24
20 19	21	23	26	27	28	25	0	24	25 24
21	23	23	26	26 26	26 26	24	23	23	25
	23	24	26	26	24	27	27 26	25	
		24 23	22	24	26	25	27		
			24	23	26	25			

DATE OF EXAM : DAY YEAR	12.01 1983	03.22 1984	05.23 1985
MEAN SENSITIVITY			
WHOLE FIELD (N: 24.1)	24.7	25.0	24.8
QUAD.UPP.NAS.(N: 23.4)	23.3	24.5	24.4
LOW.NAS.(N: 24.4)	26.6	25.9	26.0
UPP.TMP.(N: 23.5)	23.5	24.2	24.2
LOW.TMP.(N: 25.1)	25.5	25.4	24.7
ECC. 0 - 10 (N: 26.9)	27.1	27.3	26.8
10 - 20 (N: 24.9)	25.0	25.2	25.2
20 - 30 (N: 23.0)	24.0	24.3	24.2

DATE OF EXAM : DAY YEAR	12.01 1983	03.22 1984	05.23 1985
MEAN SENSITIVITY			
WHOLE FIELD (N: 24.1)	23.7	24.3	23.5
QUAD.UPP.NAS.(N: 23.4)	23.2	23.8	23.0
LOW.NAS.(N: 24.4)	24.5	24.7	23.7
UPP.TMP.(N: 23.5)	21.9	22.8	22.2
LOW.TMP.(N: 25.1)	25.3	25.8	25.2
ECC. 0 - 10 (N: 26.9)	26.5	26.7	26.0
10 - 20 (N: 24.9)	24.8	24.6	24.3
20 - 30 (N: 23.0)	22.5	23.5	22.5

FIG. 13-22

Use of indices

The use of *mean sensitivity* as an index in judging the presence of generalized depression has already been explained. If the mean sensitivity value of an individual is subtracted from his normal mean sensitivity, the *mean defect* or *mean deviation* index will be obtained. When these points are, on average, 5 dB less sensitive than normal, their defectiveness will average 5 dB. It is possible also to obtain the numeric value by determining how far each point is below the normal value (4 dB, 6 dB, 5 dB, etc.) and finding that the average defectiveness is 5dB. This is mathematically identical to taking the average of the actual thresholds determined and subtracting it from the average of the mean normal values. Some printouts give mean sensitivity or defect for each quadrant and for each zone of eccentricity separately. (The quadrant total sensitivity is equivalent, becoming mean sensitivity if divided by the number of points.)

If half the points were absolutely normal and the other half 10 dB less sensitive than normal, there would still be a mean defect of 5 dB. On the other hand, if the abnormal half were only 5 dB less sensitive than normal the mean defect would be 2.5 dB. If only three or four points were abnormal, the mean defect would be even less affected because so many of the points were entirely normal. Thus the mean defect index, relating to average defectiveness, will be affected by a widespread generalized depression (even if mild) but will not be affected as much by a local defect unless rather large or very deep, or both.

To recognize mathematically the occurrence of localized defects, there are at least two approaches already proposed. One is to calculate how often the sensitivity values deviate more widely than they should from the normal sensitivity value after it is adjusted for the mean defect value of the individual (*loss variance,* or *pattern standard deviation,* index). It is possible, in performing such calculations, to take into account the actual short-term fluctuations (RMS score) of the individual patient to obtain the *corrected loss variance* (CLV), or *corrected pattern standard deviation* (CPSD), index. A second approach is to determine to what degree the sensitivity values deviate from what would be expected based on sensitivity of the surrounding points.

FIG. 13-23. Several recognizable localized defects (circled) in locations typical of glaucoma. Note that the abnormal points are less sensitive than the normal values and also less sensitive than the surrounding points. These two characteristics are the bases for two mathematical approaches to calculating the likelihood of the presence of localized defects.

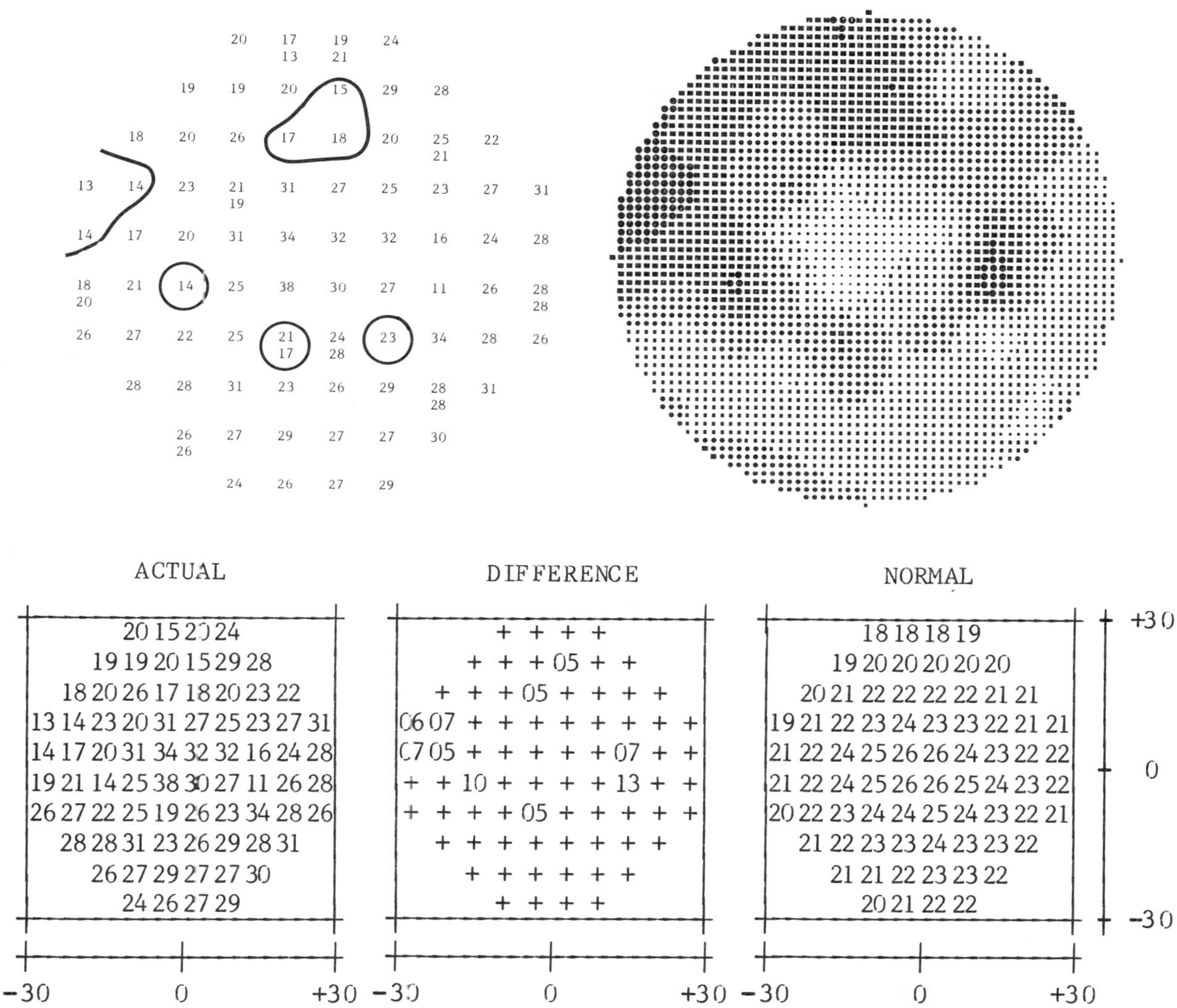
ACTUAL
20 15 20 24
19 19 20 15 29 28
18 20 26 17 18 20 23 22
13 14 23 20 31 27 25 23 27 31
14 17 20 31 34 32 32 16 24 28
19 21 14 25 38 30 27 11 26 28
26 27 22 25 19 26 23 34 28 26
28 28 31 23 26 29 28 31
26 27 29 27 27 30
24 26 27 29
DIFFERENCE
+ + + +
+ + + 05 + +
+ + + 05 + + + +
06 07 + + + + + + + +
07 05 + + + + + 07 + +
+ + 10 + + + + 13 + +
+ + + + 05 + + + + +
+ + + + + + + +
+ + + + + +
+ + + +
NORMAL
18 18 18 19
19 20 20 20 20 20
20 21 22 22 22 22 21 21
19 21 22 23 24 23 23 22 21 21
21 22 24 25 26 26 24 23 22 22
21 22 24 25 26 26 25 24 23 22
20 22 23 24 24 25 24 23 22 21
21 22 23 23 24 23 23 22
21 21 22 23 23 22
20 21 22 22
+30
0
-30
-30
0
+30

FIG. 13-23

In glaucoma some individuals appear to have a shallow generalized depression, reflected in an abnormal mean defect index, whereas others have small to moderate localized defects, reflected in the loss variance or an equivalent index (uncorrected and corrected). The localized defects may be small enough or shallow enough (or both) to have little effect on the mean defect index. As they become more advanced, however, they affect both indices.

The use of indices is just beginning and will have to undergo validation through widespread applications. Some presently defined indices may prove useful; others must undoubtedly evolve. One suggestion that has been advanced calls for a *spatial correlation* in which the abnormality of a given point is given greater weight according to any abnormality present in adjacent points. Thus two points that are adjacent and somewhat abnormal count more heavily than two equivalent points that are in separate parts of the visual field. Regardless of any developments, indices will not eliminate the need for careful analysis and judgment. The practitioner must still determine whether a localized or a generalized defect causing an abnormal index might be an artifact (see Fig. 13-43). However, indices do serve to call attention to fields that need more careful inspection.

The mean sensitivity index is used not only for recognizing the presence of an abnormality but also for comparing field examinations to recognize progression (pp. 302-329).

ADDITIONAL READING

A more detailed explanation of the preliminary indices currently proposed can be found in the following:

Bebie, H.: Computerized techniques of visual field analysis. In Drance, S.M., and Anderson, D.R., editors. Automatic perimetry in glaucoma, Orlando, Fla., 1985, Grune & Stratton, Inc., pp. 147-160.

Flammer, J.: The concept of visual field indices, Graefes Arch. Clin. Exp. Ophthalmol. **224:**389-392, 1986.

Sommer, A., et al.: Analytic approaches to the interpretation of automated threshold perimetric data for the diagnosis of early glaucoma, Trans. Am. Ophthalmol. Soc. **83:**250-267, 1985.

RECOGNIZING ABNORMALITIES WITH MANUAL KINETIC PERIMETRY
Quality of the test

The advocated technique for manual perimetry is a mixture:

First, kinetic perimetry is mixed with suprathreshold static perimetry for the purpose of detecting scotomas and verifying isopter position.

Second, detection is mixed with defect confirmation and quantitation. The technique is altered to confirm that a defect is real by rechecking locations that do not fit in with the suspected normal or abnormal isopter position. Quantitation is achieved by checking a closer cluster of points to outline the defect exactly in an abnormal region and by plotting with more than one isopter, simultaneously confirming its presence and quantifying its exact depth.

Third, an element of interpretation and differential diagnosis is mixed into the performance of the field test. The perimetrist recognizes a defect as it is being revealed and may plot isopters in specific areas that will help distinguish two different types of defects. Additionally, he represents his interpretation on the plotted diagram: a nasal step is or is not indicated on the diagram according to his interpretation of the responses. An area of inconsistent responses is represented as a shallow scotoma only if he is convinced that there is something abnormal about that region.

Thus the clinician who did not perform the test but who examines the diagram later is looking at elements of both screening and quantitation and, in addition, an element of evaluation (either correct or incorrect) furnished by the perimetrist.

As always, when the clinician interprets a field diagram, the first step is to evaluate the quality of the test. In addition to noting statements about the patient's consistency of responses and quality of fixation, he must judge the technical aspects of the field test. He may or may not have knowledge of the perimetrist's competence depending on whether the test was performed in his own office or in someone else's office. It is helpful to know from personal experience whether the perimetrist is one who may miss a small or shallow defect by being too hasty when spot-checking or one who "overcalls" a shallow scotoma if the patient happens to be a bit slow in responding.

In any event, an additional judgment about the quality of the test can be made from the diagram. The perimetrist should have noted the constancy of the patient's fixation and the reliability of his responses.* Was the correct lens used? Were central as well as peripheral isopters plotted? Is there evidence of adequate spot-checking of relevant areas? Did the perimetrist know the suspected diagnosis and check certain more relevant areas with particular care? Are the depths of any scotomas and localized depressions determined?

---

*An instructive set of examples of technical errors that can be recognized by the interpreter is given in Chapter 9 of Trobe, J.D., and Glaser, J.S.: *The Visual Fields Manual,* Gainesville, Fla., 1983, Triad Publishing Co.

Negative test

The first step in the interpretation of a negative test is to make a judgment about the thoroughness and appropriateness of the examination with regard to the nature, size, and depth of the defects being looked for. If no field defect was detected, the basic questions are "What defects (according to location, size, depth) could have escaped detection by the technique used?" and "Is the defect that could have been missed one that I am interested in?" If hemianopia was suspected, were the proper examination strategies performed to detect it? If a central scotoma was suspected, were the central five degrees tested adequately? To detect scotomas, was the relevant region explored? Were a sufficient number of points tested to detect a small scotoma? Was the stimulus used appropriate to detect shallow scotomas? Were enough points plotted on an isopter in the areas where a defect might exist?

FIG. 13-24. Limits of detectability.
A, Shallow scotomas near the isopter. These will be detected, but scotomas further inward must be deeper to be discovered. Only two of the three scotomas would be discovered with the *I-3e* stimulus. The shallower scotoma near fixation would escape detection. The interpreter must be conscious of the fact that, when spot-checking is done with only one stimulus, scotomas less than 0.5 log-unit deep might escape detection in the region of the field close to fixation (see Fig. 21-7).
B, Isopter plot based on six points. The clinician must realize that only the six points at which the patient responded to a stimulus were actually tested and that the line connecting the points may or may not be a smooth curve. Additional points must be plotted for a determination to be made that a nasal step is or is not present.

A

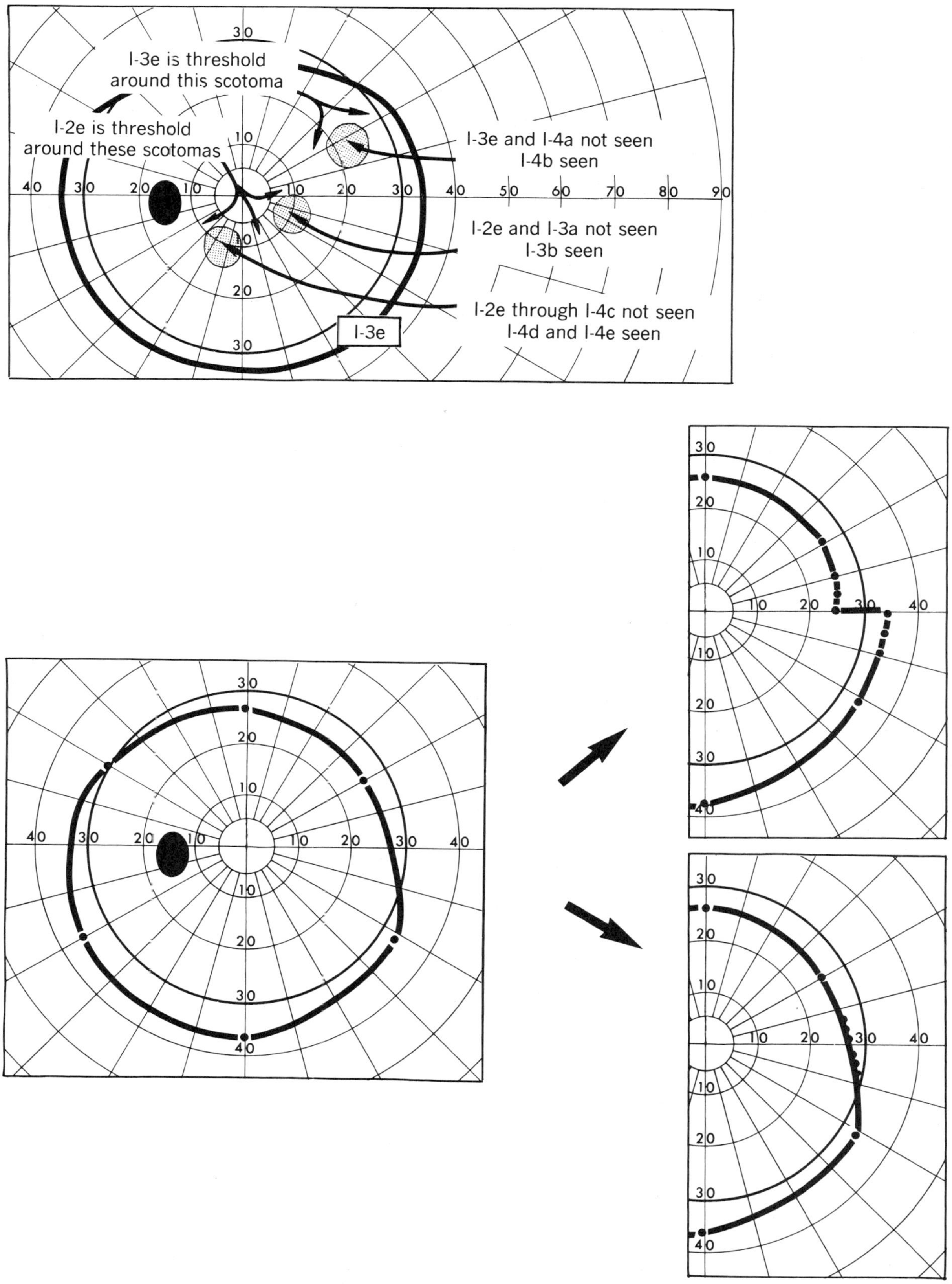

I-3e is threshold around this scotoma
I-2e is threshold around these scotomas
I-3e and I-4a not seen
I-4b seen
I-2e and I-3a not seen
I-3b seen
I-2e through I-4c not seen
I-4d and I-4e seen
I-3e

B

FIG. 13-24

Abnormal fields

The three types of defects to consider are scotomas, generalized depression, and localized depression.

Scotomas may be more immediately recognizable on a kinetic plot than on a static plot. The fact that several points around the boundary of the scotoma can be plotted kinetically immediately confirms the presence of a scotoma. Additionally, the size, shape, and location of the scotoma are obvious; and if the diagram is properly labeled, so will the depth be as well.

Generalized depression, in which sensation is reduced everywhere in the field, is represented by an inward movement of the isopters. To judge the presence of generalized depression, the interpreter needs to know the normal isopter locations with the perimeter used. Goldmann provided information on the normal isopter positions for very young individuals, and these correspond to the normal visual field shown in Fig. 5-1. More recently Johnson has provided normative data for the standard isopters at various ages (to be published).

FIG. 13-25. Normal isopter positions (mean and range) that include 95% of the undiseased normal population. The physiologic depression with age seems to be very slight up to age 50 and it accelerates thereafter. However, the *I-1e* isopter shows some constriction in earlier decades. As a rule of thumb, Goldmann's standard isopters (*I-1e* to *I-4e*) span the field out to the periphery in 20-year-olds (p. 80) and by age 70 there has been a 0.5 log-unit depression; thus the *I-4e* of a 70-year-old occupies the position of the *I-3e* in a 20-year-old, the *I-3e* occupies the former position of the *I-2e,* and so on. (Based on data courteously provided by Chris Johnson, Ph.D.)

In addition to using the normal standard position, the interpreter may compare isopter positions in the two eyes or compare the field with the previous baseline position of the isopter in the same patient on a previous occasion. In the latter case some variation in response must be allowed from one time to another equivalent to the long-term fluctuation of automated threshold static perimetry.

I-1e

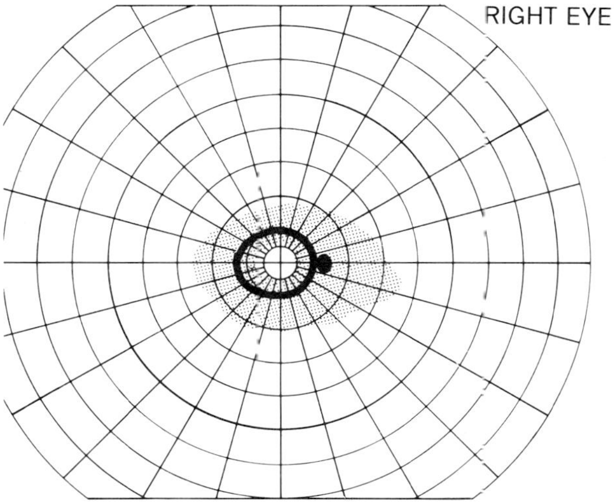

21-30

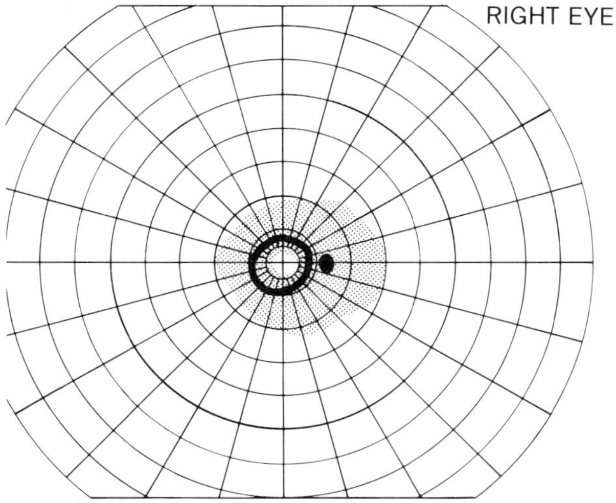

31-40

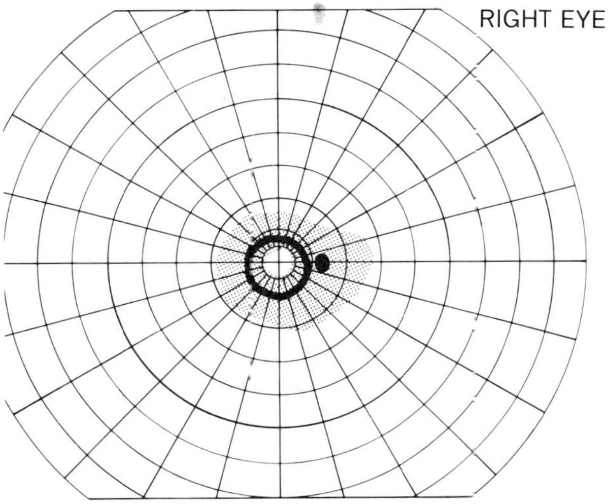

41-50

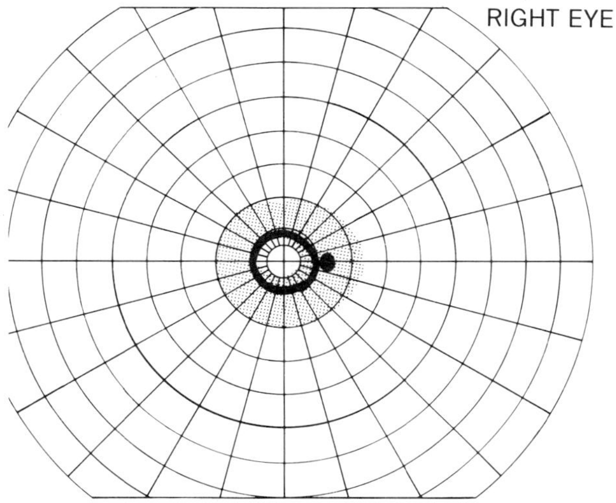

51-60

A

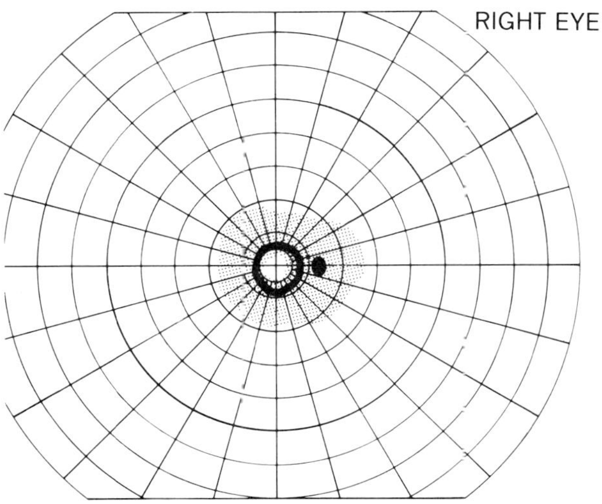

61-70

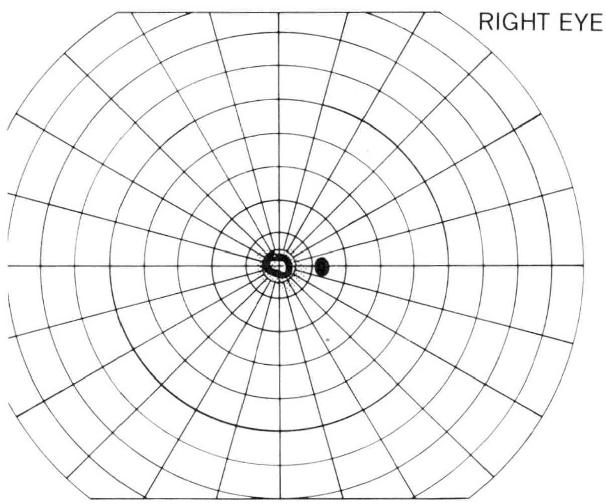

Over 70

Continued.

FIG. 13-25

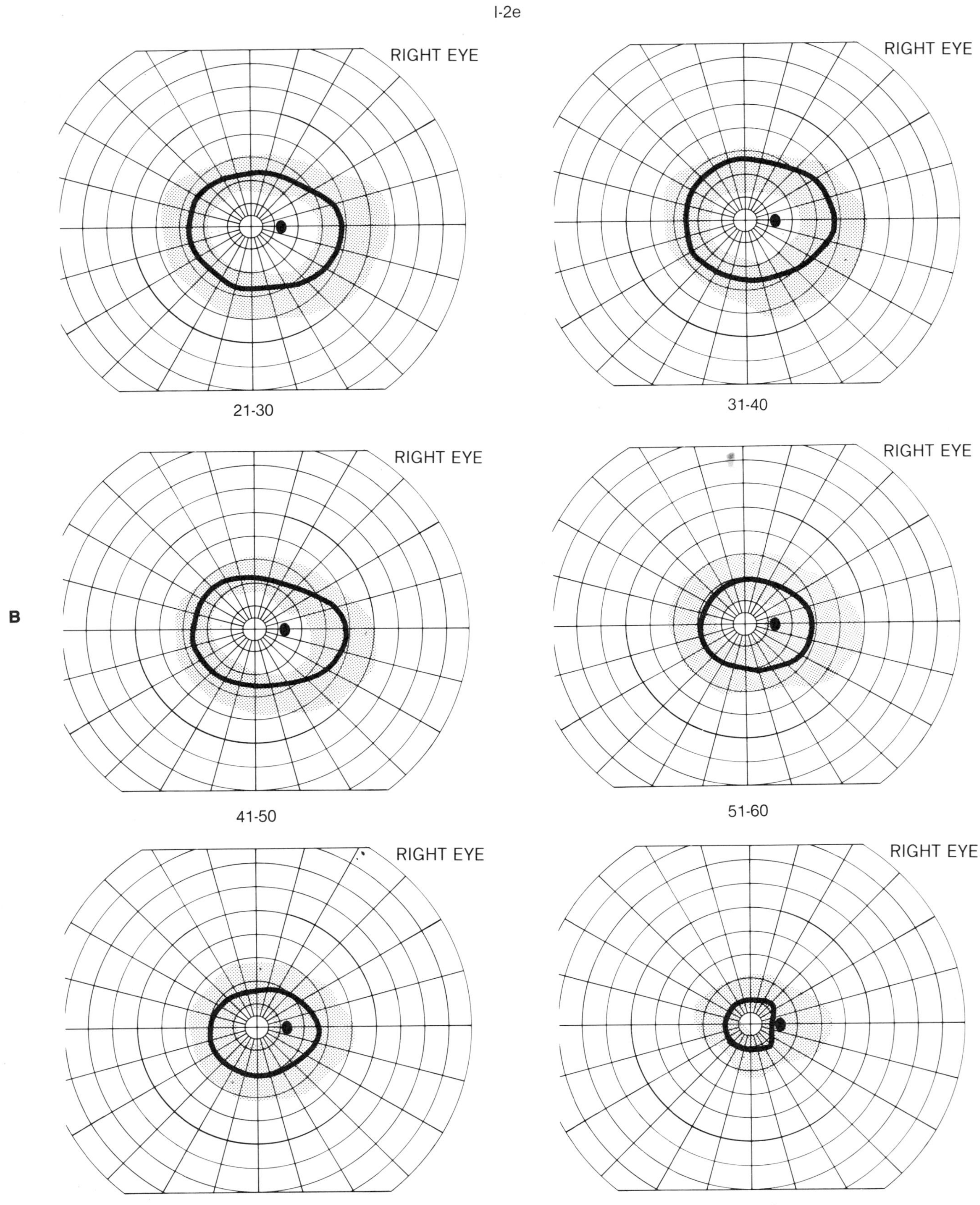

FIG. 13-25, cont'd

I-3e

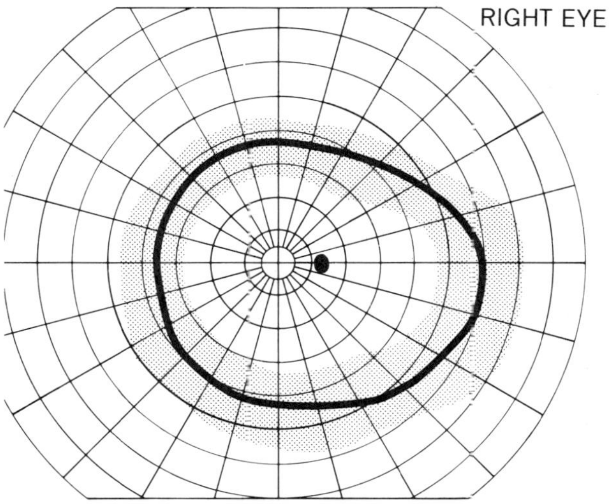

21-30

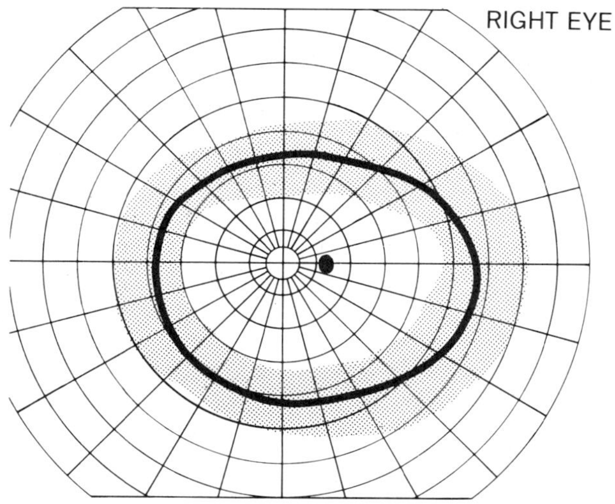

31-40

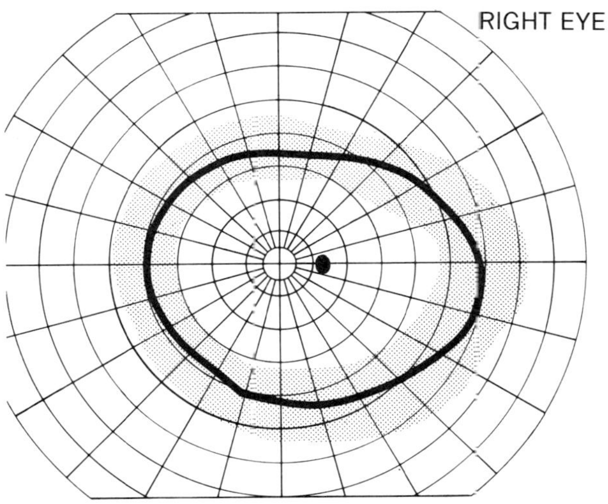

41-50

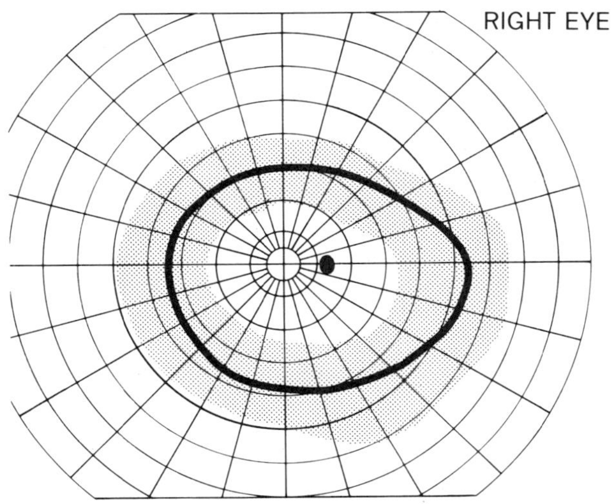

51-60

C

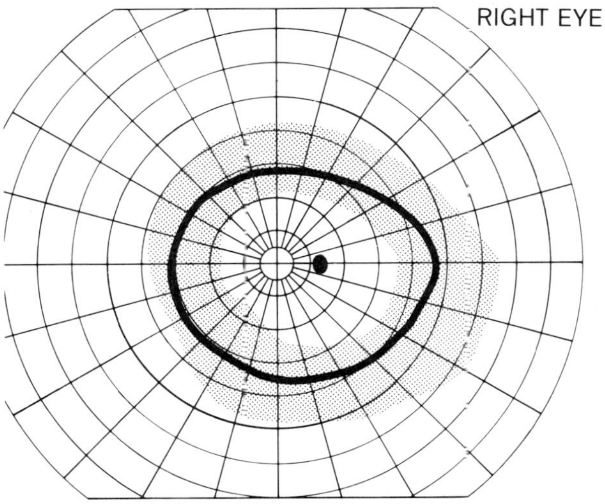

61-70

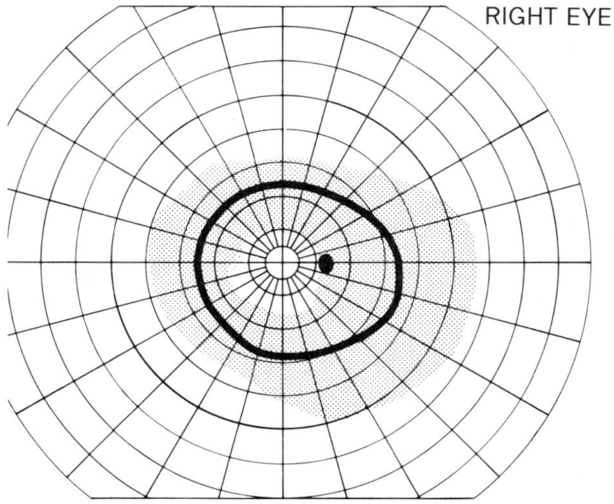

Over 70

FIG. 13-25, cont'd

Localized depression is judged not so much by comparison with the normal isopter position as by an abnormal shape to the isopter. If an isopter is of normal position and shape through most of its circumference but is deviated inward in some sector of the field, there is a depressed sensitivity in the area enclosed by the inward concavity. (EXCEPTION: Isopters may be quite irregular in a flat portion of the hill of vision, even if the field is normal.)

FIG. 13-26. Visual field in a healthy young person. Every isopter of stimuli 0.1 log-unit apart is plotted from *I-1e* to *I-3e*. Temporally 25 to 50 degrees from fixation the hill of vision is very flat. The *I-1e* and *I-2e* isopters (which differ by 0.5 log-unit) are 30 degrees apart temporally but only 15 degrees nasally. Indeed, the *I-2b* and *I-1e* isopters (only 0.2 log-unit apart) are separated by 25 degrees temporally and only 5 degrees nasally.

An irregular contour is apparent in the *I-2a* isopter (red) in the lower temporal quadrant. Enough points were plotted to ensure that the defect is reproducible with several adjacent points consistently deviated inward. The amount of reduced visual sensation is small. At point *R* the visual sensation is only 0.1 log-unit less than at point *S*. A very slight decrease in visual sensation resulting from disease might start as a shallow abnormality difficult to distinguish from this one.

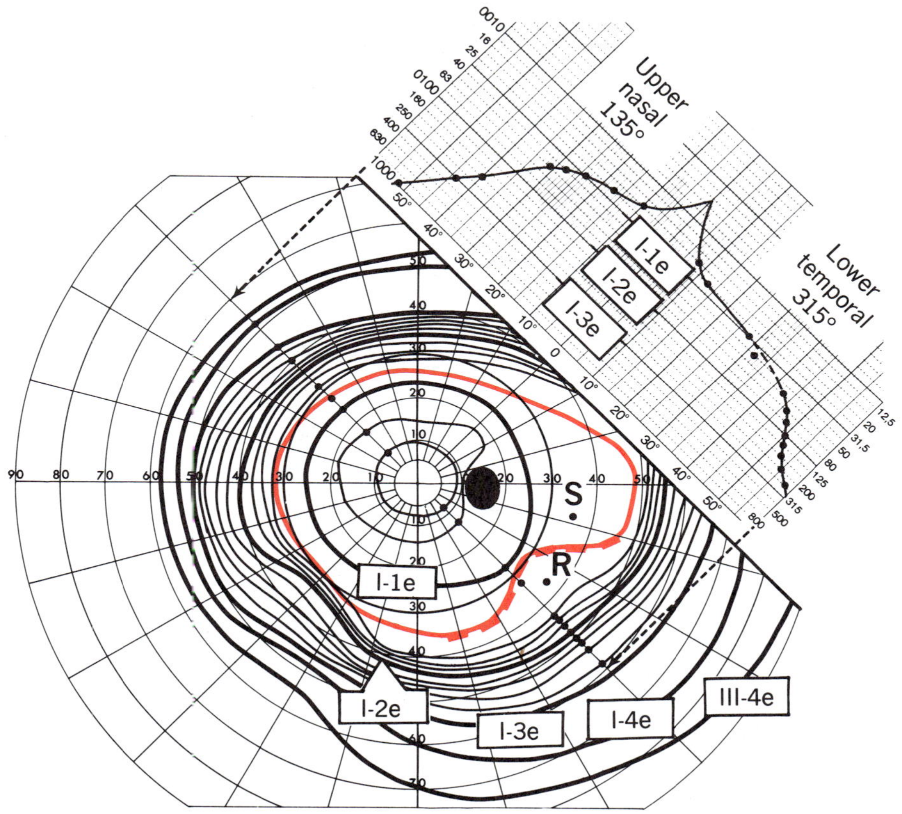

FIG. 13-26

Examples

This book contains a number of examples of both scotomas (Figs. 6-1, 6-7, 7-4, 7-7, 9-2, 9-5, and 10-3 to 10-7) and localized depressions (Figs. 7-1, 7-6, 7-9, 9-4, 9-5, and 10-3 to 10-7). In most cases in which there are well-established defects, simple acquaintance with the features of the isopter plot of the defects will allow the examiner to recognize them. Following are some examples of milder or less obvious defects.

Generalized depression is often ignored as a nonspecific finding, but it should be recognized and its diagnostic significance determined (see p. 292).

FIG. 13-27. Mild generalized depression in the left eye of a 58-year-old man. The generalized depression is recognized by comparison of the isopter positions in the two eyes, especially the *I-2e* and *I-3e*. Although the depression is small here (often, it is more striking), this subtle type occurs in eyes with a distinctly higher pressure and slightly larger cup. The slight depression is confirmed by testing with static threshold perimetry, which showed in this patient a mean sensitivity of 26.2 in the central field of the right eye compared to 24.7 in the left eye. There was no alternative explanation for this slight uniocular depression (no cataract, amblyopia, anisometropia, etc), and thus it is truly the very beginning of glaucomatous field loss. An equivalently mild generalized depression was seen in Fig. 13-22.

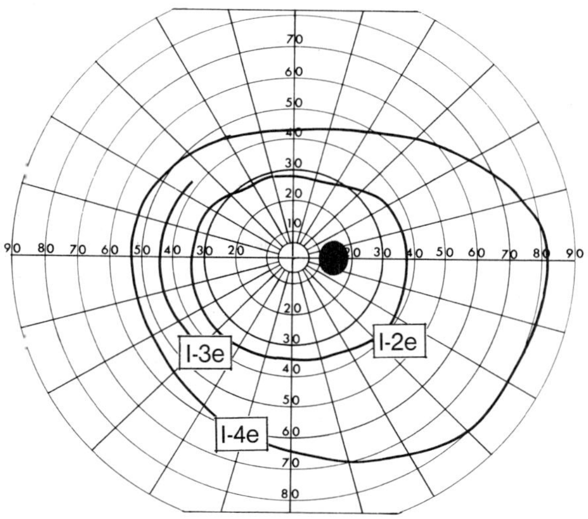

Right eye

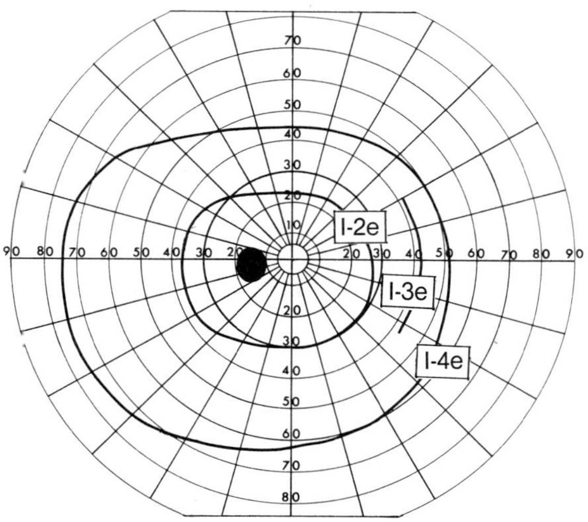

Left eye

FIG. 13-27

The following example shows that the underlying pathophysiology in all defects is depressed visual sensation and when the depressed sensation is uneven it is a bit arbitrary to separate localized scotomas and depression from generalized depression. In 1982 (and to milder degree even in 1979) the abnormality was represented by a generalized constriction of isopters without any localized defect, although in 1980 the *I-2e* isopter had shown an inferonasal localized defect. The generalized depression is recognizable on comparison of the two eyes in 1979 (and even more so in 1982) and is confirmed when the condition in the right eye is seen to progress from 1979 to 1982. Automated static threshold perimetry of this patient is shown in Fig. 13-17.

FIG. 13-28. Development of glaucomatous field loss in the left eye. In 1979 a very subtle inward movement of the *I-2e* isopter is seen as compared to the right eye, more obvious with the *I-2c* isopter. In 1980 the depression is a bit localized, with the *I-2e* isopter showing the lower nasal quadrant to be more depressed than the upper. In 1982 the entire *I-2e* isopter is constricted (now rather evenly) compared to the other eye. The feature that makes this a generalized depression is that depressed sensitivity exists everywhere—all isopters constricted inward around the entire circumference. At each location the sensitivity is less than it should be, though in 1980 one location is more depressed than others. Thus a mild localized depression can be superimposed on a generalized depression.

The amount of depressed sensitivity is judged as the degree of inward displacement of the isopters relative to their normal position. Thus, if an isopter moves inward to the position normally occupied by the isopter for a stimulus 0.5 log-unit less intense, a 0.5 log-unit depression is present. For example, a 0.5 log-unit depression is present if the I-3e isopter occupies the position that is normal for the I-2e isopter, which is 0.5 log-unit less intense.

A localized depression is most clearly represented as any distinct concavity of the isopter. Nasal steps and hemianopias that stop at the horizontal or vertical meridian are a specialized form of *concavity,* representing inward displacement of the isopter on one side of the step.

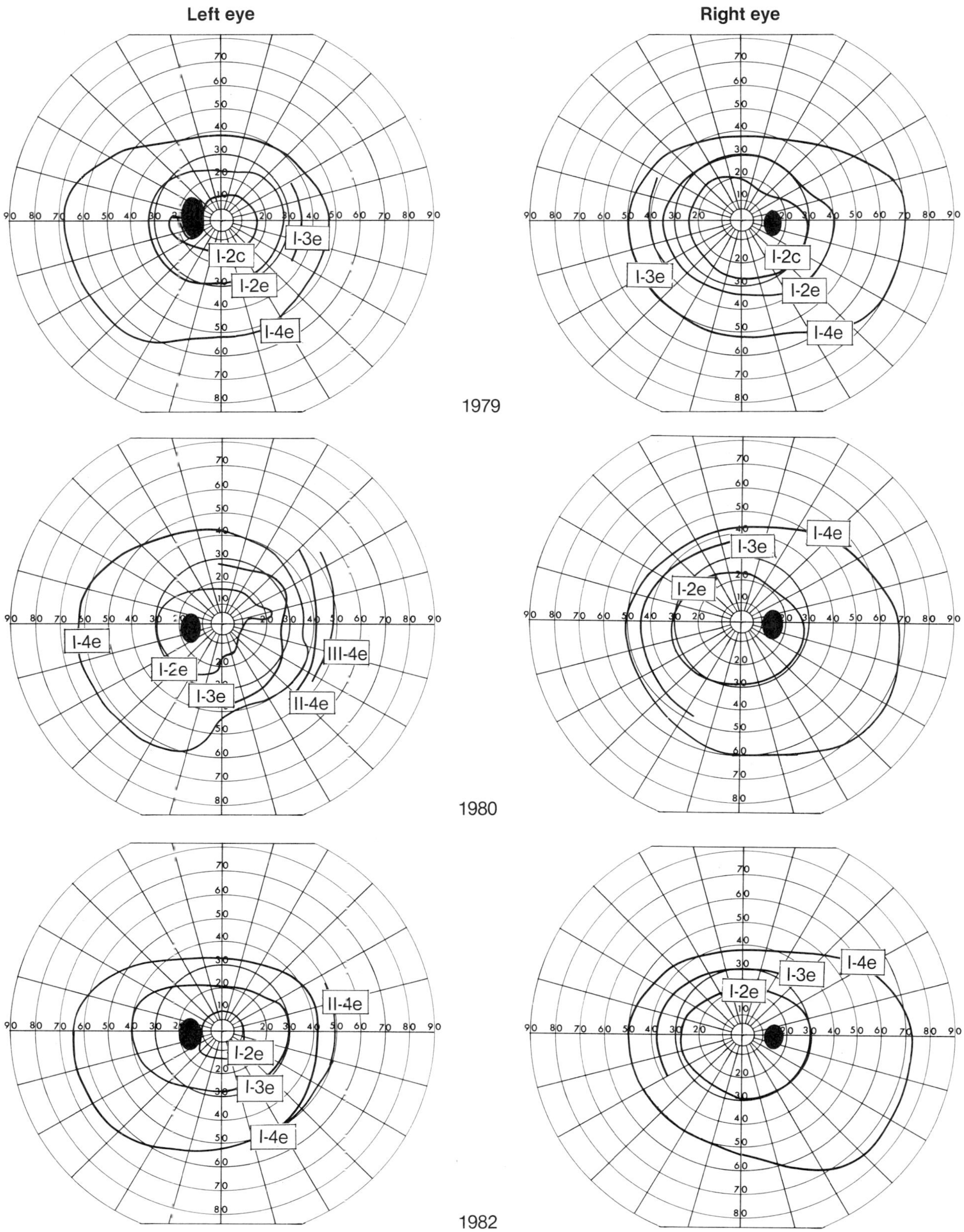

FIG. 13-28

The certainty and degree of the abnormality are at first glance judged by the number of degrees of apparent relative inward displacement. For example, a nasal step smaller than 5 degrees in width may be considered uncertain evidence of a depression but a larger step is more definitive (and more severe). However, other features must also be considered. For example, a definite step in two or three consecutive isopters represents a broad but shallow depression that may be judged real, even if the steps are only 2 to 3 degrees wide. Bear in mind also that the distance an isopter deviates inward is affected by the slope of the hill of vision in the affected region. Thus, in a very flat region of the field, a 1 dB (0.1 log-unit) relative depression might cause the isopter to move 5 or 10 degrees inward whereas, in a region of the usual slope, the same displacement would occur only with a 0.5 log-unit depression of sensitivity. It is often informative to contemplate specific points in the field and consider what the magnitude of the reduction in visual sensation might be (for example, compare points *S* and *R* in Fig. 13-26; similarly, see Figs. 7-8 and 7-9).

FIG. 13-29. Hypothetical example of a shallow depression in the arcuate Bjerrum region. In this case the *I-2e* isopter superiorly is deviated 10 degrees inward toward fixation compared to the field inferiorly. Visual sensation at point *S* is reduced (*I-2e* not visible but would be if the *I-2e* isopter were in the proper position at 23 degrees as shown by the dotted line), but the defect is not in a flat region of the field. Note that in Fig. 13-26 the inward deviation of the isopter in the flat region of the field represents at most a 0.1 log-unit reduction of visual sensitivity. In the present example, visual sensation is reduced as much as 0.4 log-unit, more than a shallow ripple in the contour of a normal hill of vision. Note also that the *I-1e* and *I-2e* isopters are close to one another but there is a wide separation between the *I-2e* and *I-3e* isopters. The defect can be accepted as pathologic if combined with an elevated IOP and mild glaucomatous cupping. Eventually, with further reduction in visual sensation, the defect could become an arcuate scotoma.

The more carefully the visual field is examined, the more likely the clinician is to find a subtle defect resulting from the early stage of a disease. The problem in interpretation is that the likelihood of finding a seeming defect in a normal field is also greater. If it is an isolated finding, it may be best not to be convinced of an apparent abnormality that is less than 0.3 or even 0.5 log-unit deep unless it is reproducible and there are other clinical signs (e.g., cupping of the disc) to confirm that there should be a pathologic defect in the area. Sometimes it is impossible to decide if a defect is really an abnormality, and the subsequent clinical course must be used in deciding whether a shallow defect is real. For example, a shallow defect can be considered real if a deeper scotoma develops in the same location as time goes on.

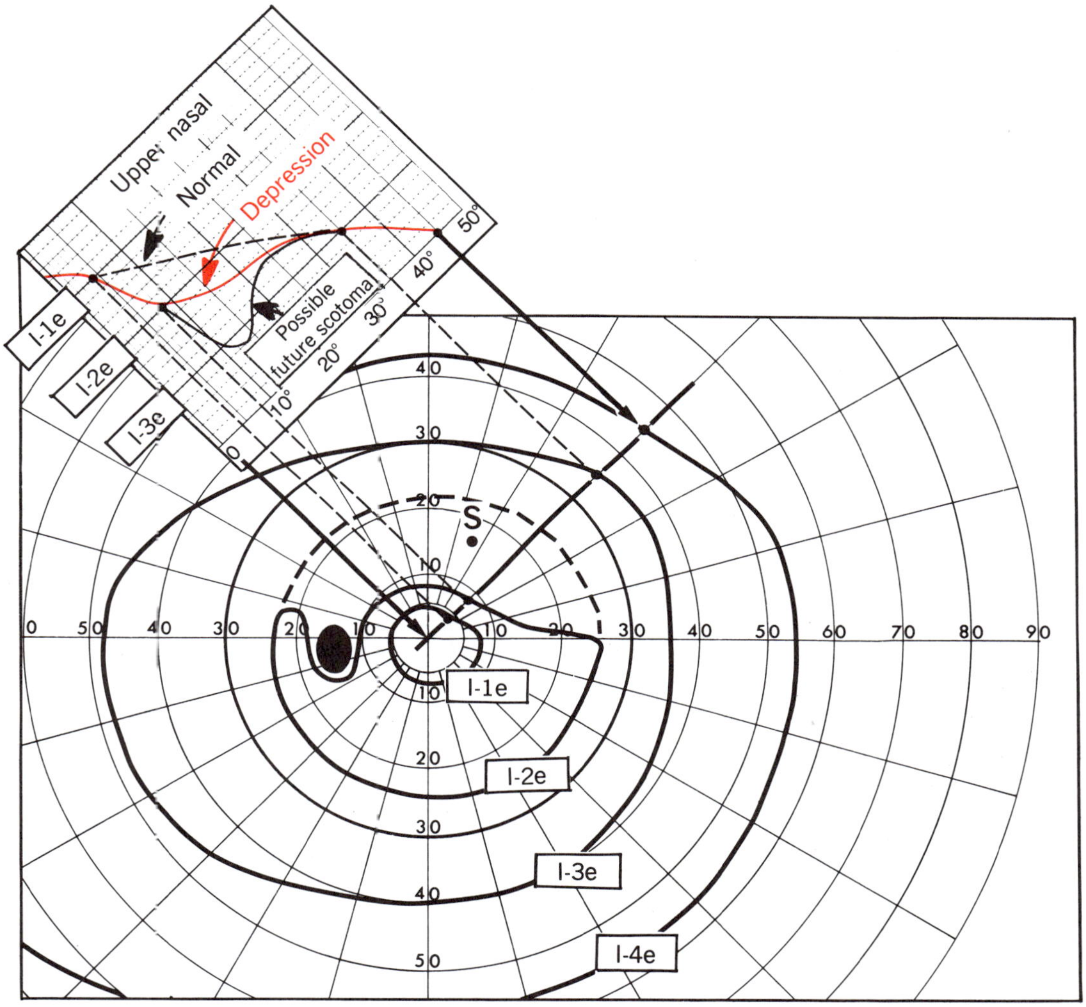
Upper nasal
Normal
Depression
Possible future scotoma
I-1e
I-2e
I-3e
I-4e
S

FIG. 13-29

In addition to looking for distinct concavities (or steps), the examiner needs to consider the shape of the isopter. Normal isopters have a more or less elliptic shape. However, if the field is distinctly flattened from above, from below, or from the nasal side, there may be a broad but localized depression even without the isopters' becoming concave in any portion of the circumference.

FIG. 13-30. Early depression in the arcuate region. The contour of the *I-2e* isopter is flattened. Inferiorly there is a wide separation between the *I-2e* isopter and the *I-3e* isopter, which is in the normal position. Thus, inferiorly there is a localized depression in the arcuate region, represented by the inward displacement of the *I-2e* isopter; peripheral to the arcuate region there is no depression. Superiorly, however, the depression may cover a broader expanse, with the *I-3e* isopter also displaced inward very slightly.

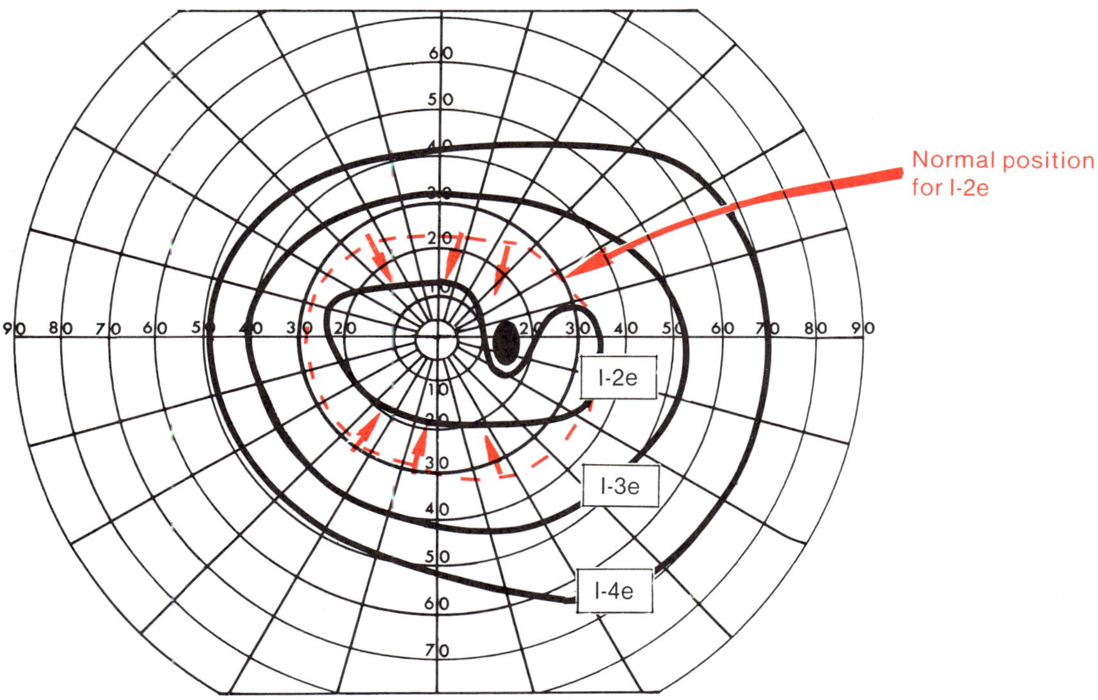

FIG. 13-30

FIG. 13-31. Flattening of isopter contour nasally in the right eye. Although the depression is generalized (all isopters have moved inward from their normal positions around the entire circumference), it is more marked nasally and the isopters are more constricted on the nasal side than in other sectors. Compare the isopter plots with the static threshold plot of this patient (Fig. 13-18).

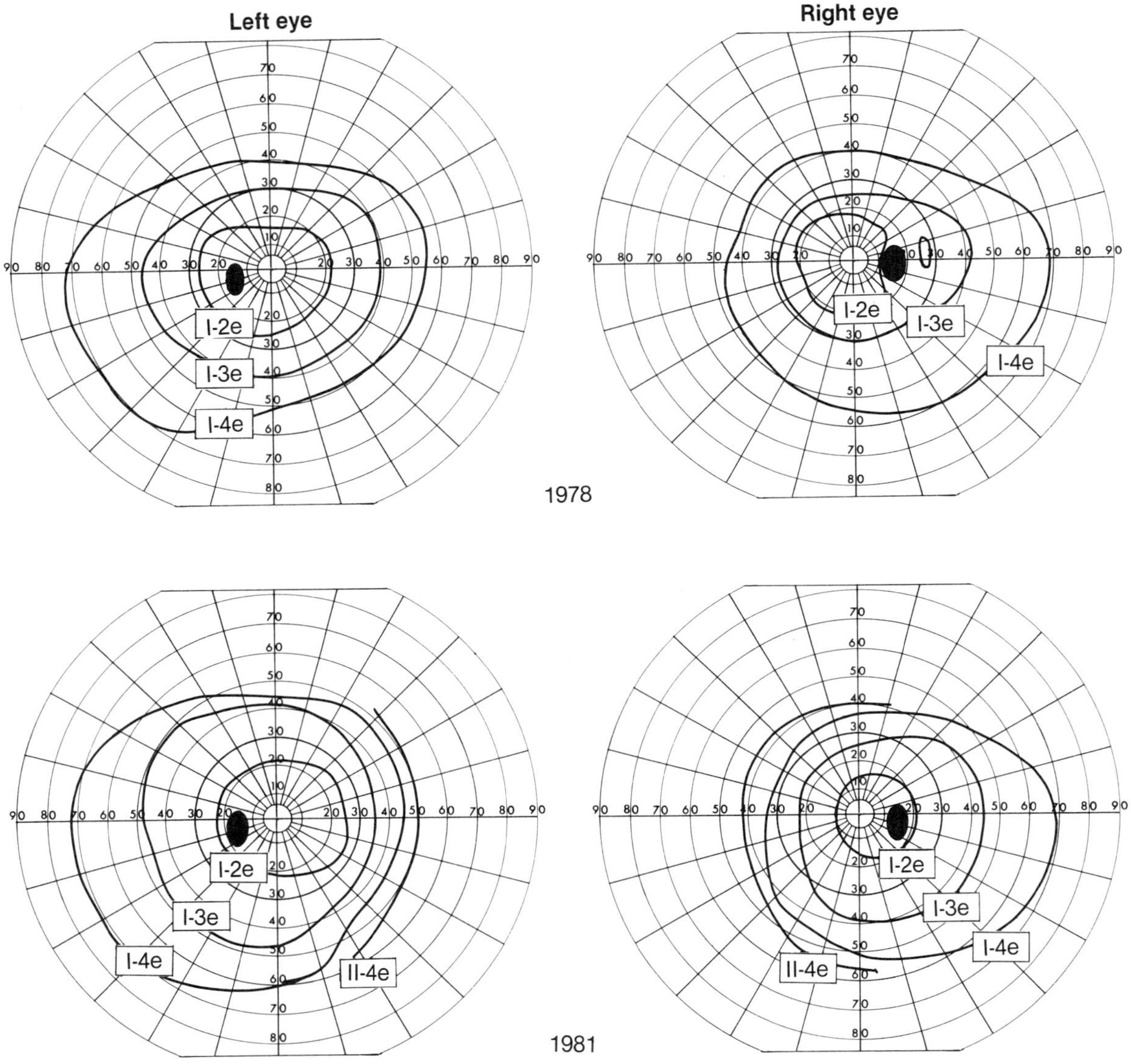

FIG. 13-31

ARTIFACTS

So far in this chapter the only question considered has been whether or not a field abnormality is present. Now we shall begin to consider what the defect represents.

The first thing to consider is that an apparent defect may be an artifact. There are many types of artifacts. Only a few of the more common representative ones are given as examples.

Edge points

Perhaps the most frequent problem in testing the central visual field is that there may seem to be an abnormality at the edge of the tested region, near 30 degrees. By manual kinetic perimetry this may be represented as an inward deviation of the isopters. By automated perimetry the edge points may be missed in suprathreshold testing or have a reduced sensitivity in static threshold perimetry.

Several factors contribute to this particular artifact:

1. The lens rim may impinge on the central 30 degrees. This will happen if the eye is not properly centered behind the lens (Figs. 12-11, 13-59, and 13-62), if the lens used is not a full-aperture design, or if the distance between the lens and the eye is too great (Figs. 12-10, 13-32, and 13-33). This artifact can also occur if the lens holder is left in place while no corrective lens is being used.
2. Superiorly, defective points can also be caused if there is a droopy upper eyelid or a prominent eyebrow, particularly if the eye is deeply set or the head is improperly positioned at the perimeter.
3. With suprathreshold testing, edge points are more likely to be missed than center points in one-level screening, since the stimulus intensity is closer to threshold near the edge than it is at the center. Even when eccentricity compensation is used along with a threshold-related strategy, the edge points may be missed if the threshold-related level is determined close to fixation and the person undergoing testing has a slope in his hill of vision that is steeper than usual.
4. With static threshold determinations, the edge points may have a seemingly low sensitivity simply because away from fixation there is both greater variability of responsiveness (short-term fluctuation) and a broader range of normal values.

FIG. 13-32. Abnormality of edge points caused by too great a distance between the lens and the eye during the field test. The lens was also somewhat decentered. As often occurs with this artifact, there is a sharp boundary between points with normal sensitivity and those with 0 dB sensitivity. However, some points at the boundary can have intermediate sensitivity values. See also Fig. 12-10.

FIG. 13-33. Same eye tested on another occasion.

FIG. 13-34. Glaucomatous defect. In this case there is no sharp boundary but a gradual reduction of sensitivity toward the edge of the central field. Comparable points well away from the edge are depressed in the upper arcuate compared to the lower arcuate region.

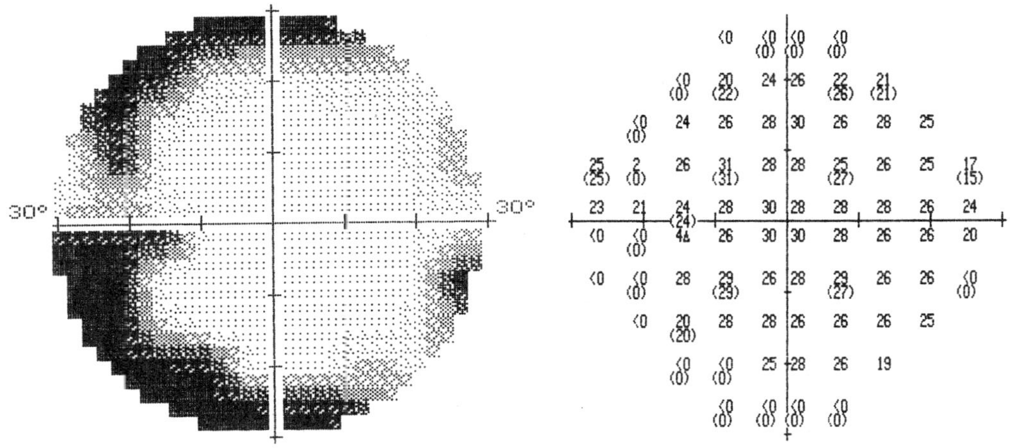

FIG. 13-32

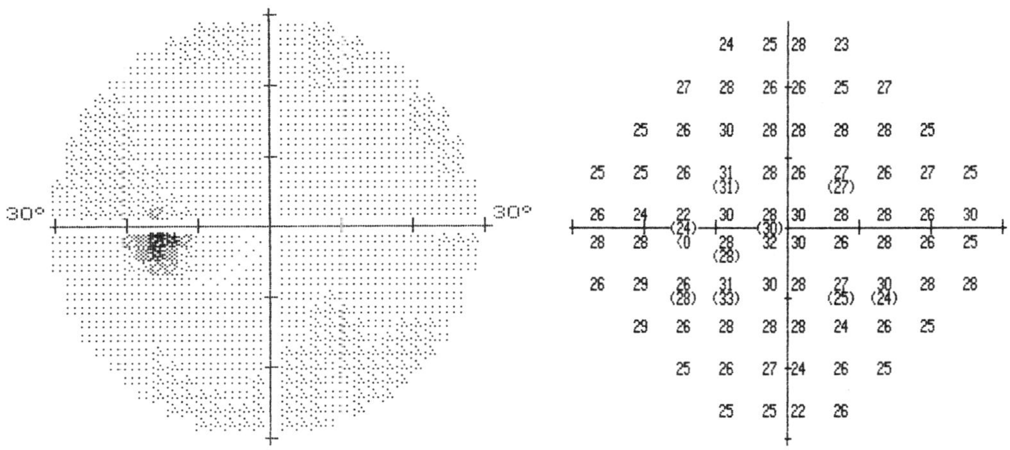

FIG. 13-33

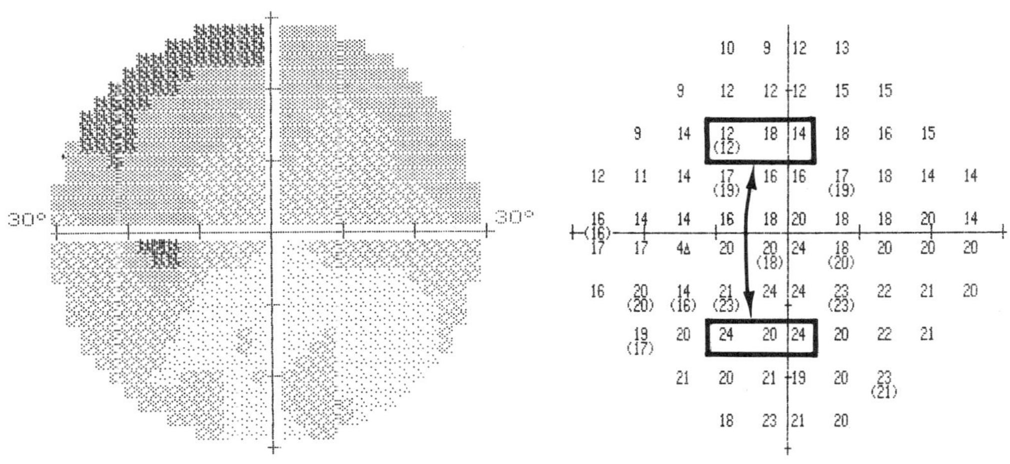

FIG. 13-34

Of course, artifacts and real defects can occur together.

FIG. 13-35. Equivocal example. There is depression of the entire upper half of the field, not just the edge, indicating a true defect. A true defect can taper into an absolute scotoma at the edge; however, the dropoff in sensitivity in this example is rather sharp at the very top.

This test was performed with a +6.00 + 1.50 × 160 correction, and only by repeating it with careful attention to lens positioning could you rule out a lens rim artifact superimposed on the true defect.

FIG. 13-36. Field with both a lens rim artifact (upper left) and true paracentral scotomas (arrows). Only the artifact disappears on repeat testing.

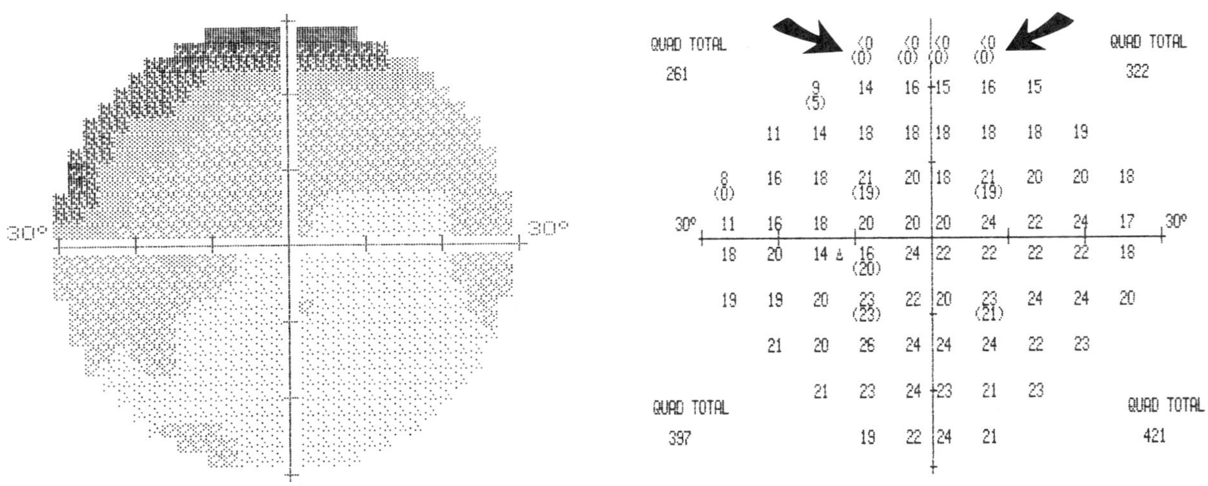

FIG. 13-35

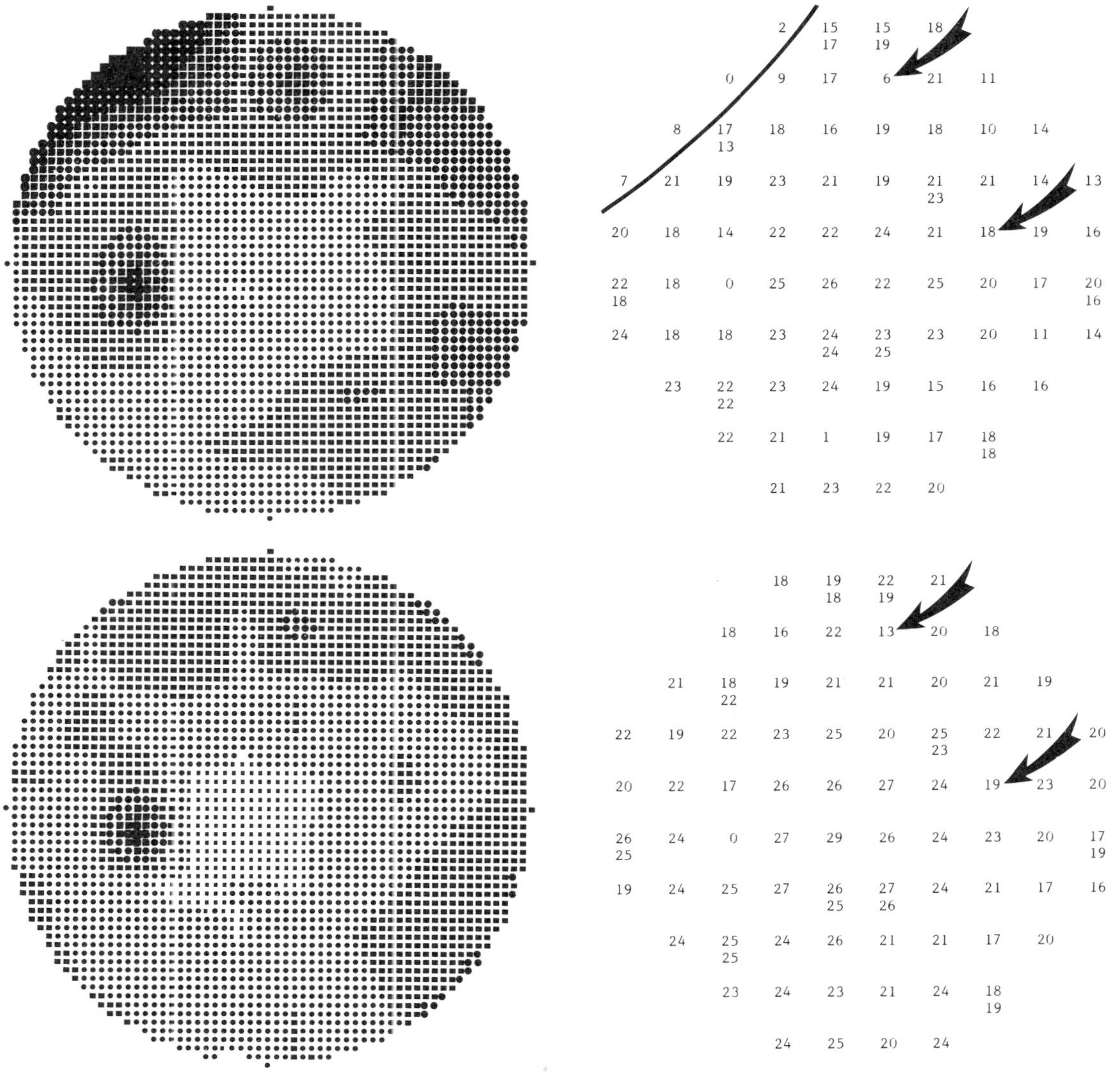

2 15 15 18
17 19
0 9 17 6 21 11
8 17 18 16 19 18 10 14
13
7 21 19 23 21 19 21 21 14 13
23
20 18 14 22 22 24 21 18 19 16
22 18 0 25 26 22 25 20 17 20
18 16
24 18 18 23 24 23 23 20 11 14
24 25
23 22 23 24 19 15 16 16
22
22 21 1 19 17 18
18
21 23 22 20
18 19 22 21
18 19
18 16 22 13 20 18
21 18 19 21 21 20 21 19
22
22 19 22 23 25 20 25 22 21 20
23
20 22 17 26 26 27 24 19 23 20
26 24 0 27 29 26 24 23 20 17
25 19
19 24 25 27 26 27 24 21 17 16
25 26
24 25 24 26 21 21 17 20
25
23 24 23 21 24 18
19
24 25 20 24

FIG. 13-36

The eyelid or eyebrow can also cause a depression superiorly (Fig. 12-3), evident on either static or kinetic perimetry. The boundary of the artifact is not sharp as with the lens rim artifact. Since glaucoma can also cause depression superiorly, the distinction is often made only by noting the patient's facial configuration or repeating the test with attention toward avoiding the artifact.

FIG. 13-37. Depressions in the superior field.
A, A prominent eyebrow or drooping eyelid may produce a relatively generalized depression superiorly all the way to the periphery of the field. It is a sloping defect, as if the upper field were shaded, in effect making every stimulus less bright.
B, Glaucomatous depression is typically more marked on the nasal side than on the temporal side and may or may not be associated with a nasal step.

When both central and peripheral fields are tested with static threshold perimetry, there may appear to be a strange ring scotoma at 30 degrees when the sensitivity values of the two field tests are combined. This may occur with strong lenses even if there is no actual obstruction of the lens rim during testing of the central 30 degrees. This artifact presumably occurs because there is some prismatic displacement of the image by the lens for points that are not at the center. Thus a spot of light in the bowl 25 degrees from the point of fixation may be intercepted by the nodal point of the eye with a different visual angle when a lens is in place. Such an artifact is equivalent to the discontinuity in isopter position experienced with kinetic perimetry (Chapter 23, p. 440).

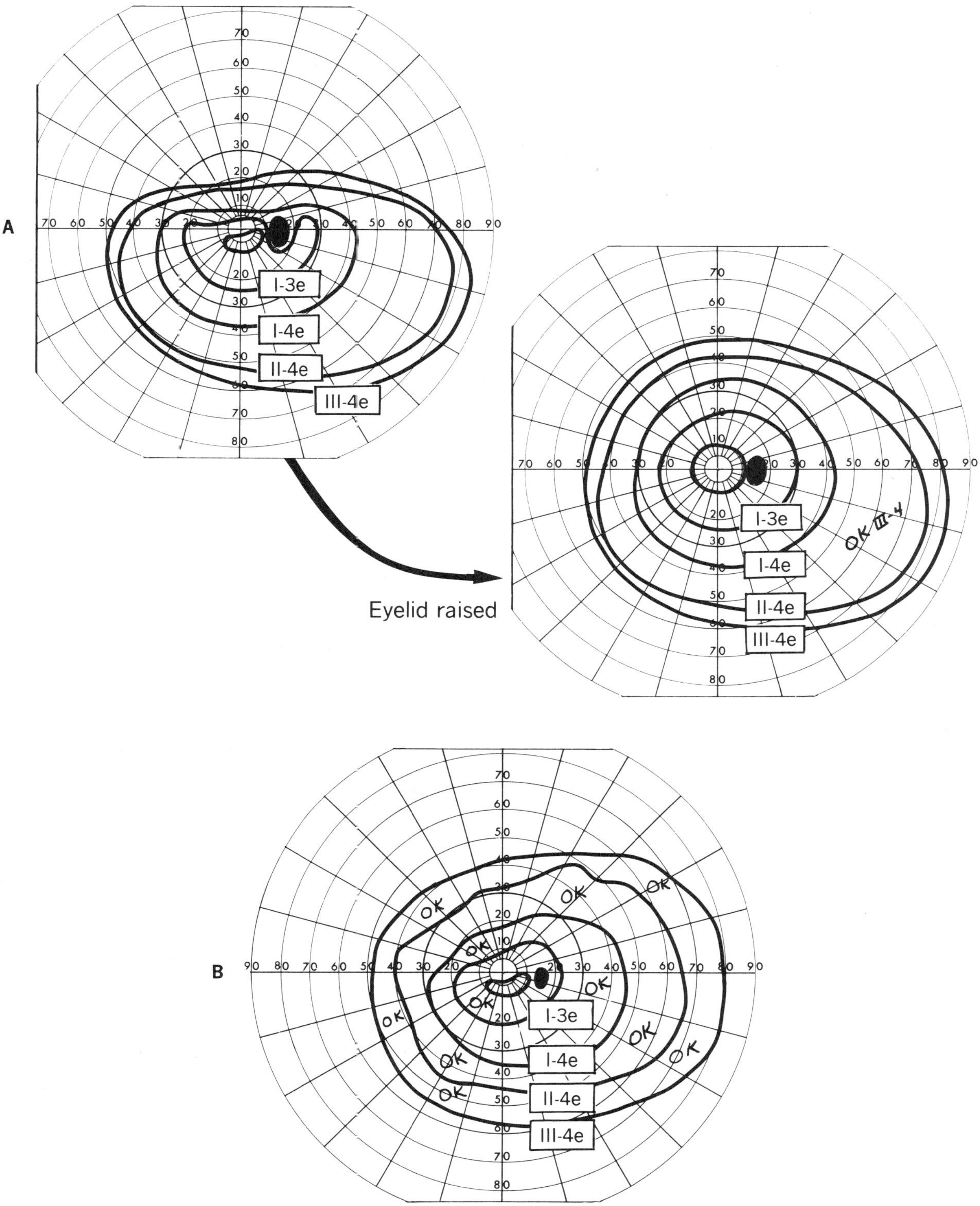

FIG. 13-37

Refraction scotomas

Another localized defect that can be a pitfall in diagnostic interpretation is the refraction scotoma, which may be either a scotoma or a localized depression, typically within a wedge-shaped zone above the physiologic blind spot. A refraction scotoma can be mistaken for an arcuate scotoma or an upper temporal hemianopia.

Usually the lens that provides the best visual acuity by bringing the fovea into focus also brings the rest of the retina into focus. A refraction scotoma results when this is not the case and the lens required to focus an eccentric stimulus on the retina away from the fovea is different from the one required to focus the fixation point on the fovea. Typically this occurs with astigmatism or myopia, when the back of the eye is not symmetric but has bulges around (and especially below) the optic nerve.

FIG. 13-38. Anatomic cause of a refraction scotoma.

The refraction scotoma appears in the zone of the visual field that corresponds to the part of the retina not in proper focus because a blurred stimulus is not as visible as a focused one. If a specific scotoma is suspected of being a refraction scotoma, the lens being used for the field testing can be varied by a −1.00, −0.50, +0.50, or +1.00 D sphere. If the test stimulus becomes visible in the region of the scotoma, there must be an improved focusing of the stimulus on the retina. If the stimulus was already in focus and the defect is a true scotoma, the scotoma would remain the same or become deeper because changing the lens would make the stimulus less visible. Remember that lenses can be used only within the central 30 degrees; thus testing for refractive scotomas in this manner is possible only within the central field.

FIG. 13-39. Refraction scotoma. Visual sensation improves in the region of the refraction scotoma with a change of the lens. At the same time, visual sensation worsens in the region around the fovea because it is being placed out of focus by the lens that brings the region of the refractive scotoma into focus. Because of this, the central isopter *(I-2e)* moves inward ("becomes smaller").

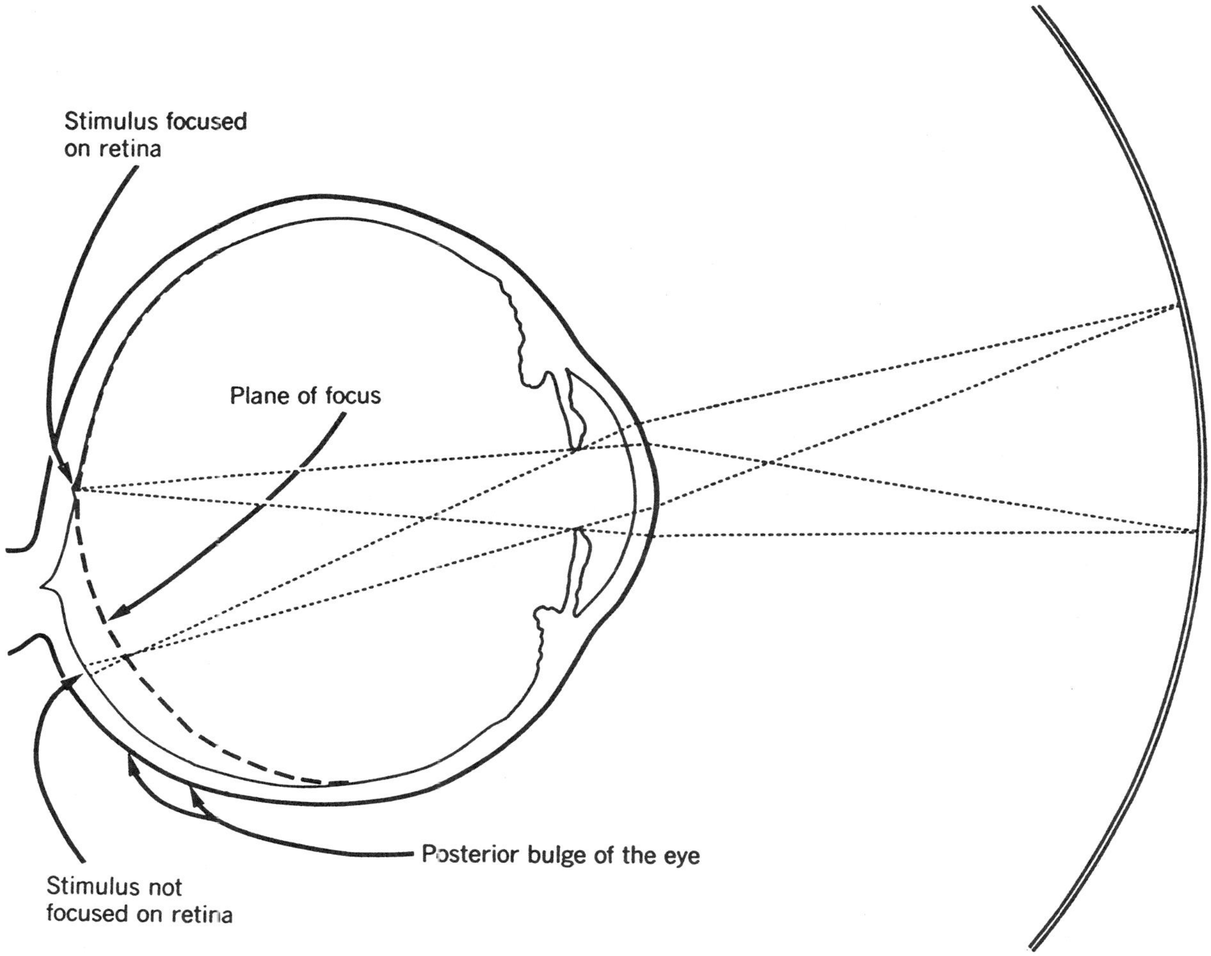

FIG. 13-38

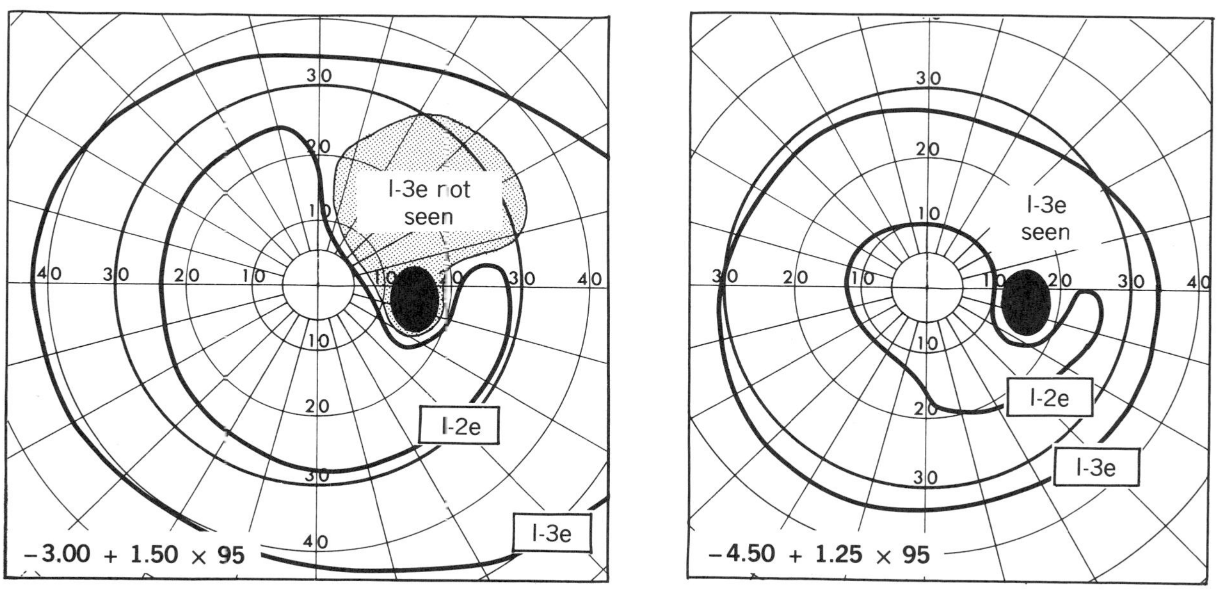

FIG. 13-39

Apart from the fact that lenses can eliminate or at least reduce the refraction scotoma, the defect is sometimes distinguished from a typical arcuate scotoma because the wedge-shaped defect goes straight upward and is only vaguely arcuate. Similarly, it may be distinguished from a hemianopia by the fact that it crosses the vertical midline and fails to show a distinct boundary at the vertical midline when tested by the usual means for confirming hemianopias. At least some refraction scotomas have been recognized to correlate with the presence of a tilted disc or a wedge of pale color in the lower nasal retina emanating from the optic disc. Such defects may be an exaggeration of the normal superior "baring of the blind spot," in which visual sensation is slightly reduced above the blind spot so the isopter curves around the blind spot without enclosing the region just above it.

FIG. 13-40. Normal or "false" baring of the blind spot. This contrasts with pathologic baring of the blind spot, in which a depression or scotoma in the arcuate (Bjerrum) region causes an isopter to skirt around the blind spot without enclosing it. Examples of pathologic baring of the blind spot can be seen in Figs. 9-2 to 9-4, 10-5 and 10-6, 21-10 and 21-11, and 23-3.

ADDITIONAL READING

For more information on refraction scotomas and tilted discs the interested reader may consult the following:

Aulhorn, E.: Visual field defects in sellar and parasellar processes, Annee Ther. Clin. Ophtalmol. **25:**424-434, 1974.

Dimitrakos, S.A., and Safran, A.B.: La dysversion papillaire. Diagnostic différentiel du syndrome chiasmatique, Ophthalmologica **184:**30-39, 1982.

Fankhauser, F., and Enough, J.M.: The effects of blur upon perimetric thresholds: A method for determining a quantitative estimate of retinal contour, Arch. Ophthalmol. **68:**240-251, 1962.

Goldmann, H.: Lichtsinn mit besonderer Berücksichtigung der Perimetrie, Ophthalmologica **158:** 362-386, 1969.

Kommerell, G.: Binasale Refraktionsskotome, Klin. Monatsbl. Augenheilkd. **154:**85-88, 1969.

Riiuse, D.: The nasal fundus ectasia, Acta Ophthalmol. (Suppl.) **126:**4-108, 1975.

Rucker, C.W.: Bitemporal defects in the visual fields resulting from developmental anomalies of the optic disks, Arch. Ophthalmol. **35:**546-554, 1946.

Schmidt, T.: Kurzes Repetitorium der klinischen Perimetrie, Ophthalmologica **149:**250-265, 1965.

Schmidt, T.: Perimetrie relativer Skotome, Ophthalmologica **129:**303-315, 1955.

Young, S.E., Walsh, F.B., and Knox, D.L.: The tilted disk syndrome, Am. J. Ophthalmol. **82:**16-23, 1976.

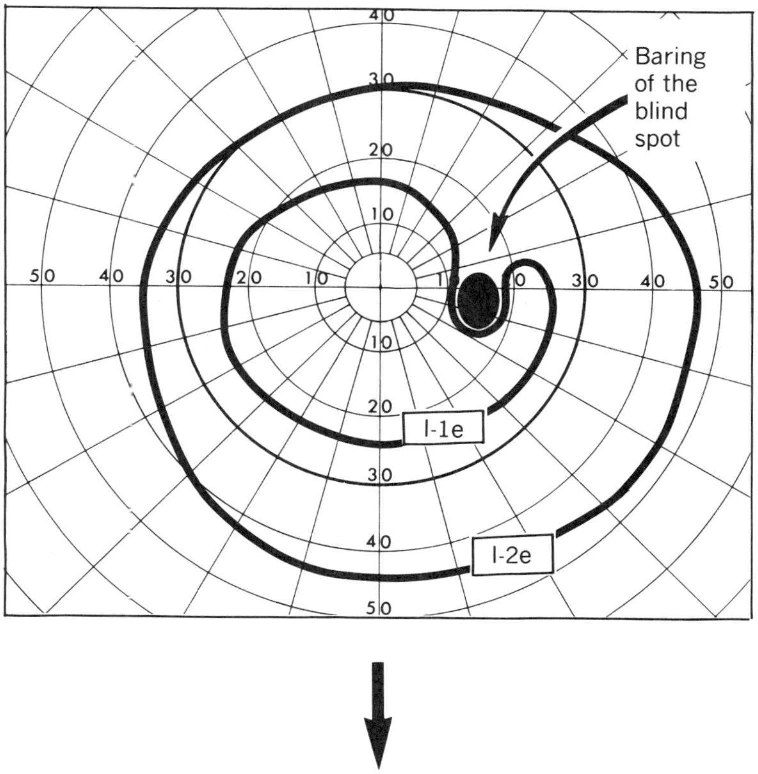

With intermediate isopters

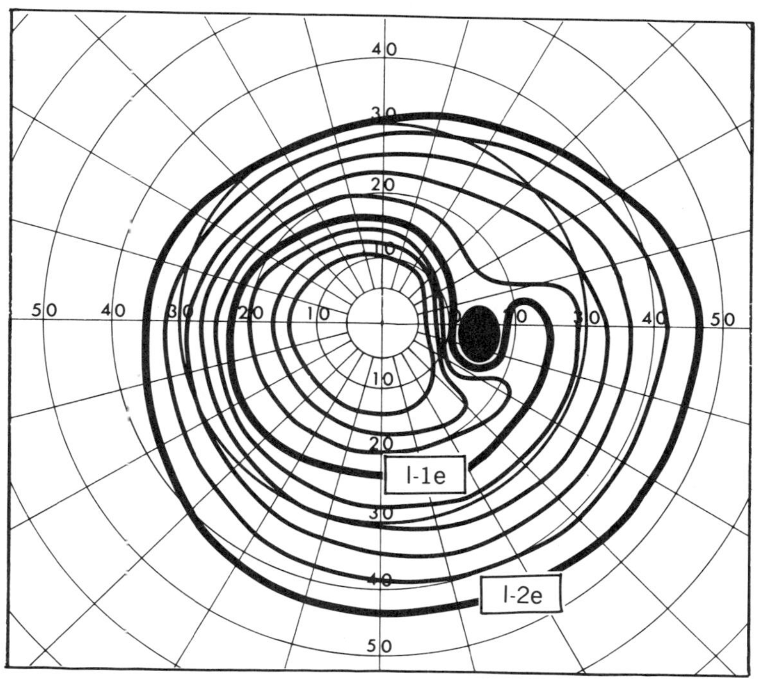

FIG. 13-40

Patient unreliability

A characteristic artifact test result is coalescent white spots (instead of coalescent scotomas, represented by dark spots) on a greyscale printout. The white areas on a numeric printout correspond to points with impossibly high sensitivities. The problem is that the patient responds even when he does not actually see the stimulus and this is reflected in a high false-positive rate on the catch trials. There may be other signs of unreliability in the field—frequent fixation losses, frequent premature replies, a high short-term fluctuation (RMS), and a high false-negative response rate. The problem can be overcome by repeating the original instructions (p. 184), explaining that it is normal not to see all presentations and that the patient should refrain from responding unless he is sure he has seen the stimulus. If this fails, performing the field is recommended because the technician can use judgment about which patient response to accept and can thereby make some determination of the field status despite the patient's unreliability.

FIG. 13-41. Unreliable field. Note the impossibly high sensitivities in some places (circled), the high rate of false-positive answers, and the poor reproducibility of repeat threshold determinations (boxes). The last corresponds to the high fluctuation (RMS) of *10.5* dB.

Number of questions: 565 Number of repetitions: 0
False positive answers (%): 57(8/14) False negative answers (%): 0(0/14)

FLUCTUATIONS (R.M.S.): 10.5 DB

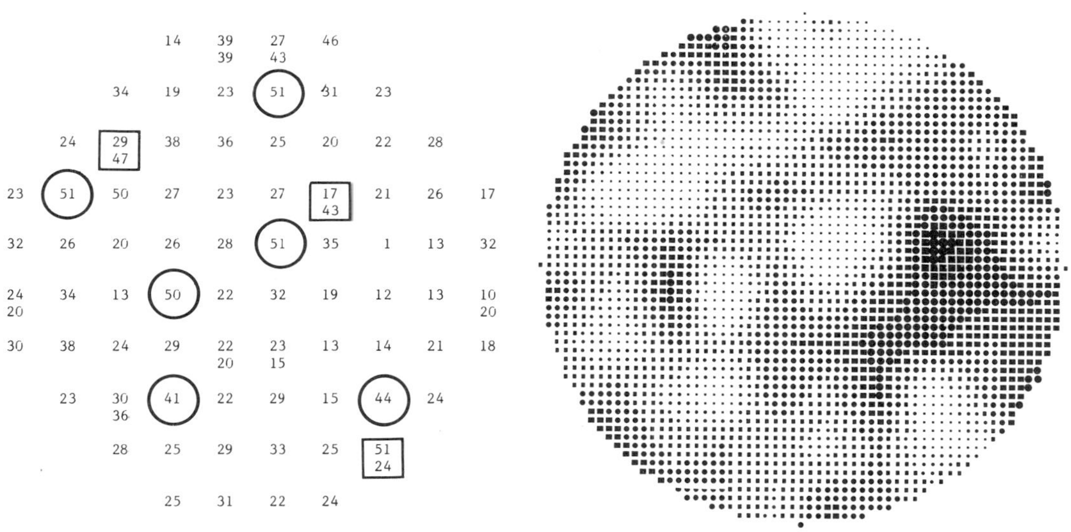

FIG. 13-41

FIG. 13-42. Similarly unreliable field. Impossibly high sensitivities appear everywhere, but especially in the lower nasal quadrant. The rate of false-positive answers is high. The reported rate of fixation losses is also high and could be due to either true losses of fixation or false-positive responses to stimuli shown in the blind spot.

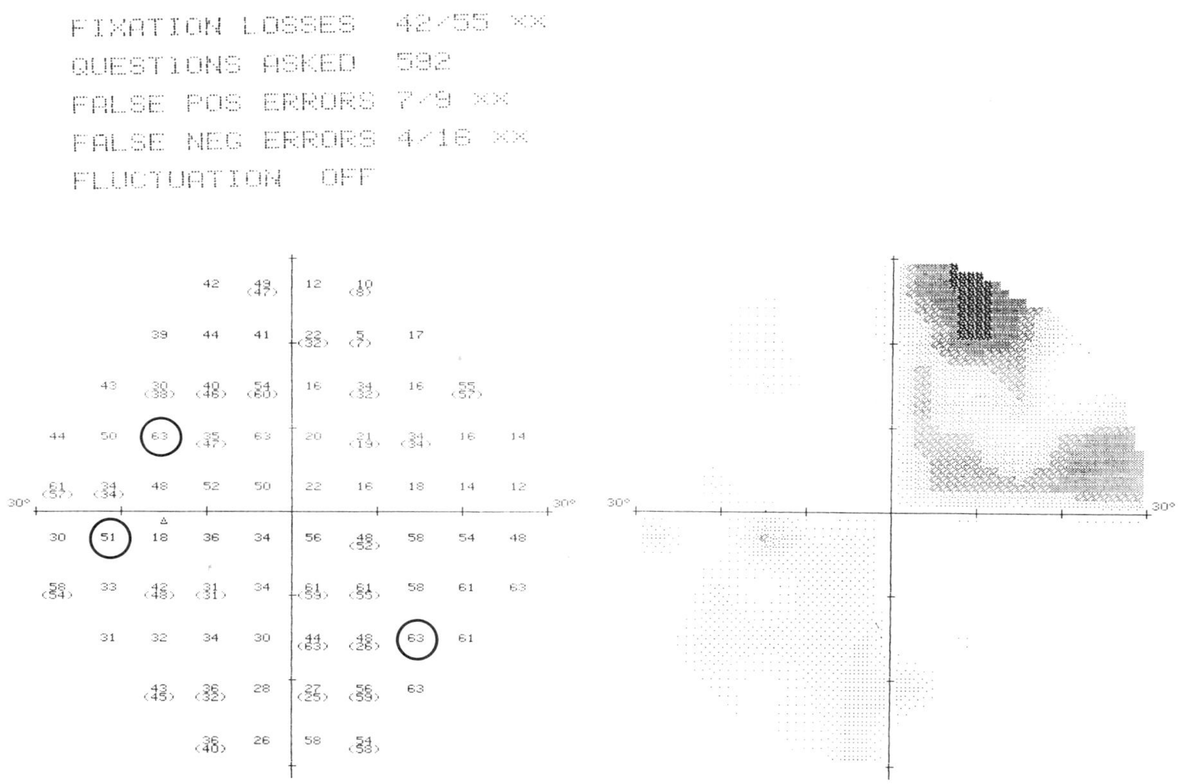

FIG. 13-42

FIG. 13-43. Less striking example of a high false-positive rate. Several locations have sensitivities higher than those recorded in the surround (inverse of a scotoma). Because of such scattered peaks, the loss variance and corrected loss variance indices, which measure unevenness of the field, are abnormally high (Octopus G1 program) in this patient who has no scotomatous loss.

Number of questions: 561 Number of repetitions: 0
False positive answers (%): 31(4/13) False negative answers (%): 0(0/14)

FLUCTUATIONS (R.M.S.): 2.0 DB LUM. INTERVAL: 4

			26	29 27	25 27	28			
		28	29	31	28	31	35		
	30	27 29	30	30	31	36	28	30	
33	29	25	31	31	31	29 35	29	28	29
30	30	26	30	36	36	27	30	33	26
28 30	30	15	37	36	32	31	30	27	26 26
30	32	30	29	30 26	29 29	31	30	27	24
	29	28 28	31	32	29	29	36	30	
		26	25	29	29	27	26 30		
			29	27	20	28			

FIG. 13-43

Other artifacts

Artifacts due to technician inexperience can often be recognized by a clinician experienced at reading field diagrams. A particularly instructive set of examples is found in Chapter 9 of Trobe, J.D., and Glaser, J.S.: *The Visual Fields Manual,* Gainesville, Fla., 1983, Triad Publishing Co. All clinicians reviewing kinetic manual perimetry results should read this chapter. Every technician should also read it to see examples of mistakes that can be made.

DIAGNOSTIC INTERPRETATION

Localized defects

Traditional diagnostic interpretation deals mainly with localized visual field defects, because the region of the field affected and the contour of the field abnormalities may pinpoint the location and nature of the lesion.

Often a diagnostic visual field test is performed to look for a specific kind of defect. The test is intended simply to confirm or to deny the presence of a particular condition. Thus, in a patient with endocrine abnormality, the examiner may be looking for a bitemporal hemianopia (caused by a pituitary adenoma) or, in a patient with glaucoma, looking for an arcuate scotoma or other type of nerve fiber bundle defect. The careful clinician will always consider whether or not the visual field findings are in keeping with the other clinical signs. For example, an arcuate visual field defect may be due to a branch retinal vessel occlusion, and the clinician may suspect this if, despite a somewhat elevated intraocular pressure (IOP), there is no cupping of the disc. Similarly an apparent central scotoma, inconsistent with a good visual acuity, is unlikely to be due to glaucoma, inviting further clinical examination if such a defect is found in a glaucoma suspect.

At other times the diagnostic visual field examination is performed to identify the cause of a visual abnormality. Thus the examining physician may try to make a distinction between types of postchiasmal lesions. For example, a congruous visual field defect with steep sharply demarcated margins would likely be due to a vascular lesion affecting the occipital cortex. Contrariwise, a homonymous hemianopic visual field defect with sloped boundaries incongruous between the two eyes would more likely be due to a tumor in the temporal or parietal lobe. Such differential diagnosis involves not only an analysis of the visual field diagram but also a consideration of the clinical circumstances, signs, and symptoms. The visual field interpretation is part and parcel of a broader differential diagnostic approach, which subject cannot be adequately covered here but will be left for the interested reader to explore in standard neuroophthalmic and visual field texts that describe the topographical characteristics of defects resulting from different types of lesions in differing locations.

For the present purpose, with regard to the analysis of localized defects, only two points will be reemphasized: First, it is worthwhile confirming a hemianopic defect by confrontation with a comparison technique (pp. 72-73). Second, the plotting of a single isopter (or the automated equivalent, suprathreshold testing at only one luminance level without quantitation of the depth of the defect) is only sometimes adequate to establish that an abnormality is a hemianopia (p. 290).

FIG. 13-44. An isopter that suggests a hemianopia. In the course of quantifying a depression (p. 390), additional isopters are drawn and one of two patterns may emerge. In a hemianopia other isopters will also show a demarcation along the vertical meridian. In a depression resulting from a prechiasmal lesion the initial isopter by happenstance may fall along the vertical meridian but other isopters will not.

In the hemianopia, depressed visual sensation is on only one side of the vertical meridian: *M* has a reduced visual sensitivity but *N* does not. In the prechiasmal lesion, depressed sensation is on both sides of the vertical meridian: *M* and *N* both are in an area of reduced visual sensation (compare with an equivalent spot in the inferior field).

Another criterion sometimes applicable is that in a hemianopia the apex of the contour of depressed isopters (if present) points toward fixation whereas in a prechiasmal lesion it may point at the blind spot.

The arc static cut (another way of obtaining the information required for diagnostic interpretation) shows that in a hemianopia there is a sharp demarcation at the vertical meridian separating the two areas, with 0.5 log-unit difference in visual sensation on the two sides. Visual sensation is reduced only on one side, not the other. In a prechiasmal lesion, however, there is depression on both sides of the vertical meridian, more marked nasally than temporally but with a gradual change in threshold as the vertical meridian is crossed.

In a hemianopia both the isopter plot and the static cut will show a steep margin along the vertical meridian (several isopters coincide). For this reason, if suprathreshold stimuli are presented just to the right and left of the vertical meridian in a hemianopia, they will be of different subjective brightnesses to the patient (more above threshold on the one side than on the other). Therefore brightness comparison testing is useful in confirming the presence of a hemianopia.

In a prechiasmal depression there is also a difference in sensation nasally and temporally but as the object passes from nasal to temporal there is a gradual increase in visibility rather than a sudden change at the vertical midline (see Fig. 3-6). Hence the technique of crossing the midline is essential in confirming the diagnostic meaning of any seeming abnormality in comparison testing.

In any event, this particular example shows that the interpreter must be on guard not to accept an inadequate field test (a single isopter) as showing the presence of a suspected defect (hemianopia) but rather must judge whether the abnormality could be due to another cause (e.g., a prechiasmal defect) demanding additional testing (Fig. 13-44) or other confirmation (pp. 175-178). Of course, the same care is required for all types of defects, not just hemianopias.

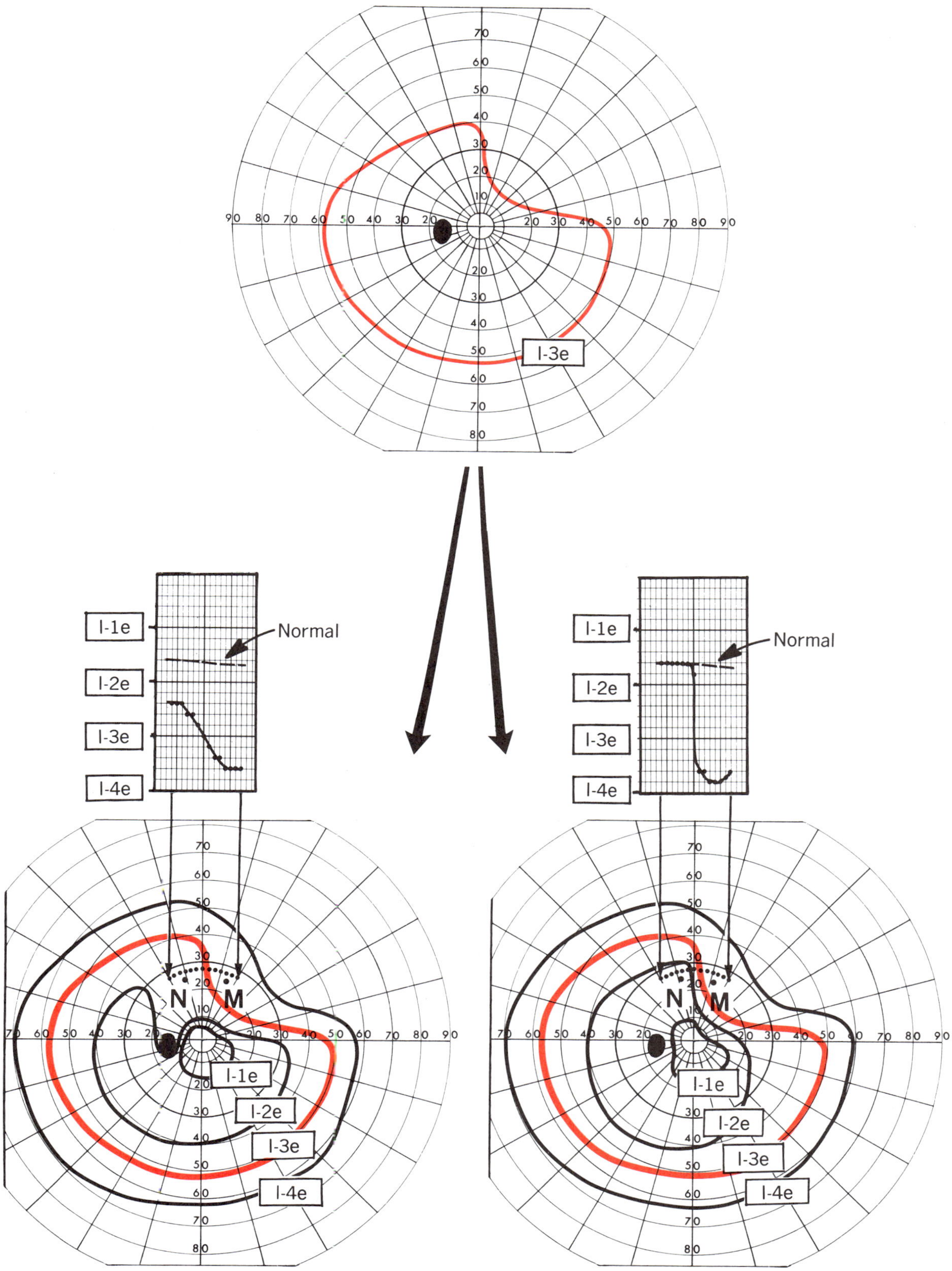
I-3e
I-1e
I-2e
I-3e
I-4e
Normal
N
M
I-1e
I-2e
I-3e
I-4e
I-1e
I-2e
I-3e
I-4e
Normal
N
M
I-1e
I-2e
I-3e
I-4e

FIG. 13-44

Generalized depression

Earlier sections of this book have dealt with the recognition of generalized visual depression from field diagrams of manual and automated perimeters. Once such a depression is recognized, the next task is a diagnostic one, to determine its cause. There is too often a tendency to dismiss the presence of generalized depression as "nonspecific," perhaps due to cataract, without bothering to check whether or not a sufficiently dense cataract is actually present. The clinician should identify the artifactual or true cause of any depression that is encountered.

Among the causes of an apparent generalized depression are the artifacts of improper instrument calibration, poor patient alertness, blurred retinal image from erroneous correction of refractive error, or (in kinetic perimetry) excessively fast movement of the target in relation to the patient's response time. Such causes should be considered especially when no other cause is identified on clinical examination, and then the test may need to be repeated to confirm that the initial test was in error.

Preretinal abnormalities typically cause generalized depression and can occur because of light scattering (corneal clouding, cataract), which reduces the contrast of the image; reduced light transmission (small pupil, brunescent cataract, vitreous hemorrhage), which places the retina in the mesopic state of adaptation; or defocusing of light (refractive error), producing a blurred image. Additionally, degeneration of the retina (myopia, retinitis pigmentosa), diffuse axon loss in glaucoma, and other lesions that affect the neural pathway diffusely can produce a general decline in sensitivity. The clinician needs to identify the cause.

FIG. 13-45. Generalized depression due to cataract. Practically all locations are depressed 5 to 10 dB from the normal value. On another occasion (right) the depression was seemingly more severe because the field examination was performed with a miotic pupil.

FIG. 13-46. Generalized depression due to glaucoma. The cause of the depression can be learned only from the clinical examination, which in this 54-year-old man showed clear ocular media but glaucomatous cupping with IOP elevation due to pigmentary dispersion.

Generalized depression plus

Sometimes it is difficult to decide whether or not a glaucomatous visual field defect is present in addition to a generalized depression resulting from age or known cataract, perhaps aggravated by a small pupil. The presence of cataract affects the center more than the periphery (pp. 126, 328); thus the field may be not merely depressed but also flattened in contour, with areas of inconsistent responses (Fig. 23-14, p. 473) that fall within the arcuate (Bjerrum) region. In this situation the presence of localized glaucomatous defects will be uncertain unless there are typical arcuate scotomas and nasal steps sufficiently deep (0.5 log-unit) not to be confused with shallow irregularities in a flattened hill of vision. A cataract can cause localized defects as well as generalized depression; thus the examiner may have to equivocate in his interpretation unless the localized defects are undeniably typical.

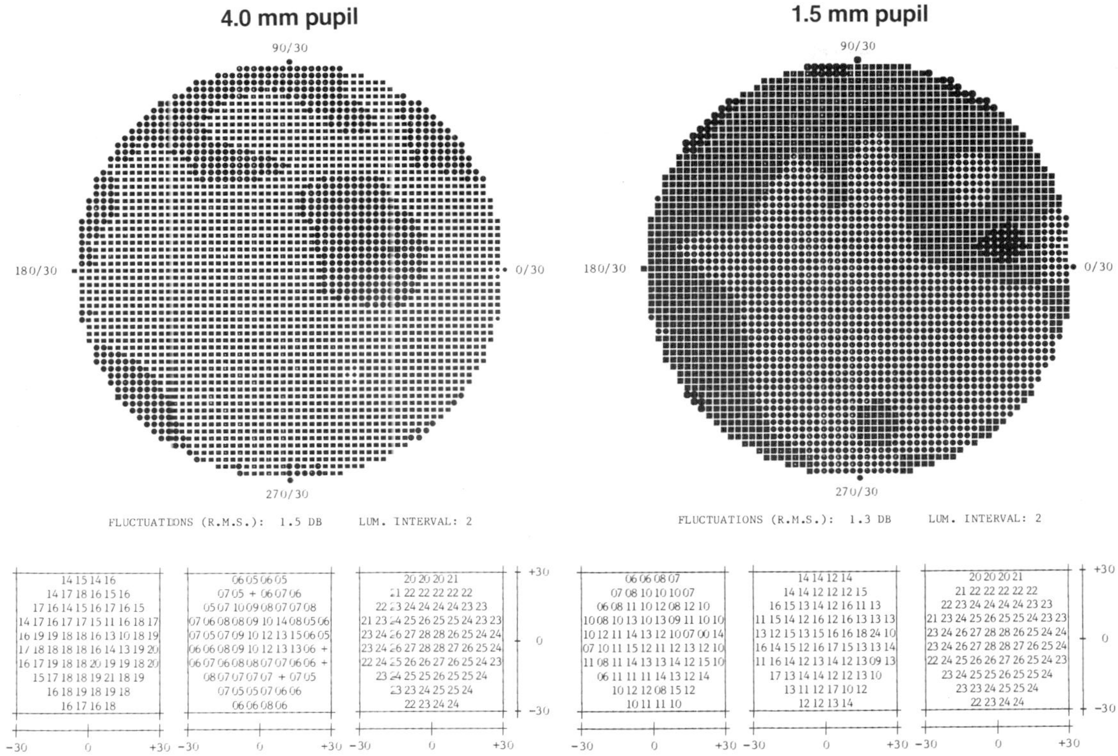

FIG. 13-45

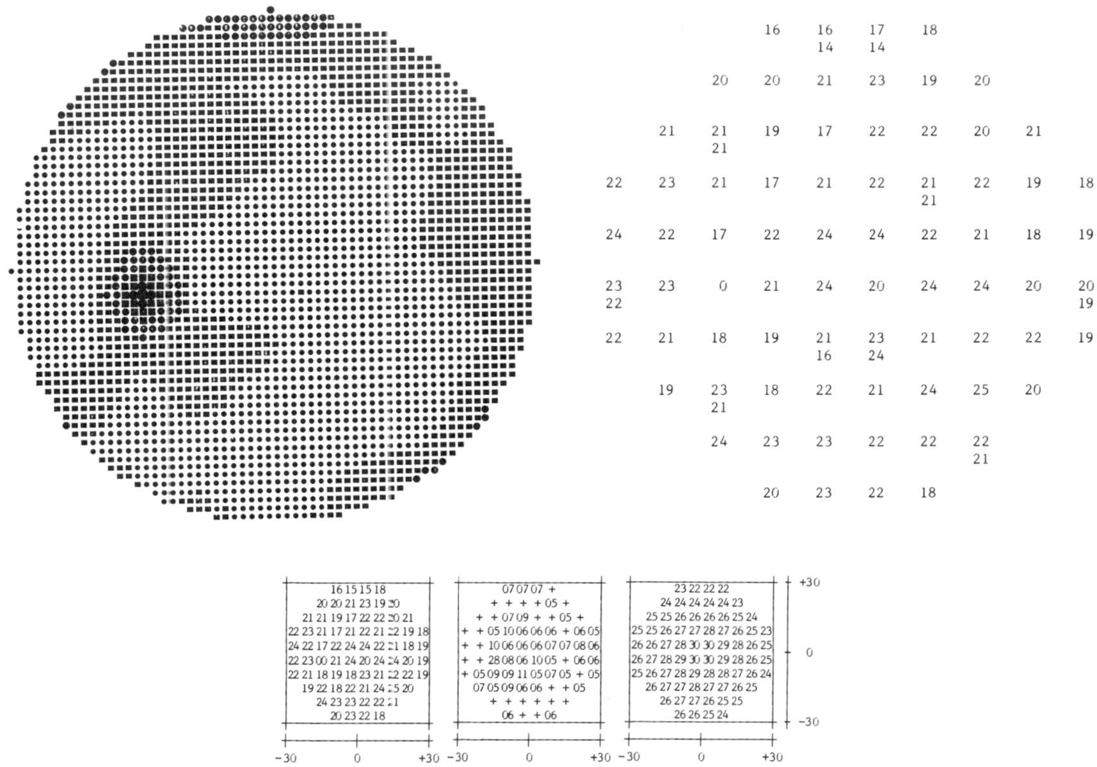

FIG. 13-46

Unexplained visual loss

In the differential diagnosis of unexplained visual acuity loss, the examiner is seeking evidence of either a generalized depression or a localized defect involving the point of fixation, e.g., a central scotoma. If neither is evident, he may search for a central scotoma occupying only the central 2 degrees that was not included in the grid of points on the suprathreshold test (or was in the region that could not be picked out with the Goldmann perimeter because of the telescope viewing port).

An automated program with a closer grid of points, a program that includes fixation itself, or both may be helpful in detecting the central scotoma. The Amsler grid, by distinguishing between a central scotoma and metamorphopsia, may point toward specific potential causes of the reduced vision. Of course, pupillary reactions and findings on ophthalmoscopy will also be revealing.

Whenever a central scotoma is present, the interpreter should look for evidence of a temporal hemianopia in the other eye and obtain additional evaluation if the field test was in any way inadequate to have uncovered such a defect.

Reduced visual acuity may result from a generalized depression, in which the point of fixation has reduced sensitivity along with all the rest of the field, or it may be due to a central scotoma, in which the reduced sensitivity at the point of fixation is surrounded by a zone of greater sensitivity. The finding of a generalized depression helps pinpoint the cause. However, the examining physician must be particularly careful when analyzing the difference-from-normal printout or the printout of a suprathreshold test with eccentricity compensation. If there is a generalized depression associated with flattening of the visual field, the greater depression of the central points than of the peripheral ones may simulate a central scotoma on these printouts by causing the central points to be missed while the more peripheral points may be seen as would happen with a central scotoma. Thus the suprathreshold test may be ambiguous when used to distinguish between generalized depression and a central scotoma.

FIG. 13-47. Flattening of the central field in early generalized depression. A central scotoma is falsely suggested by the difference-from-normal printout. An equally misleading printout can occur when a suprathreshold test is performed with eccentricity compensation (Fig. 13-9). Note that in Fig. 13-46 there is a pseudoscotoma of this type in the difference-from-normal printout affecting the central points (but also all nasal points).

ACTUAL

```
            17
         18 19 19 19 19
      19 20 20 21 20 20 20
   18 20 21 22 22 21 21 20 20
   20 22 23 23 22 22 22 22 21
20 21 22 23 23 24 22 22 22 21 21
   21 22 23 23 23 22 22 22 22
   20 21 22 22 23 23 22 21 20
      20 21 22 22 22 22 21
         20 21 22 21 21
            20
```

DIFFERENCE FROM NORMAL

```
             +
          +  +  +  +  +
       +  +  +  +  +  +  +
    +  +  +  +  +  +  +  +  +
    +  +  +  + 05 05  +  +  +
 +  +  + 05 06 08 06  +  +  +  +
    +  +  + 05 05 06  +  +  +
    +  +  +  +  +  +  +  +  +
       +  +  +  +  +  +  +
          +  +  +  +  +
             +
```

NORMAL

```
            20
         21 22 22 22 22
      23 23 24 24 24 24 24
   22 24 25 26 26 25 25 24 24
   23 25 27 27 27 27 26 25 24
23 24 26 28 29 32 28 27 26 25 25
   24 26 27 28 28 28 27 26 25
   23 25 26 26 27 27 26 26 24
      23 24 26 26 26 26 25
         23 24 25 25 25
            23
```

FIG. 13-47

Combined disease

During diagnostic interpretation the examining physician must always be careful when a patient has two conditions causing visual field defects. Some 1% of patients with a meningioma compressing the optic nerve or an infarct in the occipital cortex will also have glaucoma, as will 1% of the population without such neuroophthalmic conditions. Although any combination of two diseases may be quite rare, there are so many possible combinations among the different diseases that the examiner can expect once in a great while to encounter a patient who has two conditions simultaneously affecting the visual field. Therefore it is important to correlate the visual field findings with the rest of the clinical picture and if any discrepancy is found to explore for the possibility of a second confounding diagnosis.

PROGRESSIVE CHANGES

The nature of progression

In a chronic disease such as glaucoma, the visual field can show gradual progressive deterioration (or improvement) or the change can be episodic. With episodic progression the visual status remains stable for a while and then shows a new increment of loss, becoming stable at this new level before continuing on to the next episode of deterioration. With either episodic or continuous change there may be enlargement of a previous defect, deepening of a previous defect, the appearance of a new defect, or a generalized depression of visual sensation.

Judging the adequacy of the test

The examiner must consider whether the tests performed on two or more earlier occasions were sufficient to discover the various types of progression. In the case of manual perimetry the question is whether or not the important areas of the field were adequately explored and quantified on both occasions. In the case of automated perimetry the question is whether or not the correct program was selected.

A manual field examination should test isopters running through every portion of the field (not just the abnormal portions), with no more than 15 to 20 degrees of separation between the isopters. The spaces between isopters should be checked for scotomas in likely areas. All defects should be quantified with regard to depth and slope of the border, as taught in Part II of this book.

An automated field examination should be of the static threshold variety. Suprathreshold tests are not adequate to enable the interpreter to judge deepening of defects and generalized depression, though they may help in detecting new scotomas and enlargement of previous defects.

In the case of manual perimetry, if no progression was apparent there are several pertinent quetions: Have the abnormal areas been quantified enough to judge whether a defect is deeper than before? Were seemingly normal regions of the field tested to look for new scotomas? Were enough areas of the normal and abnormal field quantified so a generalized depression could be recognized? Conversely, when a new defect is detected, it must be asked whether that region of the field was tested adequately on the first occasion. Is this a new defect, or a newly discovered one?

Approach to field comparisons

The initial inspection of field diagrams to judge for progression is very qualitative. In observing the isopter plots of manual perimetry or the greyscale printouts of automated perimetry, the examiner looks for the appearance of new scotomatous regions and other obvious localized depressions. Enlargement or deepening of defects may be represented by movements of isopters on kinetic plots. The boundary between degrees of grey on a greyscale printout may similarly move, or there may be the impression of a greater degree of blackness in some or all portions of the field.

If the more recent field is obviously identical with a previous one, or is obviously very different, no further interpretation may be necessary. However, a detailed analysis is needed to judge suspicious changes or to recognize mild changes when two field diagrams at first glance seem the same.

For both automated and manual perimetry the **essence of the contrasting of two fields is a point-by-point comparison** of representative equivalent points in the diagrams obtained on different occasions.

To make this point-by-point comparison in manual perimetry requires thoughtful analysis. First of all, it must be realized that there is a close relationship of some scotomas and depressions (pp. 106-117) and that the same defect may be represented in several ways depending on how the test was performed. The clinician must also take into account the existence of some variability in the field from one time to another, which occurs in both manual and automated perimetry.

FIG. 13-48. Nonprogressive and progressive defects.
A, Nonprogressive defects. Note that they cover the same area and that the threshold within both is essentially identical, within the limits of variability of field testing.
B, Progressive defects. By contrast, here the visual threshold changes—becoming higher than before. However, the change is only in the defective area, not elsewhere (e.g., not in the lower temporal quadrant).

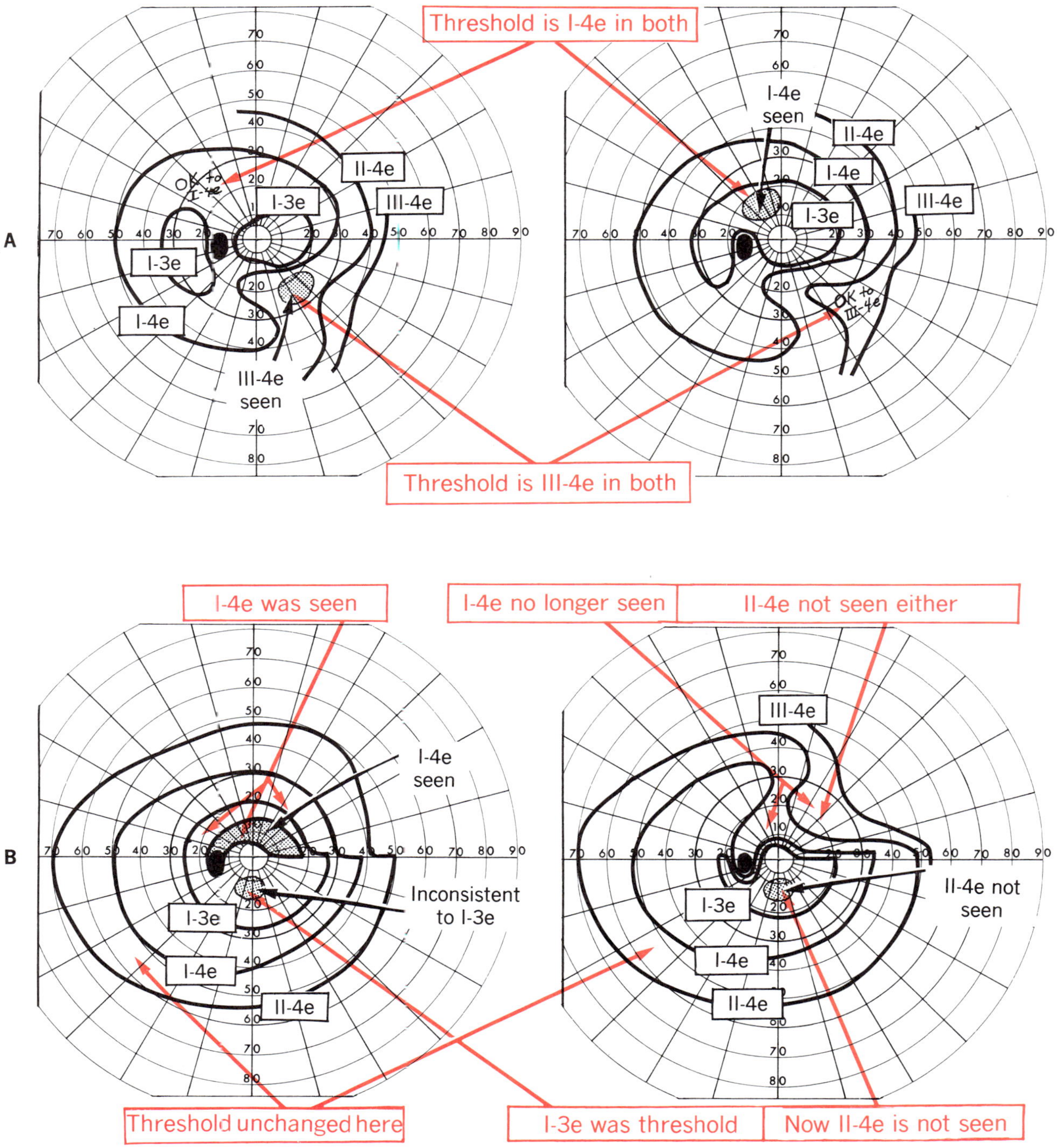
A
Threshold is I-4e in both
OK to I-4e
I-3e
II-4e
III-4e
I-3e
I-4e
III-4e seen
I-4e seen
II-4e
I-4e
I-3e
III-4e
OK to III-4e
Threshold is III-4e in both
B
I-4e was seen
I-4e no longer seen
II-4e not seen either
I-4e seen
III-4e
Inconsistent to I-3e
I-3e
I-4e
II-4e
II-4e not seen
I-3e
I-4e
II-4e
Threshold unchanged here
I-3e was threshold
Now II-4e is not seen

FIG. 13-48

In looking at the diagrams of kinetic field tests, it is tempting (and traditional) to observe the movement of isopters and to say that the field defect has progressed because a certain isopter has moved inward ("become smaller"). Thus, in Fig. 13-48 the *I-3e* isopter became smaller superiorly and this constituted a worsening of the field defect in the upper arcuate region. The practice of looking at isopter movement suffices in simple examples, but remember that the amount of isopter movement for a specific threshold change depends on the steepness or flatness of the hill of vision at that point. If isopters differing by 0.5 log-unit are 10 degrees apart in a region, then a 10-degree inward movement of an isopter represents 0.5 log-unit loss of visual sensation in that region. If the hill of vision is flatter, there is more isopter movement with the same 0.5 log-unit loss. It is best to compare representative points of interest in terms of threshold, as shown in Fig. 13-48. The visual sensation at a particular retinal location is attributable to a specific set of neurons, and progressive damage to the neurons is the underlying basis of progression. Isopters move when there is a change in visual threshold but it is the **change in threshold at a specific location** that is the relevant feature of progression.

This type of comparison is more natural with printouts of static threshold tests in automated perimetry.

FIG. 13-49. Comparison of the static threshold values on two occasions. These plots illustrate both that it is tedious to make a point-by-point comparison of two fields and that there is a certain variability in test results. Thus, because of short-term fluctuation (intratest variability) one point may seem to have worsened slightly and another to have improved when in fact neither has actually changed. It is simply an inaccuracy in the sensitivity determination.

			9	9 5	12 9	11			
		9	10	7	9	12	9		
	18	17 18	13	17	15	11	10	4	
18	21	17	20	18	24	19 15	13	9	9
20	19	14	19	22	19	20	18	11	10
21 19	20	0	23	23	23	22	24	17	18 17
10	18	18	22	24 22	23 23	23	20	17	17
	18	20 23	21	22	22	18	19	16	
		19	20	22	20	19	19 21		
			11	9	20	17			

			13	11 11	10 12	7			
		15	10	9	11	12	10		
	19	12 14	13	16	16	14	5	8	
21	19	17	14	14	17	13 15	13	7	7
21	17	17	21	20	22	20	14	12	7
21 23	20	2	26	24	26	25	20	18	14 11
16	21	21	22	24 23	23 22	21	20	7	13
	21	20 18	20	19	22	20	18	14	
		19	20	16	21	17	12 16		
			19	15	17	17			

FIG. 13-49

With automated perimetry there is help in making the comparison. A printout can be made that subtracts the sensitivity values and shows the point-by-point difference.

FIG. 13-50. Printout of the difference in static threshold at each point on the two occasions shown in Fig. 13-49. At a glance, it can be seen that some points have slightly higher threshold and others slightly lower because of the variability of measurement. One point deteriorated by 10 dB and might represent a new scotoma (this would have to be confirmed on a subsequent test). Another point, however, improved by 8 dB. Overall, there is no change.

In this type of printout any points with a drastic change will be quickly evident. However, the problem remains of deciding whether a broad region (or the entire field) is hiding a mild change within the variability. It would be impossible to perceive a sensitivity decline of 1 or 2 dB overall, because there would still be points with higher values despite the increased number with a slightly greater decline in sensitivity. To help with this, the computer can print out a table of the *average* (mean) sensitivity values for the entire field, for particular quadrants, or for specific zones of eccentricity (0 to 10 degrees, 10 to 20 degrees, 20 to 30 degrees). The averaging of several points reduces the effect of intratest variability (the points with values higher than true threshold will be balanced by those with values lower than true threshold). By the averaging method, the interpreter may be able to recognize a 2 to 3 dB (or smaller) overall decline in sensitivity of the field, even though there is 2 to 3 dB of variability in measurements (intratest variability, short-term fluctuations).

Fig. 13-51. Table of mean sensitivities of the same eye on two occasions. Sensitivities are shown for the whole field, for quadrants, and for specific zones of eccentricity.

Of course, the mean sensitivity values are not *exactly* the same; but just how much difference is "meaningful"? The answer to this question is statistical, depending not only on the mean sensitivity values but also on the intratest variability in the particular patient on these particular occasions. The comparison of two mean values can be done with a Student t-test (e.g., the Delta compare program of the Octopus perimeter). The t-test is performed on the entire field or only on points that are abnormal.

			4	4	1	- 4			
		6	0	2	2	0	1		
	1:	- 4	0	- 1	1	3	- 5	4	
3:	- 2:	0	- 6.	- 4	- 7.	- 3	0	- 2	- 2
1:	- 2.		2.	- 2	3	0	- 4	1	- 3
2:	0:		3:	1:	3:	3:	- 4.	1	- 5
6	3.	3.	0:	0:	- 1:	- 2:	0:	-10	- 4.
	3.	- 2.	- 1:	- 3.	0:	2.	- 1.	- 2	
		0:	0:	- 6.	1:	- 2.	- 6.		
			8.	6	- 3.	0:			

DIFFERENCE TABLE : MEAN B MINUS MEAN A (NEGATIVE VALUES: DECREASED SENSITIVITY)
0-0 ALL RESULTS ZERO <> LOW NORMAL VALUES
DOTS INDICATE THAT SOME (.) OR ALL (:) RESULTS ARE IN NORMAL RANGE (FULLY VALID)

CONFIDENCE INTERVAL FOR MEAN DIFFERENCE / T-TEST
(1) PATHOL. AREA (UNDOTTED) - 0.2 ± 1.2 (T-TEST: DATA DO NOT PROVE ALTERATION)
(2) WHOLE FIELD - 0.3 ± 0.8 (T-TEST: DATA DO NOT PROVE ALTERATION)

FIG. 13-50

DATE OF EXAM : DAY / YEAR	04.28 1983	08.23 1984
MEAN SENSITIVITY		
WHOLE FIELD (N: 23.1)	16.7	16.4
QUAD.UPP.NAS.(N: 22.4)	12.7	11.9
LOW.NAS.(N: 23.4)	19.7	18.1
UPP.TMP.(N: 22.5)	15.6	15.7
LOW.TMP.(N: 24.1)	18.9	20.2
ECC. 0 - 10 (N: 25.9)	21.6	21.7
10 - 20 (N: 23.9)	18.4	17.6
20 - 30 (N: 22.0)	14.7	14.6
NO. OF DISTURBED POINTS	41	47
R.M.S. FLUCTUATION	1.8	1.5

FIG. 13-51

Beginners at interpretation of field results make two types of mistakes when they get a positive t-test: *First,* they assume that a statistically significant change is a deterioration and that the patient is in trouble. They may not realize that the second field has a higher sensitivity value and, in fact, there has been a statistically significant improvement in visual sensation. Examples of statistically significant improvements due to learning effects or long-term fluctuation are given later in the chapter. *Second,* they assume that a statistically significant deterioration is due to worsening of the disease under consideration rather than to (a) an artifact, (b) some other superimposed disease, or (c) (most often) so-called long-term fluctuation (p. 310). The approach to the task of interpreting an apparent change will occupy the rest of this chapter.

To summarize how to recognize that a change has occurred (before discussing how to interpret the change): Very localized sensitivity changes may be most apparent on the kinetic plot, on a greyscale printout, or on a printout of the differences at individual points. Diffuse changes or progression in broad areas will be best recognized from a table of mean sensitivity calculations. Localized changes (new scotomas, deepening of existing scotomas) will have a less noticeable effect on the mean sensitivity value of the entire field but may be noticeable in the mean sensitivities of individual sectors or eccentricity zones.

Figs. 13-52, 13-53, and 13-54 show three examples of progressive visual field loss.

FIG. 13-52. Progressive visual loss in a case of normal tension glaucoma. A new scotoma (arrow) has appeared in the upper arcuate region near the blind spot, and the absolute defect impinging on fixation has enlarged. Deterioration of sensitivities occurred in all areas but most significantly within 10 degrees of fixation (between arrows in the summary table).

DATE OF EXAM : DAY / YEAR		05.19 1983	08.23 1984	01.16 1986	03.06 1986
MEAN SENSITIVITY					
WHOLE FIELD	(N: 23.5)	18.5	18.2	16.1	14.8
QUAD.UPP.NAS.	(N: 22.8)	17.0	17.7	14.1	13.3
LOW.NAS.	(N: 23.8)	15.4	14.1	12.2	11.1
UPP.TMP.	(N: 22.9)	20.9	20.4	18.1	16.2
LOW.TMP.	(N: 24.5)	21.1	20.9	20.2	18.9
ECC. 0 - 10	(N: 26.3)	14.0	12.8	9.9	8.7
10 - 20	(N: 24.3)	19.4	19.0	16.3	15.8
20 - 30	(N: 22.4)	19.4	19.3	17.6	16.1
NO. OF DISTURBED POINTS		33	28	36	48
R.M.S. FLUCTUATION		1.8	1.9	1.9	1.2

FIG. 13-52

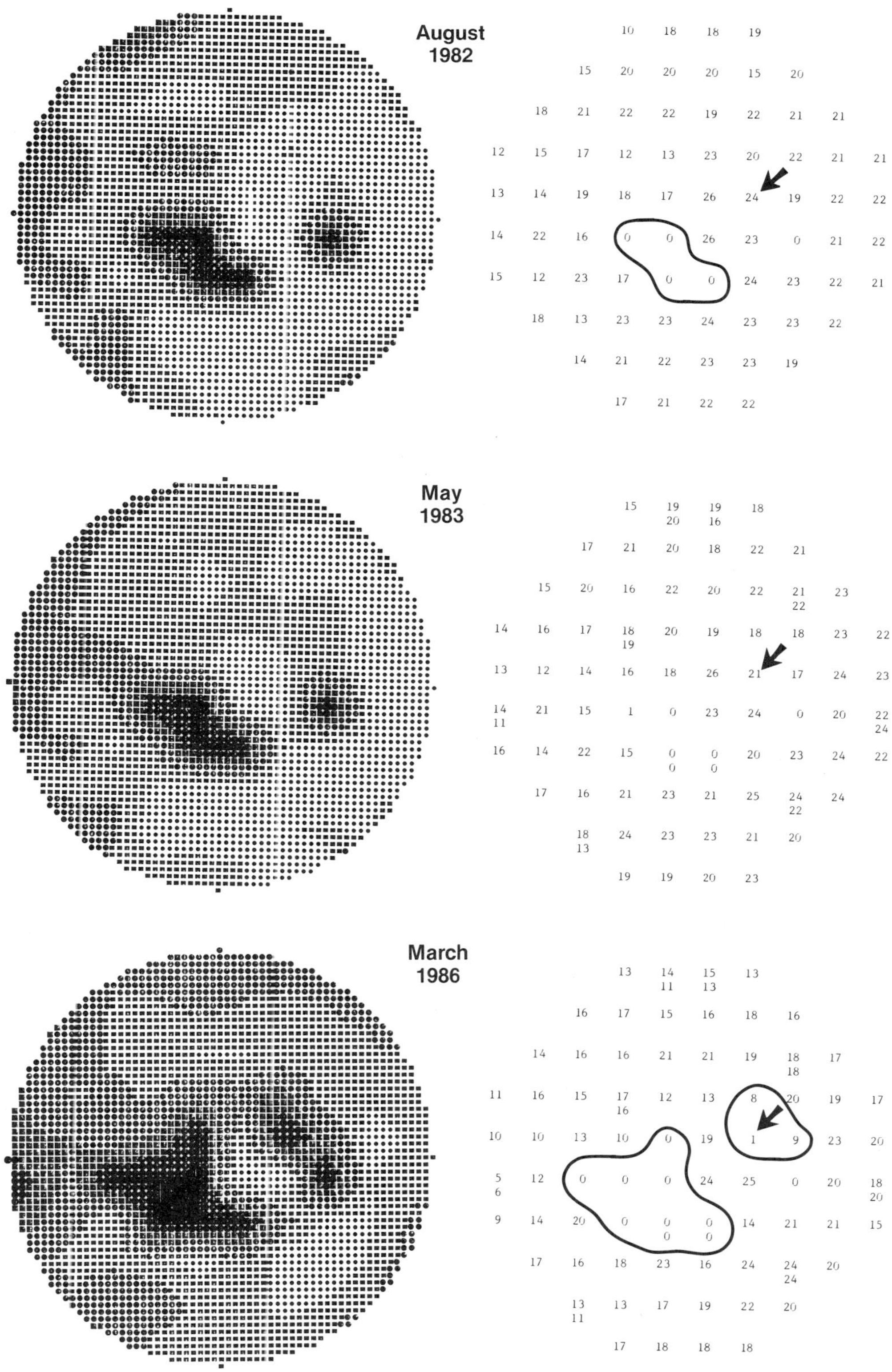

FIG. 13-52, cont'd

FIG. 13-53. Another mild example of glaucomatous progression. The most noticeable deterioration has occurred nasally (compare sensitivities on the numeric printouts and look also at the upper nasal quadrant row of the mean sensitivity table).

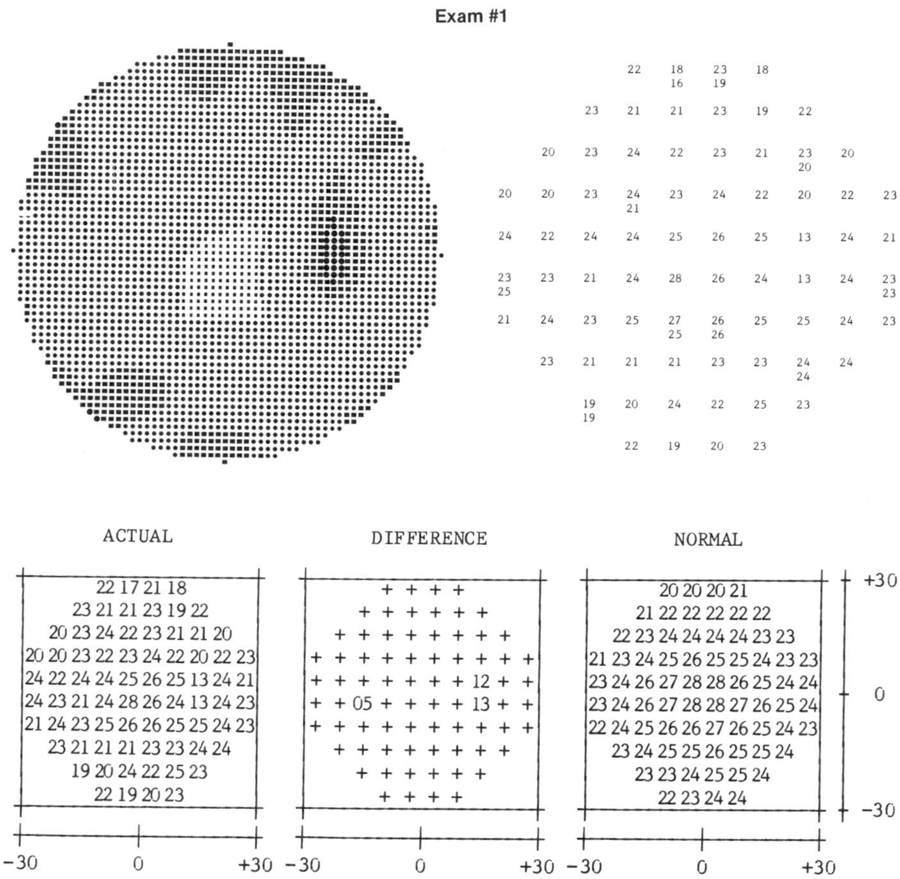

FIG. 13-53

Exam #4

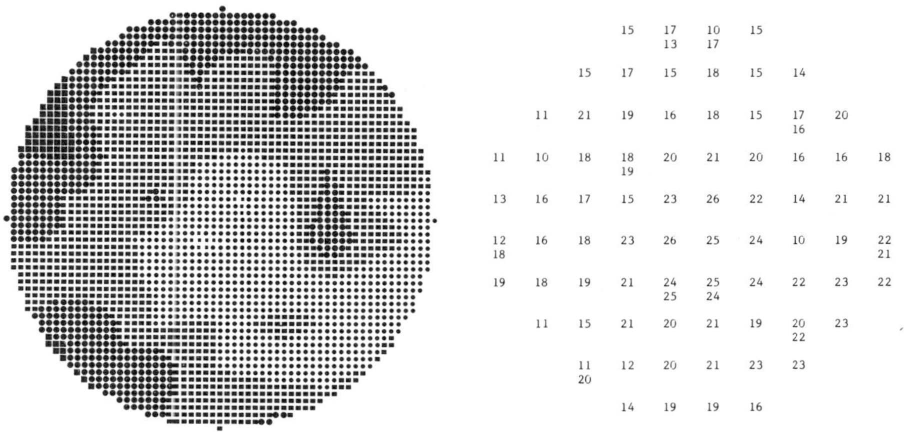

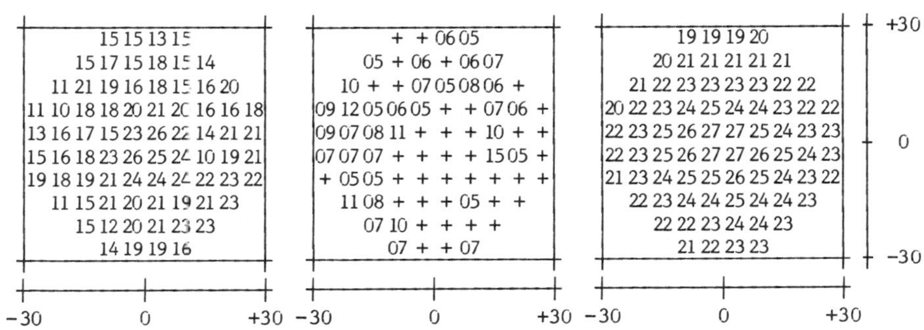

DATE OF EXAM : DAY YEAR	07.19 1984	10.31 1985	12.12 1985	03.27 1986
MEAN SENSITIVITY				
WHOLE FIELD (N: 23.5)	22.6	19.9	20.6	18.5
QUAD.UPP.NAS.(N: 22.8)	➔ 22.1	18.6	18.6	16.1 ⬅
LOW.NAS.(N: 23.8)	22.6	19.8	20.8	18.2
UPP.TMP.(N: 22.9)	21.9	19.1	20.1	18.1
LOW.TMP.(N: 24.5)	23.7	22.1	23.0	21.7
ECC. 0 – 10 (N: 26.3)	25.1	23.6	24.1	22.8
10 – 20 (N: 24.3)	22.7	20.6	21.0	19.0
20 – 30 (N: 22.4)	21.9	18.6	19.5	17.1
NO. OF DISTURBED POINTS	1	19	12	35

FIG. 13-53, cont'd

FIG. 13-54. Small central island followed with a close grid of points 3 degrees apart. The point of fixation is circled on the numeric printout. Each numeric value is the average of three determinations at that point. The area below fixation has deteriorated progressively over four successive tests.

Point of fixation

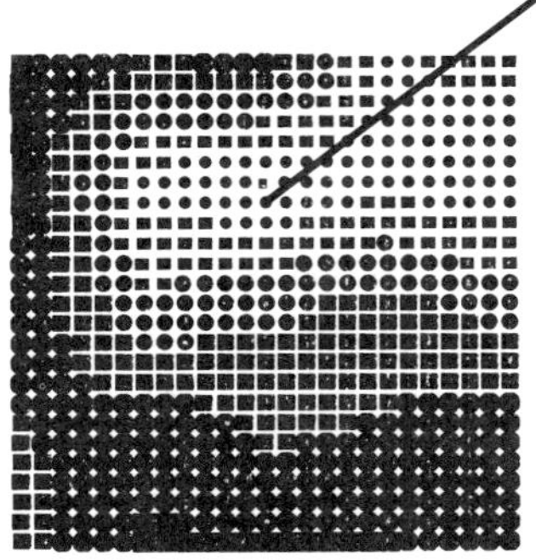

0.0	5.8	4.7	20.8	19.2
0.0	21.5	(25.5)	21.8	24.2
1.3	14.8	12.2	9.2	12.5
5.8	2.3	6.5	5.2	1.7
6.5	0.0	0.0	0.0	2.5

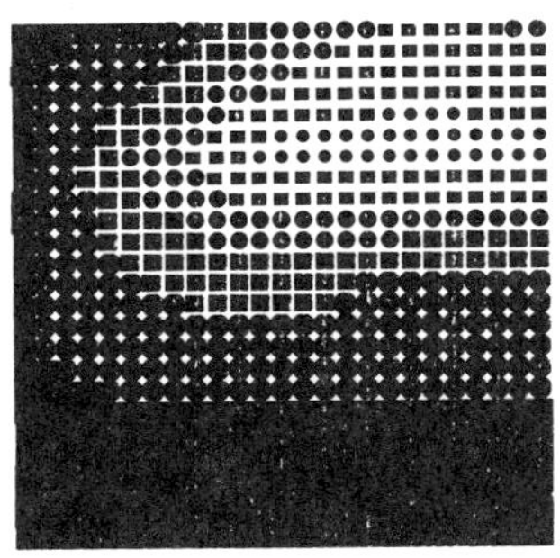

0.0	0.0	10.5	16.8	14.5
0.0	12.8	(22.5)	22.8	21.5
0.0	6.3	7.5	3.7	4.3
0.0	0.0	0.0	0.0	0.0
0.0	0.0	0.0	0.0	0.0

FIG. 13-54

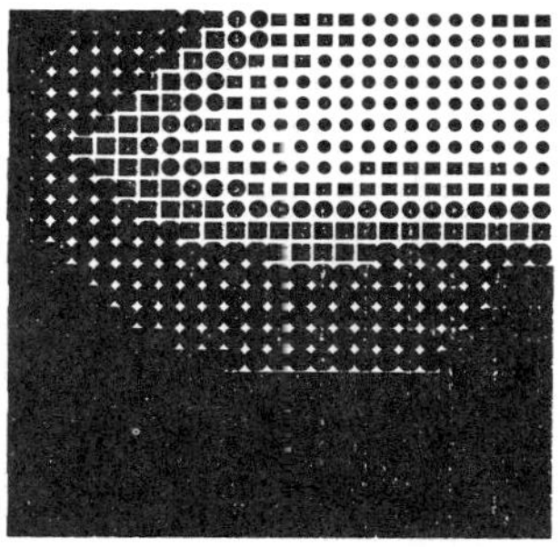

0.2	0.2	16.2	23.2	19.2
0.0	10.8	26.2	22.8	25.2
0.0	1.2	2.0	1.5	0.0
0.0	0.0	0.0	0.0	0.0
0.0	0.2	0.0	0.0	0.2

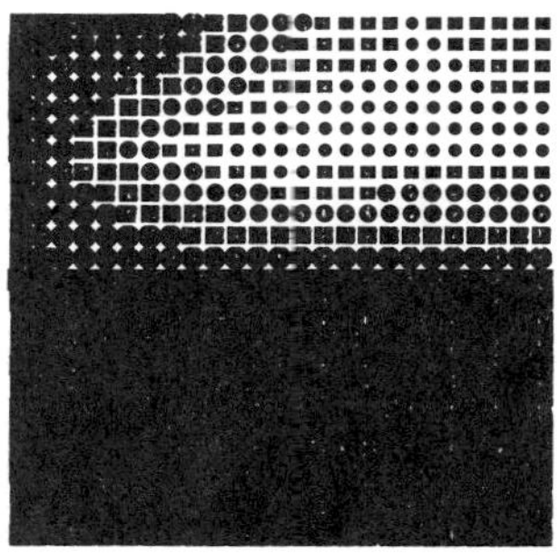

0.0	0.0	12.5	20.5	15.8
0.0	13.5	24.8	22.5	22.5
0.0	0.0	0.0	0.0	0.0
0.0	0.0	0.0	0.0	0.0
0.0	0.0	0.0	0.0	0.0

FIG. 13-54, cont'd

False progression: intertest variability

The *intra*test variability (short-term fluctuation) has already been mentioned as the unavoidable measurement uncertainty that results from the frequency-of-seeing curve, compounded by any unreliability of responses by the patient.

Over and above this type of variability, there is also an *inter*test variability (known as long-term fluctuation). The visual sensitivity may have a greater (or lesser) sensitivity than on a previous occasion, and the change may exceed what can be attributed to measurement uncertainty. The measurement is due to an actual change in the state of visual physiology from one time to another—perhaps because of such factors as fluid and electrolyte status, degree of alertness, or whatever. The point is that vision can be tested and retested on a given day and found to be at one level but on another day to be at a different level, and then on a third day to have returned again to resemble the state of sensitivity on the first day. The change may typically be 2 or 3 dB, and about 2% of the time it will be 4 dB or perhaps even a bit more.

FIG. 13-55. Table of mean visual sensitivity values. Note the variability from one time to another.

That this is a true change in visual sensitivity is indicated by the fact that the t-test often shows the change to be statistically significant, which means that the new values are due not to chance based on measurement uncertainty (intratest variability) but to the fact that over several occasions the sensitivity goes up and down and on the upswing may be statistically significantly *increased*. (Fig. 2-9 shows an example of a small but statistically significant increase in sensitivity.)

	EX1	EX2	EX3	EX4
DATE OF EXAM : DAY	06.14	06.22	07.01	03.21
YEAR	1983	1983	1983	1984
MEAN SENSITIVITY				
WHOLE FIELD (N: 24.1)	18.6	18.6	19.3	17.2
QUAD.UPP.NAS.(N: 23.4)	13.2	13.7	12.6	11.0
LOW.NAS.(N: 24.4)	21.2	20.8	21.4	18.9
UPP.TMP.(N: 23.5)	17.4	17.6	19.3	16.9
LOW.TMP.(N: 25.1)	22.7	22.7	24.1	22.1
ECC. 0 - 10 (N: 26.9)	23.8	22.8	24.6	22.2
10 - 20 (N: 24.9)	19.0	19.0	19.5	17.9
20 - 30 (N: 23.0)	17.0	17.4	17.7	15.5
NO. OF DISTURBED POINTS	36	40	33	43
R.M.S. FLUCTUATION	3.1	2.7	1.9	3.3

FIG. 13-55

The occurrence of long-term fluctuation ruins the usefulness of the t-test when comparing two field examinations. If the change is large, it is not necessary to use the t-test. If the change is small, the t-test cannot distinguish a small true change from long-term fluctuation. Therefore, when comparing two fields, the main usefulness of the t-test is that a *negative* result can be reassuring that an apparent change is *not* a conclusive finding.

The task, then, is to distinguish true deterioration from the effects of long-term fluctuation. When only two field examinations are available for comparison, you cannot conclude that a true change of mean sensitivity has occurred unless the change exceeds the 3 to 5 dB that could be due to long-term fluctuation; also changes at individual points must be greater than the combined effects of long-term and short-term fluctuations. You can justifiably be concerned that true progression has occurred if reduced sensitivity is noted at a group of points in a location typical for the disease while the rest of the field remains less affected. However, it is often difficult to be certain of a change, for two reasons: *First,* although the homogeneous component of long-term fluctuation causes a change of the same magnitude and direction at all points in the field, there is a heterogeneous component that affects some points more than others. *Second,* fluctuations, including both the long-term and the short-term variety, are of greater magnitude in abnormal regions. This has been illustrated in Figs. 13-14 and 14-1, in which the abnormal point showed a highly variable visual threshold. Therefore, when a change is suspected, particularly a small change, or when one is detected in an already abnormal region, it is often necessary to repeat the field examination in a few days to be sure.

All this variability can be discouraging when trying to compare two diagrams. Notice that in Figs. 13-52 to 13-54 the true nature of the progressive change was documented by a series of tests showing relentless deterioration (rather than the up-and-down variability evidenced in Fig. 13-55). The effect of interest variability was overcome by using a series of field tests rather than relying on only two consecutive examinations.

Another strategy is to anticipate the problem and perform a second baseline field examination a month or two after the first. Especially if there is a sizable difference, a third baseline field may be obtained. Thereafter, single visual field tests are performed at the usual intervals but, when there is a worrisome finding, are repeated a few days to a month later to confirm or deny that there has been a change compared to the baseline series. Repeat testing of any suspicious fields on a subsequent occasion and the use of a t-test to compare two or three recent tests with two or three baseline tests may allow changes smaller than the long-term fluctuation to be documented. Still another potential strategy is to use a type of regression analysis on a series of fields over many months or years; however, software for this type of analysis awaits development.

To summarize: True progression can be distinguished from long-term fluctuation when (1) the change between two occasions is drastic (say, 10 dB or more greater than the long-term fluctuation) in a typical localized defect, (2) a series of several field examinations documents a relentless downward trend that is not overcome by the upswing in long-term fluctuation, or (3) several examinations are grouped together as a baseline and compared by means of a t-test to one or a group of field exams at a subsequent time.

False progression: other causes

Apart from long-term fluctuations, there are a number of other specific explanations for a change in sensitivity. Pupil size clearly makes a difference. Certain medications affect sensitivity. The level of the intraocular pressure may play a role. Changes in mean sensitivity from one occasion to another may also occur as the patient becomes more accustomed to visual field testing (''learning curve''). On certain occasions the test results may be influenced by inappropriate centering of a correcting lens or by patient factors, such as fatigue from a sleepless night.

FIG. 13-56. Effect of pupillary size on mean sensitivities. The field examination on the left was with a 3 mm pupil and the one on the right with a 2 mm pupil. The change could be mistaken for progressive visual loss. Because the size of the pupil can affect test results, it must always be recorded at the time of the visual field examination.

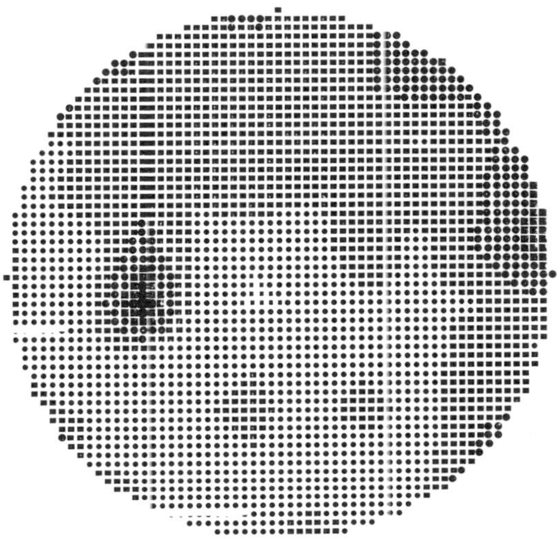

270/30

FLUCTUATIONS (R.M.S.): 1.2 DB LUM. INTERVAL: 2

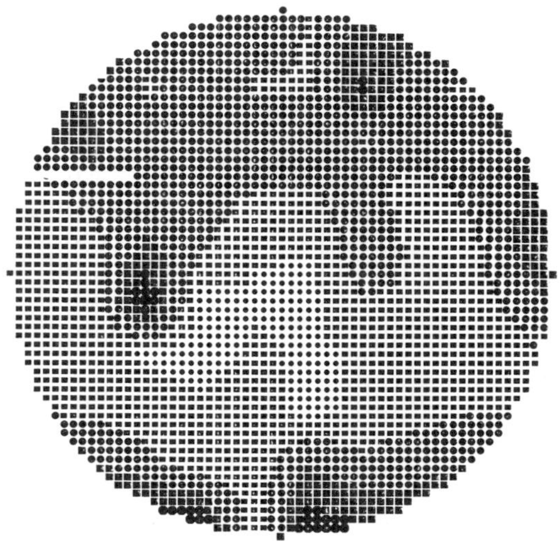

270/30

FLUCTUATIONS (R.M.S.): 1.2 DB LUM. INTERVAL: 2

ACTUAL

17 16 18 17
17 18 18 18 16 14
20 17 18 20 18 17 21 18
21 19 17 20 17 20 19 18 17 11
21 23 13 22 25 24 16 22 16 10
21 23 00 24 26 25 22 21 21 17
21 21 23 23 21 24 23 22 19 20
21 22 21 19 23 18 23 17
22 23 21 24 24 22
23 24 20 23

−30 0 +30

DIFFERENCE

+ + + +
+ + + + 05 06
+ 05 05 + 05 06 + +
− + 06 + 07 05 05 05 05 09
− + 11 + + + 10 + 07 12
− + 25 + + + + + + 05
− + + + 05 + + + + +
+ + + 06 + 06 + 05
+ + + + + +
+ + + +

−30 0 +30

NORMAL

20 19 19 19
21 21 21 21 21 20
22 22 23 23 23 23 22 21
22 22 23 24 24 25 24 23 22 20
23 23 24 25 27 27 26 25 23 22
23 24 25 26 27 27 26 25 23 22
22 23 24 25 26 25 25 24 23 21
23 24 24 25 24 24 23 22
23 24 24 23 22 22
23 23 22 21

−30 0 +30

ACTUAL

12 13 16 08
16 13 16 16 05 15
09 14 15 11 11 16 11 11
18 13 15 13 16 16 13 19 14 10
19 18 09 15 20 20 12 17 17 09
18 20 00 22 21 22 16 16 18 13
20 19 21 22 20 21 20 18 18 17
17 19 20 18 23 19 18 16
14 20 19 11 15 13
05 19 05 07

−30 0 +30

DIFFERENCE

08 06 + 11
05 08 05 05 16 05
13 08 08 12 12 07 11 10
+ 09 08 11 08 09 11 + 08 10
+ 05 15 10 07 07 14 08 06 13
05 + 25 + 06 05 10 09 05 09
+ + + + 06 + 05 06 05 +
06 05 + 07 + 05 05 06
09 + 05 12 07 09
18 + 17 14

−30 0 +30

NORMAL

20 19 19 19
21 21 21 21 21 20
22 22 23 23 23 23 22 21
22 22 23 24 24 25 24 23 22 20
23 23 24 25 27 27 26 25 23 22
23 24 25 26 27 27 26 25 23 22
22 23 24 25 26 25 25 24 23 21
23 24 24 25 24 24 23 22
23 24 24 23 22 22
23 23 22 21

−30 0 +30

FIG. 13-56

FIG. 13-57. Effect of learning on the visual field. The mean sensitivity of this patient improved considerably on the second examination and was maintained thereafter. Note also that the fluctuation (RMS) was particularly high on the first examination.

Exam #1

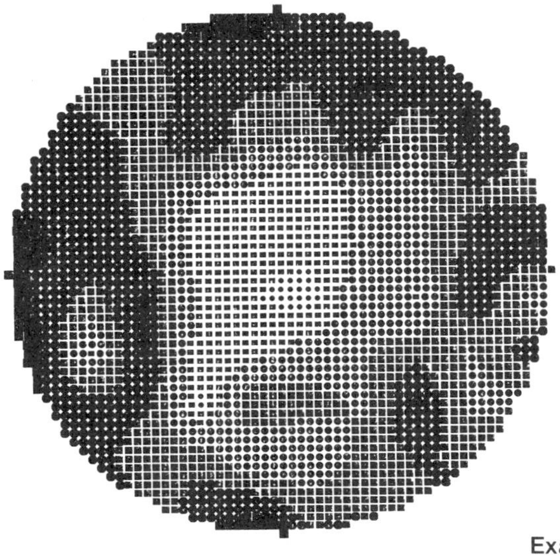

Exam #2

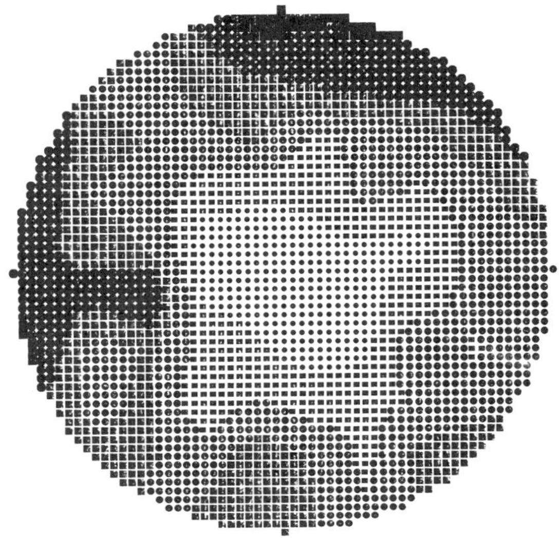

	Exam #1	Exam #2				
DATE OF EXAM : DAY	11.23	12.13	03.30	07.10	08.23	
YEAR	1983	1983	1984	1984	1985	
MEAN SENSITIVITY						
WHOLE FIELD (N: 25.1)	8.4	12.0	12.1	12.3	12.8	11.5 ± 0.
QUAD.UPP.NAS.(N: 24.4)	7.9	11.5	11.2	11.6	11.9	10.8 ± 0.
LOW.NAS.(N: 25.4)	9.7	14.4	15.0	14.3	15.9	13.9 ± 1.
UPP.TMP.(N: 24.5)	6.8	10.0	10.1	10.8	11.1	9.8 ± 0.
LOW.TMP.(N: 26.1)	9.3	12.2	12.0	12.2	12.0	11.5 ± 0.
ECC. 0 - 10 (N: 27.9)	17.7	22.3	21.4	21.9	21.8	21.0 ± 0.
10 - 20 (N: 25.9)	10.3	14.5	15.4	15.5	15.8	14.3 ± 1.
20 - 30 (N: 24.0)	5.2	8.3	8.2	8.3	9.0	7.8 ± 0.
NO. OF DISTURBED POINTS	74	71	73	72	71	72 ± 1
R.M.S. FLUCTUATION	6.3	2.2	2.0	1.7	2.8	3.0

FIG. 13-57

FIG. 13-58. Second example of the learning effect. In this case the first examination (arrow) gave a falsely high sensitivity value. Because of concern about the rapid decline in sensitivity between the first and second examinations, the test was repeated frequently for a while until the stability of the visual field was well documented. However, the mean sensitivity was never as good as on the first exam.

Exam #1

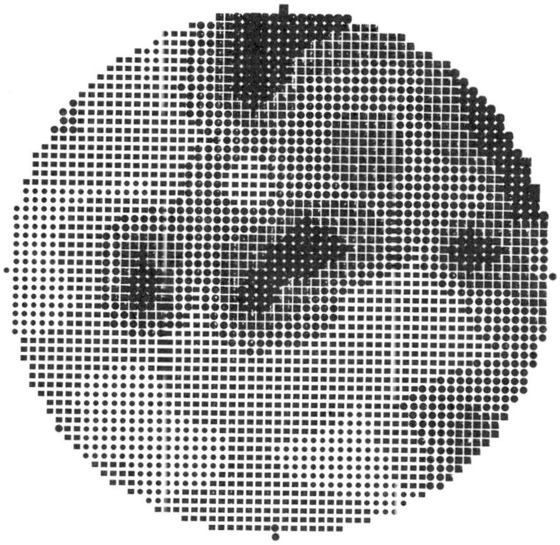

Exam #2

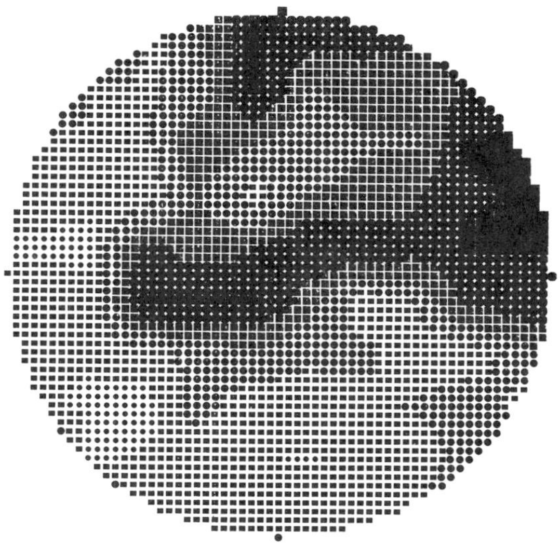

DATE OF EXAM : DAY / YEAR	09.02 1982	09.30 1982	11.23 1982	12.14 1982	03.17 1983	06.23 1983	10.19 1983	02.02 1984	07.09 1984	04.04 1985	08.22 1985	06.26 1986
MEAN SENSITIVITY												
WHOLE FIELD (N: 24.1)	14.8	12.3	12.9	13.6	14.0	13.0	12.7	12.8	13.3	13.3	13.6	12.5
QUAD. UPP.NAS. (N: 23.4)	8.9	5.5	5.7	5.9	5.4	4.8	4.5	4.0	5.3	5.3	6.8	3.9
LOW.NAS. (N: 24.4)	17.0	15.0	16.5	17.9	18.8	17.8	18.5	17.4	18.9	18.1	17.6	17.8
UPP.TMP. (N: 23.5)	14.8	12.9	13.1	12.4	13.5	11.6	11.0	12.7	12.1	12.4	12.5	11.6
LOW.TMP. (N: 25.1)	18.7	16.2	16.7	18.2	18.5	17.8	16.9	17.5	17.2	17.5	17.5	16.8
ECC. 0 - 10 (N: 26.9)	11.4	8.1	7.6	8.0	8.8	7.0	8.8	7.8	8.7	8.8	10.6	7.8
10 - 20 (N: 24.9)	16.3	13.1	13.7	15.1	14.7	14.2	13.6	14.1	14.6	14.6	14.0	13.2
20 - 30 (N: 23.0)	15.1	13.2	14.1	14.5	15.1	14.1	13.4	13.7	14.1	14.0	14.2	13.5
NO. OF DISTURBED POINTS	57	61	59	53	46	57	63	58	60	56	65	63
R.M.S. FLUCTUATION	2.7	1.9	1.8	1.2	1.9	2.1	1.2	2.2	2.2	1.4	2.1	1.2

FIG. 13-58

FIG. 13-59. Decreased mean sensitivity on the fourth examination resulting from a lens rim artifact. The cause for this decrease was uncovered by looking at the greyscale and numeric printouts and recognizing that the edge points accounted for the decline in sensitivity. Note that in the mean sensitivity table the reduction occurred in the 20- to 30-degree zone of eccentricity and in the inferior quadrants (arrows). The cause was confirmed by a subsequent examination, when care was taken to avoid this artifact.

This example illustrates that judgments cannot be made from the tabulated results alone. The tabulated results simply show that there may be an unstable field. It is wise to check the greyscale and numeric printouts of the individual fields to determine the source of the diminished overall sensitivity. It may also be useful to know whether the loss is generalized or due to a confined group of points. Consider the next example (Figs. 13-60 to 13-63), in which there is a relentless decrease in sensitivity over 2 years despite increasing therapy. Notice how continual thoughtful analysis is needed to avoid erroneous conclusions.

DATE OF EXAM : DAY YEAR	05.15 1984	11.20 1984	05.21 1985	11.26 1985
MEAN SENSITIVITY				
WHOLE FIELD (N: 25.1)	22.3	21.3	21.1	19.2 ↙
QUAD.UPP.NAS.(N: 24.4)	21.5	21.8	21.3	21.0
LOW.NAS.(N: 25.4)	21.7	21.4	21.1	18.9 ↖
UPP.TMP.(N: 24.5)	21.5	19.9	19.4	19.0
LOW.TMP.(N: 26.1)	24.3	22.1	22.8	17.9 ↖
ECC. 0 - 10 (N: 27.9)	27.2	26.4	26.4	25.5
10 - 20 (N: 25.9)	23.4	23.2	22.4	23.0
20 - 30 (N: 24.0)	20.5	19.2	19.2	16.0 ↖

FIG. 13-59

May
1984

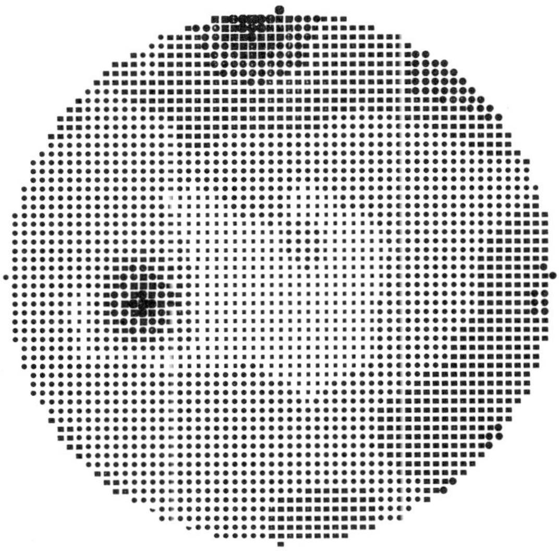

			16	3 5	19 11	20			
		20	19	17	18	19	15		
	22	19 25	20	22	21	24	24	20	
23	23	25	27	23	27	23 25	23	24	21
24	24	20	28	28	24	29	22	21	18
26 24	26	0	27	30	28	27	22	21	16 16
24	26	26	27	26 26	29 29	27	22	19	18
	23	22 24	21	22	25	21	18	18	
		24	23	21	23	21	20 20		
			23	21	18	20			

Nov.
1985

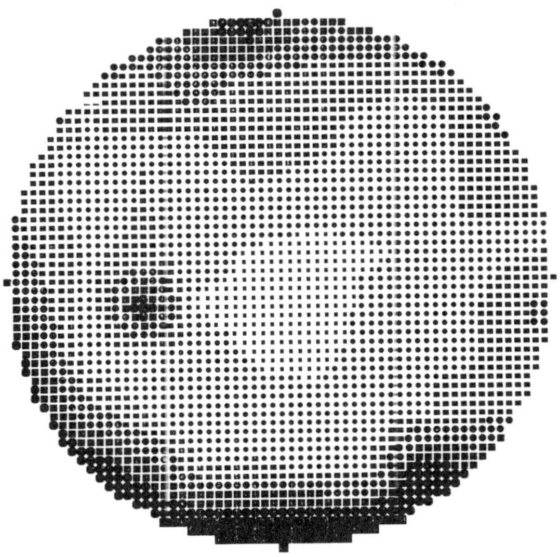

			9	2 9	16 10	11			
		18	13	20	19	20	20		
	21	21 21	22	17	19	22	24	19	
18	24	20	25	22	23	25 24	24	19	20
16	21	19	24	26	27	26	25	23	21
14 12	24	0	26	27	28	25	25	21	16 16
7	23	25	23	27 25	27 26	25	21	21	17
	13	20 21	25	23	25	24	21	18	
		8	20	20	21	22	0 6		
			0	0	0	0			

FIG. 13-59, cont'd

FIG. 13-60. Progressive reduced sensitivity in all sectors and in the whole field. The greyscale and numeric printouts show generalized further loss of sensitivity. The change from the first to the second field was attributed to long-term fluctuation, but the third field raised concern that a true deterioration might be occurring. The fourth field examination seemed to confirm the need to reevaluate this patient's treatment. However, it was recognized that the decline coincided with his increasingly vigorous use of miotics.

DATE OF EXAM : DAY / YEAR	03.03 1983	07.14 1983	11.17 1983	05.17 1984
MEAN SENSITIVITY				
WHOLE FIELD (N: 24.8)	22.6	22.2	21.7	20.4
QUAD.UPP.NAS.(N: 24.2)	20.6	21.4	20.5	19.2
LOW.NAS.(N: 25.1)	24.8	23.8	24.0	23.3
UPP.TMP.(N: 24.3)	19.7	19.0	18.2	17.1
LOW.TMP.(N: 25.8)	25.2	24.7	24.2	22.2
ECC. 0 - 10 (N: 27.7)	23.0	20.4	21.4	19.1
10 - 20 (N: 25.7)	23.8	24.9	23.9	22.2
20 - 30 (N: 23.7)	22.0	21.6	20.9	20.1

FIG. 13-60

March
1983

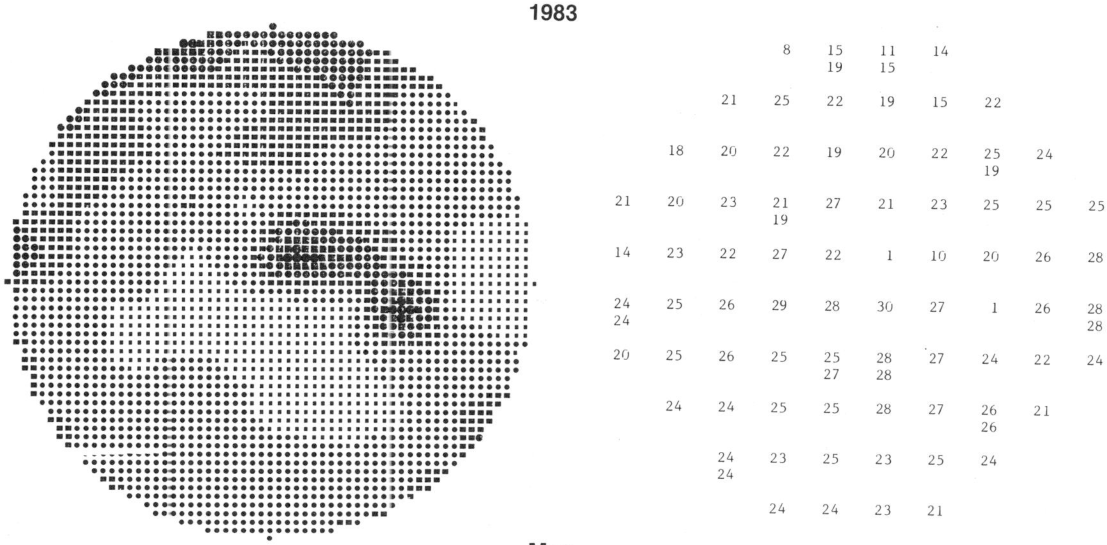

May
1984

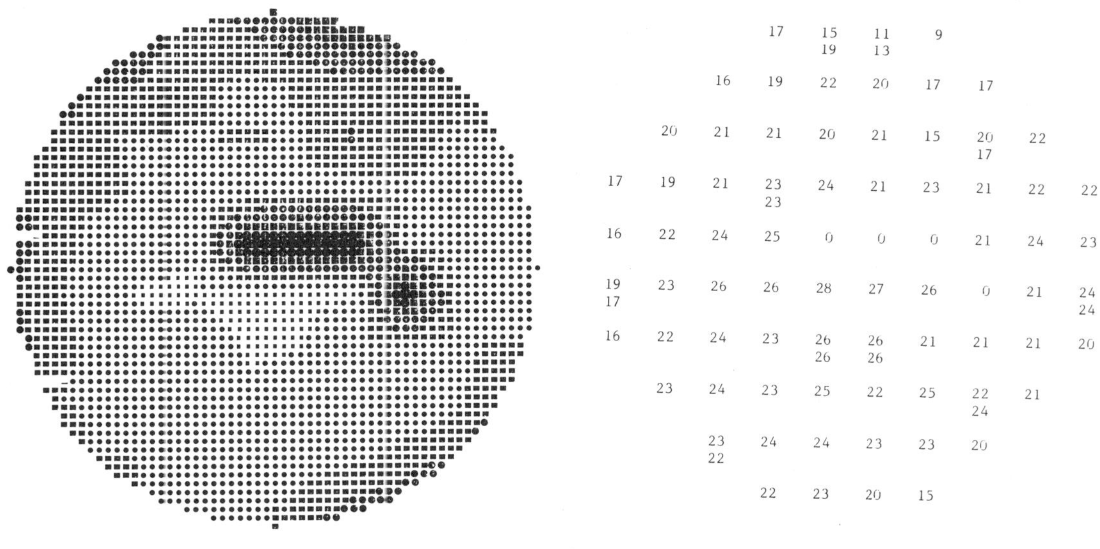

FIG. 13-60, cont'd

FIG. 13-61. Progressively smaller pupil. This correlated with the progressive loss of sensitivity shown in Fig. 13-54. Therefore, the field examination was repeated with a larger pupil.

DATE OF EXAM : DAY / YEAR	03.03 1983	07.14 1983	11.17 1983	05.17 1984
PUPIL SIZE	4.0	3.0	1.5	1.0
MEAN SENSITIVITY				
WHOLE FIELD (N: 24.8)	22.6	22.2	21.7	20.4
QUAD.UPP.NAS.(N: 24.2)	20.6	21.4	20.5	19.2
LOW.NAS.(N: 25.1)	24.8	23.8	24.0	23.3
UPP.TMP.(N: 24.3)	19.7	19.0	18.2	17.1
LOW.TMP.(N: 25.8)	25.2	24.7	24.2	22.2
ECC. 0 - 10 (N: 27.7)	23.0	20.4	21.4	19.1
10 - 20 (N: 25.7)	23.8	24.9	23.9	22.2
20 - 30 (N: 23.7)	22.0	21.6	20.9	20.1

FIG. 13-61

FIG. 13-62. Repeat examination of the patient in Fig. 13-61. The pupil was dilated for this test to check the supposition that the loss was due only to a small pupil. Unexpectedly, the overall sensitivity (arrow) did not improve. When the grey-scale and numeric printouts were examined, a new defect at the nasal edge was discovered. Indeed the sensitivity table shows the nasal sectors and the most eccentric zone (boxed values) to have become particularly reduced on this examination, which could be a new glaucomatous defect or a lens rim artifact. To confirm or deny that this is a new defect, another field examination is needed.

DATE OF EXAM : DAY YEAR	03.03 1983	07.14 1983	11.17 1983	05.17 1984	09.06 1984
PUPIL SIZE	4.0	3.0	1.5	1.0	3.0
MEAN SENSITIVITY					
WHOLE FIELD (N: 24.7)	22.6	22.2	21.7	20.4	20.0
QUAD.UPP.NAS.(N: 24.0)	20.6	21.4	20.5	19.2	18.2
LOW.NAS.(N: 25.0)	24.8	23.8	24.0	23.3	20.0
UPP.TMP.(N: 24.1)	19.7	19.0	18.2	17.1	18.2
LOW.TMP.(N: 25.7)	25.2	24.7	24.2	22.2	23.7
ECC. 0 - 10 (N: 27.5)	23.0	20.4	21.4	19.1	19.5
10 - 20 (N: 25.5)	23.8	24.9	23.9	22.2	23.9
20 - 30 (N: 23.6)	22.0	21.6	20.9	20.1	18.5

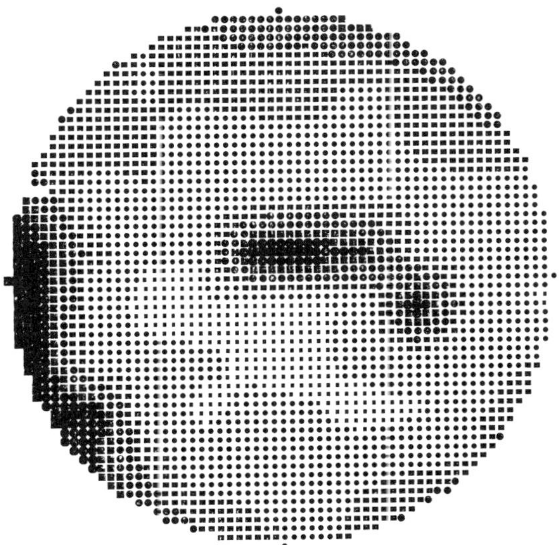

			17	13 16	12 18	11			
		21	19	19	18	22	18		
	19	19	24	22	22	23	21 19	18	
11	23	21	24 24	24	22	22	22	22	22
0	18	25	25	0	0	5	21	24	22
0 0	23	27	27	27	26	25	0	23	26 24
0	24	24	25	26 26	27 27	24	23	23	21
	0	24	26	25	25	27	26 26	22	
		16 18	24	24	24	23	21		
			17	20	24	18			

FIG. 13-62

FIG. 13-63. Return to the original sensitivity. Note that with a dilated pupil and elimination of the lens rim artifact, the greyscale and numeric printouts show the nasal defect no longer present. On four subsequent field examinations the overall sensitivity remained between 22 and 23 dB when the pupil was not constricted.

It is evident from Figs. 13-60 to 13-63 that very sensitive static threshold perimetry requires considerable analysis for correct field interpretation. Confirmation of unexpected or equivocal findings is always necessary.

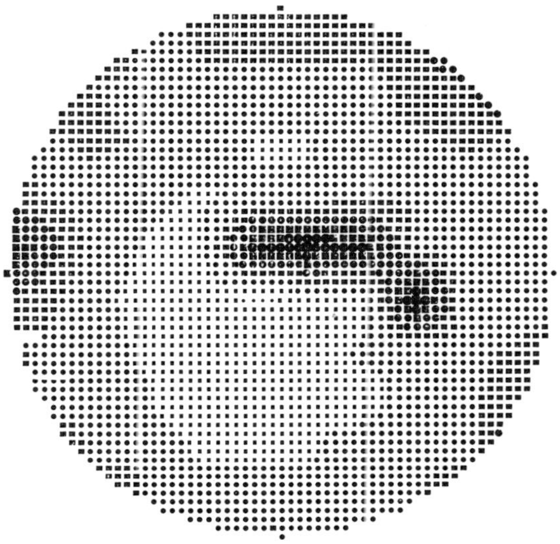

			20	16 20	16 20	19			
		23	21	22	22	22	19		
	19	21	22	26	26	21	21 22	20	
20	23	24	26 26	25	25	23	21	22	23
10	22	26	28	4	0	5	21	25	23
17 20	24	27	29	31	30	28	0	25	23 23
21	24	26	26	28 26	27 29	25	25	22	19
	24	25	28	27	27	27	24 24	21	
		23 22	26	26	26	22	23		
			22	22	23	22			

DATE OF EXAM : DAY YEAR	03.03 1983	07.14 1983	11.17 1983	05.17 1984	09.06 1984	10.23 1984	02.28 1985	02.28 1985	06.06 1985	06.06 1985	03.06 1986	03.06 1986
PUPIL SIZE	4.0	3.0	1.5	1.0	3.0	4.5	1.0	5.0	1.0	5.0	1.0	4.5
MEAN SENSITIVITY WHOLE FIELD	22.6	22.2	21.7	20.4	20.0	22.6	20.9	23.0	19.7	22.0	17.7	21.4
	20.6	21.4	20.5	19.2	18.2	21.1	19.8	22.5	19.1	21.6	15.3	19.6
	24.8	23.8	24.0	23.3	20.0	25.0	23.7	25.2	21.4	22.8	20.8	23.3
	19.7	19.0	18.2	17.1	18.2	19.7	17.7	19.6	16.9	20.0	14.3	19.1
	25.2	24.7	24.2	22.2	23.7	24.4	22.3	24.6	21.3	23.6	20.5	23.6
	23.0	20.4	21.4	19.1	19.5	21.7	19.1	21.6	19.9	22.1	16.7	20.3
	23.8	24.9	23.9	22.2	23.9	25.2	22.8	25.3	20.9	23.6	19.4	22.6
	22.0	21.6	20.9	20.1	18.5	21.8	20.6	22.4	19.1	21.3	17.4	21.2

FIG. 13-63

Differential diagnosis of progression

If the effectiveness of treatment is uncertain (e.g., borderline adequate lowering of the IOP), the visual field examination is performed to determine whether or not the pressure is adequately controlled. When progression is detected, it is a reasonable expectation that the disease being followed is the cause. However, the examining physician must be on guard because progression may be due to some other condition (perhaps a branch retinal vessel occlusion or a paramacular lesion). He must also be on guard when the progression is an unexpected finding (as might exist in a case with well-controlled pressure). The whole point in doing the field routinely is that sometimes true progression can occur despite apparent pressure control. The finding of an unexpected progression alerts the clinician to the existence of a problem: He must determine if some other condition has caused the new defect or if the defect is due to undetected poor control of the glaucoma. For example, perhaps the seemingly good pressure control is due to the fact that the patient uses his medications consistently on the day of his office visit but progressive damage occurs because the pressure is not so well controlled other times.

Particularly troublesome is the known simultaneous occurrence of another disease that can cause field loss. For example, a patient with elevated IOP may also have drusen of the optic nerve head, which can produce nerve fiber bundle defects in the visual field. The field loss may be identical to progressive glaucomatous loss. Most frequent is the simultaneous occurrence of cataract and glaucoma, leading to a progressive diffuse loss of visual field. The clinician must depend on acuity measurements, slitlamp evaluation, glare measurements, disc assessment, and other means to decide if the deterioration is in keeping with progressive opacity of the media. These tests are both difficult and critical, and he does not want to use aggressive antiglaucoma treatment (e.g., surgery) on a patient without progressive glaucomatous damage. On the other hand, he does not want to be complacent because of the existence of cataract and later (when the cataract is removed) discover that irreversible glaucomatous visual loss has occurred.

The distinction between cataractous and glaucomatous field loss may be difficult, because both are progressive and diffuse. Sometimes, however, in addition to diffuse loss, there is a more exaggerated localized loss in typical areas representing nerve fiber bundle defects. In this case the simultaneous depression of the field by cataract and the further glaucomatous loss can be recognized.

FIG. 13-64. Progressive diffuse loss of sensitivity. In this patient with declining acuity and progressive cataract formation evident by slitlamp examination, the decline was attributed to cataract because the IOP had been exceptionally well controlled. In addition, there was no progression for several years at this pressure before the cataract appeared and the disc appearance was stable (though increasingly difficult to evaluate).

1983

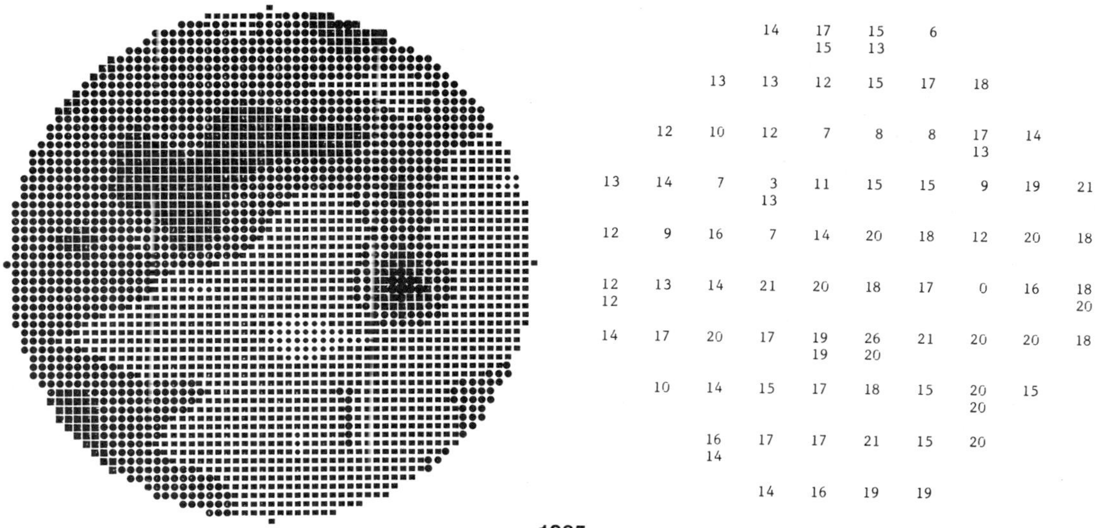

1985

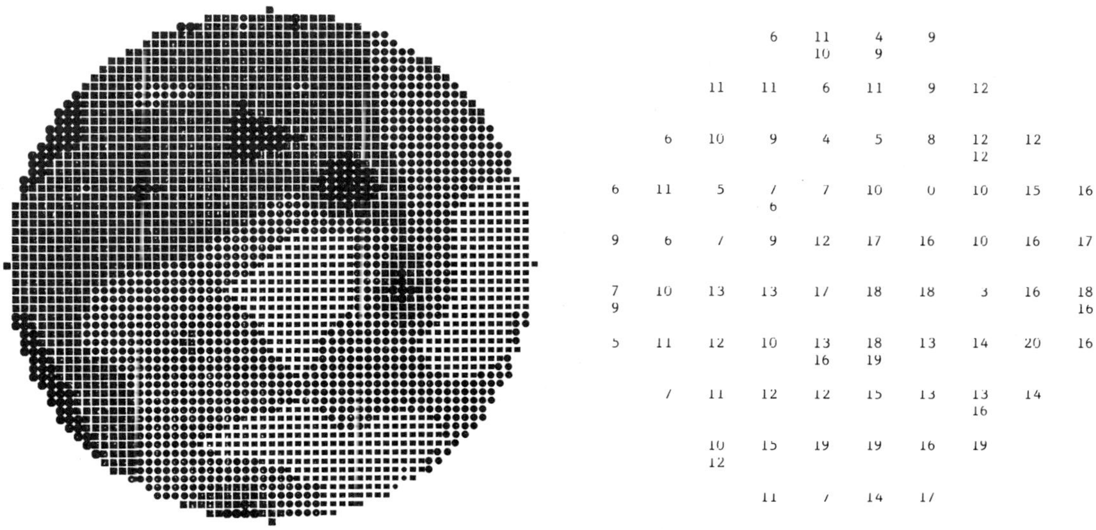

DATE OF EXAM : DAY YEAR	05.19 1983	07.19 1984	10.17 1985
MEAN SENSITIVITY			
WHOLE FIELD (N: 23.4)	15.2	13.2	11.6
QUAD.UPP.NAS.(N: 22.8)	11.6	10.1	7.9
LOW.NAS.(N: 23.7)	15.9	13.5	11.5
UPP.TMP.(N: 22.8)	15.0	12.3	11.2
LOW.TMP.(N: 24.4)	18.6	17.1	16.2
ECC. 0 - 10 (N: 26.3)	16.9	15.2	14.1
10 - 20 (N: 24.3)	13.7	11.7	9.3
20 - 30 (N: 22.3)	15.4	13.3	11.9

FIG. 13-64

The final example, from manual perimetry, illustrates how a cataract tends to reduce sensitivity everywhere in the field but perhaps to a greater degree centrally than peripherally. Glaucoma may do the same thing. However, if the arcuate or nasal areas show a distinctly greater loss than elsewhere, a localized glaucomatous loss is likely in addition to the generalized loss.

FIG. 13-65. Changes due to the development of a cataract with and without simultaneous progression of the glaucomatous defect.
B shows the baseline field. With the development of cataract, visual acuity is reduced and the entire field, **A,** becomes depressed. In a point-by-point comparison of the nasal and temporal sides, it can be seen that the reduction in sensitivity (circled numbers) varies from 0.5 log-unit in the periphery to 1.0 log-unit at the center. Note that the change in the nasal and arcuate regions is no greater than elsewhere in the field. The relationship between threshold at any point in the field and neighboring thresholds is unchanged. This kind of progression is typical of media change, but it also may occur with glaucoma. The examiner should suspect that it is glaucomatous progression if the media remain clear.

C shows how the field may appear if there is glaucomatous progression of the localized type in addition to the development of cataract. In comparing field **C** to field **B,** note that the temporal regions (left side of figure) are depressed from cataract by 0.5 to 1.0 log-unit, the same as was observed in comparing field **A** to field **B**. However, in the arcuate regions the defect has deepened by 1.0 to 1.5 log-units (circled numbers in red to the right).

The change in the *I-3e* isopter (blue) is the same when field **A** is compared to field **B** as when fields **C** and **B** are compared. If only this isopter had been plotted, it would have not been possible to distinguish whether the change was due to progressive cataract, progressive glaucoma, or both.

Cataract can cause localized changes. In cases of cataract and small pupil combined with glaucoma and with changes of uncertain nature, the diagnostic analysis is sometimes made easier by dilating the pupil and repeating the field examination.

As stated in Chapter 1, the determination of visual threshold at pertinent locations is the basis of visual field testing and interpretation for kinetic as well as static perimetry. In both, if there is a decline in visual sensation at all points of approximately equal degree a generalized depression is occurring. On the other hand, if there is a decline in visual sensation only at points that lie in the arcuate region but not elsewhere there is progressive loss of the glaucomatous type occurring. If all points are declining in sensitivity, the visual acuity test and the physical examination of the eye will be needed to distinguish cataract from glaucoma.

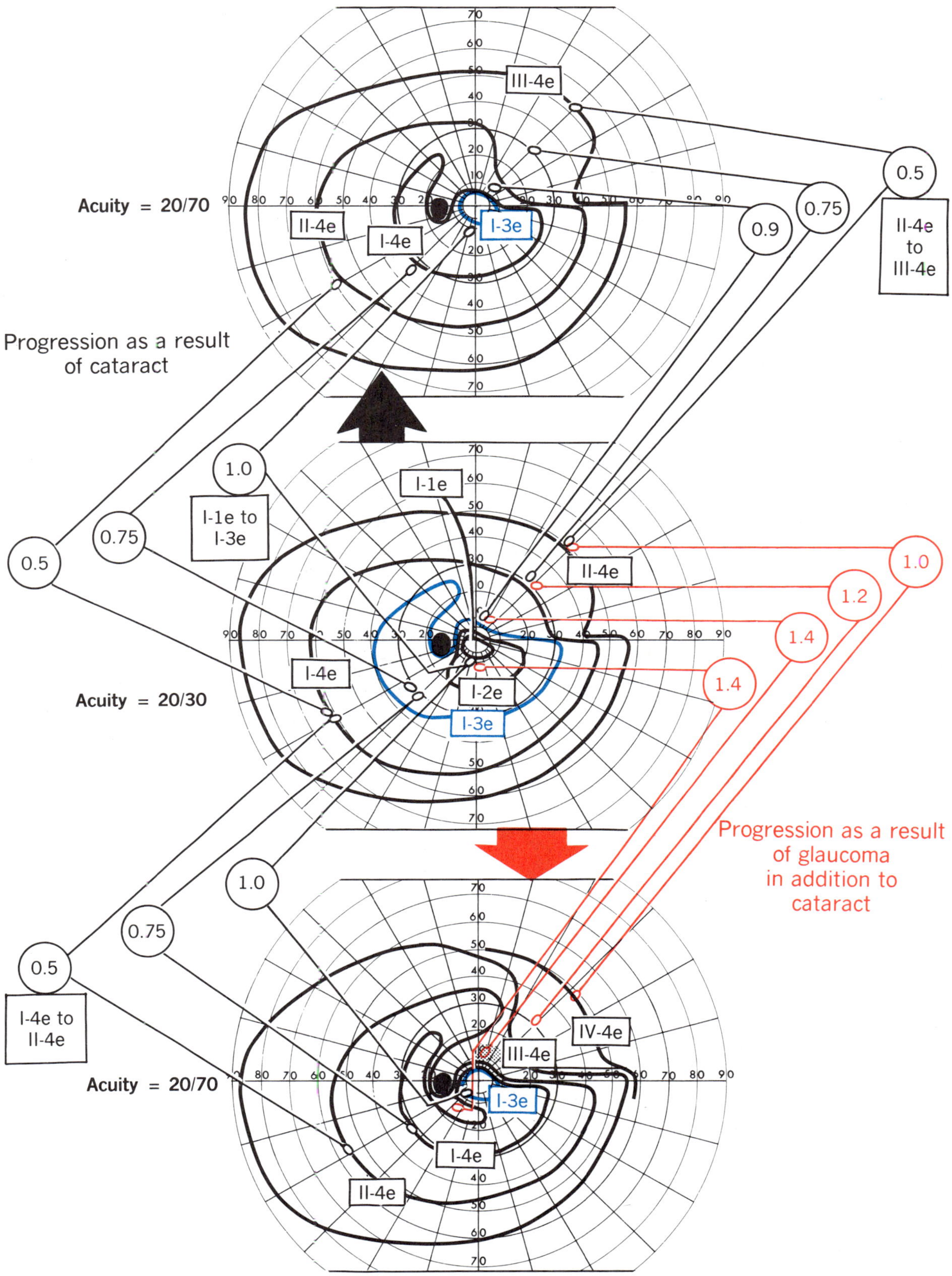
Acuity = 20/70
III-4e
0.5
0.75
0.9
II-4e to III-4e
A
II-4e
I-4e
I-3e
Progression as a result of cataract
1.0
I-1e to I-3e
0.75
0.5
I-1e
II-4e
1.0
1.2
1.4
1.4
B
I-4e
Acuity = 20/30
I-2e
I-3e
Progression as a result of glaucoma in addition to cataract
1.0
0.75
0.5
I-4e to II-4e
IV-4e
III-4e
Acuity = 20/70
I-3e
C
I-4e
II-4e

FIG. 13-65

CHAPTER 14

The basis of perimetry

In most textbooks the fundamental information is presented first and the clinical application follows. It may seem strange to many readers of this text, then, that the theoretic basis of perimetry is presented here. However, it is my belief that abstract concepts are better understood after the context has been set; also the significance of certain details is better appreciated. Actually, all of the theory has already been introduced, a bit at a time, as it became relevant, and this chapter is thus a summary (with some amplification of details) rather than an introduction.

I should comment that the physiology (psychophysics) of vision and the theoretic basis for instrument design are presented only sketchily. Just the generalities, not the details, need to be understood by the clinician who will be using, rather than designing, the instrumentation. Readers who wish to study these details of perimetry further will have to consult more extensive and more authoritative sources.

FREQUENCY-OF-SEEING CURVE AND SHORT-TERM FLUCTUATIONS

The visibility of a stimulus depends on a number of factors: its intensity, the background against which it is presented, its size, its color, whether or not it is moving, the length of time it is presented, and so on. If a given defined stimulus is not visible, one of the factors (usually the size or intensity) can be adjusted until it becomes visible. At the boundary between visibility and invisibility the patient's responses often will be uncertain or inconsistent, so a borderline stimulus is sometimes seen and sometimes not (or at least the patient may sometimes decide to respond, and sometimes not, to a stimulus that he is not sure he saw). When the stimulus is in this region of uncertain visibility, its intensity can be adjusted slightly to a level at which the patient will respond 25% of the time. At a slightly greater intensity (say, 0.5 dB more intense) he may respond 50% of the time, and at an even greater intensity he may respond 75% of the time. If the visual responses are being determined with such care, the threshold is defined as the stimulus intensity at which the *patient responds 50% of the time* (see p. 228).

In the reality of the clinical situation, threshold is estimated by using stimulus intensities 2, 3, or 4 dB apart and each stimulus is presented only once or twice. The threshold estimate is recorded as the weakest stimulus seen, or the average of the weakest seen and the strongest not seen.

In programs or strategies in which threshold is redetermined at the same point a second or third time, slightly different estimates of threshold intensity (or isopter position) will be obtained. This intratest variability of threshold estimates is called short-term fluctuation. Because of the physiologic frequency-of-seeing curve, there is always a certain minimum short-term fluctuation. Several additional factors, likewise, can affect the intratest variability: First, points with reduced sensitivity have a broader frequency-of-seeing curve (higher short-term fluctuation). Second, a patient may give frankly unreliable responses because of inattention, inconsistent decisions about responding to dim stimuli that are barely visible, poor fixation, and so on.

FIG. 14-1. Demonstration of intratest variability. A 5 × 5 grid of 25 points 3 degrees apart was tested with threshold determined three times at each location. On this printout each test point is represented by five numbers in two columns. The left column gives the three threshold estimates. The right column gives the average of the three estimates and the short-term fluctuation at each point. Note that the center point is abnormal, with a reduced threshold and a high short-term fluctuation. This high resolution grid is centered on the abnormal point in Fig. 13-14.

Short-term fluctuation is sometimes measured in the course of a clinical examination based on two (or three) threshold estimates at a sampling of locations. The purpose of measuring short-term fluctuation is to gauge the degree to which additional factors besides the normal frequency-of-seeing curve have increased intratest variability in a given examination. It serves the purpose of (1) helping to determine the reliability (reproducibility of threshold measurements) of a particular examination and (2) providing an estimate of how much a given point must deviate from the expected value before it can be confidently considered abnormal.

When the short-term fluctuation estimate (RMS score of the Octopus perimeter) is high, it is often useful to look at the actual data points where duplicate measurements were made. If both normal and abnormal points were included, the high score may simply reflect the broader frequency-of-seeing curve of the abnormal points. In this case the high score may signify not so much an unreliable examination as the fact that there are abnormal points in the field; it does mean, however, that a more generous allowance must be made in deciding whether a given point has changed from one occasion to another. In another case, even the normal points may be quite variable and the high score may reflect the patient's inability to perform the test optimally; the implication is the same, that a more generous allowance must be made before deciding that a deviant sensitivity value represents an abnormal point or that a point has changed its sensitivity from one occasion to another.

When looking at the duplicate measurements reported on numeric printouts, the examiner should recognize that (depending on the perimeter and the program used) only some may have been performed at preselected locations for the purpose of calculating the short-term fluctuation. Duplicate measurements at some locations may have been performed to determine the overall height of the hill of vision of a particular individual. Some programs make duplicate measurments whenever the first measurement has an unexpected value based on the findings at surrounding points. These duplicate measurements will more likely have large variability, and they cannot be used when judging the overall reliability of the field. Also points with 0 dB sensitivity cannot be included, because duplicate measurements will likely be the same and artificially suggest a low short-term fluctuation. In any of these situations the interpreter may have trouble coming to a valid conclusion on the meaning of duplicate values and the test variability calculation unless he learns the details of the test strategy (and the basis for calculation) in the particular program used.

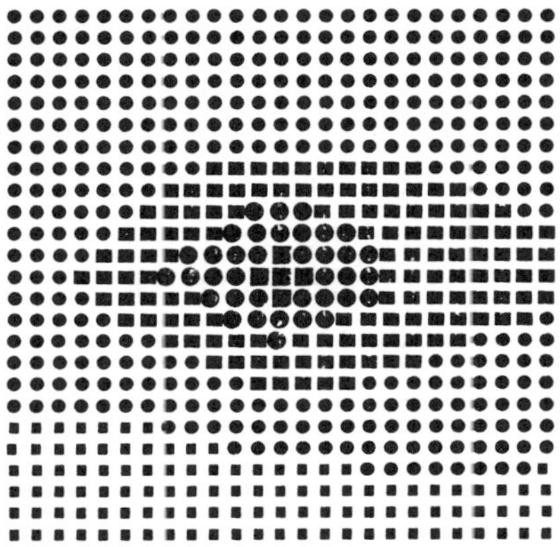

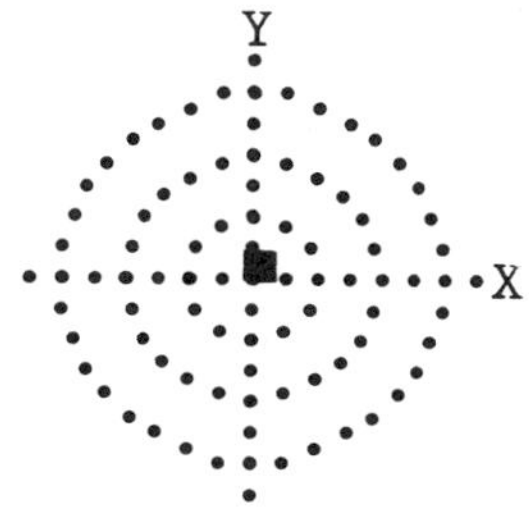

CENTRE X: + 3
Y: + 9

23.5 24.2 23.5 1.2 25.5	23.5 24.2 23.5 1.2 25.5	20.5 21.5 22.5 1.0 21.5	21.5 22.2 23.5 1.2 21.5	20.5 21.2 24.5 3.1 18.5
21.5 23.2 24.5 1.5 23.5	25.5 23.2 21.5 2.1 22.5	22.5 20.8 19.5 1.5 20.5	21.5 21.2 21.5 0.6 20.5	21.5 22.8 25.5 2.3 21.5
26.5 24.2 23.5 2.1 22.5	16.5 16.5 17.5 1.0 15.5	13.5 8.2 8.5 5.5 2.5	18.5 16.8 12.5 3.8 19.5	22.5 18.5 16.5 3.5 16.5
27.5 25.2 25.5 2.5 22.5	25.5 25.2 24.5 0.6 25.5	20.5 22.2 21.5 2.1 24.5	21.5 22.2 22.5 0.6 22.5	23.5 23.5 22.5 1.0 24.5
26.5 28.5 30.5 2.0 28.5	29.5 29.5 28.5 1.0 30.5	29.5 29.5 29.5 0.0 29.5	27.5 28.2 29.5 1.2 27.5	28.5 27.2 26.5 1.2 26.5

FLUCTUATIONS (R.M.S.): 2.1 DB LUM. INTERVAL: 2

FIG. 14-1

The zone of inconsistency affects not only static threshold determinations but also isopter position. When not considering the zone of inconsistent responses, we simply direct our attention to isopters as the boundary between seeing and nonseeing regions for the test stimulus. More accurately we consider them as narrow zones where a stimulus is sometimes seen and sometimes not seen (i.e., zones of "uncertainty"). In the purest sense, the isopter is a line (in the center of the zone) where the stimulus is seen 50% of the time.

FIG. 14-2. Visual sensation in the region of an isopter.

In kinetic perimetry the stimulus may be seen as it first enters the zone of uncertainty or it may, on second trial, be seen as it has almost passed through the zone. This can account for the patient's responding somewhat inconsistently (see p. 454).

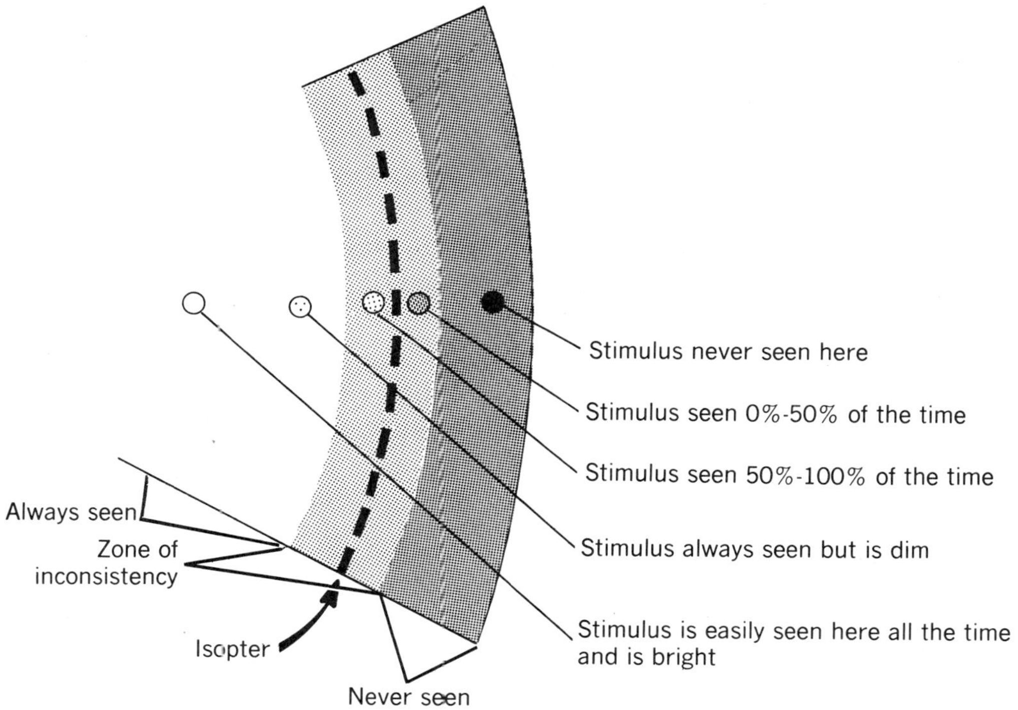

Stimulus never seen here
Stimulus seen 0%-50% of the time
Stimulus seen 50%-100% of the time
Stimulus always seen but is dim
Stimulus is easily seen here all the time and is bright
Always seen
Zone of inconsistency
Isopter
Never seen

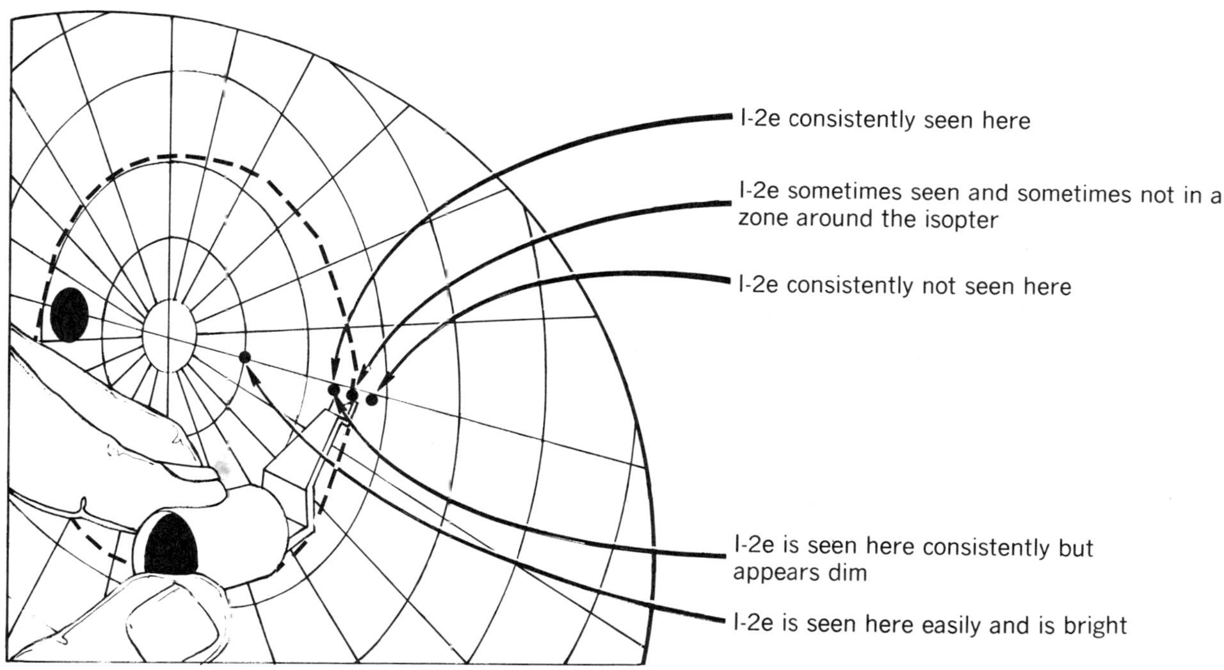

I-2e consistently seen here
I-2e sometimes seen and sometimes not in a zone around the isopter
I-2e consistently not seen here
I-2e is seen here consistently but appears dim
I-2e is seen here easily and is bright

FIG. 14-2

STIMULUS BRIGHTNESS

If the stimulus is in the threshold zone, it will seem quite dim—in fact, barely visible. When it is more intense, it will seem brighter and be easier to see with certainty. If it is even more intense, it will seem quite bright (be very easy to see). **The apparent degree of brightness is related to how much more intense than threshold the stimulus is.**

In kinetic perimetry, as the stimulus moves across the isopter, it is at first barely visible and then becomes brighter. At some point the patient believes the stimulus has appeared and he responds (p. 184).

Many patients who have previously undergone manual perimetry and are now being tested with static threshold perimetry mention that the stimulus is quite dim. They may complain that this makes the test more difficult, or they may express concern that they are losing vision because they have more difficulty seeing the stimulus on this test. They can be reassured that the nature of the new test is that whenever they see a stimulus it is made dimmer for the next presentation until the very dimmest stimulus they can see has been determined, and it is natural that the stimuli would be more difficult to see in the new test. In a similar way the patient may recognize that the stimuli are harder to see on a repeat static threshold test, and it can be explained that the computer knows what they could see on the last occasion and therefore begins by testing them with stimuli that they can hardly see.

Consider also the apparent brightness when the region of the isopter is explored with static spot-checking. A short distance inside the isopter the test object should be seen almost every time it is presented. A short distance outside the isopter it should never be seen. In the region right at the isopter there should be a zone within which the stimulus is sometimes not seen and sometimes seen (but dimly). Here the responses may be both inconsistent and sometimes delayed, with a long response time. This region is the zone of uncertainty, the zone of inconsistency, or the threshold zone.

The fact that apparent brightness relates to how much more intense than threshold a stimulus is has two other implications for suprathreshold testing in manual perimetry: *First,* when suprathreshold static spot-checking is performed in the paracentral region where a stimulus is comfortably suprathreshold the stimulus may seem reasonably bright to the patient. If it is presented within a shallow scotoma, it may appear dimmer even though being visible. If the patient can recognize that the stimulus is dimmer, it may represent a shallow scotoma; and the alert perimetrist will explore this area more carefully if the patient volunteers that the stimulus is dim at a particular location (p. 458). *Second,* if the scotoma is of a depth that the presumably suprathreshold stimulus happens to be close to threshold, the patient may give inconsistent responses in one region (Figs. 13-6 and 23-8) because the stimulus happens to be within the zone of uncertainty surrounding the threshold value at that location.

In comparison testing (e.g., confrontation fields) we are making use of the fact that the subjective sense of brightness depends on how far above threshold the stimulus is. Thus a stimulus can appear less bright (and of different coloration) in a region where sensitivity is reduced because its intensity exceeds the threshold stimulus value by a lesser amount than it does in the normal portion of the visual field.

BACKGROUND INTENSITY AND RETINAL ADAPTATION

The background illumination affects visual threshold. For one thing, it determines the state of the light- versus dark-adapted retina. The dark-adapted retina can perceive very weak stimuli, but the improvement in sensitivity with dark adaptation is not the same at every point on the retina. The hill of vision becomes flatter with dark adaptation, and thus the foveal peak of sensitivity is lost. Indeed, with profound dark adaptation the fovea (packed with cones) does not gain the same sensitivity as the surrounding region (richer in rods) and in essence a physiologic type of central scotoma is produced. However, in most clinical circumstances the visual field test is not being performed under dark-adapted (scotopic) conditions so this scotoma is not present.

The background illumination plays another role besides establishing the level of retinal adaptation. The visibility of a stimulus of given intensity depends on the background against which it is being viewed. In a typical projection perimeter, there is a certain background intensity (I_b) and onto the surface is projected a spot with a certain additional intensity (I_p). The total intensity of light in the projected spot is $I_b + I_p$ (although in classic notation I_p is represented by ΔL, the difference between the total intensity of the spot and the background).

When the background illumination is always kept constant (as in the usual clinical setting, where the background of a given perimeter is properly calibrated to the same value each time the perimeter is used), threshold can be expressed simply as I_p, the intensity of the projected spot. The threshold I_p will be different for differing values of I_b.

When the background illumination is not standardized, threshold cannot be expressed simply as I_p, because the threshold value of I_p changes whenever I_b changes. It is the relationship between stimulus intensity and background that determines visibility, so threshold is expressed as the ratio I_p/I_b ($\Delta L/I_b$). The ideal would be that threshold, expressed as such a ratio, could always be the same while there were changes in background and under conditions that altered the intensities of both I_p and I_b before light reached the retina. For example, if the electric supply to a perimeter varied a bit, changing proportionately both the background intensity and the stimulus intensity, the threshold value I_p/I_b would remain the same. It would also be ideal if threshold values of two perimeters with differing background intensities could be compared when each was expressed as I_p/I_b. Finally, it would be desirable if as the pupil changed size the threshold stimulus value could remain unchanged because retinal illumination from the background and from the projected stimulus was changing in proportion.

Weber's law says that this ideal circumstance (the threshold expressed as I_p/I_b remaining constant) does occur under photopic conditions when the retina is fully light-adapted. Remember that the level of light adaptation depends on the amount of light reaching the retina, which in turn depends not only on the background illumination in the perimeter bowl but also on the size of the pupil (and on any absorption of light that may occur in the ocular media). Thus the threshold value expressed as I_p/I_b will be unchanged by pupillary size only if the retina is still fully light-adapted when the pupil is small. To achieve the "ideal" conditions may require background illumination stronger than any currently in use. Some data suggest that 100 *trolands** of retinal illumination (which occurs when 25 asb is viewed through a 4 mm pupillary diameter) may be enough to ensure photopic adaptation, but other data show that 100 asb may be necessary (especially if the pupil is smaller). In any event, as seen in Chapter 13, pupillary size certainly can affect retinal sensitivity under the conditions of clinical testing. However, the effect may be somewhat less with perimeters that use a background of 31 rather than 4 asb.

STIMULUS SIZE AND SPATIAL SUMMATION

Because of spatial summation, a large stimulus is more easily seen than a small one. Thus, if a threshold stimulus is of a certain area and luminous intensity, it can be made suprathreshold by increasing its area. Decreasing the luminous intensity by an appropriate amount will bring it back to a threshold stimulus. The two stimuli are related by the formula

$$A^k \times I = C$$

where A is the area of the stimulus, I is the luminous intensity, and C is a constant representing visual threshold at that location. The value for the exponent k varies with retinal position from 0.55 to 0.9. Goldmann decided to use an approximation value for k of 0.8 when deciding how much to increase the area of the stimulus to be equivalent to a 0.5 log-unit increase in intensity. In addition to varying with retinal position, the relationship is inconstant because (1) there is increasing spatial summation with dark adaptation, (2) individual differences exist from one person to another, (3) the value of the exponent k varies a bit with the size of the stimulus, and (4) the equivalence may be different in diseased visual regions from that seen in normal retinal regions.

The variability of the area-intensity relationship means that the stated equivalence of two stimuli is only an approximation. For example, the III-2e (4 mm^2, 100 asb), II-3e (1 mm^2, 315 asb), and I-4e (0.25 mm^2, 1000 asb) stimuli are indeed roughly equivalent but are not precise substitutes for one another under all conditions and in all retinal locations.

---

*Troland: light reaching the retina through a 1 mm^2 pupillary area from a source that is 1 candela per square meter.

REFRACTIVE ERROR AND RETINAL BLUR

Visibility of a stimulus is optimal when it is well focused on the retina. The blurred image of a spot is larger than the focused spot but overall is less intense (with the same total amount of light entering the eye). Additionally, the sharp boundary between background intensity and stimulus intensity, which contributes to visibility, is lost. The effect of blur is greater with small-sized stimuli presented near the fovea but is less with stimuli presented in the periphery (where spatial summation of the enlarged size is more efficient) and with larger stimuli (for which the blurred boundary is proportionately less compared to the overall stimulus size). Thus it is more important to correct a refractive error in the central field than in the peripheral field. Actually, for the peripheral field, refractive correction is almost inconsequential except possibly in the presence of large refractive errors. Exact correction of refractive errors is a bit less important with automated perimeters that use a size III stimulus rather than the previous standard of manual perimetry (size I). Nonetheless, an improperly corrected refractive error will influence results in the central field, even with a size III stimulus.

TEMPORAL SUMMATION AND STIMULUS DURATION

By virtue of temporal summation, a static stimulus presented for 0.02 second is more visible than one presented for 0.01 second. However, after a certain time, temporal summation is complete. For example, if a stimulus is presented for 1 second and is not seen, it will not become visible regardless of how long it is left on. Although the limits depend on other factors (background illumination, target size, etc.), it can be said roughly that the amount of temporal summation begins to decline after 0.06 second and is largely complete by 0.1 second; but under some conditions there may be additional summation up to 0.5 or even 1.0 second. In manual perimetry (in which stimulus duration is not rigidly defined) 0.5 second for static spot-checking and static threshold determinations is recommended to ensure that none of the stimuli are cut short before temporal summation has been completed. With automated perimetry a stimulus duration of 0.1 or 0.2 second is more common. Temporal summation seems to be mostly complete by this time; but, in any event, the stimulus duration does not vary from one presentation to another. (The stroboscopic flash of the Friedmann Analyser is clearly shorter than the time required for complete temporal summation, although the threshold values are reproducible because the duration of the flash is the same every time.) The reason for choosing a 0.1 or 0.2 second duration instead of a somewhat longer presentation is that this does not allow enough response time for the patient to move his eyes to look at the stimulus after he thinks he has seen it.

KINETIC AND STATIC STIMULI

As the stimulus moves across the retina, there is a type of summation that makes kinetic stimuli somewhat more visible than static ones. This is particularly striking in disease conditions in which Riddoch's phenomenon is observed. However, if the stimulus is moved slowly enough, the threshold intensity for kinetic and static stimuli is so close that static spot-checking can be used to confirm the position of an isopter.

STRATEGIES OF AUTOMATED TESTING

The designers of automated instruments are continually striving for improvements that will shorten the time it takes for the examination while also enhancing the detection and definition of abnormalities. It would be impossible within the confines of this chapter to discuss all the variations or to predict new ones that will be used in the near future. It would also serve no purpose, since the details of the strategy are largely ''transparent'' (not obvious to the user) and anyway not under user control. However, some aspects are of interest to the intellectually curious and knowledge of how the perimeter works may occasionally help in understanding the results that are obtained. Therefore, although the user of an automated perimeter will have to read elsewhere for the details of how his particular instrument is programmed, still some generalities can be provided here to supplement what was explained on pp. 46-51.

A pattern of points is often chosen to detect a particular disease. In screening a population for glaucoma, the points selected generally lie along a circular (arcuate) pattern in the central field, with additional peripheral points nasally (and perhaps also temporally) above and below the horizontal. It is appealing, both practically and commercially, to use the locations originally selected by Armaly for manual glaucoma screening. However, patterns with more numerous points have become popular. The test can be made more sensitive thereby, with very little additional expenditure of time, because much of the time is utilized getting the patient set at the perimeter, and even doubling the number of points tested adds only a small proportion to the total amount of time used. These patterns are intended primarily for suprathreshold testing. Virtually all suprathreshold programs now check by repeat presentation any missed responses. Compensation of the stimulus intensity for eccentricity can be incorporated into the computerized program and does not use up any additional test time.

With static threshold perimetry a pattern of points evenly spaced 6 degrees apart is often used. The central field is blanketed by approximately the same number of points as in the Armaly pattern, but the points are evenly distributed without artificially concentrating near the center (which may or may not be advantageous). One benefit of an evenly spaced grid is that interpolated values can be given to a large number of intermediate points so a greyscale printout can be constructed.

Two such grids with a 6-degree resolution offset from each other by 3 degrees horizontally and vertically are offered. One includes points lying exactly on the horizontal and vertical meridians as well as on fixation. The other includes rows of points 3 degrees above and below the horizontal meridian and columns of points 3 degrees to the right and left of the vertical meridian. Some clinicians have found it helpful to know the visual threshold at the point of fixation, and the advantage of the former pattern is that it includes this. The advantage of the second pattern is that it offers threshold values at points straddling the vertical and horizontal meridians, which is often helpful in evaluating a field for nasal steps and hemianopias. Some programs also now offer a pattern that straddles the meridians and, in addition, determines threshold at the point of fixation. It is even possible to test both patterns (at the expense of doubling the test time) and to combine the results into one printout. However, if the examiner is willing to spend the additional time in field testing, it is not clear whether that time would be better spent (1) improving the spatial resolution by testing each pattern once or (2) increasing the accuracy of the visual threshold determination by testing one of the patterns twice.

A recently introduced static threshold program (the G1 of the Octopus) has returned to the idea of concentrating attention in the diagnostically more relevant regions of the field. However, it may take some work to provide a greyscale representation of results with its printout. Also on the horizon are strategies that will automatically determine a closer grid of points (greater spatial resolution) where an abnormality *is* present, but details need to be worked out so it will be possible to get helpful additional information without adding too much time to the examination.

Whatever pattern of points is used for threshold testing, the determination consists of first presenting a stimulus and later presenting additional stimuli that are either more intense or less intense than the previous depending on the patient's response to the earlier presentation at that location. The boundary between visibility and invisibility is established by a bracketing technique in which care is taken to confirm by repeat presentations the *seen* and *not seen* stimuli on two sides of the boundary.

Because it is not known ahead of time exactly what the threshold will be at each point, it typically takes at least six stimulus presentations for a determination of threshold to be made at each point. The total length of time for the test depends on how many stimulus presentations (''questions'') are needed before the threshold is defined. This, in turn, depends on how far away from actual threshold the initial stimulus presentation is. To save time, there must be some strategy for guessing at threshold. Three methods are currently used for this purpose: In the *first* a stimulus is presented that is the normal threshold for that location. This starting point may be optimal for fields that, in fact, are normal. However, for fields that are abnormal it makes sense to start with the threshold determined at each point on an earlier occasion and use the *second* method, in which the perimeter accesses information about the previous field examination. In the *third* method (''prethresholding'') threshold is determined accurately by repeat presentations at four points (one in each quadrant) starting with a presumed normal level. Points adjacent to these initial locations are then thresholded by using as a start the threshold determined at the nearby location.

FIG. 14-3. Use of prethresholding. Threshold was first determined at four selected points (arrows), and it turned out that the strongest stimulus was not seen (threshold equal to 0 dB). The surrounding points were then tested with the maximum stimulus, and it was quickly determined that at most of these points also the strongest stimulus could not be seen. Several central points were the only ones showing good sensitivity. This test was conducted in 7 minutes 34 seconds with 243 questions.

FIG. 14-4. Another example in which the third strategy was used. In this example the depressed sensitivities were quite irregular, with multiple scotomas; thus they often were different from those at adjacent points, whose thresholds were used to begin the thresholding process. This examination was more lengthy (19 minutes 37 seconds) and required 665 questions.

It should be noted that, in addition to influencing the test time, the value chosen for the initial presentation to determine threshold also influences (biases) the final threshold value obtained. This is especially true for patients who have a high frequency of false-positive and false-negative errors. Thus, if the starting presentation is too far from actual threshold, the patient is likely to give a false response before the bracketing strategy can reach actual threshold and the falsely obtained threshold estimate will likely be closer to the starting stimulus intensity than it should be. In this situation entire quadrants may have higher or lower thresholds than they should. An example of this was seen in Fig. 13-42, in which the patient's inconsistency caused the four initial threshold determinations to be different from each other (and presumably also from the true threshold values) and the entire quadrant of threshold values to be influenced by the combination of the strategy used and the patient's unreliability.

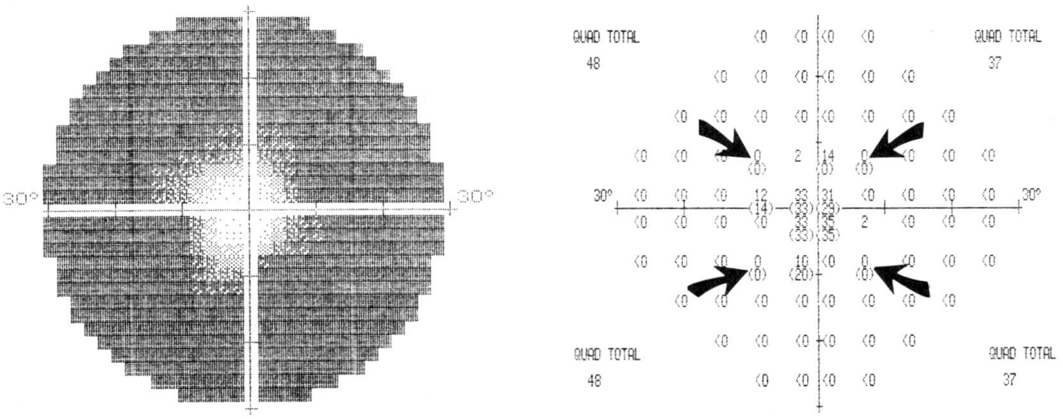

FIG. 14-3

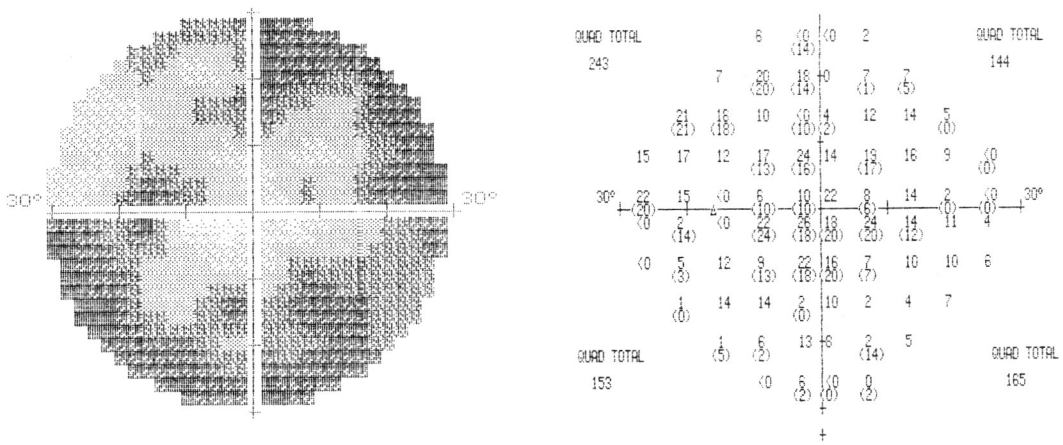

FIG. 14-4

ADDITIONAL READING

Aulhorn, E., and Harms, H.: Early visual field defects in glaucoma. In Leydhecker, W., editor: Glaucoma: Tutzing symposium, Basel, 1967, S. Karger, pp. 151-186. *An unusually lucid presentation of the underlying considerations in perimetry with glaucoma as the example. This article is well worth the hour it will take to read and absorb.*

Aulhorn, E., and Harms, H.: Visual perimetry. In Jameson, D., and Hurvich, L.M., editors: Visual psychophysics: handbook of sensory physiology, vol. VII, no. 4, New York, 1972, Springer-Verlag, Inc., pp. 102-145. *Authoritative encyclopedia of information about the psychophysical basis of perimetry.*

Bedwell, C.H.: Visual fields. A basis for efficient investigation, London, 1982, Butterworth Scientific.

Fankhauser, F.: Problems related to the design of automatic perimeters, Doc. Ophthalmol. **47:**89-139, 1979.

Fankhauser, F., and Jenni, A.: Programs SARGON and DELTA: two new principles for automated analysis of the visual field, Albrecht von Graefes Arch. Klin. Exp. Ophthalmol. **216:**41-48, 1981.

Fankhauser, F., et al.: Three years of experience with the Octopus automatic perimeter, Doc. Ophthalmol. Proc. Ser. **14:**7-15, 1977.

Fankhauser, F., et al.: Octopus programs SAPRO and F: two new principles for the analysis of the visual field, Albrecht von Graefes Arch. Klin. Exp. Ophthalmol. **216:**155-165, 1981.

Gloor, B., et al.: Glaukomgesichtsfelder-Analyse von Octopus-Verlaufsbeobachtungen mit einem statistischen Programm, Klin. Monatsbl. Augenheilkd. **177:**423-436, 1980.

Greve, E.L.: Single and multiple stimulus static perimetry in glaucoma: the two phases of perimetry, Doc. Ophthalmol. **36:**1-355, 1973. *A major thesis on many details of modern perimetry.*

Häberlin, H., et al.: Researches on adaptive high resolution programming for automatic perimeter: principles and preliminary results, Int. Ophthalmol. **2:**1-9, 1980.

Heijl, A.: Computer test logics for automatic perimetry, Acta Ophthalmol. **55:**837-853, 1977.

Heijl, A., and Krakau, C.E.T.: An automatic static perimeter, design and pilot study, Acta Ophthalmol. **53:**293-310, 1975.

Jenni, A., et al.: Neue Programme für das automatische Perimeter Octopus, Klin. Monatsbl. Augenheilkd. **197:**536-544, 1980.

National Research Council, Committee on Vision, Assembly of Behavioral and Social Sciences: First interprofessional standard for visual field testing, Report of Working Group 99, Adv. Ophthalmol. **40:**173-224, 1980. *Detailed discussion of variables that influence clinical visual field testing and their standardization.*

Tate, G.W., Jr.: The physiological basis for perimetry. In Drance, S.M., and Anderson, D.R., editors: Automated perimetry in glaucoma. A practical guide, Orlando, Fla., 1985, Grune & Stratton, Inc., pp. 1-28. *A recent review with extensive list of original references.*

Tate, G.W., Jr., and Lynn, J.R.: Principles of quantitative perimetry: testing and interpreting the visual field, New York, 1977, Grune & Stratton, Inc. *This general clinical visual field text book concentrates on the physiology and psychophysics underlying visual field testing, and the technique of performing visual fields. It is worth reading in order to become better acquainted with the various basic and technical factors that influence visual field testing.*

PART TWO

TECHNIQUE OF MANUAL PERIMETRY

Part I of this book has covered the general principles of perimetry as they apply to both manual and automated techniques. The remainder will deal with the technical skills required for manual perimetry. The emphasis is on the Goldmann bowl perimeter, but the same principles pertain to the tangent screen and other manual methods.

The exact technique used is of prime importance in manual perimetry. In the end, the perimetrist who chooses the right technique and strategy at the right time is more important than the instrument. Also important is the perimetrist's ability to put the patient at ease and obtain the best results the patient can give.

> Perimetry is done by the perimetrist, not the perimeter.
>
> TRAQUAIR

> There is no such thing as Goldmann perimetry, only a Goldmann perimeter.
>
> GOLDMANN

> I would like to emphasize that perimetry, esecially kinetic, is an art.
>
> GOLDMANN

CHAPTER 15

Operation of the Goldmann perimeter

Modern perimeters consist of a hemispheric bowl evenly illuminated inside. The patient looks at a central fixation point while test spots of light of varying size and intensity are projected at various places within the bowl and the patient communicates whether or not they are visible.

The most common type of manual bowl perimeter is the Goldmann—of which there are several models, all very similar, made by several manufacturers (Haag-Streit Co., Topcon, Inc., Marco Equipment, Inc.). The Goldmann perimeter 940, made by Haag-Streit, will be described; and persons now learning to use a manual perimeter should consult the instructions provided by the manufacturer, which will include such things as the method for changing the light bulb and the fuse.

CARE OF THE PERIMETER

The inside of the bowl must stay clean and evenly white, without smudges, scratches, or pencil marks. Therefore, do not touch the bowl with anything except the brush used to clean it. Never hold a pencil when you are placing or removing the lens holder or you may accidentally write on the bowl surface. Also, do not allow the lens holder to scrape against the side of the bowl.

If more than an hour will elapse before the next usage, and especially overnight, place a dust cover over the perimeter. A soft brush that looks like a shaving brush is provided for dusting out the inside of the bowl as needed. This brush is not for use on the outside of the perimeter because it may pick up oil or grease. The outside of the perimeter must be kept dusted, of course, but with something else.

A special cleaning compound is available for use inside the bowl, which should be cleaned about once a year depending on usage and care. Rarely will the inside of the bowl ever need repainting, but if necessary this should be done by the manufacturer's service representative.

INSERTION AND ALIGNMENT OF PAPER

There are two knobs to loosen the chart plate. When these are given half a turn, it is possible to insert the paper into a narrow slit. At the bottom of the chart paper are four short vertical lines near the center. One of these is taller than the others and in line with the vertical meridian passing through the center of the circular chart. This taller mark should be placed exactly within the V-notch in the frame at the bottom. Be sure, also, that the paper is level with the two lateral V-notches. Then turn the knobs back to hold the paper in place.

FIG. 15-1. Inserting field chart paper into the Goldmann perimeter.

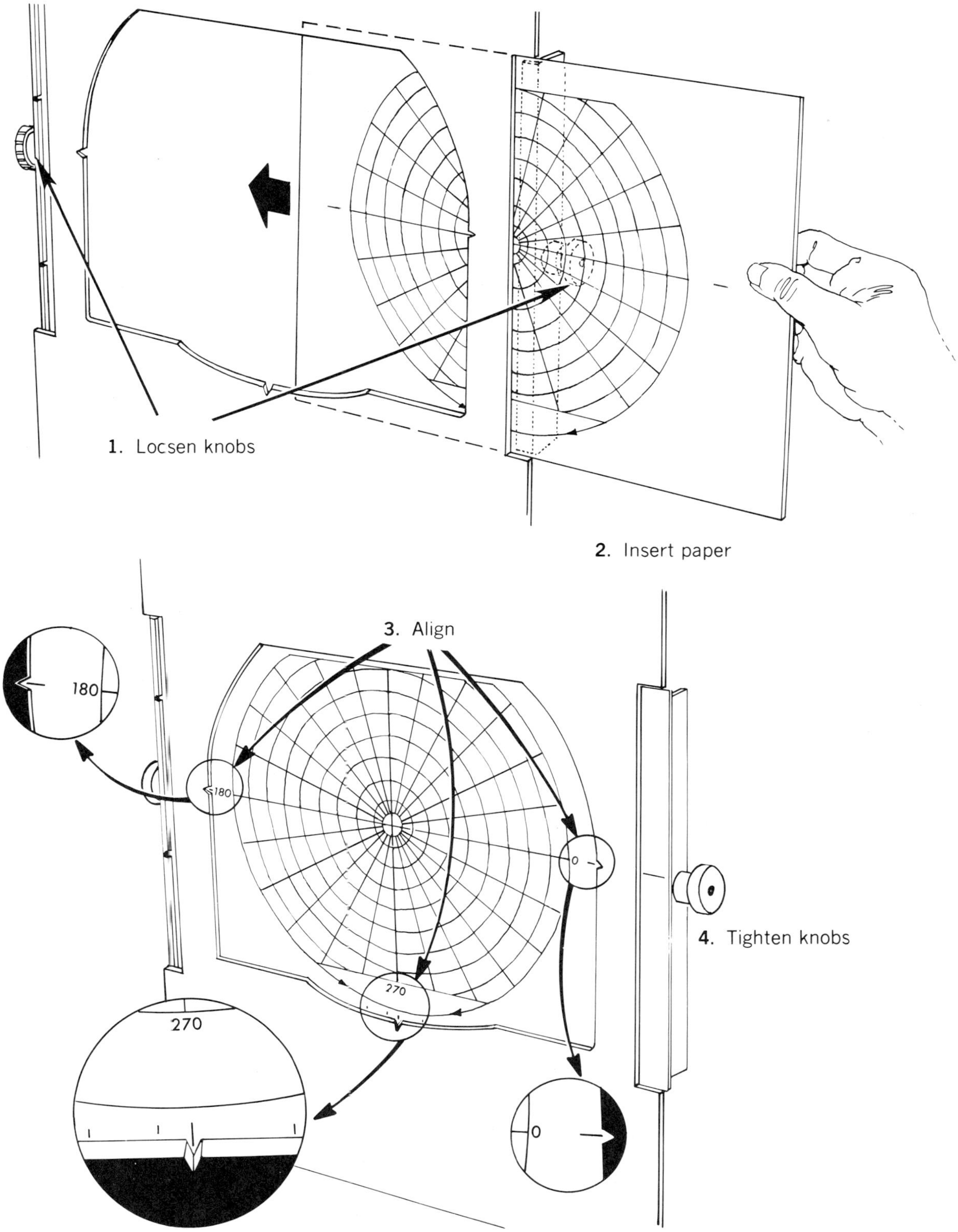
1. Locsen knobs
2. Insert paper
3. Align
180
0
270
4. Tighten knobs

FIG. 15-1

CONTROL OF PROJECTED LIGHT STIMULI

On the back of the perimeter is a set of levers to control the size and intensity of the projected test stimuli.

FIG. 15-2, A. Controls for the size and intensity of stimuli on the Goldmann perimeter. The three levers provide control of

Size: *0, I, II, III, IV,* and *V* (V is the largest.)

Intensity (coarse adjustment, 0.5 log-unit steps): *1, 2, 3,* and *4* (4 is the brightest.)

Intensity (fine adjustment, 0.1 log-unit steps): *a, b, c, d,* and *e* (e is the brightest.)

Recent models have an extended range of intensity by means of an additional lever with major jumps (2 log-units) in intensity. The single bar setting is 2 log-units dimmer, and the double bar 4 log-units dimmer, than the setting with no bar (which is the most intense).

With all the levers pushed to the right, the stimulus is the largest and brightest possible. With all levers pushed to the left, it is the smallest and dimmest possible.

Size I is the standard size of test stimulus used, and perimetry can be performed with various stimulus intensities. The larger sizes are used *only* when the most intense stimulus of size I (I-4e) is not adequate and a stronger one is required. Similarly, size 0 is used only when a weaker stimulus is needed than can be obtained with size I and all the intensity filter levers are to the left. This sometimes happens on instruments without the extended range of intensity (see p. 34 for further details).

The stimulus is turned on and off during visual field testing with a knob at the right side of the perimeter near the bottom. This knob can be twisted clockwise and counterclockwise and can also be depressed or elevated.

FIG. 15-2, B. Controls for turning the stimulus on and off.

Left, When the knob is twisted to one position, the stimulus is on with the knob depressed and off with the knob released.

Right, When the knob is twisted to the alternate position, the stimulus is off with the knob depressed and on with the knob released.

Except for rare occasions, during visual field testing the knob must be set so it is in the depressed position for the stimulus to be on. The main exception is during calibration of the instrument, when you want the stimulus to be on without having to hold the knob down. So you can know whether the stimulus is on or off, there is a tiny aperture (the stimulus indicator) below the plate with the levers to control the size and intensity of stimuli. Light is visible through the aperture when the test stimulus is on, but the aperture is dark when the stimulus is off.

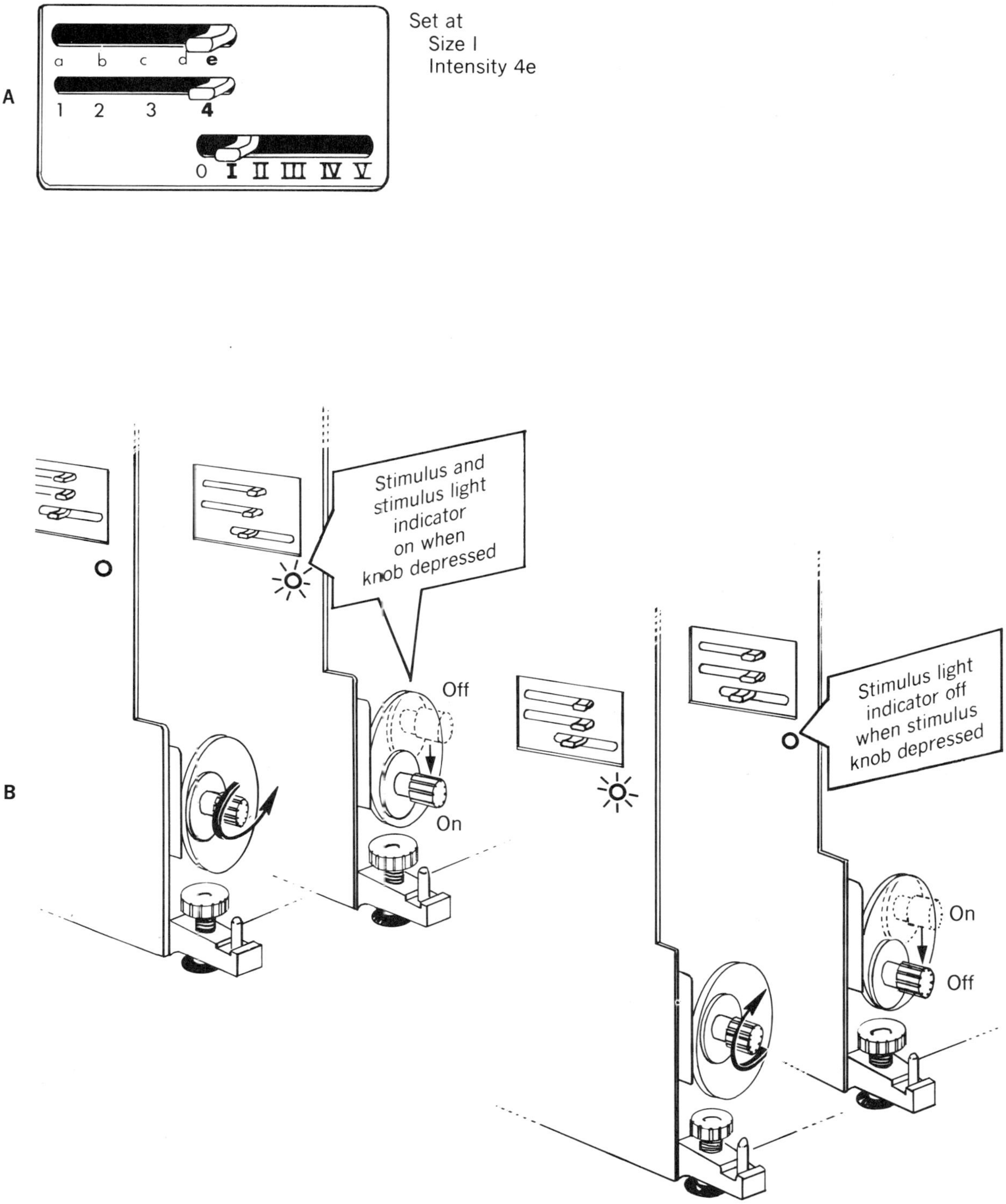
A
a b c d e
1 2 3 4
0 I II III IV V
Set at
Size I
Intensity 4e
B
Stimulus and stimulus light indicator on when knob depressed
Off
On
Stimulus light indicator off when stimulus knob depressed
On
Off

FIG. 15-2

The position of the stimulus inside the bowl is controlled by the pantograph handle. With the handle on the left side of the field chart, the projected stimulus will be inside the bowl to the patient's left.

FIG. 15-3. Pantograph handle on the Goldmann perimeter.
A, When to the left, the handle covers somewhat more than the left half of the field (unshaded portion) but cannot go beyond a curved line to the right of the vertical meridian on the chart.
B, To test the right half of the field, pass the handle to the other side by moving it carefully around the bottom of the chart.
C, After passing the handle along the pathway indicated by arrows on the chart, begin testing the right half of the field.

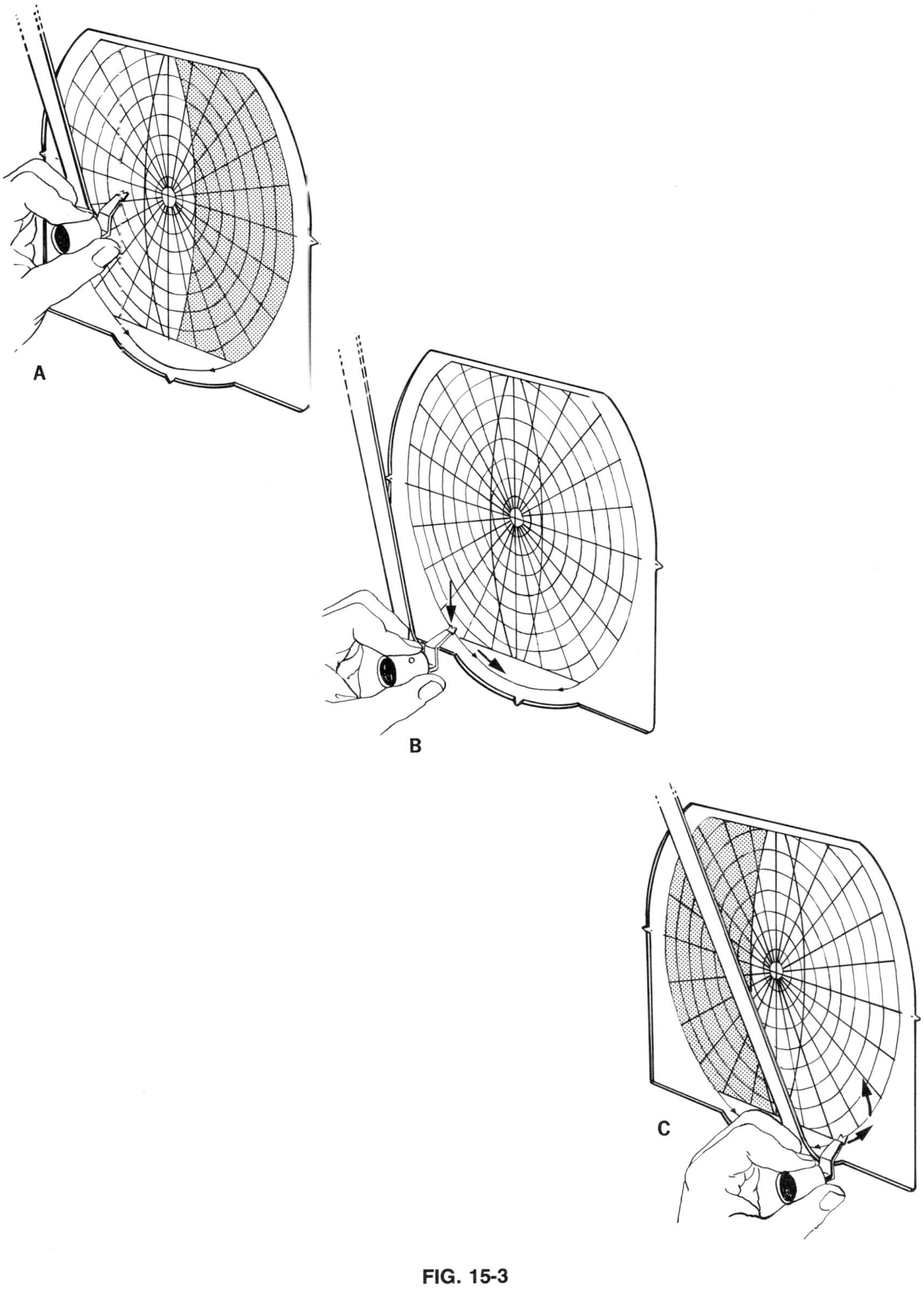

FIG. 15-3

POSITIONING THE PATIENT

Only one eye is tested at a time, and the other eye is covered. The perimeter comes with a translucent white occluder designed to provide the theoretic advantage of avoiding dark adaptation of the covered eye. It will then be ready for visual field testing when the testing of the first eye is completed. This was deemed important because field testing is performed under light-adapted (photopic) conditions. However, in actual practice if a black patch is used as an occluder the eye soon becomes light-adapted again when uncovered.

When the eye not being tested is covered and the patient's chin and forehead are in the appropriate position, the head can be moved up or down as well as right or left with the large chin rest control knobs at the bottom of your side of the perimeter. You can determine by looking through the telescope whether the eye is centered. (The image will be upside down.) The telescope can be focused by pulling the eyepiece in or out. When the telescope is focused, a reticle is visible that is subdivided in millimeters for the purpose of measuring the diameter of the patient's pupil. If the patient's eye is not in focus while the reticle is in focus, it usually means that his head is not fully forward against the forehead rest.

With the patient's eye properly positioned, he can see a small fixation point in the center of the bowl. If you position yourself in front of the fixation point, you will see that this is actually a small mirror mounted on a small pillar reflecting light from the light bulb above the patient's head. A larger mirror behind the small one and controlled by a lever at the base of the telescope on your side is for patients with poor vision who cannot see the small mirror. However, you should use the small mirror whenever possible for more accurate fixation and for better control of accommodation.

FIG. 15-4. Controls on the Goldmann perimeter for centering the patient's position.

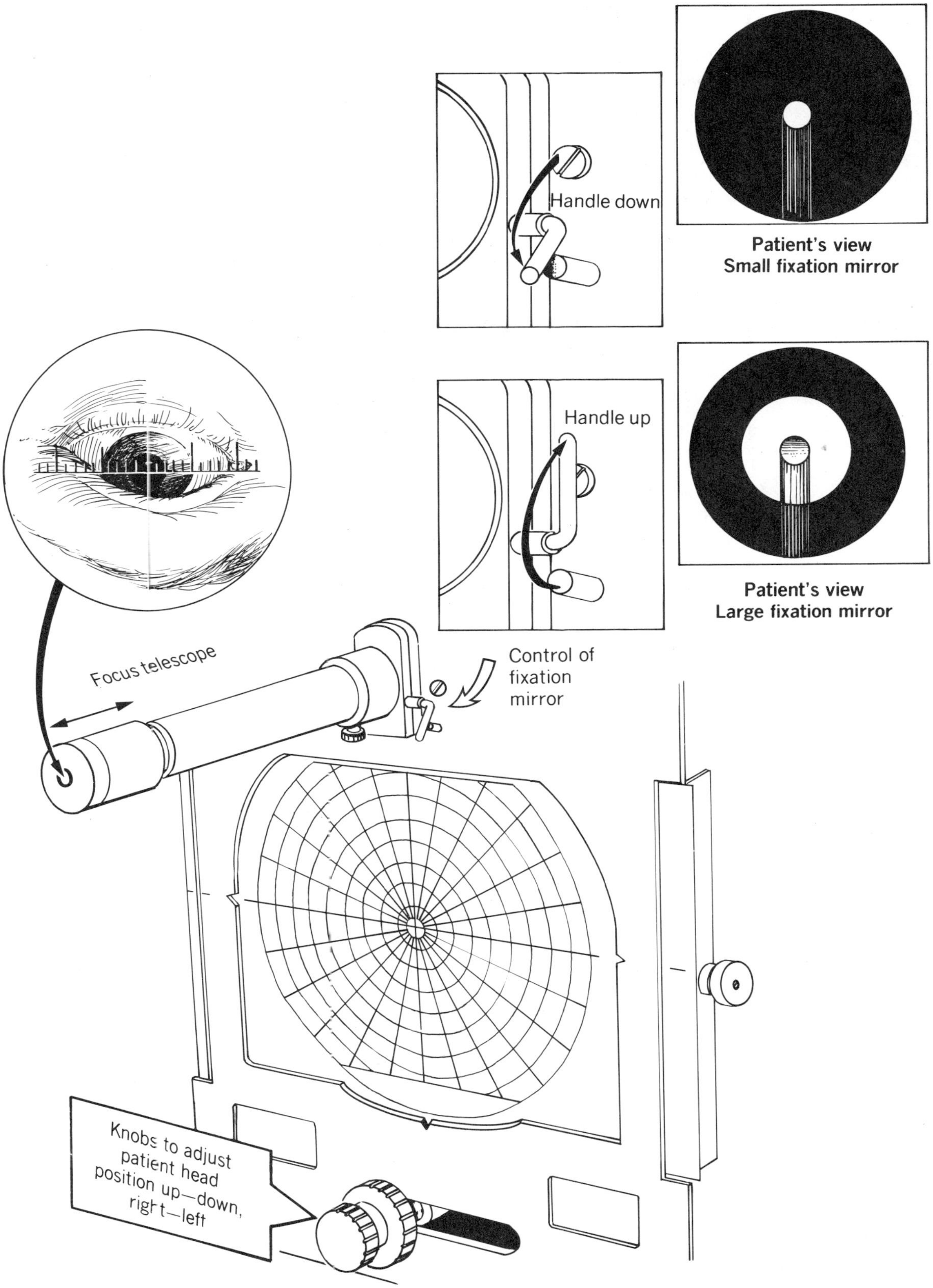

Handle down
Patient's view
Small fixation mirror
Handle up
Patient's view
Large fixation mirror
Focus telescope
Control of
fixation
mirror
Knobs to adjust
patient head
position up—down,
right—left

FIG. 15-4

LEVELING THE PERIMETER

The perimeter should be leveled. When it is level, its projection arm if released will automatically come to rest (by gravity) in the port at the side of the perimeter bowl. This prevents the patient from hurting himself or damaging the projector arm by sitting back at the end of the test and bumping his head on the extended arm. It also prevents harm to the arm if someone bumps it when the perimeter is not in use.

FIG. 15-5. Leveling controls on the Goldmann perimeter. Two knobs control feet at the bottom front of the perimeter. On the left side is a bubble level.

CONTROL OF ILLUMINATION FOR THE OPERATOR

Because the test is performed in a darkened room, provision must be made for you to see. Light bulbs inside the machine illuminate the field chart from behind, and light shines on the table through adjustable panels.

FIG. 15-6. Light for the operator. On the side of the Goldmann perimeter to your left are two rheostats. The closer one controls the intensity of light behind the chart paper. On each side of the perimeter beneath the chart paper are sliding metal door panels that can be opened to varying degrees to let some of the light behind the chart fall on your side of the table so you can see the pencils and anything else on the table.

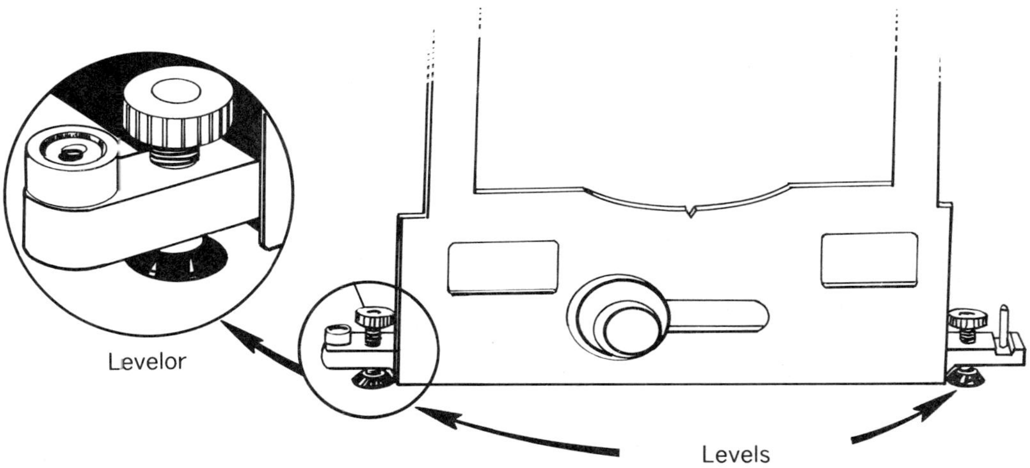

FIG. 15-5

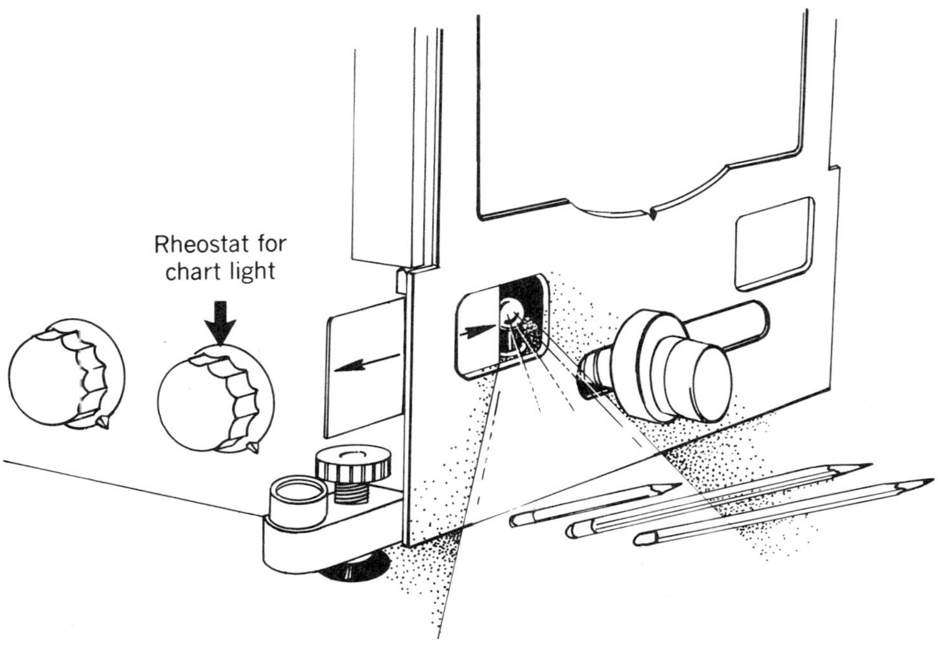

FIG. 15-6

LENS HOLDER

For optimum visibility the test stimuli must be in focus on the retina. Therefore the patient may need corrective lenses to be able to give consistent responses.

FIG. 15-7. Lens holder for the Goldmann perimeter.
A, Post for storing the lens holder when not in use.
B, Placing the lens holder in position for use. When placing the lens holder in position, be sure not to have a pencil in your hand, which could scratch the inside of the bowl.

By turning the knob on the base of the lens holder, you place the lens as close to the patient's eyelashes as possible. The lens is used for examining the central 30 degrees of the visual field but is removed for examination of the peripheral field. Optical correction for the entire visual field would be ideal; however, as a practical matter, the rim of the lens gets in the way, and therefore a lens cannot be used outside 30 degrees. Fortunately, there is less need for a sharply focused retinal image in the peripheral field than in the central field.

When placing lenses in the lens holder, put the spherical ones in the back (toward the patient) and the cylinders in front (away from the patient).

It is important to use full-aperture lenses with a narrow metal rim around the glass, not lenses with a broad metal rim around a smaller glass.

The use of corrective lenses is described in Chapter 12.

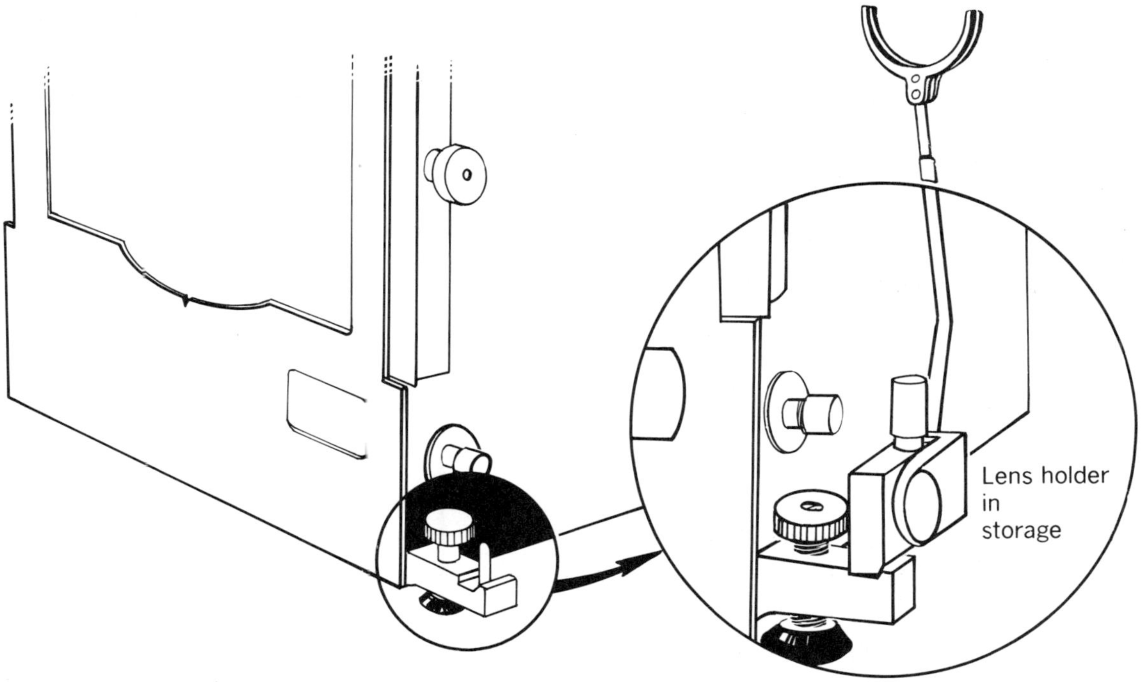

A

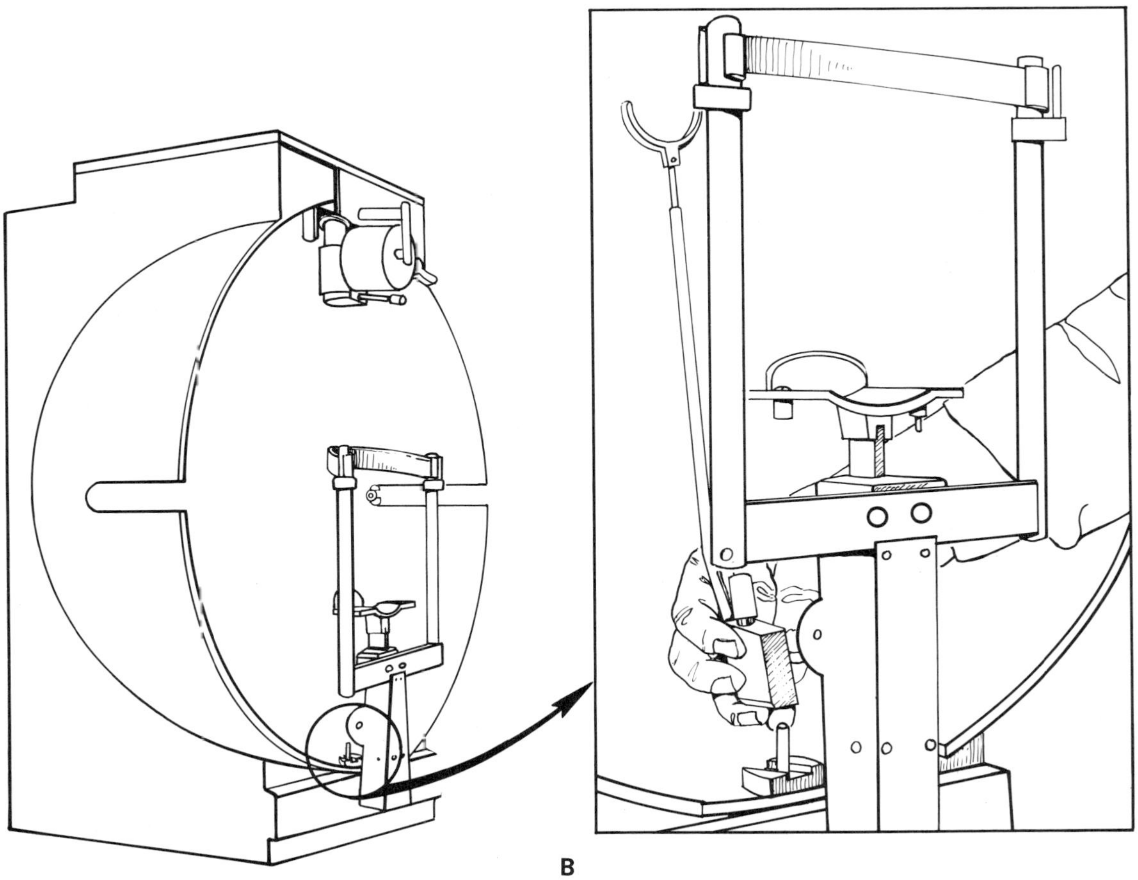

B

FIG. 15-7

CHAPTER 16

Calibrating the Goldmann perimeter

The perimeter should be calibrated often—perhaps at the beginning of each day or whenever you are not certain if someone else may have turned the knobs while dusting or while looking for the on-off switch. Calibration is fast and easy. If you have to look up how to do it, you are not doing it often enough!

For the perimeter to be calibrated, it is necessary that the intensities of both the projected stimulus and the background be adjusted.

The first step is to make certain that the room lights are off and the door to the room is closed. There must be no stray light inside the perimeter bowl. The stimulus switch should be turned so the stimulus is on without the knob's being depressed, just the opposite of when the perimeter is being used for field testing.

FIG. 16-1. Setting the perimeter for calibration. Move the pantograph handle to a position at 70 degrees on the right side and lock it. Set the stimulus control at the largest and brightest *(V-4e)*, with all levers to the right. Turn the stimulus switch so it does not have to be depressed when the projected stimulus is on. After the calibration is complete, be sure to reset the knob to the proper position for field testing.

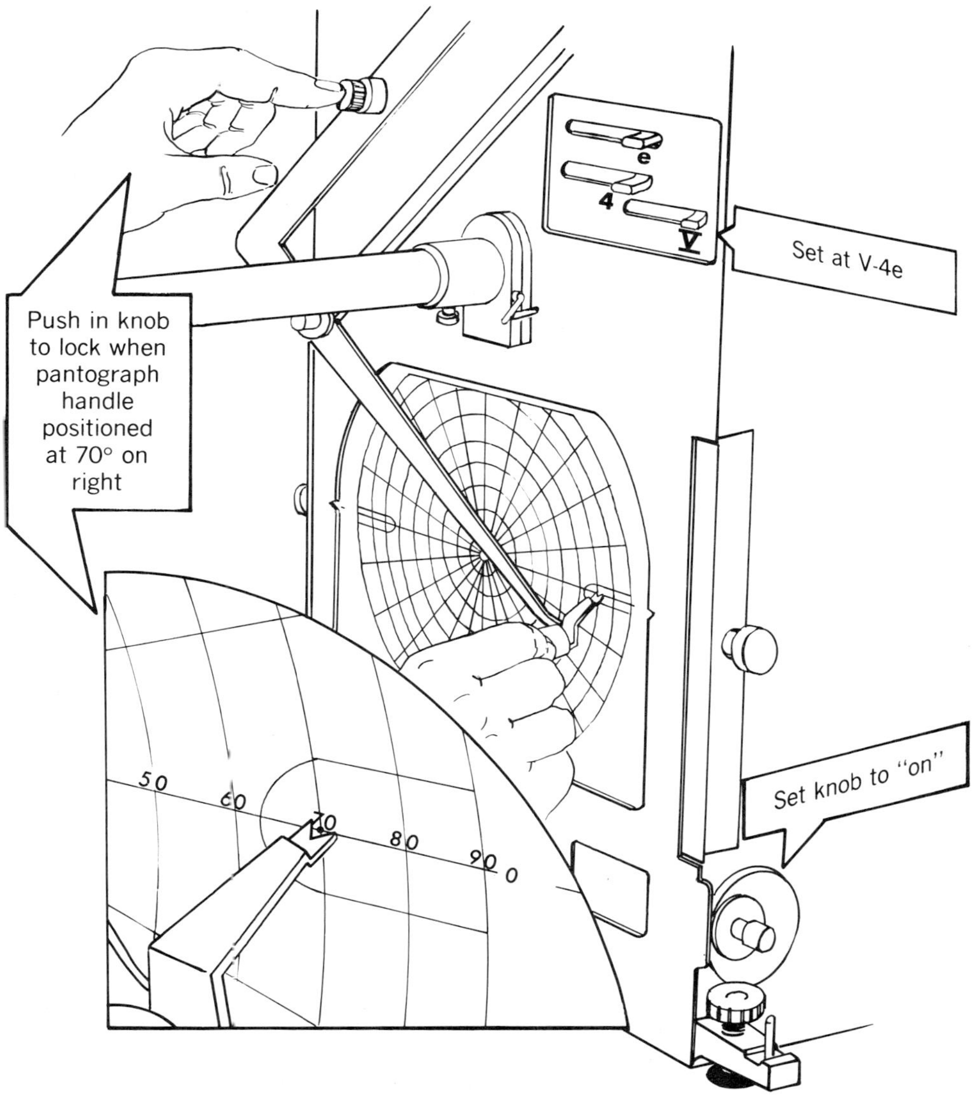

e
4
V
Set at V-4e
Push in knob to lock when pantograph handle positioned at 70° on right
Set knob to "on"
50
60
70
80
90
0

FIG. 16-1

CALIBRATION OF THE STIMULUS

FIG. 16-2. Adjusting the stimulus. Insert the light meter and raise the flaglike photometer screen out of the way so the projected stimulus will shine into the meter. With the stimulus control on the largest and brightest *(V-4e)* setting, adjust the rheostat until the light meter registers 1000 asb. There is a special light operated by a push button just below it to help you see the light meter in the darkened room.

If the intensity will not go high enough to show a reading of 1000 asb, replace the light bulb of the perimeter after making sure that the stimulus is set for V-4e, that it is turned on, and that it is shining onto the light meter without obstruction. Sometimes the reason for diminished intensity is simply that the bulb has turned black on the top, in which case you can merely turn it over (inverting top and bottom) instead of replacing it.

The light meter should be protected from constant exposure to bright light and also from physical abuse when not in use, usually by merely placing it carefully in the drawer.

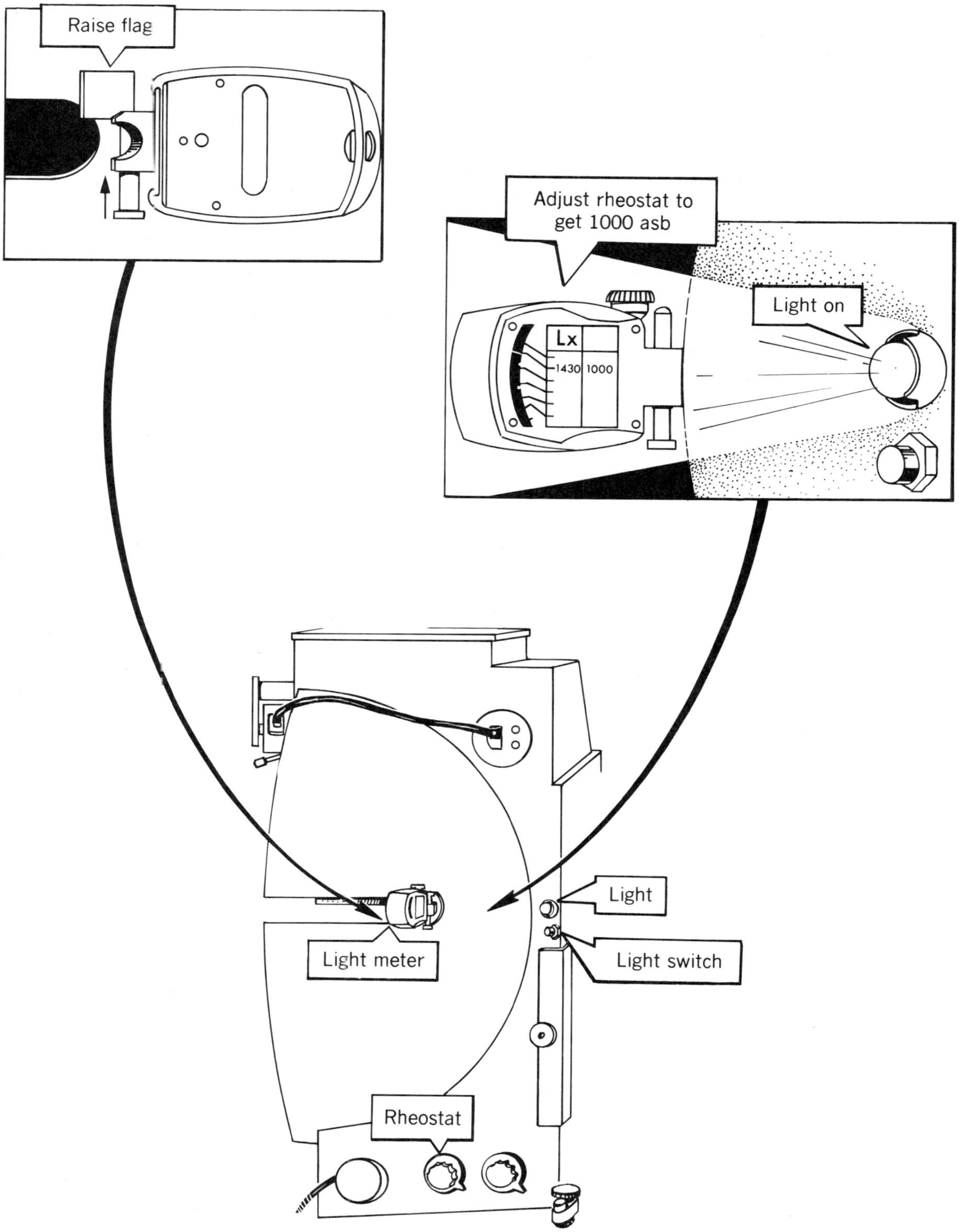
Raise flag
Adjust rheostat to get 1000 asb
Light on
Lx
1430
1000
Light
Light switch
Light meter
Rheostat

FIG. 16-2

CALIBRATION OF THE BACKGROUND

To calibrate the background, use a dim but large (V-1e) stimulus. This will reduce the intensity of light to 32.5 asb, 1.5 log-units less than the 1000 asb of a V-4e stimulus.

FIG. 16-3. Adjusting the background to 32.5 asb. Lower the flaglike photometer screen so it intercepts the projected stimulus. By looking through one slot at the edge of the hemisphere and through the hole of a ring at the other slot, you can see the projected stimulus. Adjust the lamp shade until the intensity of the ring (representing the background illumination) is equal to the 32.5 asb of a stimulus projected onto the photometer screen, as seen through the hole.

When calibration is complete, put the light meter away, turn the stimulus switch so the stimulus will be *off* with the switch not depressed, and unlock the pantograph handle so the arm will swing into its position of rest and be out of the way.

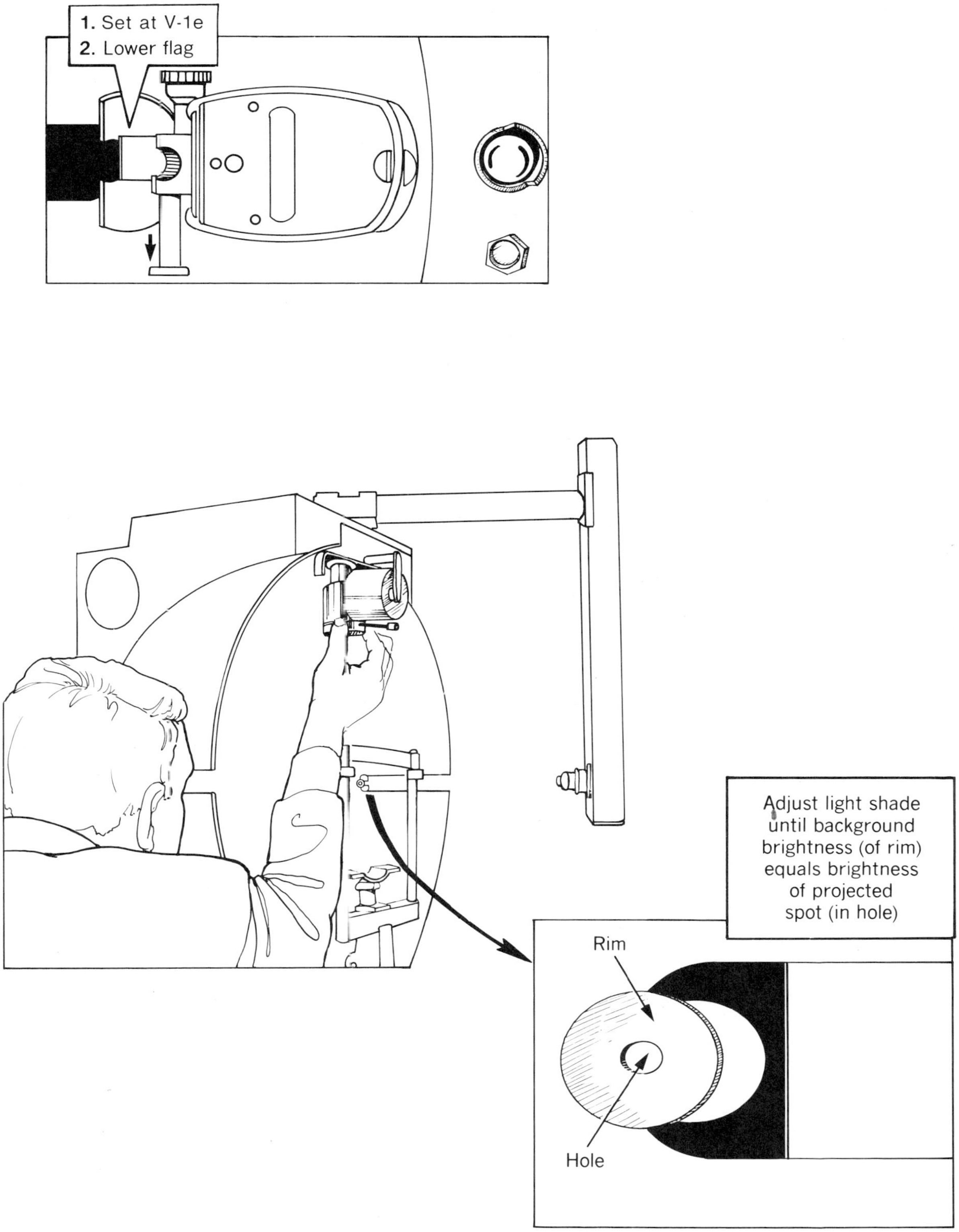
1. Set at V-1e
2. Lower flag
Adjust light shade until background brightness (of rim) equals brightness of projected spot (in hole)
Rim
Hole

FIG. 16-3

CHAPTER 17

Plotting isopters kinetically

In Chapter 1 the principles of kinetic perimetry were introduced, and the beginning perimetrist should read that chapter before proceeding with this one. Chapters 4 and 5 are also appropriate preludes to this chapter.

The method of plotting normal isopters is illustrated with the Goldmann perimeter. However, the principles and sequence can be adapted to any other visual testing apparatus, including the tangent screen. You may wish to attempt the sequence on a volunteer with normal sight first to help yourself become acquainted with the mechanics of the instrument.

FIG. 17-1, A. Setting the levers to the desired stimulus size and intensity. For example, *I-2e* is appropriate for a person with normal sight. Turn the knob of the shutter switch so the projected stimulus comes on when the switch is depressed but is off when the switch is not depressed (see Fig. 15-2).

Turn off all room lights and close the door of the room. There must not be any stray light. Cover the eye not to be tested. Position the patient's head so the uncovered eye is properly centered in front of the fixation target when you look through the telescope and adjust the large knobs near the bottom of the perimeter to move the head sideways or up and down. Note the size of the pupil and record it on the chart.

FIG. 17-1, B. Projecting the stimulus. With your left hand, move the position of the test stimulus until it is near fixation (e.g., at 5 degrees). Depress the shutter switch with your right hand, which is holding the pencil, so the patient is able to see the object when it is turned on. Make a mental note of the approximate reaction time from when the stimulus is turned on to when the patient pushes the buzzer.

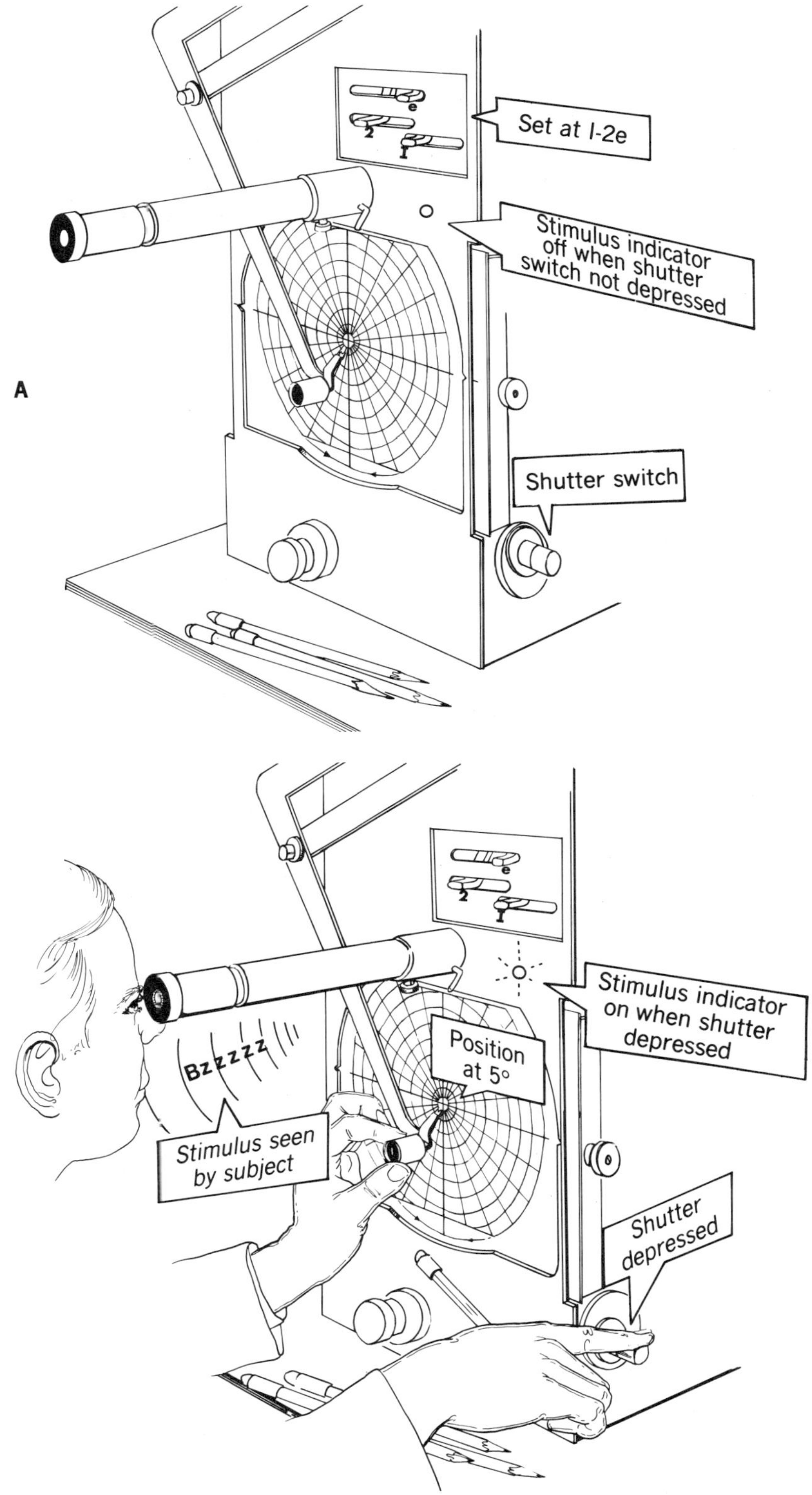
A
Set at I-2e
Stimulus indicator off when shutter switch not depressed
Shutter switch
B
Stimulus indicator on when shutter depressed
Position at 5°
Bzzzzz
Stimulus seen by subject
Shutter depressed

FIG. 17-1

After confirming in this way that the test object is visible near the center of the field, lift your right hand off the shutter switch so the projected spot will be off.

FIG. 17-2. The plotting procedure.
A, With your left hand, move the pantograph handle to the peripheral portion of the field (e.g., 60 degrees). Turn on the projected stimulus by depressing the shutter switch with your right hand. Wait about a second (or twice the patient's reaction time) to be sure that the object is not seen at the periphery of the field. If it is seen at 60 degrees, use a weaker stimulus (such as the *I-1e*). But be sure that this weaker stimulus is visible at the center of the field before turning your attention again to the periphery of the field.
B, After waiting a second to make sure that the object is not visible at the periphery, move the stimulus inward at a speed of about 3 to 5 degrees per second. Keep the stimulus on by holding the shutter switch in a depressed position with your right hand. As the object moves toward the center, look through the telescope at the patient's eye to be sure he is maintaining fixation.

It is important to be looking at the eye just prior to the patient's response so you can tell if he is maintaining fixation at the very instant he responds. If he happens to look away momentarily toward the object and then respond that he saw it, this response must be ignored. It is no good for you to look at fixation after the patient has responded. He may have been looking in the direction of the stimulus when he saw it, but by the time you look through the telescope he will have regained his proper fixation and you will not realize that he looked away for a split second.

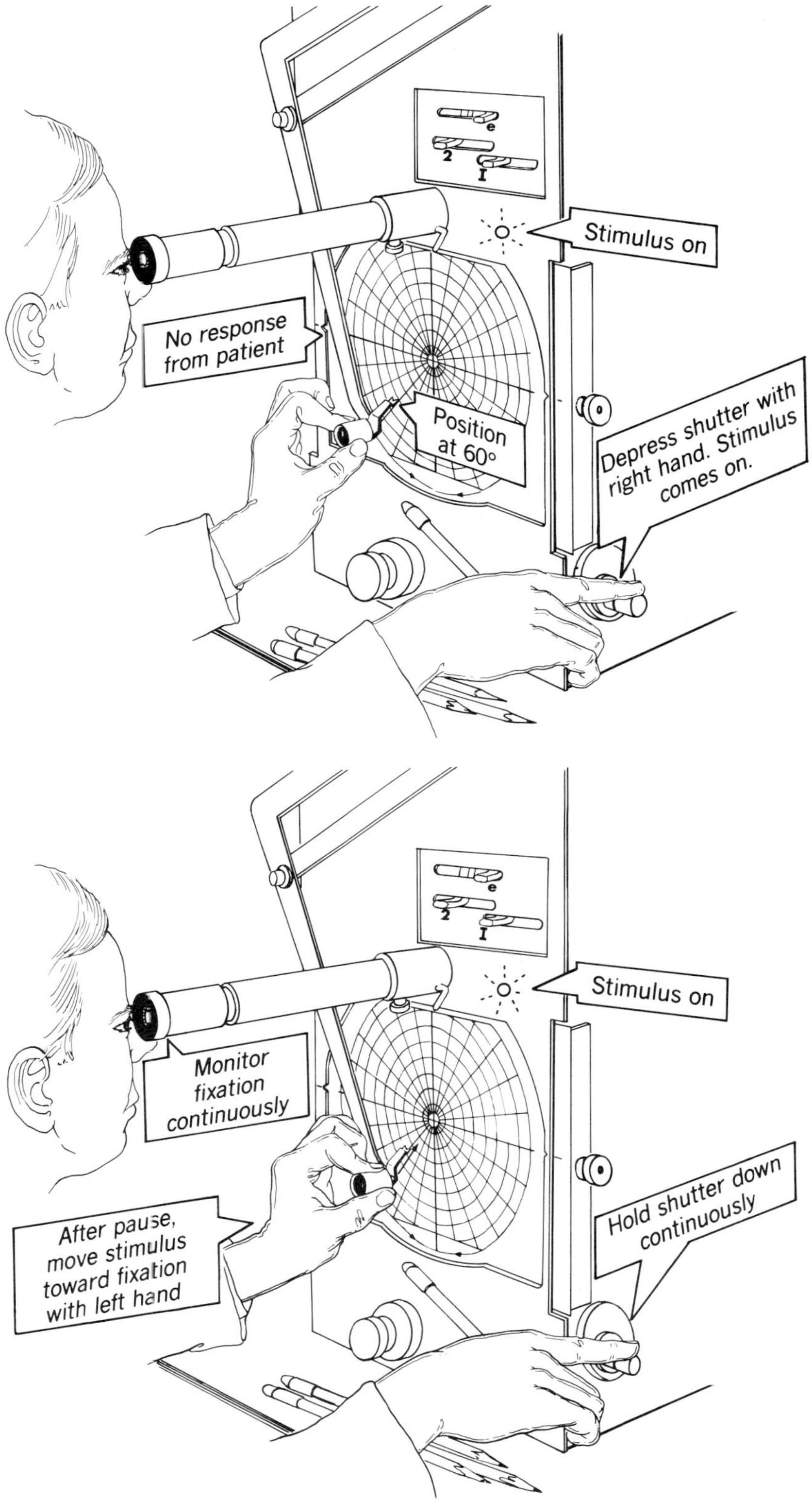
A
Stimulus on
No response from patient
Position at 60°
Depress shutter with right hand. Stimulus comes on.
B
Stimulus on
Monitor fixation continuously
After pause, move stimulus toward fixation with left hand
Hold shutter down continuously

FIG. 17-2

FIG. 17-3. Continuing the procedure.

A, As soon as the patient responds without having shifted fixation, stop moving your left hand.

B, Then lift your right hand off the shutter knob, which turns off the stimulus.

C, Use the pencil in your right hand to mark the position at which the object became visible.

From the patient's perspective the sequence of events is as follows: the test object becomes visible, he responds, the test object disappears.

A

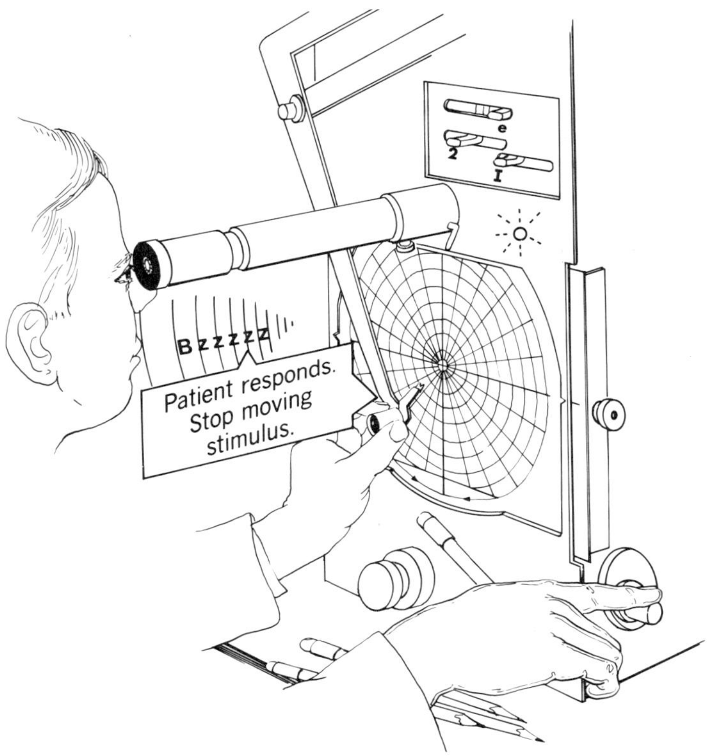

FIG. 17-3

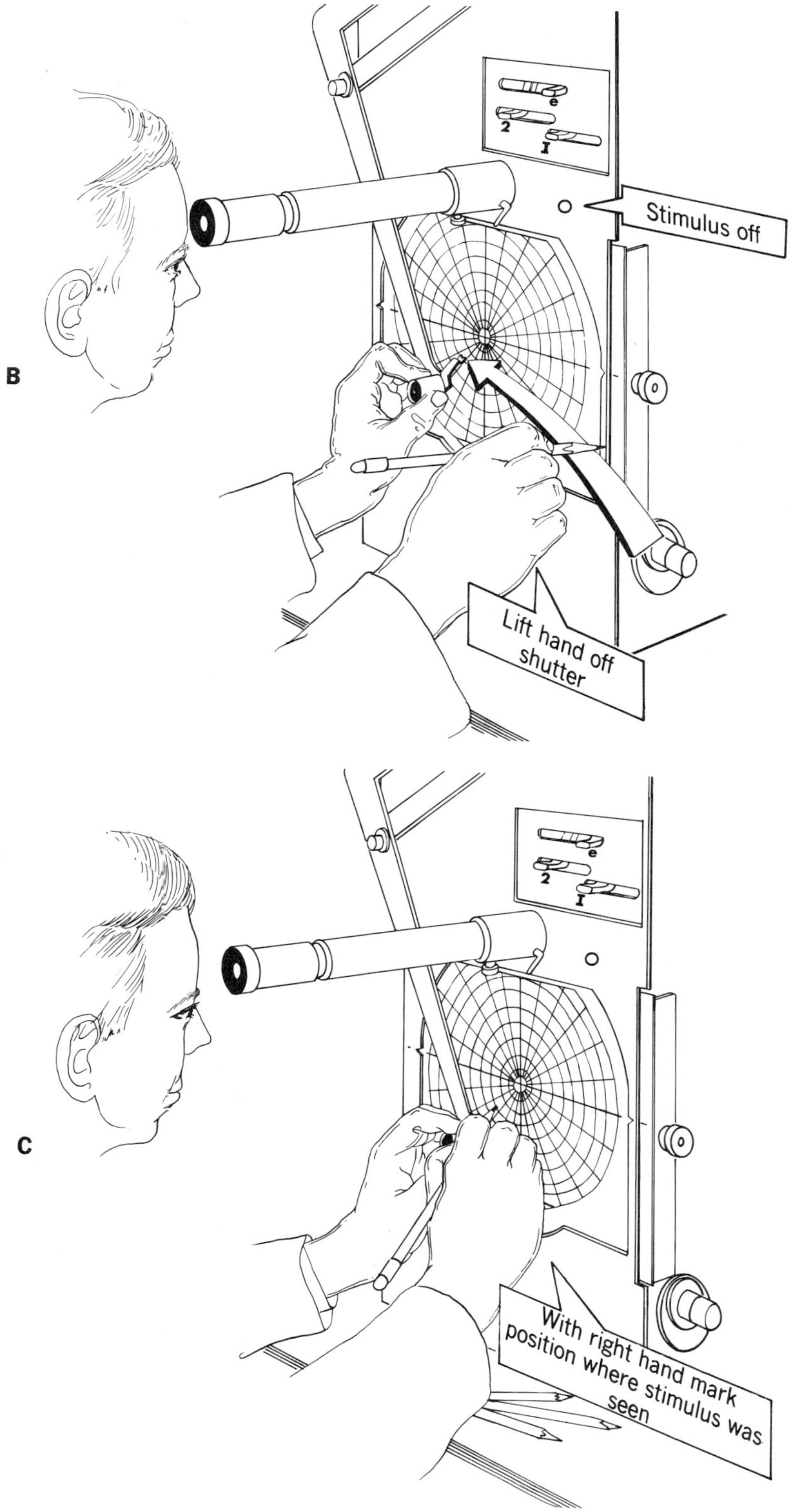

FIG. 17-3, cont'd

FIG. 17-4. Continuing the procedure.
A, Next, with your left hand, move the projected stimulus outward by 10 or 15 degrees and shift to an adjacent meridian.
B, Again, depress the shutter with your right hand. After a 1-second wait to be sure the object is not visible, move it toward the center. If the stimulus is seen before it is moved, turn it off, move it more peripherally, and start again. When the patient responds, release the shutter switch with your right hand and mark the position where the stimulus became visible.

This process is repeated around the entire circumference. From the patient's perspective the sequence is as follows: the stimulus is seen, he responds, the stimulus disappears, he waits for the next stimulus to appear.

A

B

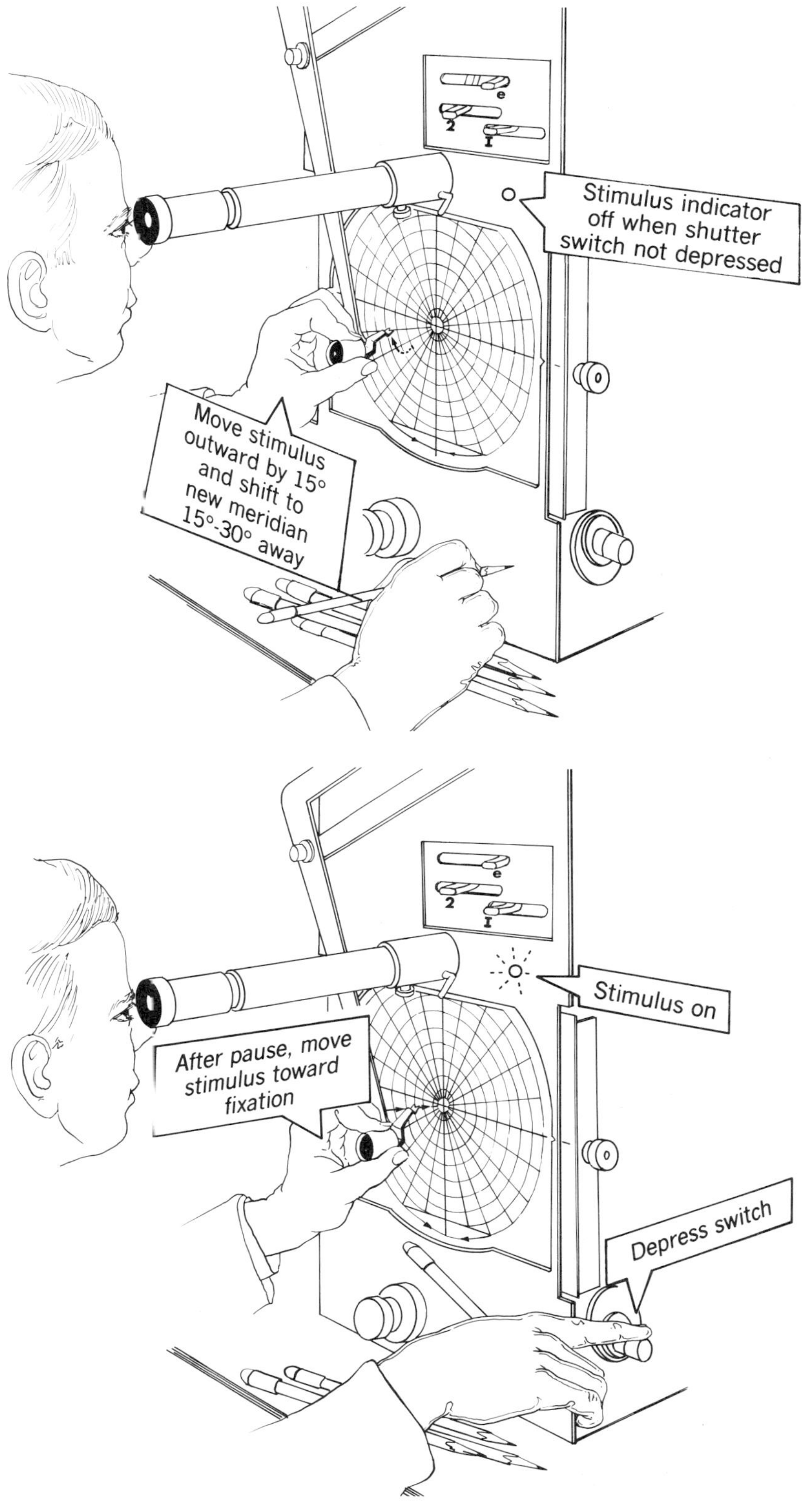
Stimulus indicator off when shutter switch not depressed
Move stimulus outward by 15° and shift to new meridian 15°-30° away
Stimulus on
After pause, move stimulus toward fixation
Depress switch

FIG. 17-4

When the I-2e threshold points are completely plotted, draw a line connecting all of the dots. Then set the test stimulus at I-4e and repeat the entire procedure.

FIG. 17-5, A. Repeating for a second isopter. Complete the isopter for *I-2e* and begin plotting the *I-4e* isopter.

After this is completed, repeat the entire procedure testing the patient's other eye.

FIG. 17-5, B. Field diagram. Label each diagram completely to include the following:
Name of the patient—first and last
Date—include the year
Evaluation of the quality of the test
Name of the perimetrist
Size of the pupil
Stimuli used
Eye tested

Other data that should always be recorded on a field diagram are the visual acuity, the lenses used, and which isopters were tested with lenses (see Chapter 12). In addition, the IOP is often given on the field chart (see also Chapter 23 and pp. 380 and 443).

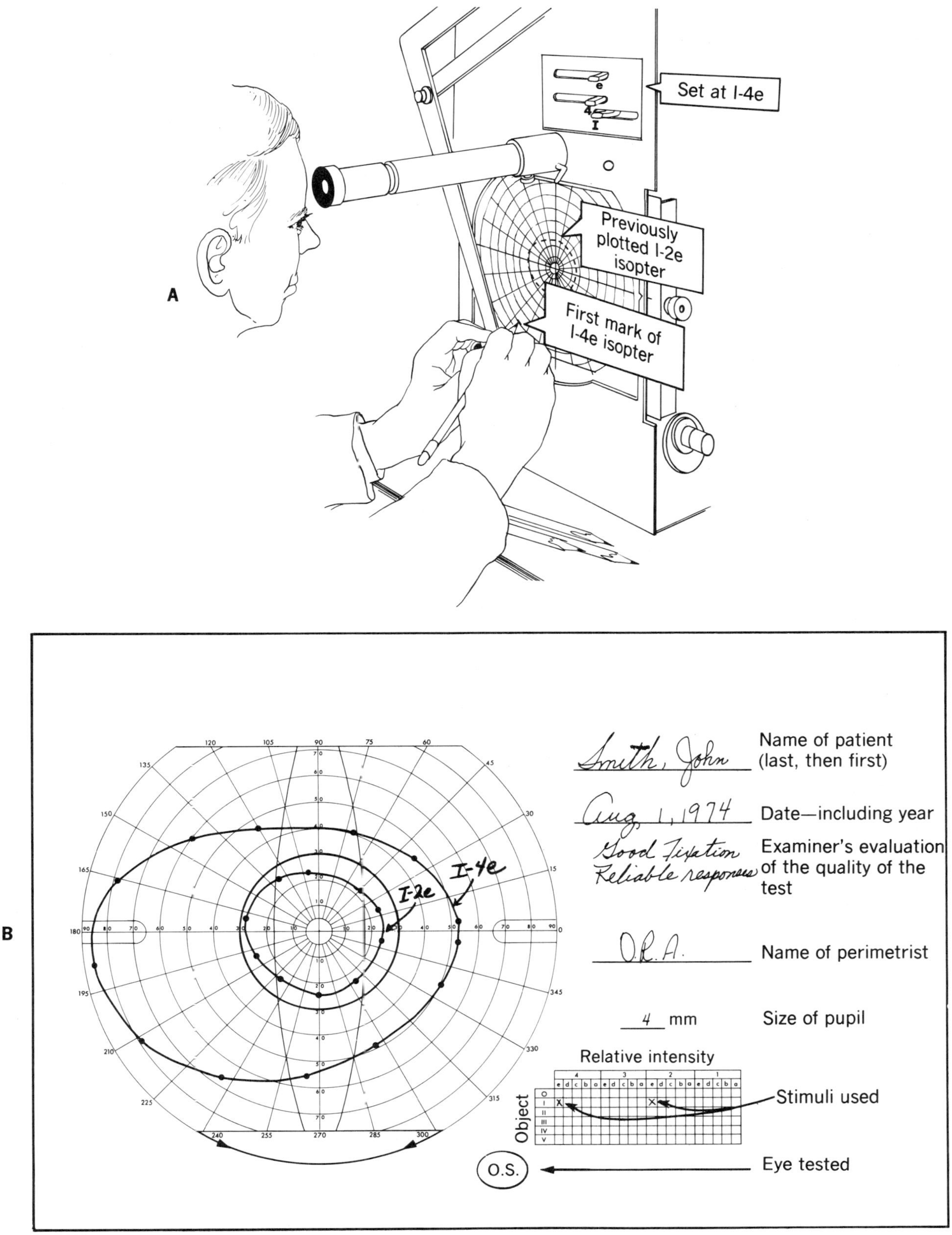
A
Set at I-4e
Previously plotted I-2e isopter
First mark of I-4e isopter
B
I-4e
I-2e
Smith, John
Name of patient (last, then first)
Aug. 1, 1974
Date—including year
Good fixation
Reliable responses
Examiner's evaluation of the quality of the test
O.R.A.
Name of perimetrist
4 mm
Size of pupil
Relative intensity
Object
Stimuli used
O.S.
Eye tested

FIG. 17-5

CHAPTER 18

Scotoma detection

The basic principles of scotoma detection by suprathreshold testing are given in Chapter 6, which should be read before proceeding with this chapter.

The technique described here outlines the physiologic blind spot and looks for abnormal scotomas after the isopter has been plotted by kinetic perimetry. It is a good idea to plot the I-2e and I-4e isopters and then practice the ensuing steps on a volunteer.

The location of the physiologic blind spot is between 10 and 15 degrees from fixation, just below the horizontal meridian on the right side for the patient's right eye and on the left side for his left eye. Most often the I-4e stimulus, which is the smallest but most intense, can be used to plot the blind spot; however, a stronger one may be required if the I-4e isopter is too small and fails to enclose the blind spot. With the stimulus set at I-4e but turned off, move the pantograph handle to the expected position of the blind spot.

FIG. 18-1, A. Finding the blind spot by static spot-checking. After positioning the pantograph handle with your left hand, depress the shutter switch with your right hand to turn the *I-4e* stimulus on. If the patient sees the stimulus, turn it off, move to another spot (but stay between 10 and 15 degrees, somewhat below the horizontal meridian), and try again. If a blind spot cannot be found, check to see if you forgot to cover the eye not being tested and if you are searching the correct side (right side for the right eye, left for the left eye).

Note the sequence: The patient responds when he first sees the stimulus. After he responds, the stimulus disappears and he waits for another. In this way, static spot-checking seems no different to the patient from the procedure used for kinetic isopter plotting.

FIG. 18-1, B. Plotting the size of the blind spot. With the pantograph handle in a position where the stimulus is not seen, depress the shutter switch with your right hand, turning the stimulus on. After pausing for a second to be sure that the stimulus is indeed not seen, move the handle downward to find the lower boundary of the blind spot.

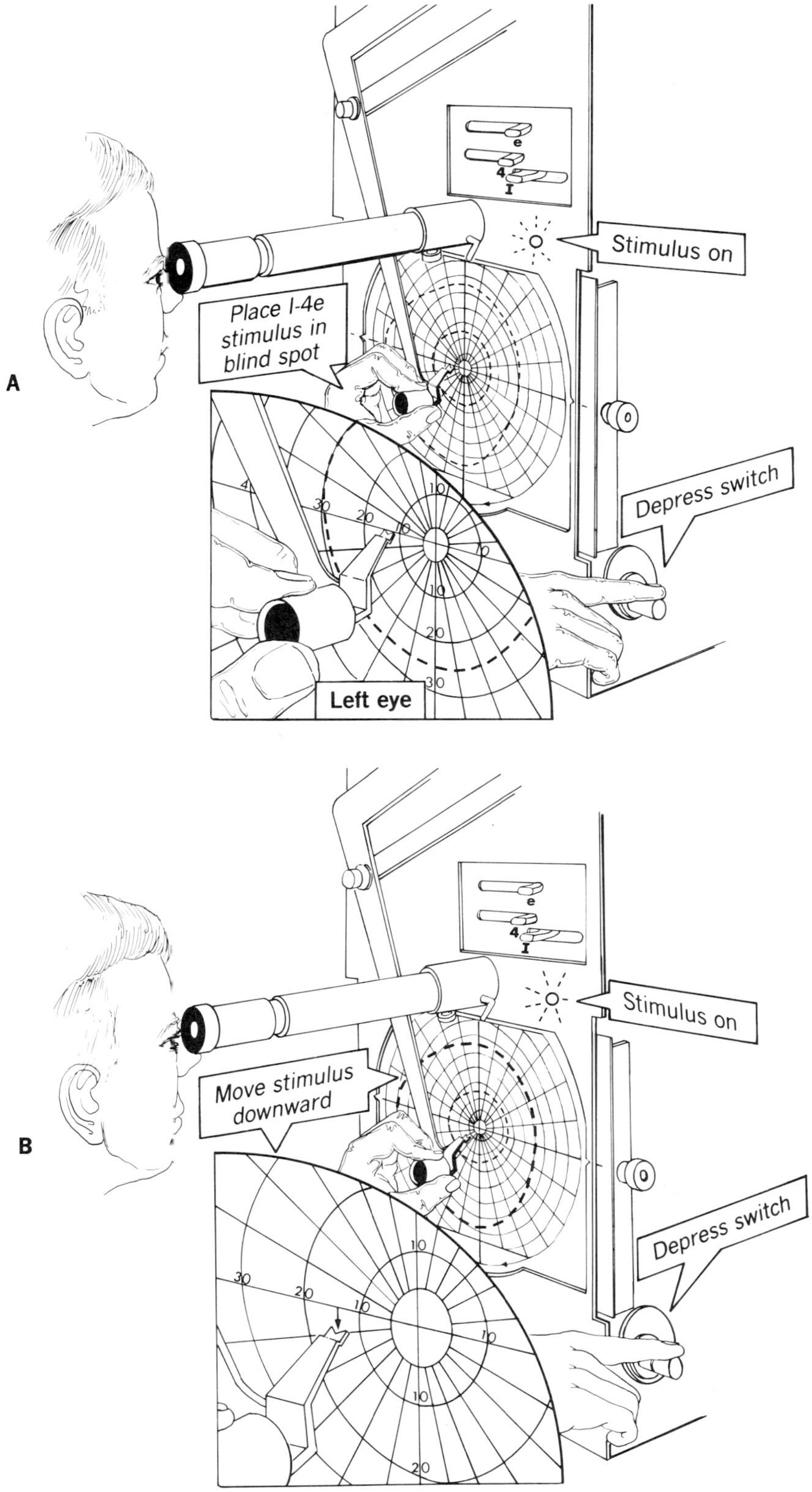
A
Stimulus on
Place I-4e stimulus in blind spot
Depress switch
Left eye
B
Stimulus on
Move stimulus downward
Depress switch

FIG. 18-1

FIG. 18-2, A. Continuing to plot the blind spot. When the patient responds by sounding the buzzer, remove your right hand from the shutter and mark the position with a pencil.

After the lower boundary of the blind spot is found (the stimulus is still off), move the pantograph handle back to the presumed center of the blind spot. Then turn on the stimulus and, after a pause to be sure it is not seen, move it upward until it is seen. Repeat the process until the boundary is plotted at the top and bottom, to the right and left, and in the four oblique directions.

FIG. 18-2, B. Plotting the boundary of the blind spot. Next, join the eight pencil marks and shade in the blind spot.

This constitutes the procedure for plotting the boundary of a scotoma, in this case the physiologic blind spot. From the patient's perspective the procedure continues to be exactly the same when plotting the boundary of a scotoma as when plotting an isopter or doing static spot-checking: The stimulus is turned on without his knowing (because it is in an area where he does not see), it becomes visible as it moves, he responds, it disappears, he waits for the next presentation.

Remember: In plotting isopters, always move the stimulus from a nonseeing area to a seeing area. This rule applies both to plotting the usual isopters and to plotting the boundary of scotomas.

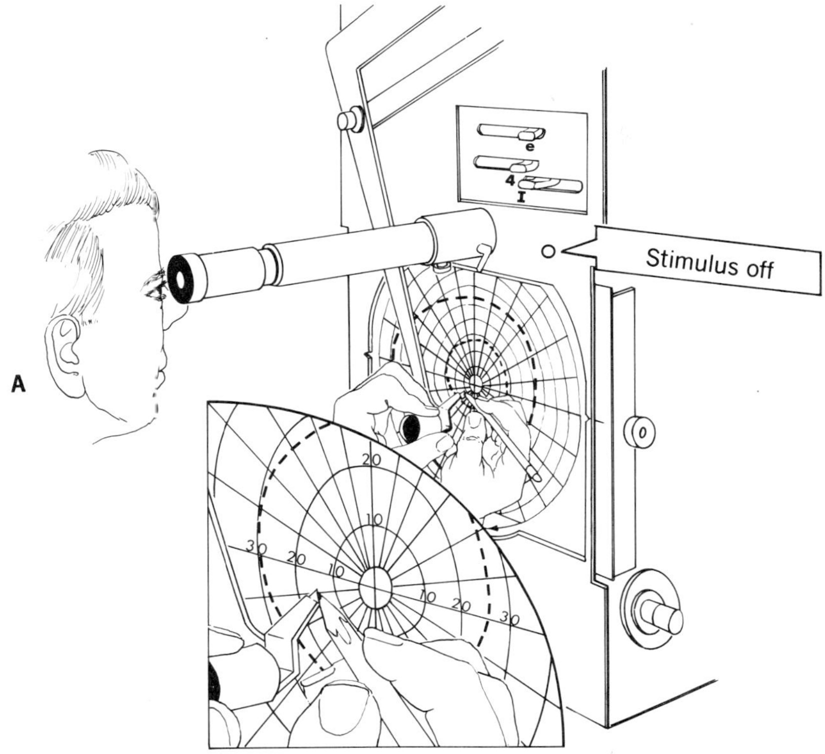

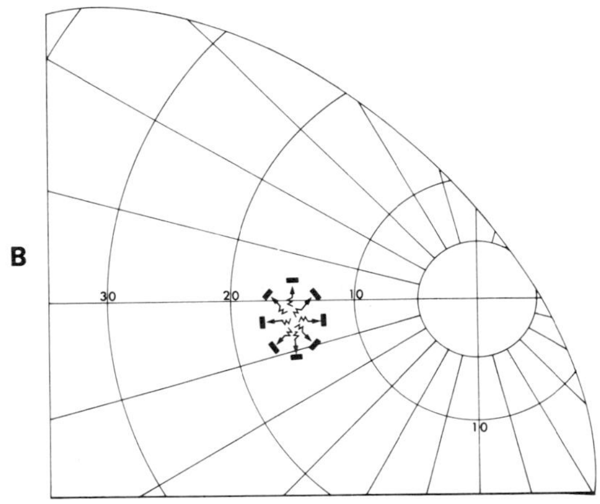

FIG. 18-2

After the isopters are plotted and the blind spot is outlined, search the area within the isopters by static suprathreshold spot-checking to find any scotomas.

FIG. 18-3. Static spot-checking inside the I-2e isopter with the I-2e stimulus. Present the stimulus at several locations within the isopter. It should be visible everywhere. The technique here is to position the projected stimulus with your left hand and depress the shutter switch with your right hand. When the patient responds, or after about a second if he does not respond, lift your hand off the shutter, move the stimulus to a new location with your left hand, and once again depress the shutter to test a new spot. This is repeated until the entire area within the isopter has been searched. So the patient does not know when the stimulus will be presented, try to depress and elevate the switch gently and silently. Also an irregular rhythm helps (see p. 400).

From the patient's perspective, the sequence remains as follows: a stimulus appears, he responds, it disappears, he waits for a new stimulus to appear in a new location. Thus the procedure seems to him exactly the same whether you are plotting an isopter, outlining the blind spot, or checking for scotomas. This is important, because it means that the patient needs only one set of instructions, which apply to the entire test.

Check the area inside the I-2e isopter with the I-2e test stimulus for scotomas. The region between the I-2e and I-4e isopters should also be checked with the I-4e test stimulus. It is not necessary to use the I-4e within the I-2e isopter, however, because this area has already been checked with the I-2e. Since the I-2e stimulus was determined to be visible everywhere, the brighter (I-4e) stimulus will certainly be seen also. Label the diagram as shown.

FIG. 18-4. Proper labeling of a field diagram. The areas in question were spot-checked and the appropriate stimulus was seen. Either "O.K. to I-2e" or "1-2e seen" is satisfactory. However, such notations alone may be disadvantageous in that there is no indication of the number of spots checked or their precise location. In some offices and clinics therefore the standard practice is to mark with an *X* every spot that is tested and found to be all right. In other offices the *X* is used to indicate spots where the stimulus was not seen. If *X*s are used as symbols, it is well in addition to mark the diagram "I-2e seen" or "I-2e not seen" to clarify the meaning of the symbol. What to do with the spot not seen is the subject of the next chapter.

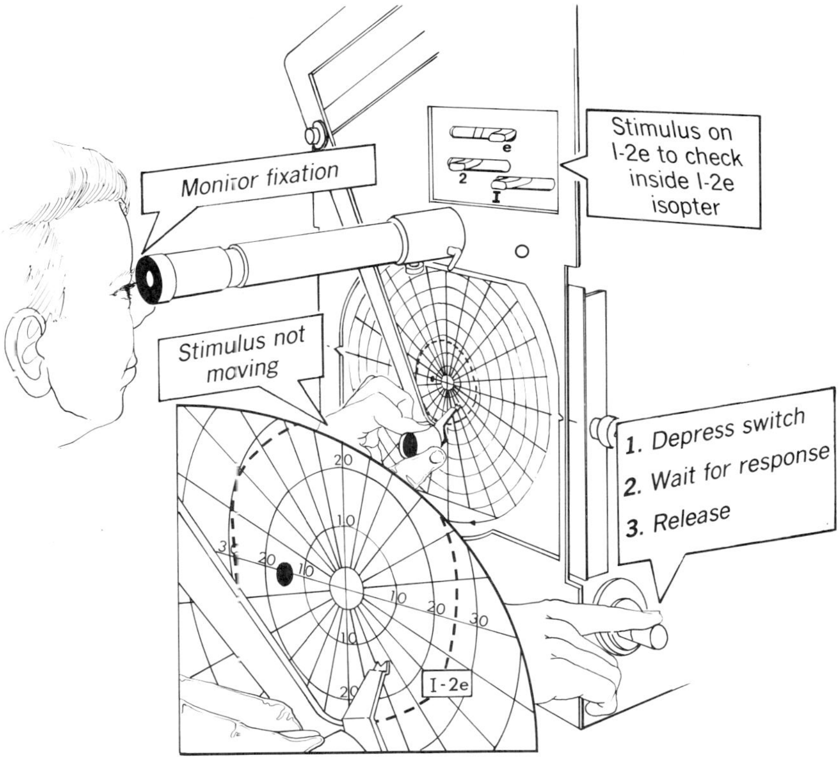

FIG. 18-3

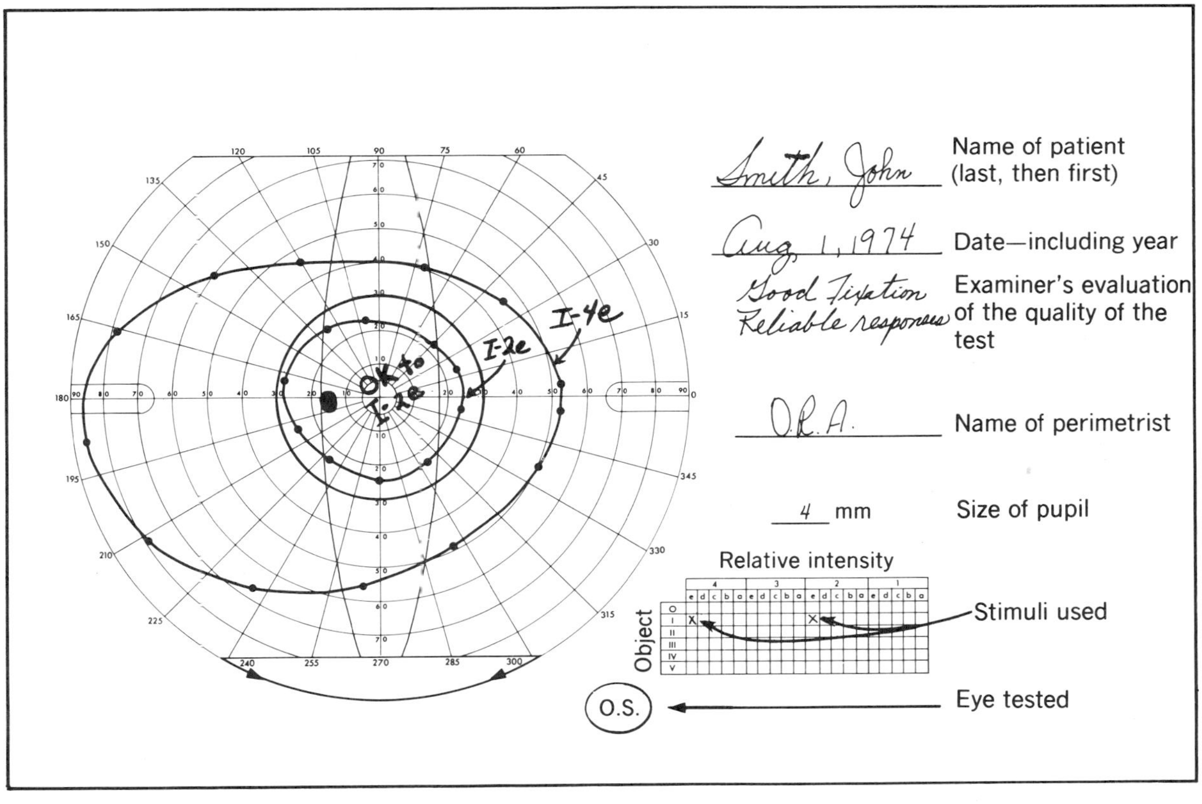

FIG. 18-4

CHAPTER 19

Scotoma quantitation

REVIEW

A scotoma is a region in which sensitivity to light is less than in the area immediately surrounding it. On an isopter plot a scotoma is represented as an area within an isopter where the test stimulus is not seen. When a scotoma is found, its boundary is plotted. Then the depth and slope or steepness are measured, or quantified:

DEPTH—Determine the threshold or that the strongest available stimulus is invisible.

SLOPE OR STEEPNESS OF THE BOUNDARY—Plot the boundary with several stimuli or at least with both the weakest and the strongest stimuli for which the scotoma is present.

FIG. 19-1. Comparison of isopter and profile plots of shallow and deep scotomas with sloping and steep margins.
A, Shallow scotoma within the *I-2e* isopter. The *I-2e* stimulus is not seen but the *I-3e* is. This is compared to the physiologic blind spot, an absolute scotoma within which the strongest available stimulus *(V-4e)* is not seen.
B, Moderately deep scotoma with sloping margins. The size of this scotoma is smaller for stronger stimuli *(I-4e)* than for weaker stimuli *(I-2e)*. Note on the right the physiologic blind spot, a steep-walled scotoma that is essentially the same size for all stimuli.

A scotoma is said to be *shallow* if a slightly stronger stimulus is visible, *deep* if only a very strong stimulus is visible, of *maximum luminosity* if the strongest stimulus on the testing apparatus is not visible, and *absolute* if no stimulus is visible. In addition, a scotoma that is the same size for all test stimuli has *steep margins* and one that is larger for weaker stimuli has *sloping margins*.

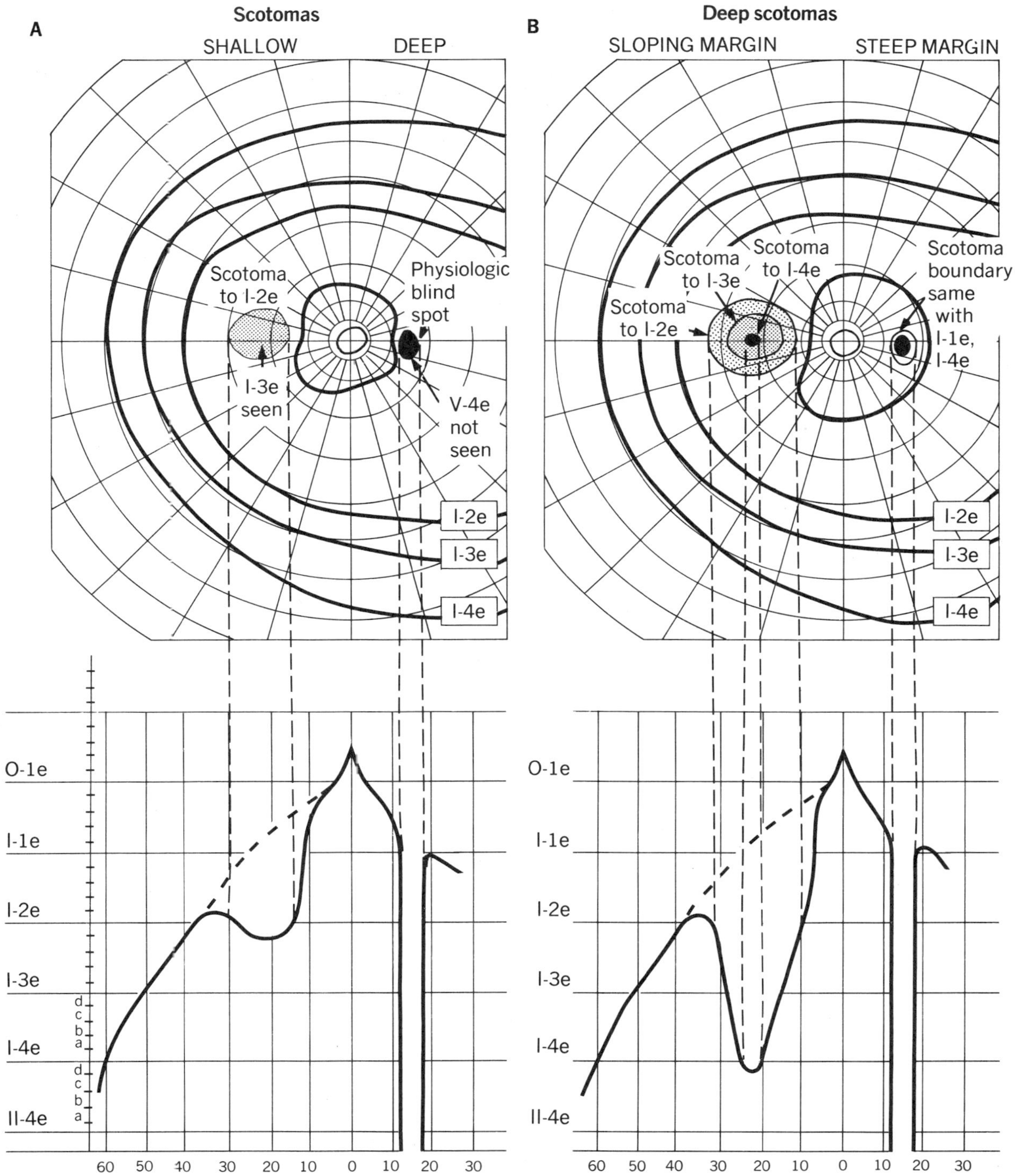
A
Scotomas
SHALLOW
DEEP
Scotoma to I-2e
Physiologic blind spot
I-3e seen
V-4e not seen
I-2e
I-3e
I-4e
B
Deep scotomas
SLOPING MARGIN
STEEP MARGIN
Scotoma to I-3e
Scotoma to I-4e
Scotoma to I-2e
Scotoma boundary same with I-1e, I-4e
O-1e
I-1e
I-2e
I-3e
I-4e
II-4e
d
c
b
a
60 50 40 30 20 10 0 10 20 30

FIG. 19-1

STRATEGY

Once a scotoma is discovered in a certain location, it must be quantified with regard to its boundary, depth, and slope.

FIG. 19-2. Outlining the boundary of a scotoma. When a stimulus is not seen, and hence a scotoma is discovered in a specific location, move the stimulus until it becomes visible at the boundary of the scotoma. Then move it in the opposite direction until the opposite boundary is encountered. Subsequently the outline is determined in all directions. By this method you are determining the scotoma's boundary kinetically.*

The boundary line is the isopter for a specific test stimulus and separates the region where the stimulus is visible from the region where it is not visible. However, the isopter of a scotoma encloses an area within which the stimulus is *not* seen rather than within which it *is* seen. Note the important practical point that, in either instance, **the isopter is plotted by moving the target from a place where it is not seen toward a place where it is seen.** This makes for more consistent responses than the alternative—moving from a seeing to a nonseeing region and asking the patient to say when it disappears. Moreover, it keeps the instructions and sequence of events the same in all stages of the examination: the patient responds whenever he sees a stimulus and then he waits for another.

---

*You can also determine the boundary by spot-checking numerous adjacent locations until the entire extent of the scotoma becomes evident as a cluster of spots where the stimulus is not visible. However, the kinetic plotting of a boundary is usually more efficient in manual perimetry.

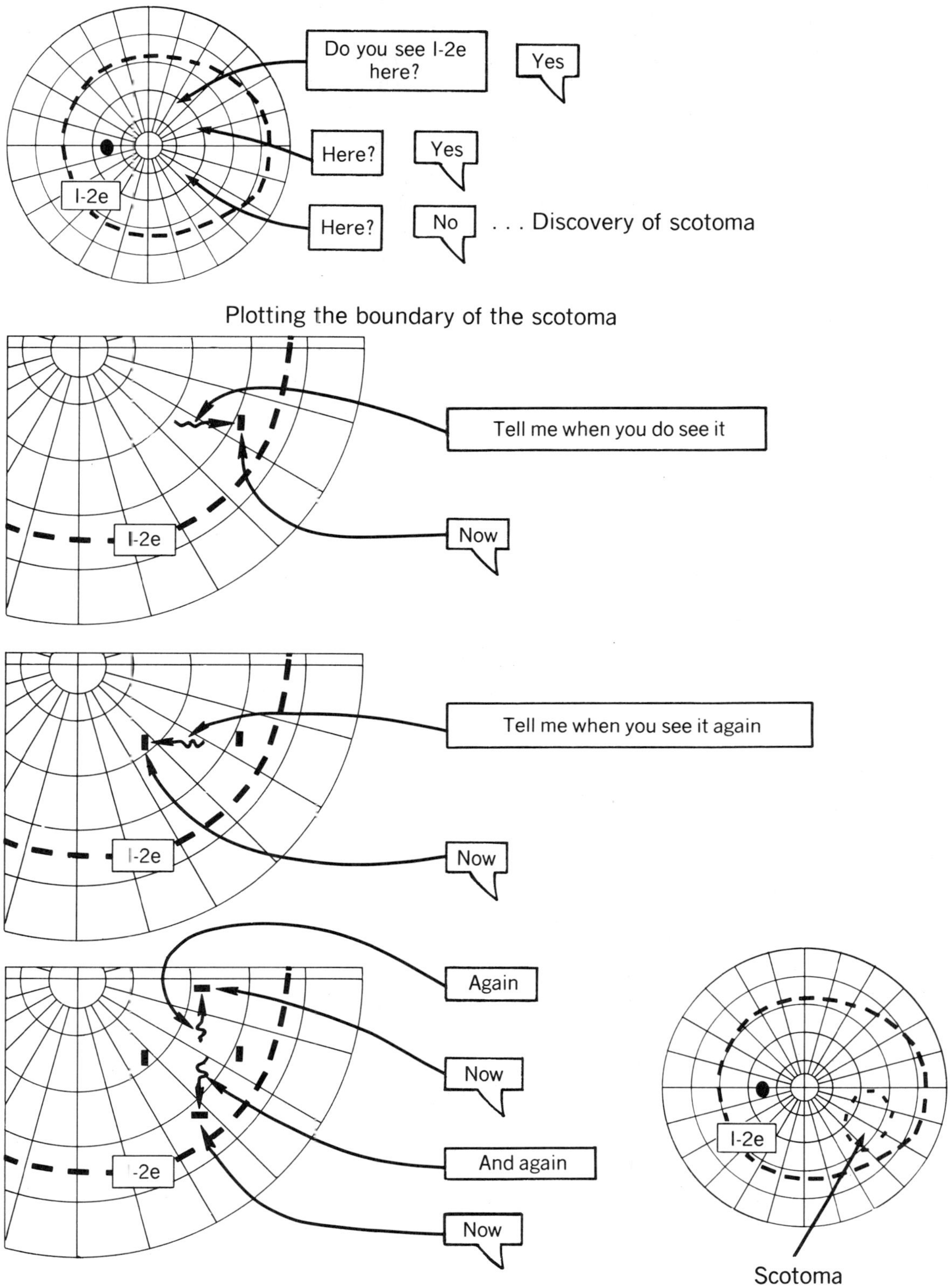
Do you see I-2e here?
Yes
Here?
Yes
Here?
No
. . . Discovery of scotoma
I-2e
Plotting the boundary of the scotoma
Tell me when you do see it
Now
I-2e
Tell me when you see it again
Now
I-2e
Again
Now
And again
Now
I-2e
Scotoma

FIG. 19-2

FIG. 19-3. Determining the depth of a scotoma. At the apparent geometric center of the scotoma, which is usually but not always the deepest part, increase the stimulus until it becomes visible. Label that spot with the threshold value (e.g., *II-4e seen*). It is assumed that if a field diagram is labeled "II-4e seen" then II-4e is the weakest stimulus visible—just as when visual acuity is said to be 20/70 we mean that the 20/70 letters are the smallest the patient can read correctly.

This is STATIC THRESHOLD PERIMETRY. The stimulus is not moving *(static)* and the *threshold* (weakest stimulus visible) is determined. However, the threshold value is simply written on an isopter chart, not represented on a profile graph.

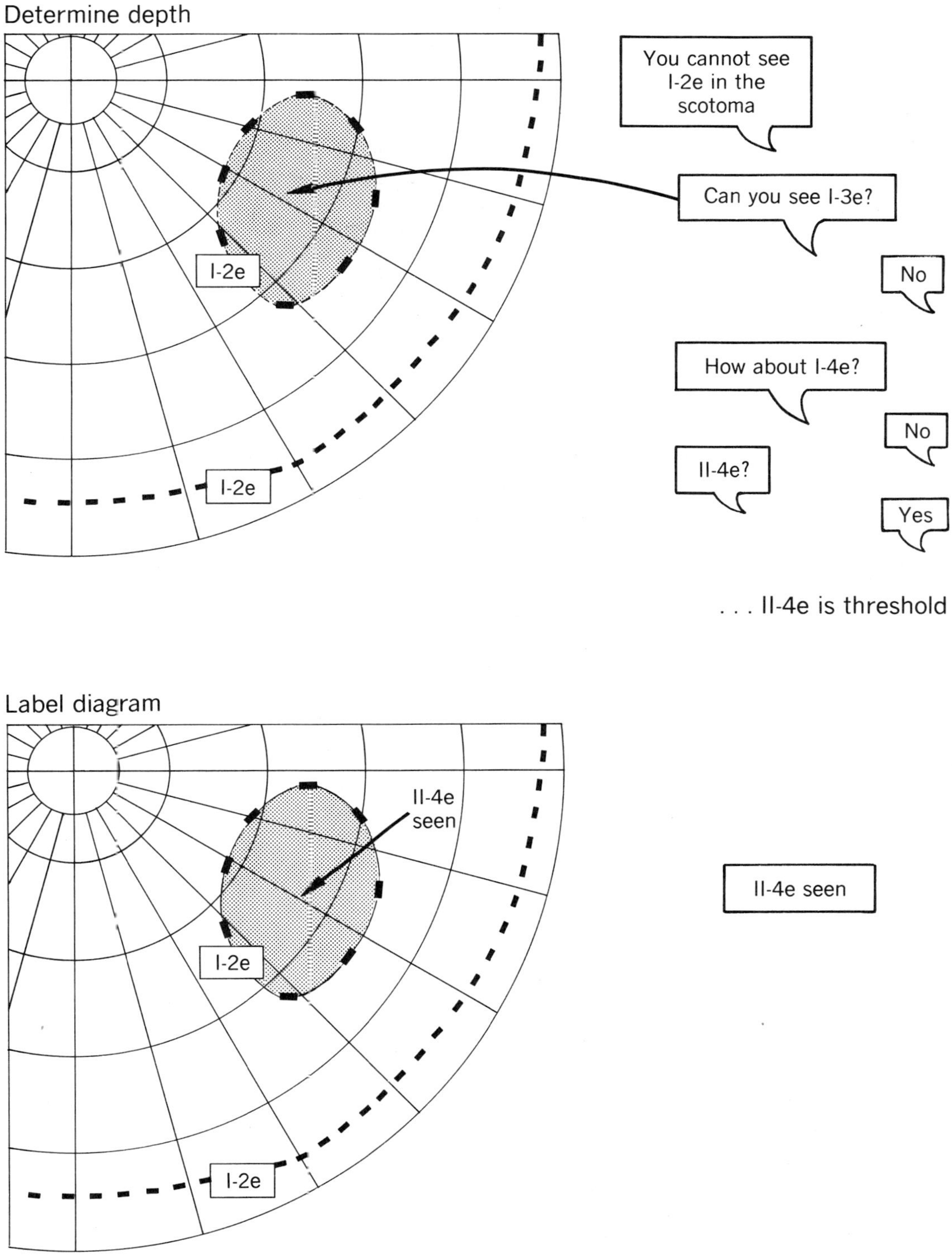
Determine depth
You cannot see I-2e in the scotoma
Can you see I-3e?
No
How about I-4e?
No
II-4e?
Yes
. . . II-4e is threshold
I-2e
I-2e
Label diagram
II-4e seen
II-4e seen
I-2e
I-2e

FIG. 19-3

Unless the scotoma is very shallow, you will determine its slope in kinetic perimetry by plotting the boundary with at least two isopters—one representing the weakest and one representing the strongest stimulus for which the scotoma is present. Usually the weakest has already been plotted because it is the boundary of the scotoma to the stimulus that was used in discovering the scotoma. The strongest is just a bit weaker than threshold. On occasion, you will find it appropriate to plot additional boundary lines for complex scotomas with regions of varying depth and slope.

FIG. 19-4. Determining the slope of the boundary. Note that in this example the *I-2e* isopter represents the boundary. Threshold of the center (depth) is *II-4e,* the weakest stimulus seen. The next weakest *(I-4e)*, which is the strongest stimulus not seen, is the second isopter plotted.
A, Sloping wall. The area enclosed by the *I-4e* boundary is smaller than that enclosed by *I-2e*.
B, Steep wall. The area enclosed by the *I-4e* boundary is almost as large as the area enclosed by *I-2e*.

To help identify the scotoma, shade in the nonseeing area enclosed by the boundary isopters. In this way you can distinguish isopters that form boundaries of the scotoma (pp. 88 and 96) from ordinary isopters.

Another way to quantify the depth and slope of scotomas is by static threshold perimetry, either as a *static cut* through the scotoma (p. 470) or using a *scatterplot* (p. 478).

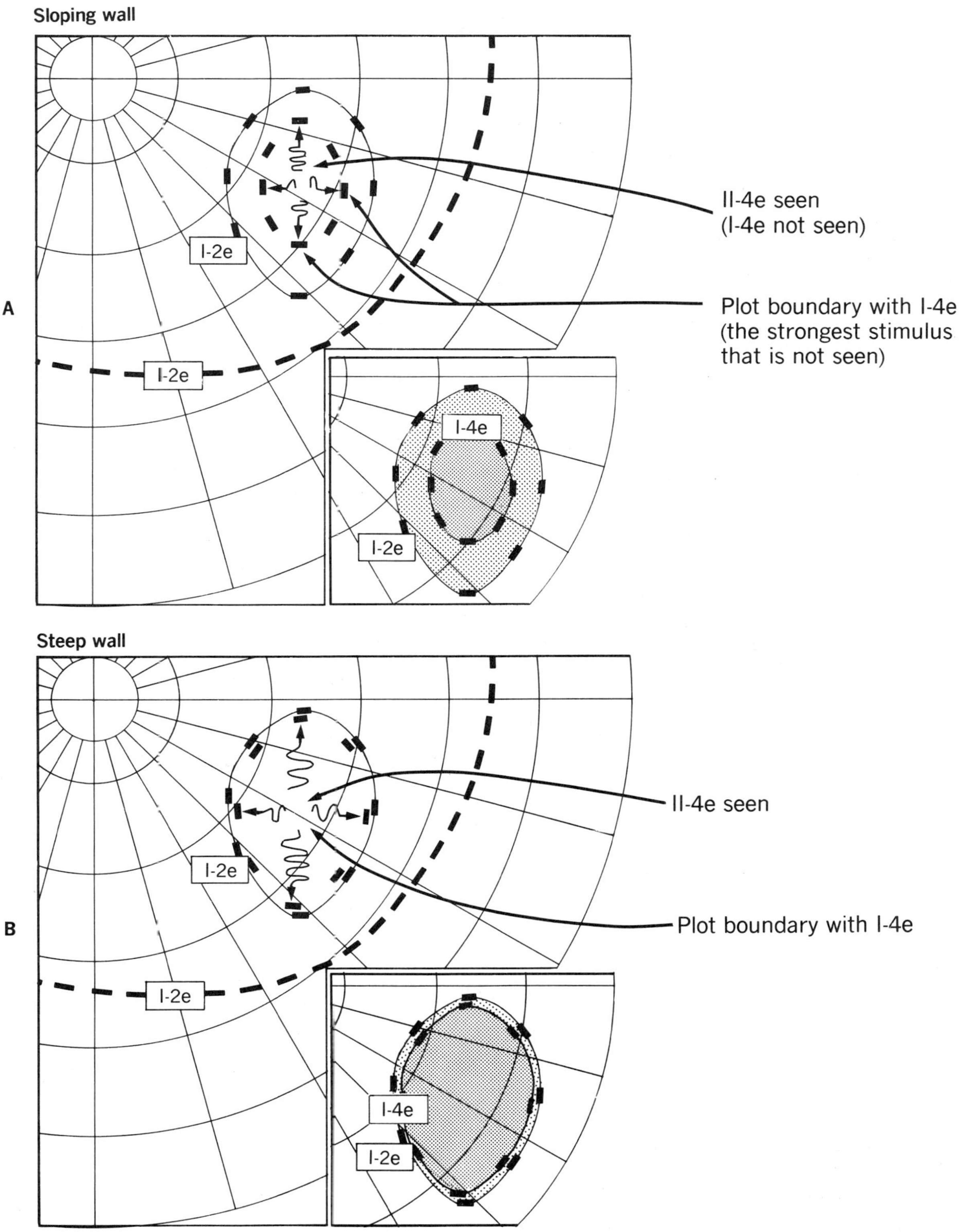
Sloping wall
A
I-2e
I-2e
I-4e
I-2e
II-4e seen
(I-4e not seen)
Plot boundary with I-4e
(the strongest stimulus
that is not seen)
Steep wall
B
I-2e
I-2e
I-4e
I-2e
II-4e seen
Plot boundary with I-4e

FIG. 19-4

CHAPTER 20

Quantifying depressions

STRATEGY

As discussed in Chapter 7, visual sensation can be reduced in an area without producing a scotoma. Such reduction is called a depression and is represented by an inward deviation of the isopter.

If while plotting an isopter you discover a localized depression, you must measure it quantitatively. As with scotomas, the basic rule is to measure the depth of depressed visual sensation in this location. To be specific, in discovering a depression along the isopter for I-2e, you are determining that I-2e is not seen in a certain location where it should be seen but now you must determine what *is* seen.

In any abnormal region, whether a scotoma or a depression, the question is not what is *not* seen but rather what *is* seen or what the visual threshold is.

FIG. 20-1. First step in quantifying a localized depression. Determine, first, what is seen. Plot the isopter for a stronger stimulus, in this case *I-3e,* which may show the boundary to be, **A,** normal, **B,** slightly depressed, or, **C,** markedly depressed inward.

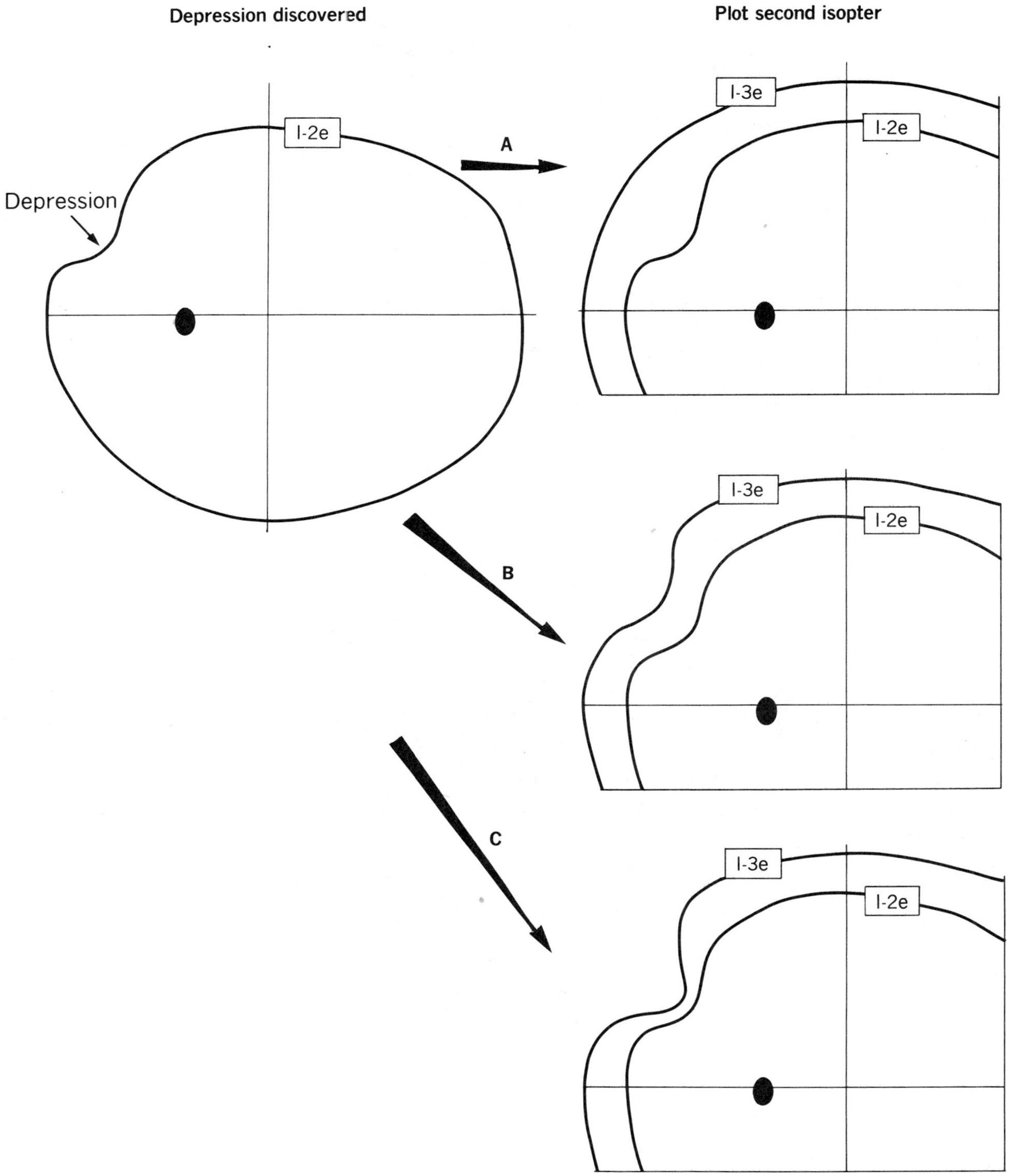
Depression discovered
Plot second isopter
Depression
I-2e
A
B
C
I-3e
I-2e
I-3e
I-2e
I-3e
I-2e

FIG. 20-1

FIG. 20-2. Subsequent steps in quantifying a localized depression.
A, If the newly plotted isopter for a stronger stimulus does not have an inward deviation, this is evidence of reduced visual sensation between the two isopters, specifically in the concavity of the inward deviation of the weaker isopter. With static spot-checking, you need to search this area with a stronger stimulus *(I-3e)*. You may or may not find a scotoma. If one is found, its depth and slope must, of course, be quantified in the same manner as described in Chapter 19.
B, If the second isopter *(I-3e)* shows an inward deviation of approximately the same degree as the initial one, you have discovered an area of reduced visual sensation in relation to that isopter and must now plot an even stronger isopter *(I-4e),* continuing to plot progressively stronger isopters until (1) an isopter shows no evidence of depressed visual sensation, (2) the extreme periphery of the visual field is reached, or (3) all the stronger stimuli available have been used. Then the spaces between each isopter can be explored for scotomas and if any are found they can be quantified.
C, If the newly plotted isopter is steeply deviated inward, you should plot in the same way isopters for consecutively stronger stimuli, searching the spaces between isopters for scotomas with the appropriate stimulus.

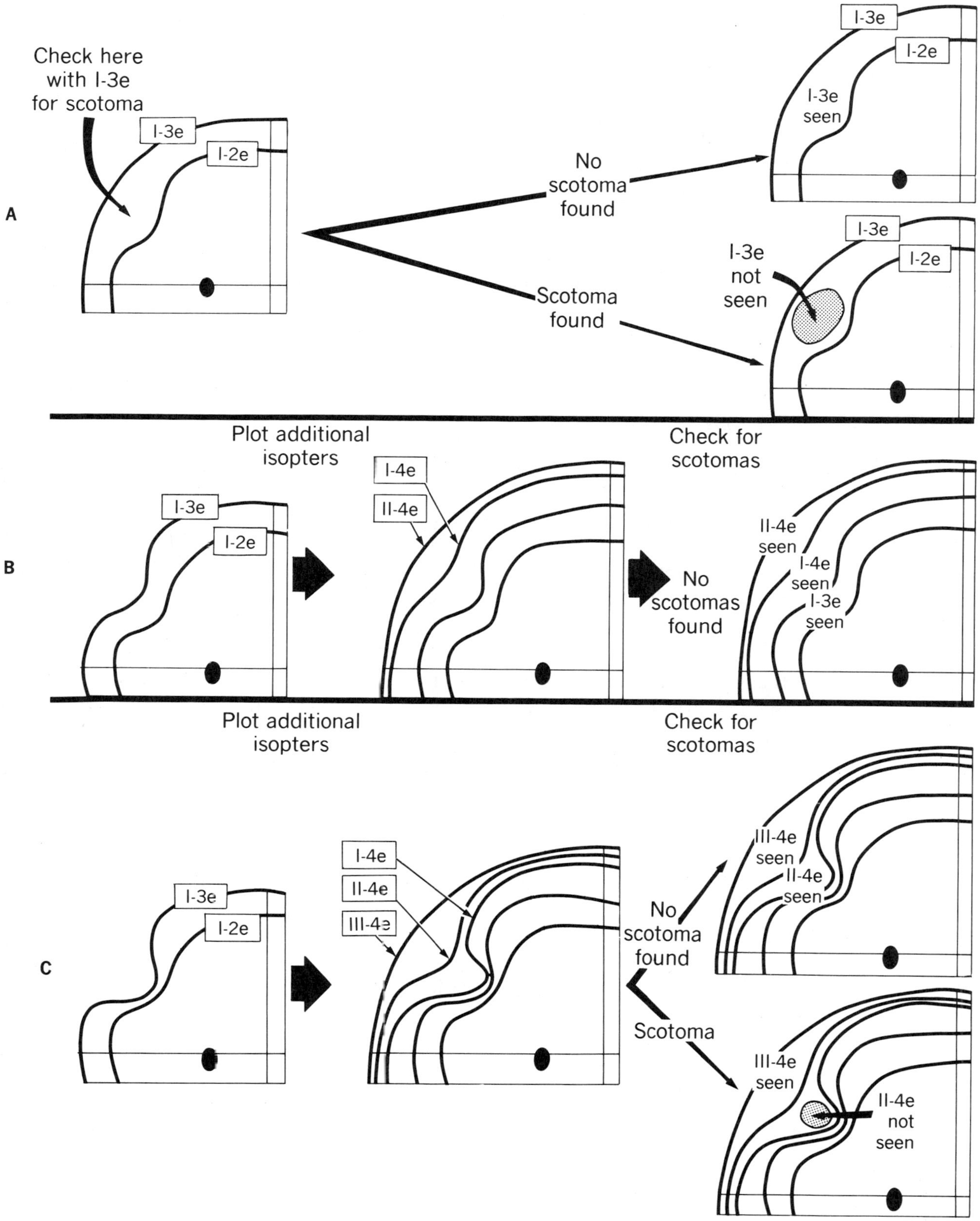
A
Check here with I-3e for scotoma
I-3e
I-2e
No scotoma found
Scotoma found
I-3e seen
I-3e not seen
B
Plot additional isopters
I-4e
II-4e
No scotomas found
Check for scotomas
II-4e seen
I-4e seen
I-3e seen
C
Plot additional isopters
III-4e
No scotoma found
Scotoma
Check for scotomas
III-4e seen
II-4e seen
II-4e not seen

FIG. 20-2

FIG. 20-3. Final step in quantifying a localized depression. It is also necessary to plot isopters for weaker stimuli inside the depressed area until one with a normal contour is found or else the center of the visual field is reached. In this example, *I-1e* and *0-1e* are plotted within the abnormal *I-2e*. Thus, when a depression is discovered, you have to plot isopters for both stronger and weaker stimuli.

Thus the principle of quantitative perimetry is to plot multiple isopters in the abnormal region to be quantified, checking for scotomas between isopters and quantifying any that are found. If none are found when spot-checking with a certain stimulus, e.g., I-4e, label the region "I-4e seen" or "O.K. to I-4e" (see also Fig. 18-12).

FIG. 20-4. Correctly labeled isopter plot of a localized depression. Within the depression, visual threshold is obvious at every location. Some of the isopters are plotted only in the depressed area, illustrating the principle that abnormal regions need to be quantified more carefully than normal regions.

GENERALIZED DEPRESSION

A generalized depression is characterized by an inward deviation of the isopter along its entire circumference (Chapter 8). To quantify the abnormality, follow the same principle as with localized depressions: plot isopters toward the periphery of the field until the outside boundary of the depression is reached, the extreme periphery of the field is reached, or the strongest available stimulus has been used without reaching the periphery. Then plot additional isopters toward fixation until a normal one is obtained or until the center of the field is reached. As the isopters are being plotted, spot-check the spaces between them for scotomas. If any are found, quantify their depth and slope. If none are found, mark the spot to show that the stimulus was seen, thereby indicating the approximate visual threshold in that region.

When plotting an abnormal field, be sure that all areas of the field are blanketed (Fig. 1-7) and fully quantified (Figs. 8-2, 13-65, 20-3, and 23-1).

Plot additional isopters

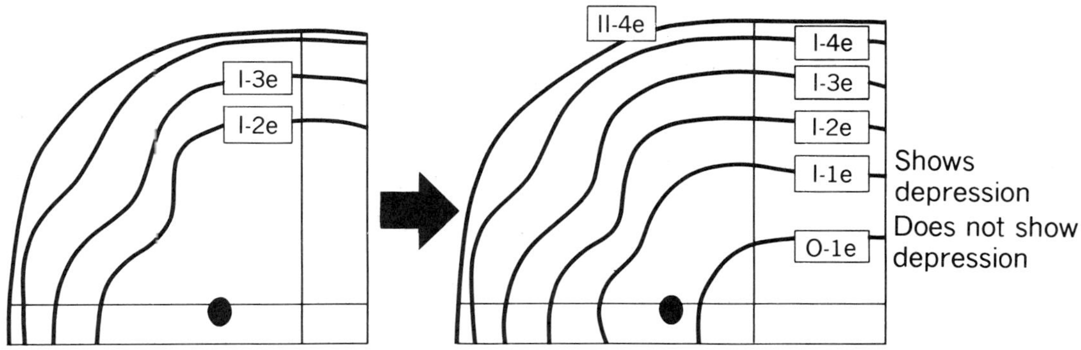

FIG. 20-3

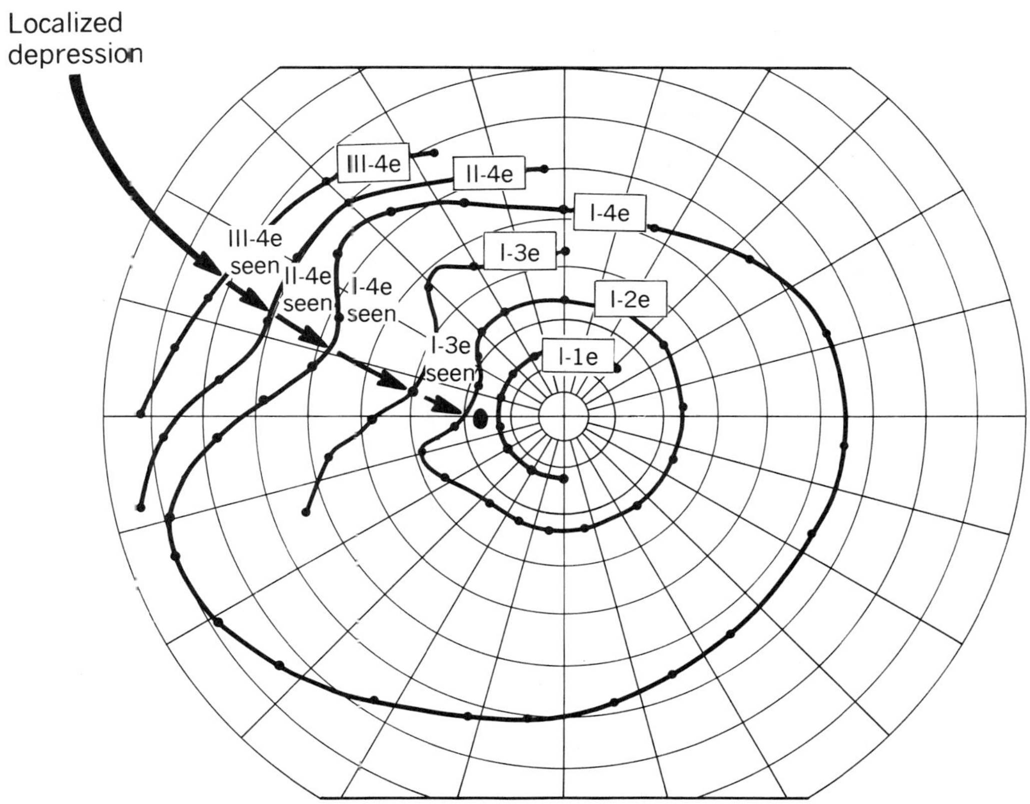

FIG. 20-4

CHAPTER 21

The basic glaucoma field examination

SCREENING

A screening examination is intended to determine whether or not a visual field defect is present. The technique must be sensitive (able to detect most of the defects present), specific (not too many false-positives), and not too time-consuming. In general, 10 minutes per eye should be the maximum spent in ruling out the presence of a defect. The 10-minute time limit for screening avoids fatigue to the patient and makes the test results, especially of the second eye, more reliable.

The trick to saving time while retaining sensitivity in screening for abnormalities is to concentrate your effort on the regions where the abnormalities are most likely to be. For this reason it is always necessary to know why the field examination is being performed (e.g., suspected glaucoma or brain tumor) and to concentrate on the region where field defects first appear in the condition suspected. It is therefore necessary to know both where the defects are likely to occur and how best to detect them.

FIG. 21-1. Visual field defects in glaucoma. The earliest visual field defects will almost always be found in the central region (paracentral scotoma, arcuate scotoma, nasal step) or in the nasal periphery (depression producing a nasal step). If there are no abnormalities in these regions (outlined in red), you are not likely to find any elsewhere.

For glaucoma you can examine carefully the central area and the nasal horizontal meridian, which are the regions most likely to be affected (Chapter 10). If no abnormalities are found, you will probably not find any in the broad crescent above, below, and temporal to the central 30 degrees. The area needing special attention is only about one fourth of the total visual field.

There are a number of strategies to use in exploring the field for glaucomatous abnormalities. The next several pages show one of these techniques, which should be mastered completely before learning the several others (discussed in Chapter 22). In the method described here, the central field is tested first and then the peripheral field. Some clinics reverse the sequence, however.

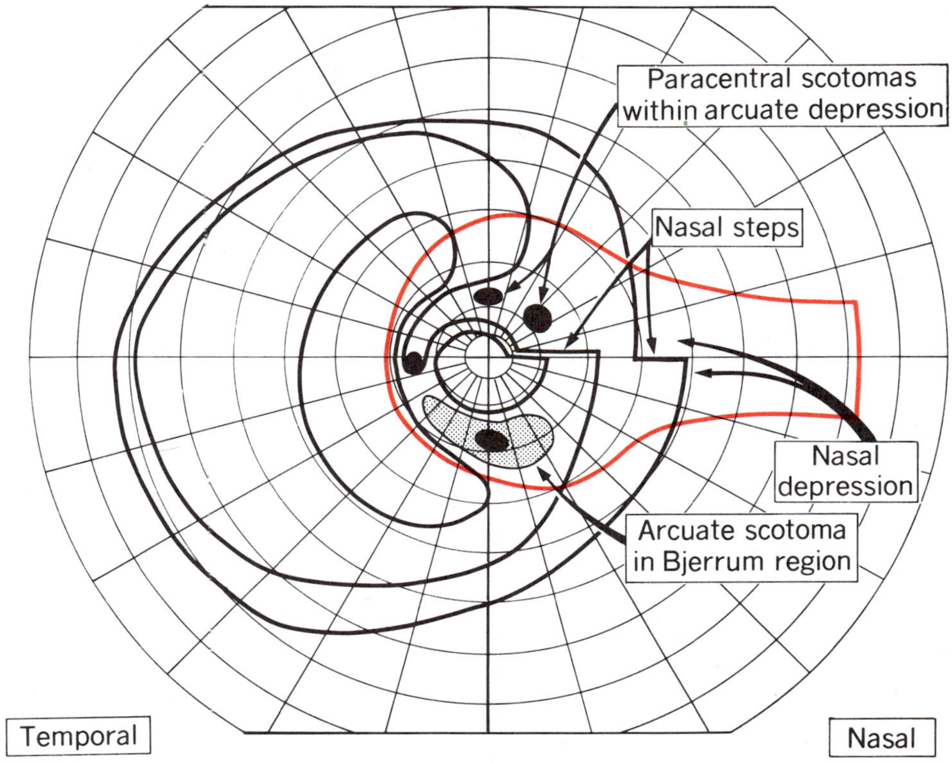
Paracentral scotomas
within arcuate depression
Nasal steps
Nasal
depression
Arcuate scotoma
in Bjerrum region
Temporal
Nasal

FIG. 21-1

Central field

After selecting the appropriate corrective lenses (Chapter 12), you may begin by educating the patient and plotting the physiologic blind spot with the I-4e stimulus. At the same time, you should determine which test stimulus will form an isopter that encloses most of the central 20 to 30 degrees of the field, including the physiologic blind spot. If the choice of stimulus is not obvious, determine threshold at 20 to 25 degrees temporal to fixation, just above and below the horizontal meridian, and just outside the location of the physiologic blind spot.

FIG. 21-2. Two methods for determining threshold at 20 to 25 degrees.
A, Static perimetry. Position the stimulus as shown and increase it until it first becomes visible.
B, Kinetic perimetry. Bring several stimuli in from the periphery so you can determine which one forms an isopter at 25 to 30 degrees.

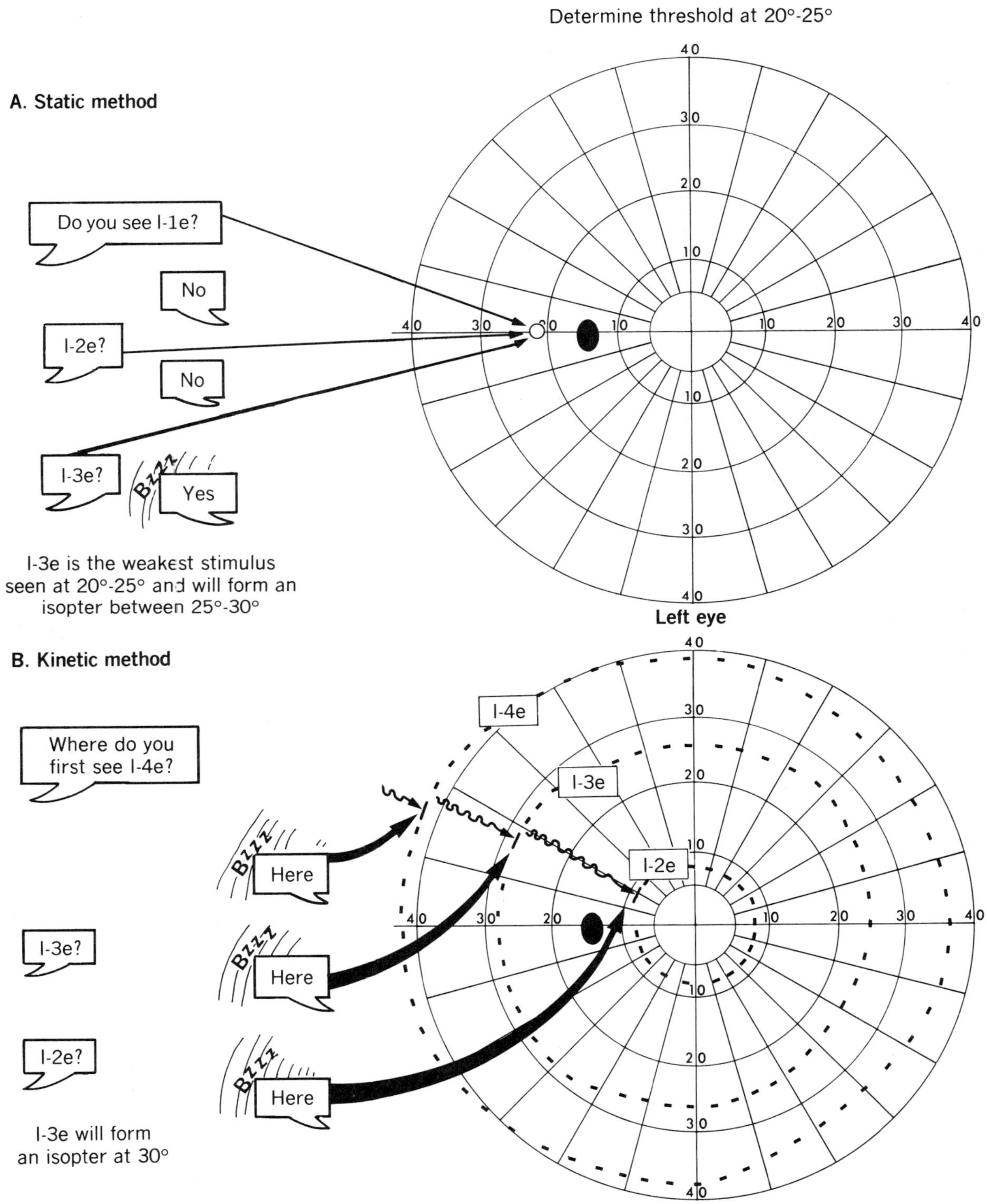
A. Static method
Determine threshold at 20°-25°
Do you see I-1e?
No
I-2e?
No
I-3e?
Bzzz
Yes
I-3e is the weakest stimulus seen at 20°-25° and will form an isopter between 25°-30°
Left eye
B. Kinetic method
Where do you first see I-4e?
Here
I-3e?
Here
I-2e?
Here
I-4e
I-3e
I-2e
I-3e will form an isopter at 30°
10
20
30
40

FIG. 21-2

Plot an isopter with the selected stimulus, paying particular attention to the area just above and below the horizontal meridian on the nasal side to look for a nasal step.

FIG. 21-3. Plotting an isopter with the selected stimulus.

With that same stimulus, explore the entire area within the isopter for scotomas by presenting the stimulus at 75 to 100 locations.

FIG. 21-4. Exploring for scotomas. The exploration for scotomas by suprathreshold static spot-checking concentrates on the two arcuate (Bjerrum) regions, indicated in red. It is the single most important step in glaucoma defect detection.

Testing of many points is necessary because early scotomas may be quite small and they will not be found if the spots tested are too widely distributed. The area explored should include the entire inner 20 degrees of the visual field and also 20 to 30 degrees on the nasal side. Be sure to test in the region just above and below the physiologic blind spot. Some offices and clinics use a regimented plan in which there are 4 spots tested inside 5 degrees, and then 72 spots where the 5-, 10-, and 15-degree circles cross the 24 meridians, for a total of 76 spots (Chapter 22). It is wise also to test at 20 degrees and 25 degrees nasally. Thus, 76 spots are an absolute minimum and perhaps 100 spots should be the average number checked.

It is important that the stimulus appear and disappear in each location, with the patient responding each time that it appears. This is easily accomplished with the projection perimeter but can also be performed at the tangent screen. Scotomas will be missed if you make the mistake of leaving the stimulus on continuously, moving it around, and asking the patient to tell you when it disappears.

Present the stimulus in a somewhat irregular rhythm to make sure that the patient is actually responding to it and not simply sounding the buzzer rhythmically at 1-second intervals. If the patient does not respond to a stimulus in a certain location, retest that location. Occasionally a stimulus will be missed even by a person with a normal visual field. However, areas where the response is inconsistent or slower than elsewhere must be explored with extra care because these may indicate a shallow scotoma. Further details will be given later on the technique of static spot-checking and how to deal with inconsistent responses (Chapter 24).

After completing this step, label the field chart to indicate that this stimulus was seen everywhere inside the isopter.

Plot the isopter

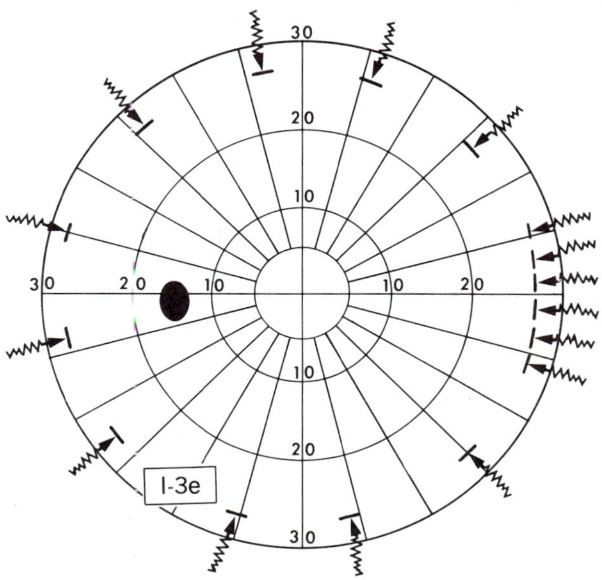

Plot carefully on nasal side especially

FIG. 21-3

Check for scotomas

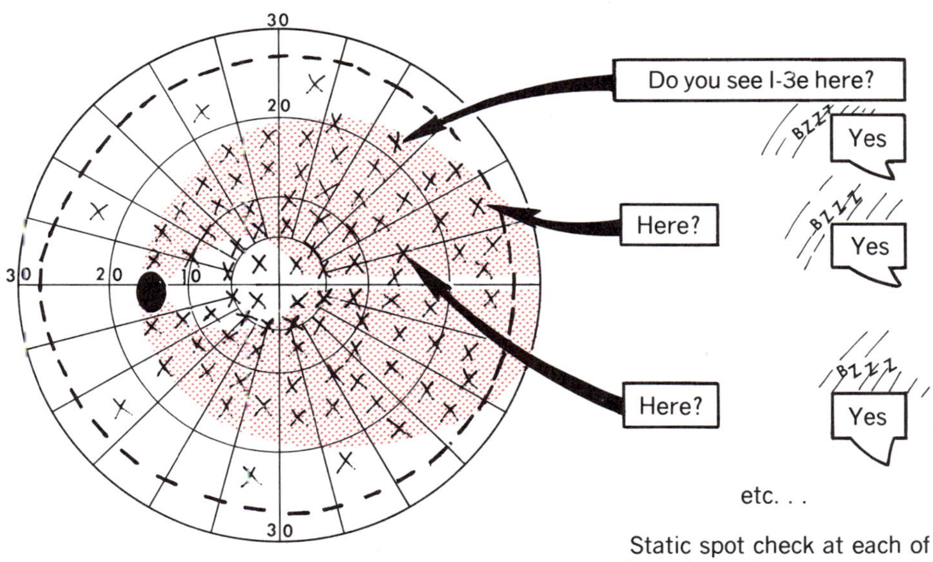

Static spot check at each of 75-100 locations covering the entire central field inside the isopter

FIG. 21-4

It may happen that a single stimulus is not sufficient for exploring the area inside 30 degrees. Suppose that there is a significant area inside 30 degrees that does not lie within the isopter plotted in the previous step, e.g., if the isopter extends to 25 degrees temporally and surrounds the blind spot but only to 10 to 15 degrees superiorly and nasally. In that case you cannot explore the area outside 15 degrees superiorly and nasally for scotomas with this stimulus because only the area inside the isopter can be tested. Therefore you will plot the next larger isopter to surround the area within 30 degrees that has not been explored. This isopter, however, is used only in sectors where the weaker stimulus was not usable. The idea is to explore the entire central 25 degrees for scotomas and not leave any regions unexplored.

FIG. 21-5. Use of two stimuli to test the central 25 degrees.

Testing for paracentral scotomas is the single most important component of screening for glaucomatous defects, and the two key principles are (1) selecting the correct test stimulus and (2) exploring the entire central area that might be involved in glaucoma with a sufficient number of test points.

FIG. 21-6. Scotoma for the I-3e isopter, which encloses the inner 35 degrees. This would not have been detected if you had (incorrectly) chosen the *I-4e* test stimulus, whose isopter is at about 45 degrees, to look for scotomas.

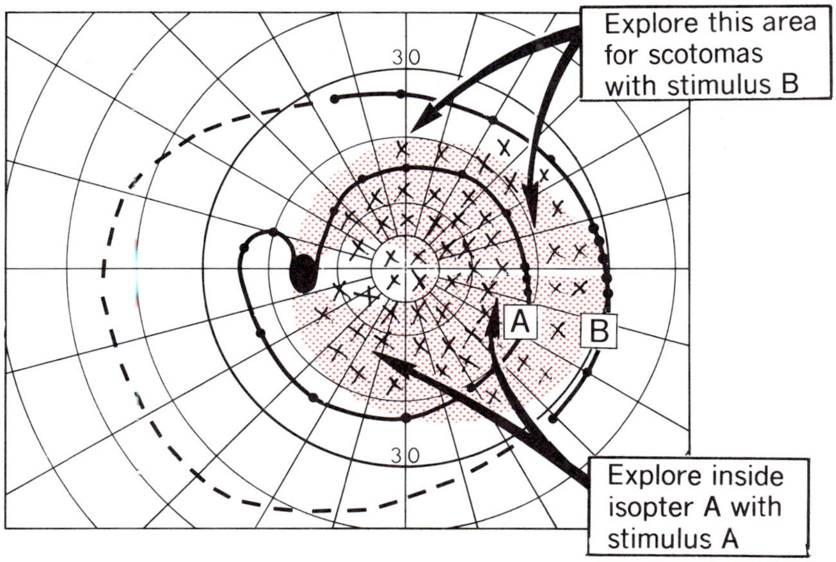

FIG. 21-5

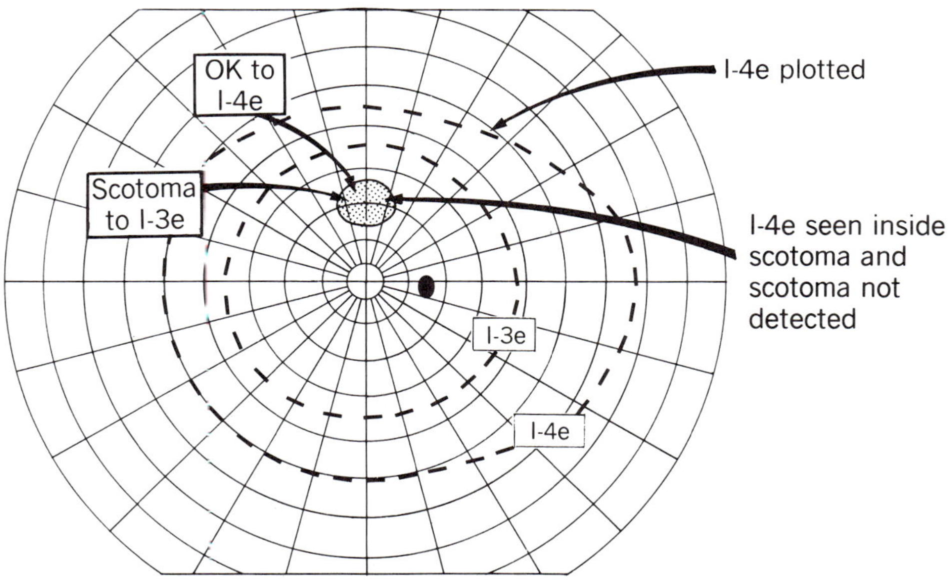

FIG. 21-6

It is possible that some scotomas will be missed even when the correct stimulus is used.

FIG. 21-7, A. Shallow scotoma near fixation. The *I-2e* isopter encloses 15 degrees, and the *I-3e* isopter 25 degrees. There may be a scotoma at 5 degrees where the *I-2e* isopter is not seen but the *I-3e* isopter is still visible. Such an early scotoma would have been missed with the method described here, in which the *I-3e* stimulus is used because it is threshold at 25 degrees. However, you would have missed only the early very shallow scotomas, not the more established deeper ones.

In the usual screening setting, although some small or shallow scotomas may be missed, the larger deeper ones will not. Sometimes it is acceptable to miss small shallow scotomas, as long as the more important ones are detected. However, at other times (e.g., in the presence of considerable elevation of the IOP or clear evidence of damage to the optic disc) there may be extra reason to test more thoroughly. For example, it is possible to select a stimulus and plot an isopter at 10 to 20 degrees, to explore within this isopter for scotomas, and then to plot a second isopter between 20 and 30 degrees. The space between the two isopters may be searched with this second stimulus. The extra time needed with the additional step is related to the plotting of the second isopter. The number of spots checked for scotomas is exactly the same, but half the locations are tested with one stimulus and half with another.

FIG. 21-7, B. Strategy to avoid missing a shallow scotoma.

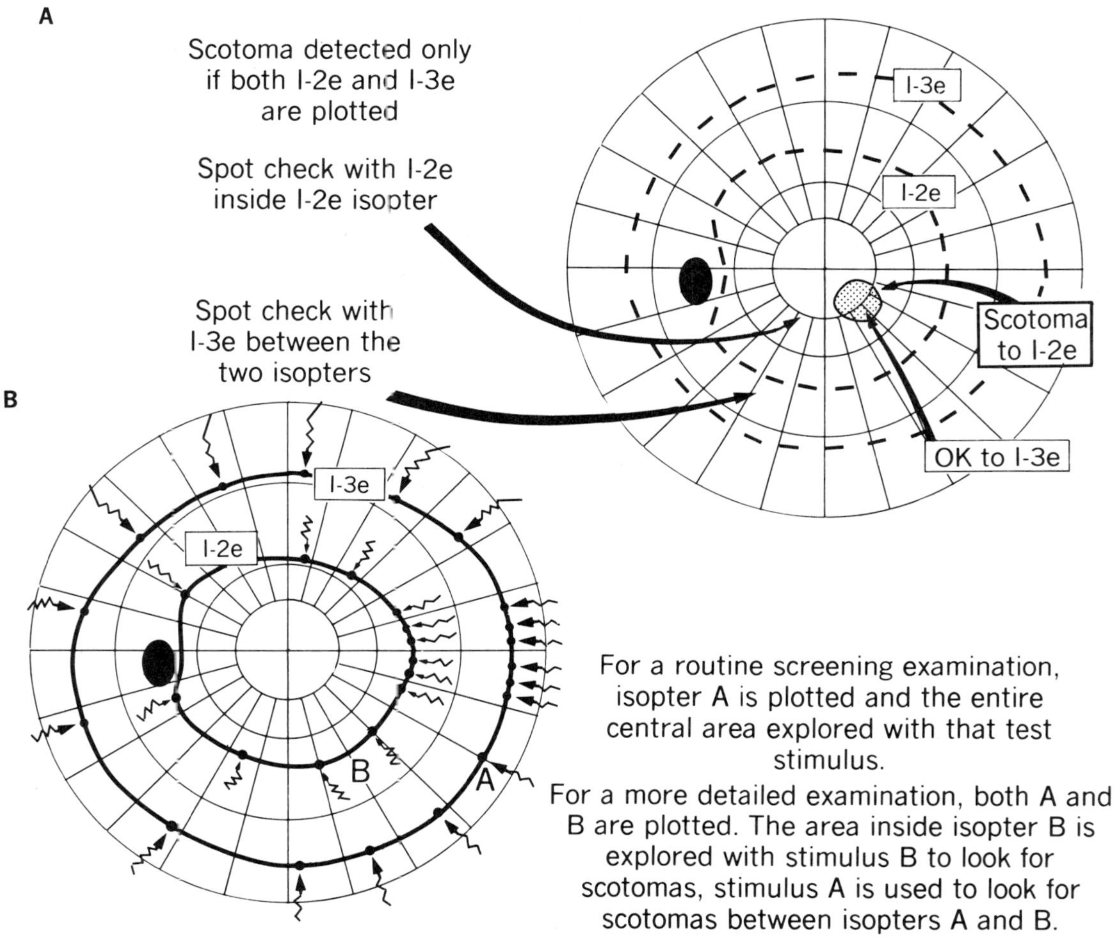
A
Scotoma detected only if both I-2e and I-3e are plotted
Spot check with I-2e inside I-2e isopter
Spot check with I-3e between the two isopters
I-3e
I-2e
Scotoma to I-2e
OK to I-3e
B
I-3e
I-2e
B
A
For a routine screening examination, isopter A is plotted and the entire central area explored with that test stimulus.
For a more detailed examination, both A and B are plotted. The area inside isopter B is explored with stimulus B to look for scotomas, stimulus A is used to look for scotomas between isopters A and B.

FIG. 21-7

Peripheral field

After exploring the central 25 degrees for scotomas, remove the corrective lens (unless it is a contact lens, in which case it should be left in) and search the nasal side of the field for a depression or nasal steps. The manner of plotting the isopters is important. Depression of light sensitivity is detected simply by determining inward deviation of the isopters. When depression occurs nasally in glaucoma, it is typically unequal above and below by 5 to 10 degrees or more, producing a nasal step where the isopters cross the horizontal meridian. To detect a nasal step, plot three or four points just above and three or four just below the horizontal meridian nasally. This applies to all isopters, including the first one that was plotted in preparation for exploring the central field.

FIG. 21-8. Testing for a nasal depression or steps.
A, Plot an additional isopter with a stimulus stronger than the one used to look for paracentral scotomas. It is not necessary to explore the entire isopter, because the main interest is in the nasal field. Instead, plot the isopter for each stimulus only just above and just below the horizontal meridian nasally to look for nasal steps. It is important that three to four points be plotted close together just above the horizontal meridian and three to four just below the meridian.
B, Use successively stronger stimuli at intervals of 0.5 log-unit or equivalent (e.g., *I-3e, I-4e, II-4e* or *I-2b, I-3b, I-4b*) to plot across the horizontal nasal meridian at about 10-degree intervals, beginning with the isopter used to explore the central field. As progressively stronger stimuli are used, each isopter will be farther out than the previous one until the absolute nasal periphery of the visual field is reached (i.e., until a stronger stimulus does not increase the size of the field).
C, Now you have explored the keyhole-shaped area in which most glaucomatous defects are found (Fig. 21-1).

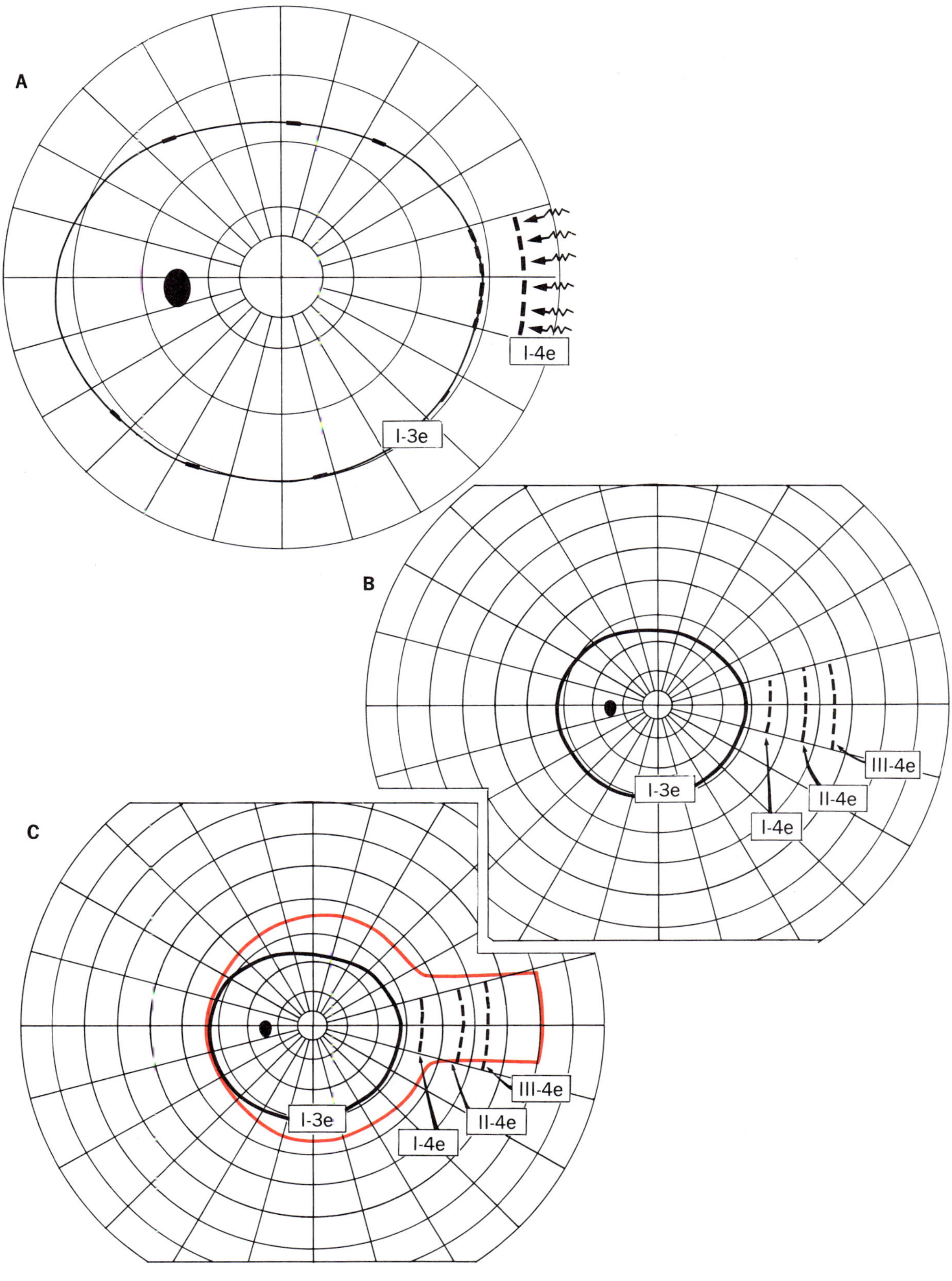

FIG. 21-8

When the periphery is reached, plot the weakest stimulus that is visible at or just within the absolute periphery all the way around. This will usually be the stimulus that forms an isopter at or barely outside 50 degrees. When mapping this isopter, you should plot a sufficient number of points to pick up a wedge-shaped depression that sometimes occurs in the temporal field.

FIG. 21-9. The peripheral isopter.
A, In plots of progressively stronger stimuli, note that *IV-4e* coincides with the previously plotted *III-4e*.
B, Therefore you would choose the *III-4e* to plot the peripheral isopter because it is the weakest stimulus at or just inside the absolute nasal periphery.

If you strongly suspect the existence of a scotoma, you may explore inside each isopter although this is not part of the standard screening procedure. In addition, you may explore the temporal field by plotting the isopters all the way around and checking for scotomas. Of course, you will always be very suspicious of any irregularity in the contour of the isopters or of any area where the patient's responses are somewhat slow or inconsistent and you will explore these with careful plotting of additional isopters searching for scotomas.

Remember: The reason for plotting the *weakest* stimulus at the periphery is that a strong stimulus might be visible in a relatively peripheral defect, whose presence would be missed thereby. (Consider what would happen if only the *III-4e* isopter were plotted in Fig. 20-4.)

A

B

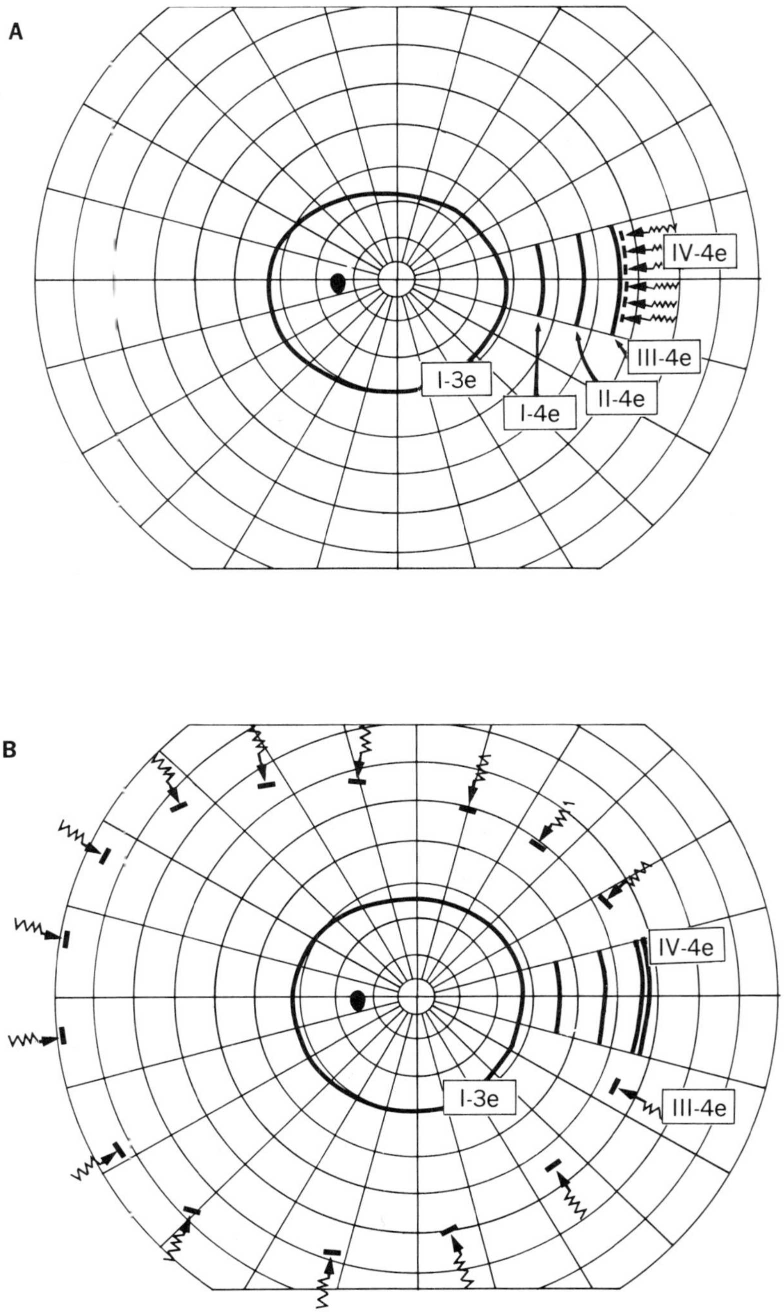

FIG. 21-9

QUANTIFYING AN ABNORMAL FIELD

If abnormalities are discovered, they must be quantified (by means of the methods outlined in Chapters 19 and 20). The 10-minute limit for screening is lifted. On encountering an abnormality during a screening examination, you will, of course, plot its boundary and quantify its depth and slope before proceeding to screen the remaining areas for other defects. Thus the technique becomes both a screening for defects and an assessment of any that are found.

FIG. 21-10. Quantifying a scotoma.
A, When a scotoma is discovered, you first will determine its extent and depth.
B, Plot the boundary of the scotoma kinetically with the stimulus used to discover it by moving the stimulus from the center outward and having the patient report when it becomes visible.
C, Quantify the scotoma's depth. Threshold can be determined at the center by testing with progressively stronger stimuli until one becomes visible.
D, With the strongest test stimulus that is still invisible, again plot the boundary to determine its slope. The boundary may be the same as it was with the weaker stimulus, or it may be smaller.

Quantifying a scotoma

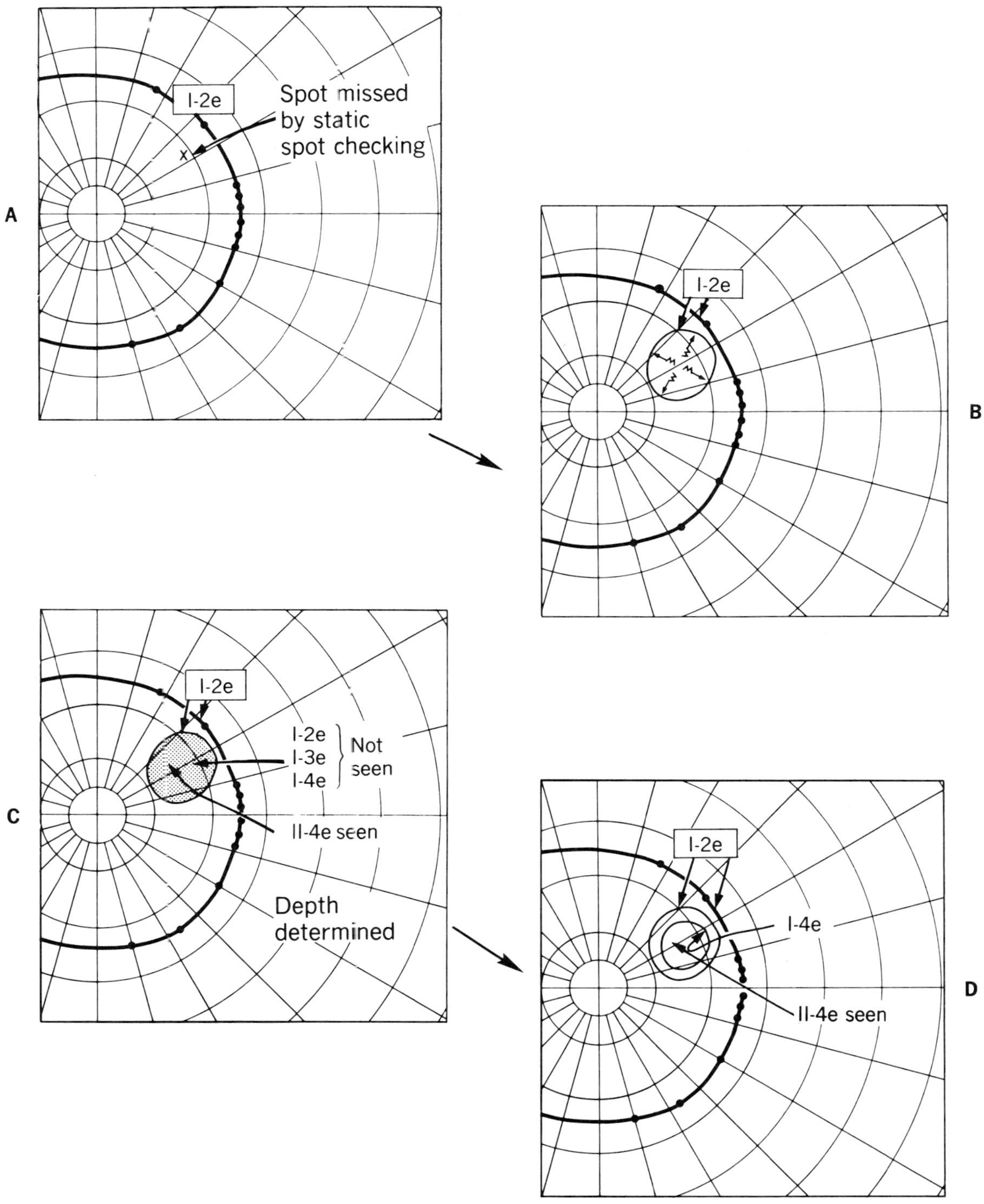

FIG. 21-10

FIG. 21-11. Quantifying a nasal step. When a nasal step is discovered, you can confirm its presence by moving the stimulus across the horizontal meridian and noting that it becomes visible at the horizontal meridian as it passes from a position outside to a position within the isopter. (The step may not be *exactly* at the horizontal meridian.) Then, because a nasal step represents a depression, you will quantify it just like any depression (Chapter 20). Plot additional isopters inward toward fixation and outward toward the periphery to see how far the abnormal region extends. Where the isopters separate because only one has a nasal step, this may be a scotoma.

When a depression is discovered on the temporal side (a wedge-shaped deviation of the isopter), this depression must also be quantified. (The quantitation of temporal wedge defects is illustrated in Fig. 20-4.) Plot isopters for stronger stimuli in 0.5 log-unit steps through the involved region until the absolute boundary is reached or until the strongest available stimulus has been plotted. Also plot the isopters for weaker stimuli in 0.5 log-unit steps until the inner boundary of the depression or the physiologic blind spot is reached.

The screening examination concentrates on the most likely areas for the occurrence of the *first*, or earliest, visual field defect in glaucoma (e.g., paracentral scotomas, nasal steps, peripheral depression). Other regions are left unexplored in a screening examination because they are unlikely places for the first defect to occur. However, these areas can have defects later and **as soon as the examination discloses defects in the most likely areas it becomes necessary also to look in all other regions of the field.** This means plotting isopters in 0.5 log-unit steps, or approximately every 15 to 20 degrees in the entire peripheral field and every 10 to 15 degrees in the central field, and checking for scotomas between the isopters.

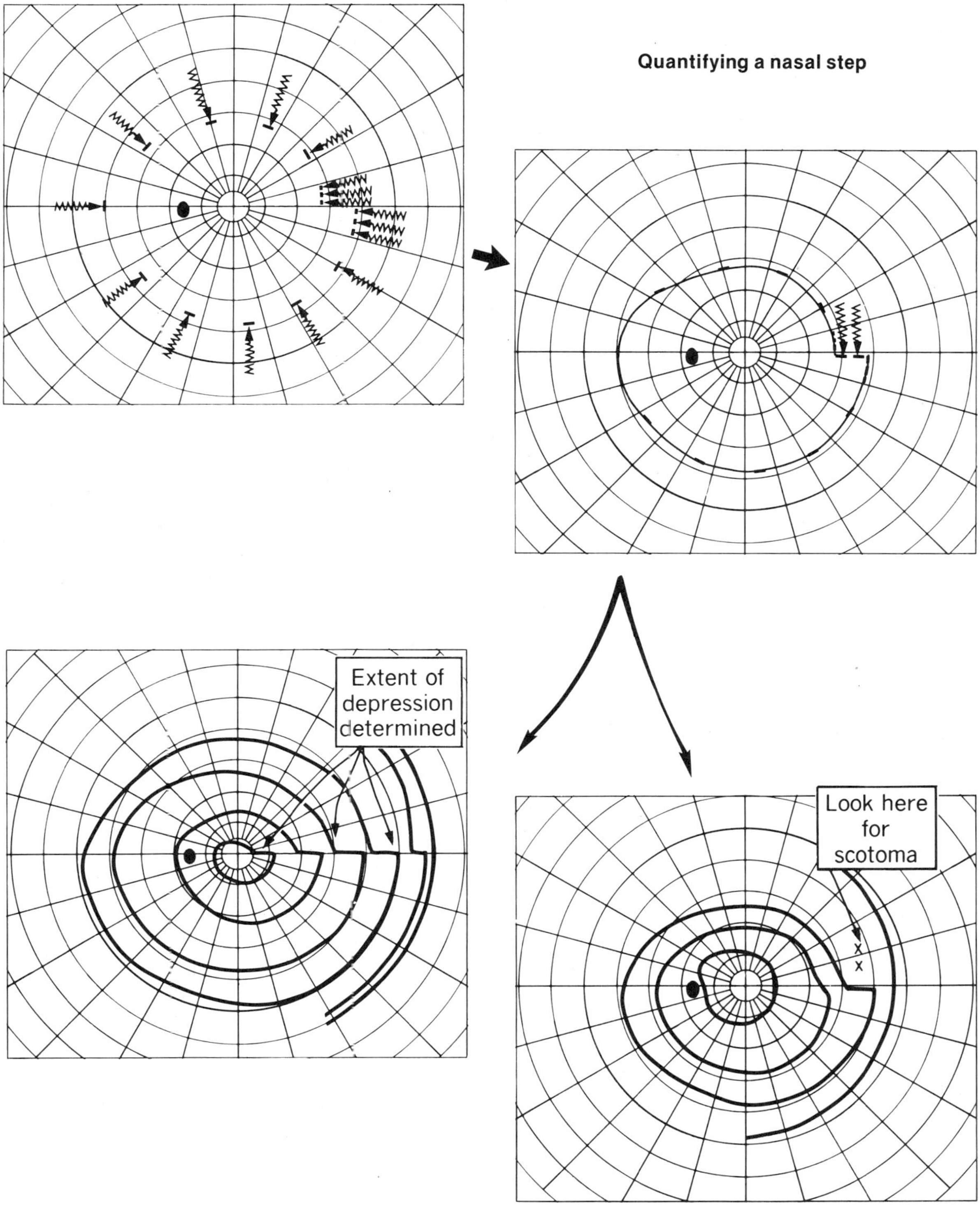
Quantifying a nasal step
Extent of depression determined
Look here for scotoma

FIG. 21-11

TANGENT SCREEN FOR GLAUCOMA

The same method of kinetic plotting of isopters and suprathreshold static spot-checking can be used at the tangent screen. A difference would be that the tangent screen is employed only to test the central field. Fewer than 10% of patients with an abnormal field will have defects *only* in the periphery, however, so if the central field is absolutely normal you can be more than 90% certain that there will be no defects in the peripheral field either. Moreover, the central field certainly will be involved by the time the visual loss has become functionally significant. Thus, the central field is the most important part of the glaucoma field examination.

If the tangent screen is to be used, the basic principles of target selection and spot-checking many spots will be followed. Plot the isopter for the smallest test object that is visible at 25 to 30 degrees and spot-check many places statically. The static spot-checking is done by turning the wand as illustrated in Chapter 13. Quantify any scotomas by plotting their boundary and determining their depth (how large the object must be to become visible) and slope. Frequently overlooked with the tangent screen is the need to plot several isopters in abnormal regions to quantify the depression fully, whether localized (nasal steps) or generalized. For example, if isopters become constricted in one examination compared to a previous examination, you may have to plot with progressively larger stimuli until the edge of the tangent screen is reached.

CHAPTER 22

More about testing for glaucoma

In Chapter 21 an approach to the visual field is described that includes screening, diagnosis, and quantitation for glaucoma all at one time. This approach certainly applies to the usual clinical setting, where the diagnostic screening examination is performed with patients who already have some sign of glaucoma, e.g., an elevated IOP or an abnormality of the optic disc. In such a setting the likelihood that a defect will be present is greater than in an unselected group of people, and a careful method requiring moderate expenditure of time is warranted. Moreover, if a defect is found, it needs to be described quantitatively, since the progress of the glaucoma patient must be checked at intervals to judge the adequacy of the treatment. It makes sense to use a strategy and an instrument that will allow for a quantitated examination as soon as a defect is discovered.

The technique presented in Chapter 21 is basic and good and, for several reasons, should be mastered by everyone who performs visual field examinations.

First, in the usual clinical practice in which glaucoma patients abound, it is the most frequent examination performed. *Second,* with slight modification (e.g., checking for steps along the vertical meridian or checking for brightness differences across the vertical meridian) it can be used for field defects other than glaucoma. Even without modifying the method, you may be able to recognize when some type of defect other than glaucoma is present. The major problems with using this technique for nonglaucomatous defects are that

1. It is inefficient when there is no need to examine as many regions of the field or to be quite so quantitative.
2. Some important defects, especially central scotomas, will escape detection because the strategy is not directed toward these defects.

A *third* reason why the glaucoma technique in Chapter 21 is a good basic one is that for general use it represents a suitable compromise between accuracy and efficient use of time. It is fairly rapid, as long as no field efects that need quantitation are present, and hence it serves as a good screening test.

In this chapter are described the original Armaly method to screen for glaucoma, the modifications by Drance, and other variations of field examinations for glaucoma.

BASIC ARMALY-DRANCE TECHNIQUE

Armaly described the basic method of suprathreshold static spot-checking to detect scotomas, and he simplified it to a rapid technique for use in his scientific study of glaucoma in the general population. He called his method "selective perimetry." Drance studied the accuracy of the technique and made certain modifications. Both Armaly and Drance have, through the years, used several variations; but the basic nature of the technique, as it has evolved, includes the steps described in the ensuing pages.

Static spot-checking

Static spot-checking is the single most important component of the glaucoma screen. The first step is to select the stimulus for spot-checking.

The stimulus can be simply a standard one, e.g., 1w/1000 at the tangent screen or I-2e on the Goldmann perimeter or it can be 2w/1000 or I-3e if the weaker stimulus forms an isopter smaller than 20 degrees. However, it is better to determine the approximate visual threshold at 25 degrees and use that stimulus.

FIG. 22-1. Stimulus selection. Determine the visual threshold at four locations where the horizontal and vertical meridians cross the 25-degree circle. Traditionally for this you will use (in 0.5 log-unit steps) the I-1e, I-2e, I-3e, I-4e, and II-4e. More often the selected stimulus will be I-2e, less often I-3e, etc. Therefore choosing a target usually is a matter of determining that *I-1e* is not seen and *I-2e* is. A more compulsive and more time-consuming method would be to determine threshold to the nearest 0.1 or 0.2 log-unit.

Practice varies with regard to using (1) the strongest of the four threshold stimuli, which is the weakest that can be seen in *all* four locations, (2) the weakest of the four threshold stimuli, which is the weakest that can be seen at *any* of the four locations, or (3) the threshold at 25 degrees temporally (near the blind spot), which would ignore the other three locations. The easiest, and perhaps the best overall, is simply to use the stimulus that is threshold at 25 degrees temporally, without bothering to determine the threshold at the other three points.

There is no "best" way for choosing the stimulus. It all depends on the clinical setting. The weaker stimulus, seen only at one of the four locations, has the advantage that it will allow detection of shallow scotomas. However, it will be barely visible even in normal regions of the field. Therefore the patient may miss seeing it once in a while, falsely giving the impression that there is a scotoma.

For example, with a certain weak stimulus you might find that 5% of those screened falsely appeared to have a scotoma but the field turned out to be normal on more careful examination. This 5% false-positive rate could cause a problem when screening a group of people in a retirement center where only one in 200 might have glaucoma. The weak stimulus that yielded 5% incorrect diagnoses would yield 10 false diagnoses in 200 people along with one correct diagnosis. This might be acceptable if you had the time and facilities to perform a more detailed ocular examination, including a thorough field examination, to sort out the 10 false-positives (normals) from the one true-positive (glaucoma). Usually, however, in such a setting you would rather use a slightly stronger stimulus to get fewer false-positives—knowing that some shallow defects might not be detected, but also that the defects *not* detected would be milder and not of as much consequence as the deeper defects that *were* detected.

The situation would be different among a group of patients with other signs of glaucoma, perhaps 20% or more of whom really did have a field defect. The proportion of 20 true-positives (those with a defect) to 5 false-positives (normal people who just *seem* to have a defect) when a weak stimulus was used would be acceptably high. Moreover, the extra effort to sort out the true-positives from the false-positives would be worthwhile in this group, which overall would be at greater risk than the general population of developing glaucoma and in whom you would be anxious not to miss detecting a shallow defect.

See Chapter 13 for further discussion of this problem.

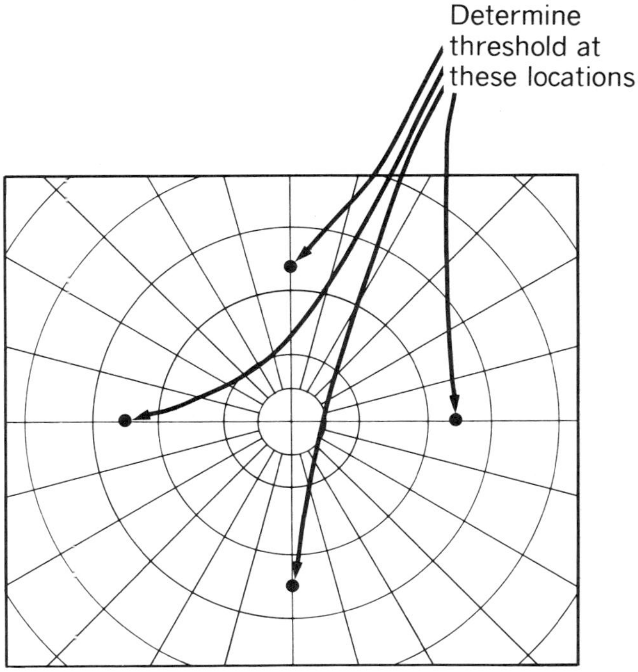

FIG. 22-1

Once the stimulus is selected, static spot-checking is performed at 76 locations (every 15 degrees along the circles 5, 10, and 15 degrees from fixation where the circles intersect the meridians, and at four locations inside the 5-degree circle).

FIG. 22-2. Static spot-checking at 76 points. The standard technique when testing manually is a 1-second presentation of a selected stimulus once, and only once, at each location in an orderly sequence—e.g., around the 5-degree circle, then around the 10-degree circle, then around the 15-degree circle. Some automated methods will present the stimulus in a random sequence but still only once at each location. Be sure to mark the location of each missed point.

If four or more adjacent points are missed, an arcuate scotoma is likely present and the field is likely abnormal. If the only purpose is to determine whether or not a field defect probably exists, the screening test can be terminated as soon as a definite defect is detected. You can then do a more thorough diagnostic test later. Or you may proceed immediately to plot isopters and quantitative defects as outlined in Chapter 21.

If fewer than four adjacent spots are missed, be sure to check any missed points a second time with the same stimulus (p. 46). A paracentral scotoma is probably present at any spots where, on the second presentation, the stimulus is again not seen; but you may ignore any spots where the stimulus is seen on the second presentation. (In some clinics, points that were missed only on the first presentation are considered significant if several are clustered together.) Any time the criteria show that the field is probably abnormal, you can terminate the screening examination and defer the quantitative examination for another occasion; or you may proceed immediately to determine the depth of the scotoma and outline its boundary kinetically.

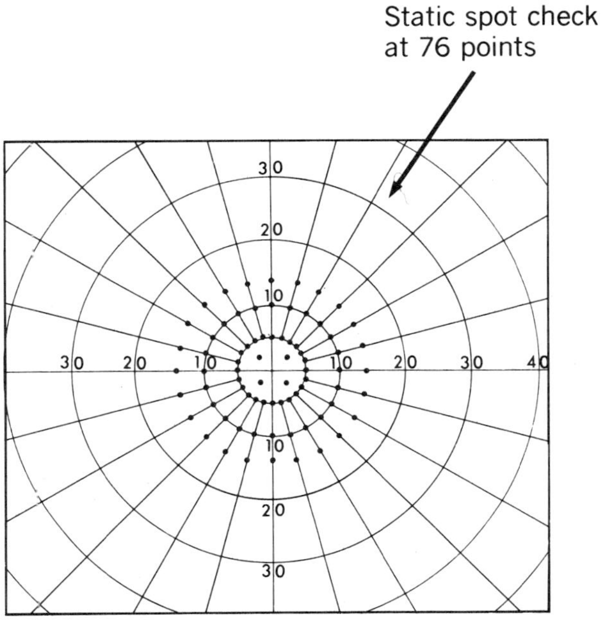
Static spot check
at 76 points
30
20
10
30
20
10
10
20
30
40
10
20
30

FIG. 22-2

Kinetic plotting in the central field

You will be using the stimulus selected for static spot-checking to plot the blind spot kinetically by moving the stimulus in eight directions outward from the center of the blind spot. Actually, this step is usually performed prior to the static spot-checking. In addition to detecting arcuate field defects, you will be ensuring that everything is in order; if the blind spot cannot be plotted, something may be wrong (p. 376). The same stimulus is also used to plot an isopter.

FIG. 22-3. Checking the central field kinetically.

First, plot the blind spot.

Then, use the selected stimulus to plot part of an isopter on the nasal side to look for a nasal step. Plot eight points at 5, 10, 15, and 30 degrees above and below the nasal horizontal meridian. (A 10-degree nasal step is considered diagnostic by itself. A 5-degree nasal step may also be significant but is usually considered a definite diagnostic sign only if there is a concomitant paracentral or arcuate scotoma.)

Finally, use the selected stimulus to plot two points kinetically on the temporal side of the field 30 degrees above and below the horizontal meridian. (These two points, along with the eight nasal points, give a partial representation of the isopter. However, the two temporal points are marginally informative and you may omit them, especially if using the Drance method of checking the temporal field statically.)

In some descriptions of the Armaly-Drance technique the entire isopter is plotted by determining points kinetically along every 15-degree meridian; but if the purpose is only to screen, you can reduce this to eight points nasally and perhaps two points temporally as a method of saving time. The rest are not needed except to help with interpretation if the results of static spot-checking suggest the presence of an abnormality.

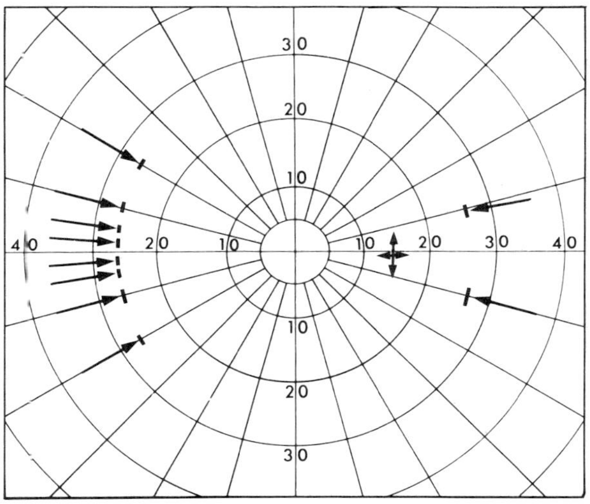

FIG. 22-3

Kinetic plotting in the peripheral field

To check the peripheral field, you need to plot the location of an isopter at eight points nasally to look for a peripheral nasal step—similar to plotting the central isopter but using a stronger stimulus. A more complete method would involve plotting the entire isopter.

In the original technique, when the I-2e is used routinely to plot a standard central isopter, the I-4e is used to plot a peripheral isopter. In a more refined technique, the weakest stimulus seen nasally at 55 degrees either above or below the horizontal meridian is used for the peripheral field. If no stimulus is seen at 55 degrees nasally, the absolute periphery of the field is determined with the V-4e and threshold is determined 5 degrees inside this.

FIG. 22-4. Checking the peripheral field kinetically.

A, Position at which threshold is determined (55 degrees nasally) for selection of the peripheral stimulus.

B, Selection of a stimulus if *V-4e* is not visible at 55 degrees nasally. You need to find the absolute nasal periphery of the field with the *V-4e* and then determine threshold 5 degrees inside the periphery.

C, Plotting the peripheral field with the selected peripheral stimulus. In this example, *I-2e* was used to plot the central isopter and *I-4e* to plot the peripheral isopter. At a minimum, you should search for a nasal step by plotting eight points nasally (solid arrows). However, you may also do, in addition, a complete plot of other meridians around the periphery (dashed arrows).

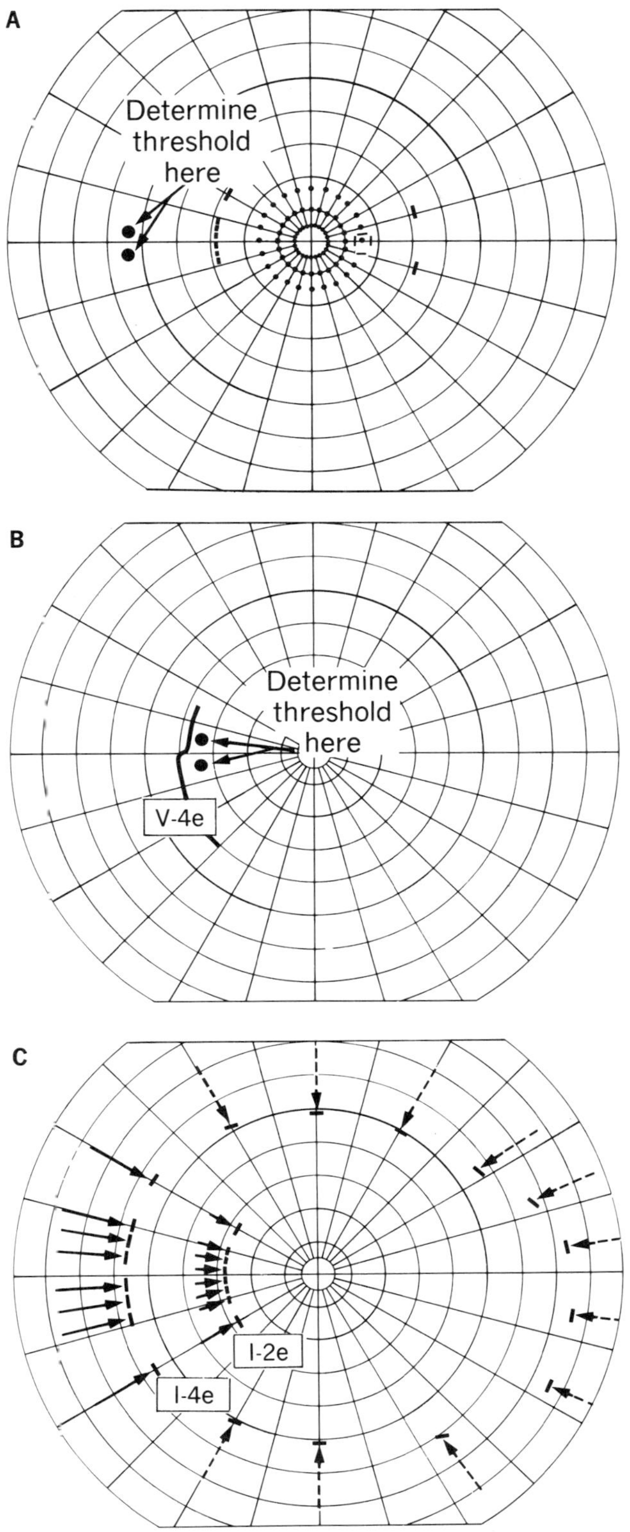
A
Determine threshold here
B
Determine threshold here
V-4e
C
I-2e
I-4e

FIG. 22-4

Summary

To review, the sequence of testing in the basic Armaly-Drance technique is as follows:

1. Select a stimulus for the central field by determining threshold at 25 degrees temporally, adjacent to the blind spot. Alternatively, also, you can (a) take into account the threshold 25 degrees above, below, and nasal to fixation when selecting a stimulus or (b) simply use the I-2e routinely.
2. With the selected stimulus:
   a. Plot the blind spot.
   b. Check statically 76 points.
   c. Plot the isopter at least nasally (eight points) and temporally (two points). Additional points all the way around are optional.
3. Select a stimulus for the peripheral field by determining threshold at 55 degrees nasally above and below the horizontal (or simply use an I-4e) or, if necessary, determine threshold 5 degrees inside the absolute nasal periphery.
4. With the peripheral stimulus, plot eight points of the isopter nasally and (optional) two points temporally, or the whole isopter.

ADDITIONAL READING

For those interested, the original descriptions of the method and its modifications can be found in the following references, listed in *chronological order* so the reader can follow the historical development:

Armaly, M.F.: Ocular pressure and visual fields: a ten-year follow-up study, Arch. Ophthalmol. **81:**25-40, 1969.

Armaly, M.F.: Visual field defects in early open angle glaucoma, Trans. Am. Ophthalmol. Soc. **69:**147-162, 1971.

Rock, W.J., et al.: A modification of the Armaly visual field screening technique for glaucoma, Can. J. Ophthalmol. **6:**283-292, 1971.

Armaly, M.F.: Selective perimetry for glaucomatous defects in ocular hypertension, Arch. Ophthalmol. **87:**518-524, 1972.

Drance, S.M., et al.: A screening method for temporal visual defects in chronic simple glaucoma, Can. J. Ophthalmol. **7:**428-429, 1972.

Rock, W.J., et al.: Visual field screening in glaucoma: an evaluation of the Armaly technique for screening glaucomatous visual fields, Arch. Ophthalmol. **89:**287-290, 1973.

Application

The Armaly-Drance technique is an accurate and rapid (7 minutes per eye) method for determining whether or not a glaucomatous field defect is present. It can be easily taught to someone who is not a fully trained perimetrist and utilized to screen large numbers of people. The regimented sequence of stimulus presentations can be achieved easily with an automated perimeter.

Confirmation that the defects are real (diagnosis) and quantitation (for later checking) can be accomplished subsequently. If the Armaly-Drance technique is performed manually with the Goldmann perimeter and followed immediately by quantitation, it is essentially that described in Chapter 21. One difference, however, is that the technique in Chapter 21 allows freedom to decide on the number and location of points to explore and to recheck areas with combined static and kinetic stimuli. This will allow a good perimetrist to do a better job (sometimes at the expense of taking longer) or a poor perimetrist to do a poorer job (e.g., not checking enough points carefully). One advantage of a regimented system, whether manual or automated, is its usefulness in a research study. A regimented method ensures that every field examination is uniformly consistent, even if performed by different people or in different clinics.

Thus the Armaly-Drance screening method is useful in a wide variety of clinical situations:

1. By itself in screening large numbers of people, perhaps by relatively inexperienced perimetrists (manually or with an automatic perimeter), with the plan being to perform on a subsequent occasion the definitive diagnostic and quantitation steps on people with possible defects
2. As the first visual field technique to teach those in training before going on to quantitation steps
3. As the essential base of a full quantitative field examination (Chapter 21) (Experienced perimetrists must realize that, despite the freedom that comes with experience, they must not spot-check fewer than the prescribed 76 points centrally, lest they do a poorer job than a novice who simply follows directions.)
4. As the basic screening program for automated perimeters
5. In research studies when it is important that all fields be performed identically, either manually or with automated perimeters

Refinements and variations

It is tempting to try to improve on the basic technique for better sensitivity in picking up mild defects. However, each ''improvement'' may at the same time complicate the technique and lengthen it.

1. The number or distribution of spots to be checked in the central field is sometimes altered. Because of the shape of the arcuate regions involved in glaucoma (Fig. 21-4), it is logical to check the nasal field at 20 and 25 degrees in addition to the prescribed 5, 10, and 15 degrees.

FIG. 22-5, A. Additional nasal points (large dots). Of course, it is not abnormal to miss these points if the isopter falls between 20 and 25 degrees without producing a nasal step.

For any pattern it is important to check a sufficient number of spots, including the area near fixation. With too few points, it becomes possible for a small scotoma (e.g., 5 degrees in diameter) to escape detection because it falls between the points checked (Fig. 13-1).

2. In searching for nasal steps, an additional isopter may be plotted nasally (eight points) with a stimulus that forms an isopter at approximately 40 to 45 degrees (e.g., I-3e or the threshold stimulus at 40 degrees nasally). This will yield a total of three isopters plotted at approximately 25 to 30 degrees, 40 to 45 degrees, and 50 to 55 degrees across the nasal meridian.

FIG. 22-5, B. Exploration of the nasal field with three nasal isopters instead of two. Note the similarity to the basic method (described on p. 406).

3. Instead of an isopter plotted kinetically across the horizontal meridian nasally, an arc static cut across the meridian at 25, 40, and 55 degrees could be used to look for nasal steps. A 0.5 log-unit difference above and below would be significant.

FIG. 22-5, C. Arc static cut. The threshold is *I-4e* at three points above the horizontal meridian and *I-3a* at three points below the nasal meridian. Because there is more than 0.5 log-unit difference, a nasal step is present. In this example the nasal step is also shown kinetically with the *I-3e* stimulus to demonstrate that the two methods are equivalent (see also Fig. 23-15).

4. In Drance's second modification of the Armaly technique, additional attention is given to the temporal field. Suprathreshold static spot checking is performed at 24 midperipheral points along the 30-, 40-, and 50-degree circles.

FIG. 22-5, D. Location of the 24 temporal points checked in Drance's modification of the testing technique.

The stimulus used is the weakest seen at 30 degrees from fixation superiorly, 35 degrees from fixation inferiorly, or 55 degrees from fixation temporally.

FIG. 22-5, E. Locations where threshold is checked temporally. The threshold stimulus at these points is used for static suprathreshold spot checking of the temporal field at the points indicated in Fig. 22-5, *D.*

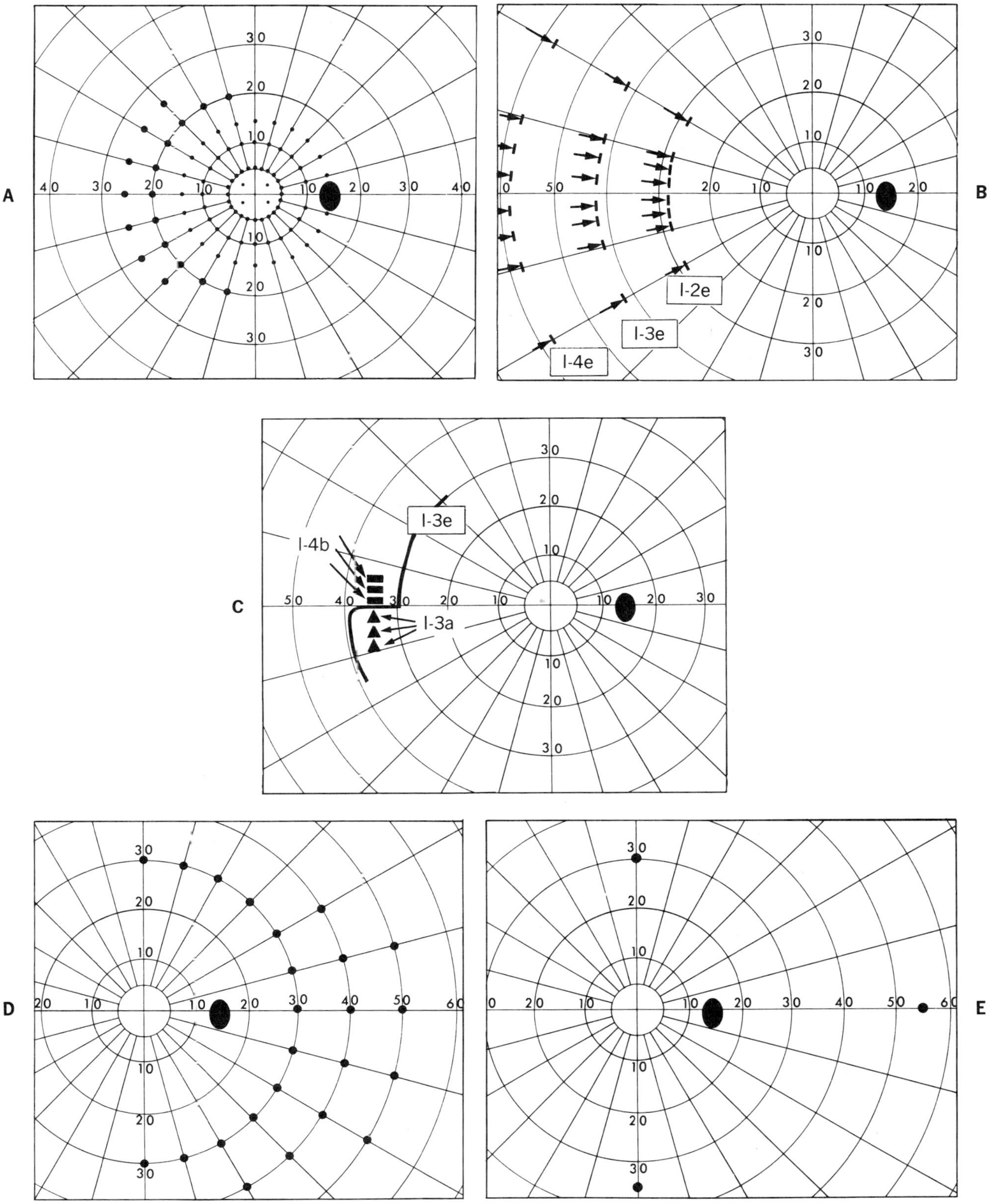

FIG. 22-5

5. As noted earlier (p. 404), when a stimulus that is threshold at 25 degrees is used for spot-checking, a shallow scotoma near fixation may be missed because the stimulus is too strongly suprathreshold close to fixation. To overcome this problem, when extra sensitivity is required, the central 10 to 15 degrees is spot-checked with a stimulus that forms an isopter at 10 to 15 degrees and the usual slightly stronger stimulus is used elsewhere in the central field (Fig. 21-7, *B*).

To spot-check for shallow scotomas near fixation without plotting several isopters, Drance's department now uses the following method:

a. Threshold is determined along the horizontal meridian 5 degrees temporal to fixation.
b. A stimulus 0.2 log-unit brighter than this is used to check the 5-degree circle and four points within the 5-degree circle. For example, if the threshold is I-1b, then I-1d is used.

FIG. 22-6, A. Checking the central 5 degrees. Threshold is determined at *A* and a stimulus 0.2 log-unit more intense is used for spot checking along the circle 5 degrees from fixation.

c. Similarly, threshold is determined 10 degrees temporal to fixation and a stimulus 0.2 log-unit brighter is used for the 10-degree circle.

FIG. 22-6, B. Checking the 10-degree circle with a stimulus 0.2 log-unit more intense than the threshold at *B*.

d. Finally, the 15-degree circle is checked with a stimulus 0.2 log-unit brighter than threshold 20 degrees temporal from fixation (the 15-degree location cannot be used to determine threshold because it usually will fall within the blind spot).

FIG. 22-6, C. Checking the 15-degree circle with a stimulus 0.2 log-unit more intense than the threshold at C.

See pp. 484-486, on which there is a discussion of the Friedmann Analyser, for another approach to this problem.

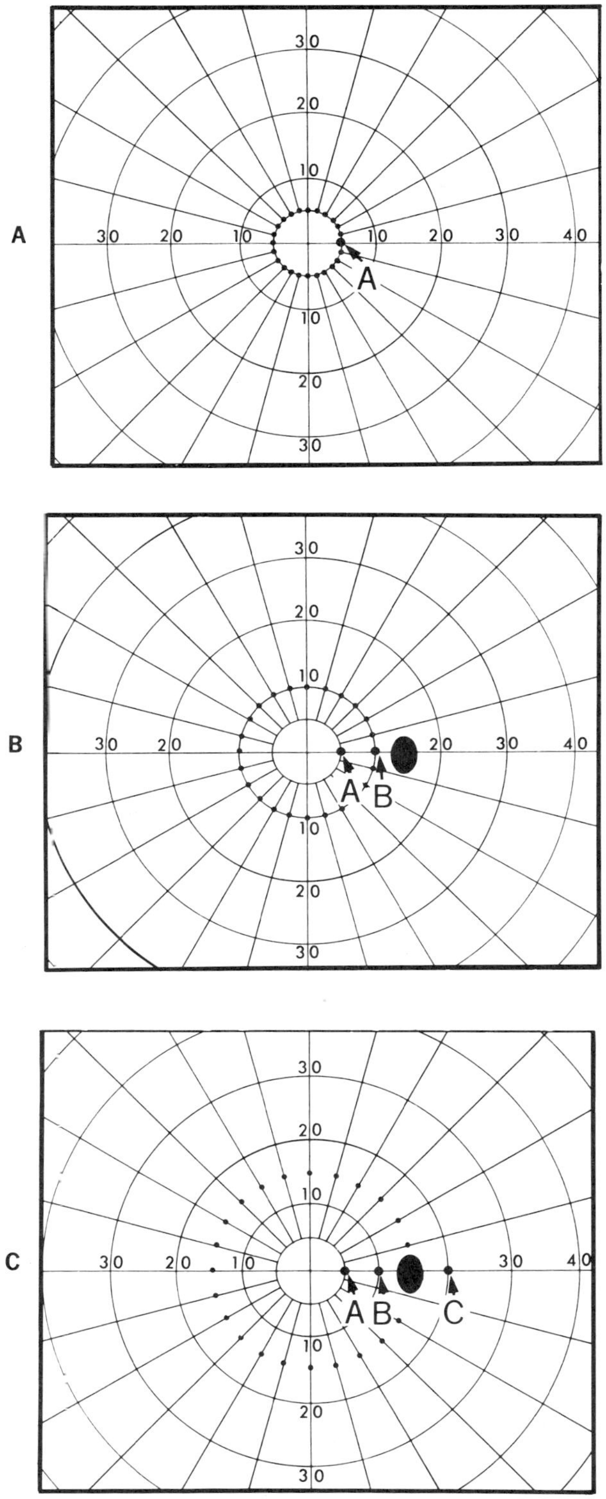

FIG. 22-6

GRID PERIMETRY

Haag-Streit now has a chart for the Goldmann perimeter designed to facilitate static suprathreshold and threshold perimetry in a pattern of points that mimics what is done by automated perimetry.

FIG. 22-7. Field chart for grid perimetry. In each quadrant, at 30 degrees (arrows) are points where threshold was determined prior to suprathreshold perimetry.

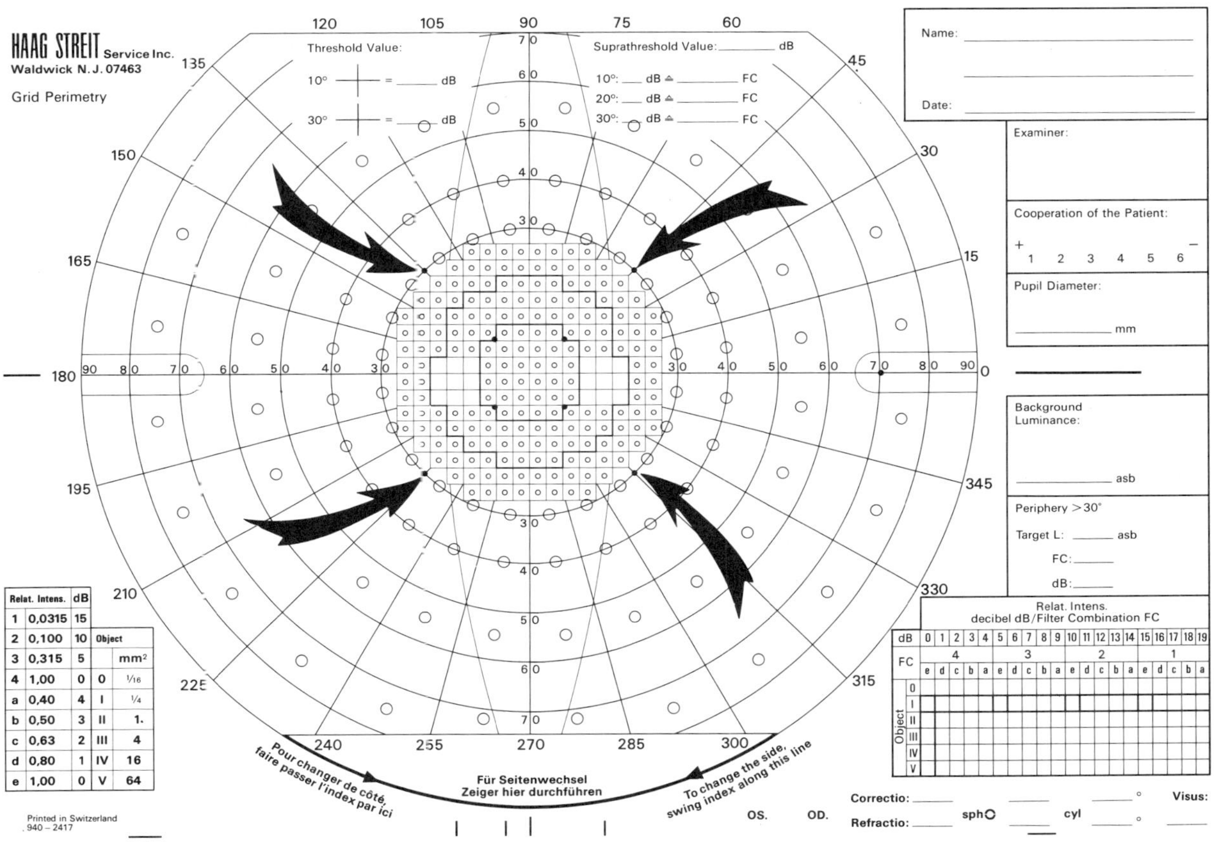
HAAG STREIT Service Inc.
Waldwick N.J. 07463
Grid Perimetry
Threshold Value:
Suprathreshold Value: dB
Name:
Date:
Examiner:
Cooperation of the Patient:
Pupil Diameter:
Background Luminance:
Periphery >30°
Relat. Intens.
decibel dB/Filter Combination FC
Für Seitenwechsel
Zeiger hier durchführen
To change the side, swing index along this line
Pour changer de côté, faire passer l'index par ici
Correctio:
Refractio:
Visus:
Printed in Switzerland

FIG. 22-7

FIG. 22-8. Suggested pattern of 104 points to be tested for glaucoma screening. Different patterns or grids of points may be used for different purposes. Alternatively, every square may be tested, but then there may be too many points for the screening examination.

For suprathreshold perimetry the first step is to determine threshold at four points, one in each quadrant, 30 degrees from fixation. Starting with the I-2a stimulus, increase the intensity in 1 dB steps (I-2a, I-2b, I-2c, etc.) until the weakest visible stimulus has been determined (''method of limits,'' see pp. 48 and 462). The average of the four points (e.g., 1-2c = 12 dB) is considered threshold at 30 degrees (unless of the four points, two or more are apparently abnormal and require a stimulus 4 dB more intense than the average; in that case, consider the weakest stimulus at any of the four points to be the 30-degree threshold).

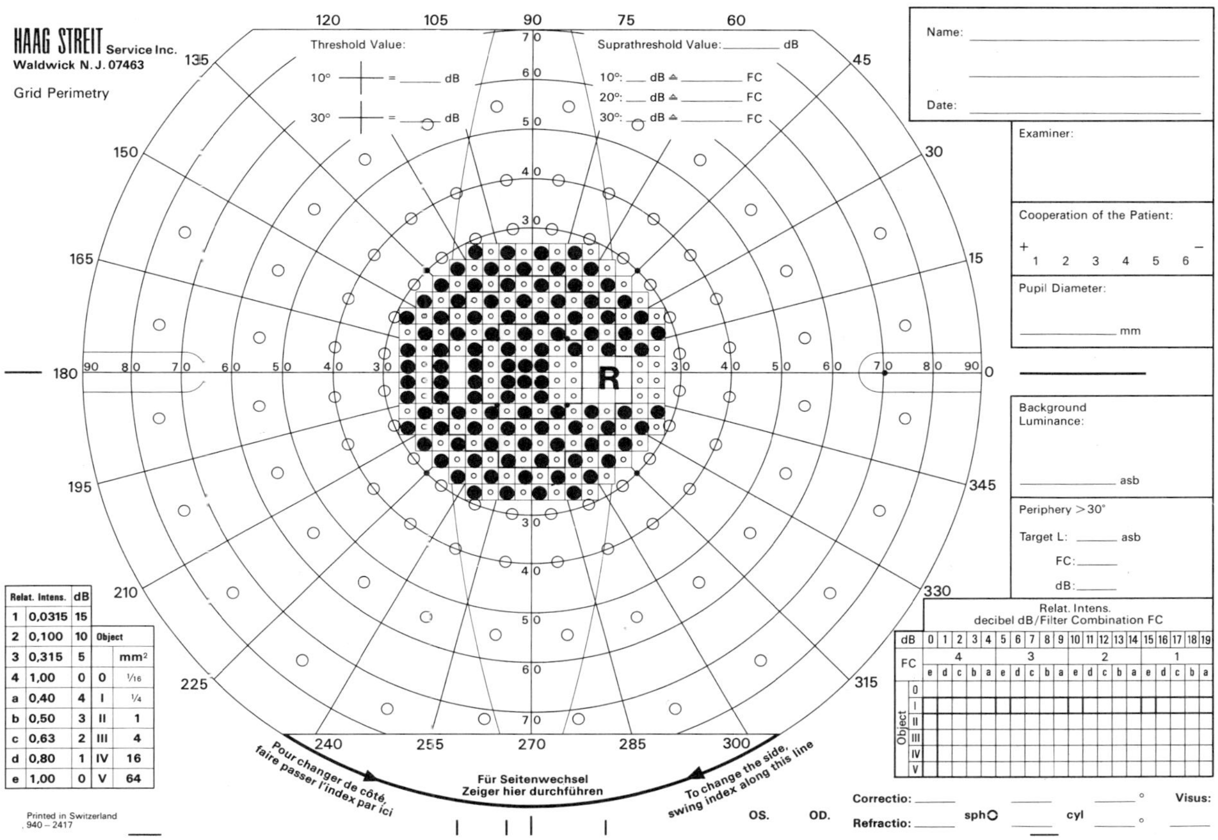
HAAG STREIT Service Inc.
Waldwick N. J. 07463
Grid Perimetry
Threshold Value:
10° = dB
30° = dB
Suprathreshold Value: dB
10°: dB ≙ FC
20°: dB ≙ FC
30°: dB ≙ FC
Name:
Date:
Examiner:
Cooperation of the Patient:
+ 1 2 3 4 5 6 −
Pupil Diameter:
mm
Background Luminance:
asb
Periphery >30°
Target L: asb
FC:
dB:
Relat. Intens. decibel dB/Filter Combination FC
Relat. Intens. dB
1 0,0315 15
2 0,100 10
3 0,315 5
4 1,00 0
a 0,40 4
b 0,50 3
c 0,63 2
d 0,80 1
e 1,00 0
Object mm²
0 1/16
I 1/4
II 1
III 4
IV 16
V 64
R
Pour changer de côté, faire passer l'index par ici
Für Seitenwechsel Zeiger hier durchführen
To change the side, swing index along this line
OS. OD.
Correctio: sph cyl Visus:
Refractio:
Printed in Switzerland 940 – 2417

FIG. 22-8

After the 30-degree threshold is determined, you may use either of two techniques:

The first would be to test the region from 20 to 30 degrees with a stimulus 3 dB more intense than the 30-degree threshold, the region from 10 to 20 degrees with the 30-degree stimulus, and the region from 0 to 10 degrees with a stimulus 3 dB less intense than the 30-degree threshold. In this way the threshold-related eccentricity-compensated strategy of automated perimetry (see Chapter 2) could be achieved, each point being tested with a stimulus about 3 dB more intense than the expected threshold at its location.

A more exacting method would be to determine a 10-degree threshold in addition to the 30-degree threshold (at the four points indicated on the chart). The area from 0 to 10 degrees might be tested with a stimulus 3 dB more intense than the 10-degree threshold, the area from 20 to 30 degrees with a stimulus 3 dB more intense than the 30-degree threshold, and the region in between (from 20 to 30 degrees) with the average of the two.

Present each stimulus for 0.5 second, and pause 1 or 2 seconds for a response. In a simple screen, mark points that are seen with a dot and those that are missed with a cross.

Semiquantitation of defective areas can be achieved as follows:

If the patient sees the stimulus, place a dot in the center of the square (to indicate that the location was tested).

If he fails to see the stimulus, draw a semicircle in the square.

If he fails to see it on subsequent retesting of that location, complete the semicircle into a circle.

Then test the spot with a maximum stimulus (e.g., I-4e, 0 dB).

If he fails to see this, fill in the circle.

Thus an open circle indicates a confirmed relative defect, and a filled circle an absolute defect. (This notation is modified from the one recommended by F.W. Fisher.*)

A spatially adaptive strategy would be that whenever there was an abnormal area all the grid squares in the seemingly abnormal region would be tested, not just the ones included in the grid pattern that had been selected for screening. Spatial resolution could then be further refined by testing not only the center of each square but each corner as well.

For the particularly hardy examiner (and patient), actual thresholds can be determined at the most relevant abnormal points, using the method of limits (pp. 48 and 462). At the abnormal point you increase the stimulus by 1 dB steps until one is seen, and you write the threshold value (in decibels) in the grid square.

---

*Schwellenangepasste überschwelle Raster perimetrie am Goldmann-Perimeter, Klin. Monatsbl. Augenheilkd. **185:**204-211, 1984; Zur freien statischen Schwellenperimetrie am Goldmann-Perimeter, Klin. Monatsbl. Augenheilkd. **186:**310-314, 1985.

STATIC CUT FOR GLAUCOMA SCREENING

A static cut in the 45- to 225-degree and 135- to 315-degree meridians is sometimes performed for glaucomatous screening. Such a pair of cuts, if performed by themselves, may not be more time consuming than other screening strategies. At present, however, this method is not widely used because in only a few offices or clinics are the personnel facile with static perimetry. The use of some automated devices may make such static cuts more easily available.

Obviously, a pair of static cuts provides very accurate information about visual threshold along the two meridians but it will not detect scotomas that lie elsewhere (see Fig. 1-9). The basic premise is that only rarely will there be a scotoma someplace without there being also a disturbance along the entire arcuate region that would be detected by the two static cuts. As always, a screening test shows only whether or not the field is abnormal; it does not necessarily demonstrate all the abnormalities.

FIG. 22-9. Hypothetical pair of static cuts for glaucoma screening. This field is abnormal, but not all the defects are detected. For example, the scotoma inferiorly is missed. The 45- to 225-degree cut shows the upper nasal depression, and the 135- to 315-degree cut shows the scotoma above the blind spot.

The criteria devised by Greve are that the defect must be 3 degrees wide and 0.5 log-unit deep. Because of the appearance in a static profile plot, he calls these "wedge-shaped defects." However, he does not use the static cut as the primary screening method.

ADDITIONAL READING

To supplement the references already given on pp. 424 and 435, additional information about the distribution of glaucomatous field defects and screening strategies can be found in Appendix B.

Greve, E.L.: Single and multiple stimulus static perimetry in glaucoma: the two phases of visual field examination, Doc. Ophthalmol. **136:**1-355, 1973.

Greve, E.L., et al.: A critical phase in the development of glaucomatous visual field defects, Doc. Ophthalmol. Proc. Ser. **19:**127-135, 1979.

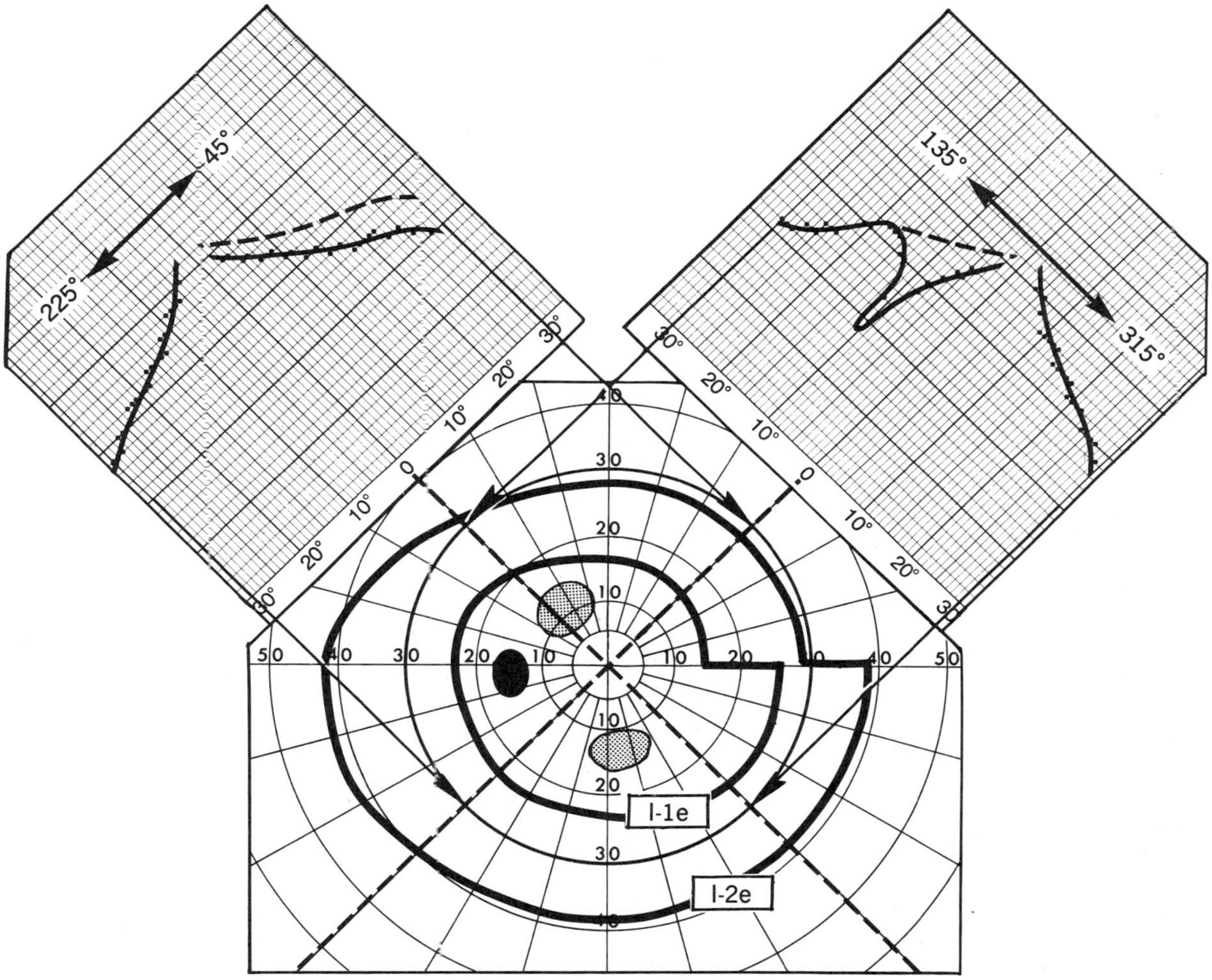

FIG. 22-9

CHAPTER 23

Advanced perimetric technique

BASIC STEPS IN PERIMETRY

Before proceeding to this chapter, please read Chapter 1, the first part of Chapter 2, and most of Chapters 3 through 10. Also review the important details of perimetric technique covered in Chapter 12. The present chapter begins with a statement of the basic manual perimetric technique, some of which is a review of Chapter 12 and the preceding chapters in Part II.

With the Goldmann perimeter the visual field examination is performed in a darkened room. The doors are closed so there will be no stray light shining in the bowl to create a nonstandard background illumination or cause uneven illumination or shadows within the bowl. The intensity of the projected stimulus and of the background should be calibrated frequently (Chapter 16), especially if someone else has used the perimeter since you last used it.

As you may recall (from Chapter 12), it is important to educate the patient about his task and to establish a pattern of good fixation and consistent responses. If he has not had a field evaluation before, confrontation testing will teach him that he is supposed to report what he sees without looking directly at it. Confrontation testing will also give you a general idea of the kind and severity of any major field defects that may be present.

At the perimeter it is wise to start with the patient's better eye if he has not been tested previously. Show him a large object near fixation, a small object near fixation, a large object farther from fixation, and so on, until he understands that there will be several types of stimuli in various locations. This process of using several sizes of objects and making them appear and disappear in various areas can be continued until the patient's responses are consistent. **During the entire introductory phase, note the consistency of responses, the response time, and the general size of his visual field for various stimuli.** Finally, map the blind spot as a check on whether or not he is ready to proceed. In outlining the absolute boundary of the physiologic blind spot, it is a good idea to use a small bright object (I-4e). If looking for depressed sensation (''enlarged blind spot''), outline the blind spot with a weaker stimulus. This may not be necessary if static spot-checking with an appropriate test object is being done in the region around the blind spot. Of course, a stimulus stronger than I-4e will have to be used to outline the blind spot if the field is so depressed that the I-4e isopter does not enclose the position of the blind spot by a reasonable margin of 5 degrees or more.

It is important to choose the appropriate test stimuli, the areas of the field in which to concentrate your effort, and the strategy of the field examination. These decisions are based on the characteristics of the suspected field defect (i.e., the reason for which it was decided to perform a visual field test) as well as on the responses obtained during the phase of educating the patient.

For example, knowing the location of a retinal lesion will enable you to determine the correct area to search for a corresponding scotoma. Knowing that an optic nerve lesion is suspected as the cause of reduced acuity will allow you to be particularly careful in seeking a central scotoma. Knowing that the IOP is elevated will lead you to look especially for paracentral scotomas and nasal steps (Chapters 21 and 22). Knowing that a pituitary tumor is suspected will induce you to search for a hemianopia.

This approach saves both time and energy of the patient and you, and it makes the test more sensitive by concentrating on areas where a visual field defect is most likely. You can therefore be more confident when no defect is found that indeed there is no defect, because you are sure that the right areas of the field have been checked carefully.

The small fixation mirror (Fig. 15-4) is used whenever it can be seen by the patient, and the large mirror only when the small one cannot be seen. The small mirror holds a steadier fixation and it automatically stimulates the appropriate degree of accommodation, so the fixation spot and the rest of the bowl will be in correct focus on the retina.

It is important to monitor fixation continuously. Be especially careful that you are looking through the telescope as the test object is moved inward kinetically so you are monitoring the eye at the time just before the patient responds and you can be sure that he has not looked away for an instant.

Corrective lenses (Chapter 12) may be used inside 30 degrees, but loose corrective lenses should not be used outside 30 degrees. Be careful that, when testing outside 30 degrees, you remove both the lens and the lens holder. A common mistake is to believe that certain stimuli require correction and others do not. This is false. Correction is required for all stimuli inside 30 degrees, but trial lenses are not needed outside 30 degrees for any stimuli. The exception, of course, is contact lenses, which may be used outside 30 degrees.

ISOPTERS THAT CROSS FROM CENTRAL TO PERIPHERAL

The need for a corrective lens inside 30 degrees does not relate to which isopters are being plotted. Thus, if an isopter has part of its course inside 30 degrees, that part is plotted with a lens in place and the part outside is plotted without the lens. You will find that it is more convenient for you and more comfortable for the patient if each isopter inside 30 degrees is plotted until it begins to leave the central zone and then, after the lens is removed, the remainders of all the isopters are plotted. When the lenses are removed, the lens holder must also be removed because it, like the rim of the lens itself, can interfere with visibility of the stimulus outside 30 degrees inferiorly.

Sometimes the isopter shifts slightly when the lens is removed because of the prismatic effect of the edge of the lens and because the visibility of the stimulus is altered by whether or not it is in focus. When this happens, the segment of the isopter plotted with the lens in place does not join exactly with the segment plotted without the lens. The break in continuity does not hamper interpretation of the visual field diagram and is simply indicated with a double slash.

FIG. 23-1. Isopters plotted with correction inside 30 degrees and without correction outside 30 degrees. The portions plotted while the lens is in place are in red for illustrative purposes. Ordinarily only a double slash mark, not color coding, is used to indicate which part of an isopter was plotted with a corrective lens and which was plotted without a lens.

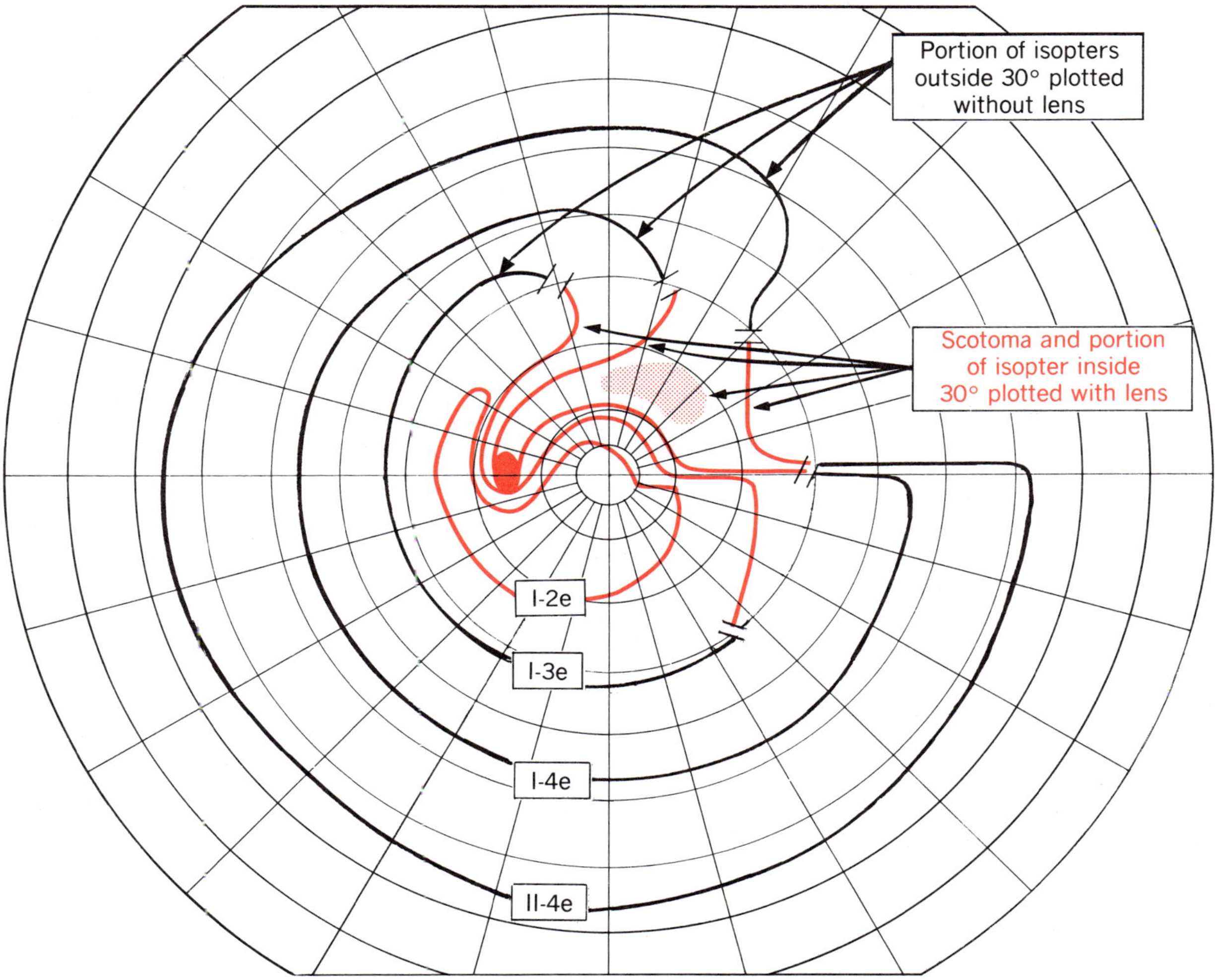
Portion of isopters
outside 30° plotted
without lens
Scotoma and portion
of isopter inside
30° plotted with lens
I-2e
I-3e
I-4e
II-4e

FIG. 23-1

STANDARD STIMULI

Except for very special purposes, only standard stimuli are used: 0-1, I-1, I-2, I-3, I-4, II-4, III-4, IV-4, and V-4. With each of these, the brightness of any of the subdivisions (a through e) may be used.

This selection of stimuli derives from the fact that size I is the standard for Goldmann perimetry and is used with the entire range of 20 light intensities (from 1a through 4e). The larger sizes, II through V, are utilized only if the strongest stimulus of standard size, I-4e, is too weak in a region of the field being tested.

At the other end of the range, if I-1a is too strong for testing near the very center of the field there are two ways to achieve a weaker stimulus:

The first is to use a 2 log-unit filter (represented by a single bar), beginning the series again at I-4e. Thus, in 0.5 log-unit steps, in descending order of intensity, the stimuli are I-3e, I-2e, I-1e, I-$\overline{4e}$, I-$\overline{3e}$, ... In 0.1 log-unit steps and descending order of intensity, the stimuli would be I-1c, I-1b, I-1a, I-$\overline{4e}$, I-$\overline{4d}$, I-$\overline{4c}$, ... If the I-$\overline{1a}$ stimulus is still not sufficiently weak, a 4 log-unit filter (represented by a double bar) is used, again beginning at the top of the series with 4e. Thus, in 0.1 log-unit steps, in descending order of intensity, the stimuli would be I-$\overline{1c}$, I-$\overline{1b}$, I-$\overline{1a}$, I-$\overline{\overline{4e}}$, I-$\overline{\overline{4d}}$, I-$\overline{\overline{4c}}$, ...

The second way, for perimeters that are not equipped with either a 2 or a 4 log-unit filter, is to use the reduced size, 0, but only with intensities 1e through 1a. Thus, in descending order of stimulus strength, the stimuli would be I-1c, I-1b, I-1a, 0-1e, 0-1d, 0-1c, 0-1b, and 0-1a. In terms of visibility, 0-1e is roughly equivalent to I-$\overline{4e}$, 0-1d is roughly equivalent to I-$\overline{4d}$, and so on:

I-1b	I-$\overline{4b}$ = 0-1b
I-1a	I-$\overline{4a}$ = 0-1a
I-$\overline{4e}$ = 0-1e	I-$\overline{3e}$
I-$\overline{4d}$ = 0-1d	I-$\overline{3d}$
I-$\overline{4c}$ = 0-1c	. . .

REPRESENTING THE STIMULI

It is useful to have a color code for the various stimuli, with dense colors for the strong stimuli and light colors for the weak ones:

V-4 black	I-4 red
IV-4 brown	I-3 orange
III-4 purple	I-2 blue
II-4 green	I-1 yellow
	0-1 pink

When this system is used, the isopters are drawn and a check mark is placed in the appropriate box in the lower right-hand corner of the field diagram. A region can be marked "O.K." in the appropriate color, indicating that it was searched with that test object by static spot-checking and no scotomas were found. Thus, "O.K." in blue indicates that the region was checked by static spot-checking with the I-2 test stimulus and this test stimulus was seen throughout this region. If the same color code is used routinely, it makes comparing successive field tests easier when looking for progressive change.

To represent scotomas, you color in the nonseeing areas to a particular test stimulus. Thus the scotomatous region might be colored red within the region where the I-4 was not seen; the surrounding larger area where the I-2 was not seen would be colored blue; and the center would be marked "II-4 seen," indicating that this was the threshold value in the location where the I-4 was not seen. If plotting the blind spot with the I-4 test stimulus, you color it red. For a steep-walled scotoma you outline its boundary with the weakest stimulus and fill in with the color of the strongest stimulus to which there is a scotoma. Areas of inconsistent or slow responses are marked with cross-hatching in the appropriate color, indicating which stimulus has elicited inconsistent responses.

LABELING THE CHART

You must be able in some sense to interpret the responses of the patient and be sure that the visual field chart correctly reflects what has transpired while the field test was being administered. Only you can know what actually has occurred during the testing, and this information must be transmitted on the field chart. Areas of inconsistent responses must be so labeled—do not just draw in an isopter where you think it might be without indicating that there was some question about its location or that there were inconsistent responses in a particular portion of the field. This information could be very important.

The consistency of the responses, the steadiness of fixation, whether or not the patient was particularly slow in responding generally, and the overall reliability of the field should be indicated. Obviously it is important to know whether the patient had inconsistent responses everywhere in the field (indicating a flat hill of vision or an unreliable field) or had inconsistent responses only in one place (indicating a localized abnormality). It is important to know these things if diagnostic and therapeutic decisions are going to be made on the basis of the visual field—especially in clinics where over a period of years the patient may be cared for by several different physicians, where the perimetry is not performed by the physician only, or where the perimetrist may not be the same person each year. The nonphysician perimetrist has a special obligation not only to be knowledgeable but also to record accurately the results so the physician can make adequate diagnostic and therapeutic decisions. Labels such as "I-4e seen but I-3e not seen" or "depression still present when eyelid taped up" show that the perimetrist was alert, knew to do these extra steps, and actually did them.

Of course, the field chart must also be labeled with the patient's name (first and last), the date (including the year), your name, whether the eye was right or left, the correction used, the visual acuity, the pupil size, and (if customary) the intraocular pressure.

NONSEEING TO SEEING

An important general rule in kinetic perimetry is that the test stimulus be moved from nonseeing areas to seeing areas. This applies to the plotting of ordinary isopters as well as to the plotting of scotoma boundaries and permits the greatest consistency of responses because it is physiologically easier for the patient to recognize when something *appears* than when something *disappears*.

Moreover, the technique of moving the object from a nonseeing to a seeing area establishes the signal pattern that the patient responds whenever he sees the object. This pattern also occurs during static suprathreshold spot-checking and static threshold perimetry, in both of which the patient is expected to respond each time he sees the stimulus. It would be confusing if during kinetic perimetry the patient were asked to respond when he did not see the stimulus but during static perimetry to respond when he *did* see it.

FIG. 23-2. Kinetic perimetry. To plot an isopter, turn the stimulus on in a region that you think is nonseeing and then pause a second to make sure that indeed it is not seen. Once certain that it is not seen at the position where you turned it on, move the stimulus inward toward the seeing area. As soon as the patient responds, turn it off. If the stimulus is kept on, the patient may be confused, not knowing whether or not you expect him to respond again.

The rate of movement of the stimulus should not be great—about 1 degree per second in the central field for careful plotting of isopters and the boundary of scotomas, 2 to 3 degrees per second in the intermediate part of the field for ordinary isopter plotting, and up to 5 degrees per second in the most peripheral field. It is important to guard against moving the stimulus too fast. If you have had previous experience at the tangent screen, be particularly cautious to move slowly within the 30 degrees of the central field, remembering that the perimeter chart is miniaturized compared to the tangent screen and you, likewise, must move in miniature. Keep the speed even slower than normal if the patient has a long response time and occasionally spot-check the position of the isopter by static technique inside and outside the isopter.

The rate of movement should be steady until the patient responds. Avoid slowing down when approaching the expected position of the isopter, for this increases the time that the stimulus remains in the area where you think the isopter will be and thereby introduces a bias that the responses will occur where you expect the isopter to be rather than where it really is.

It is a great time saver if the stimulus is turned on close to the expected position of the isopter (i.e., 5 to 10 degrees away) so there is a short path of movement, for only 1 or 2 seconds, before the stimulus is seen. With a short path, a long wait by the patient between stimuli is avoided. Also there is less temptation to move the stimulus too fast, which could result in a careless determination of the isopter's location. Moreover, with slow movement the stimulus approximates a static presentation and the isopter position is closer to what would be obtained if threshold were determined statically.

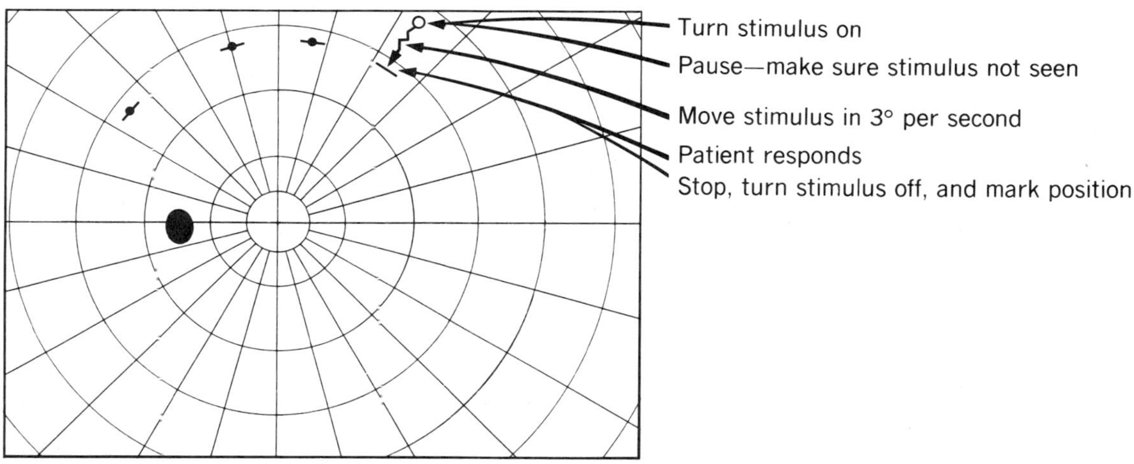
Turn stimulus on
Pause—make sure stimulus not seen
Move stimulus in 3° per second
Patient responds
Stop, turn stimulus off, and mark position

FIG. 23-2

The danger in starting close to the expected position of the isopter is that you may inadvertently already be within the seeing zone when you first turn on the stimulus. This makes it important that you pause before beginning to move the stimulus (Fig. 23-2) to make absolutely certain that it is not seen before you begin to move it. If you move the stimulus immediately and have started inside the seeing zone, the patient will likely respond several degrees inside where you started the kinetic paths and you will think you are plotting an isopter when in fact the true isopter is much more peripheral. Also, if the patient responds the very instant you start to move it, you are too close to the isopter and need to back up a little further into the nonseeing area.

You should not allow too much time to elapse between sightings by the patient. If an isopter is being plotted and a stimulus does not become visible for several seconds, the stimulus should be moved into a position where it is known to have been seen, allowing the patient to respond and thereby reassuring him that the test is still in progress and he need not fear that he has missed something he should have seen. It also reassures you that the patient is still alert and responding when he does see the stimulus. Then, continue moving the stimulus along the path in the area being tested until it becomes seen.

FIG. 23-3. Alternative method. If the patient does not respond at the expected position, move the stimulus rapidly toward the seeing area until he sees it and does respond. This gives him the needed reassurance of not having to wait too long and also saves you time by letting you know the approximate location of the isopter. Then you can back up a short distance along the same path using slower movement to obtain the precise location of the isopter. This method saves time if there are large irregular field defects.

STATIC SPOT-CHECKING

Similarly, during static spot-checking, if you find three or four consecutive presentations that the patient cannot see, put the stimulus in an area where you know he can see, allow him to respond, and then return to exploring the apparent defect. This will reassure you that the machine continues to function properly and that the patient is paying attention; and, equally important, the patient will not become tense waiting for a stimulus that seems delayed in coming. In fact, if you handle this situation with finesse, the patient may not even be aware that there are spots he is not seeing.

Practice depressing and releasing the shutter switch silently, so the patient will not have an audible clue to when the stimulus is being presented. Also, when spot-checking or when plotting the isopter, do not present the stimulus rhythmically, for example every second, or the patient may simply respond every second, even when he does not see the stimulus, or perhaps even continue to respond after you stop presenting the stimulus. The rhythm should be somewhat irregular, with no more than 10 normal presentations before a pause or break in the pattern.

Remember also that it is important to check *many* spots when looking for scotomas. Resist the temptation to cut corners by checking only a few spots.

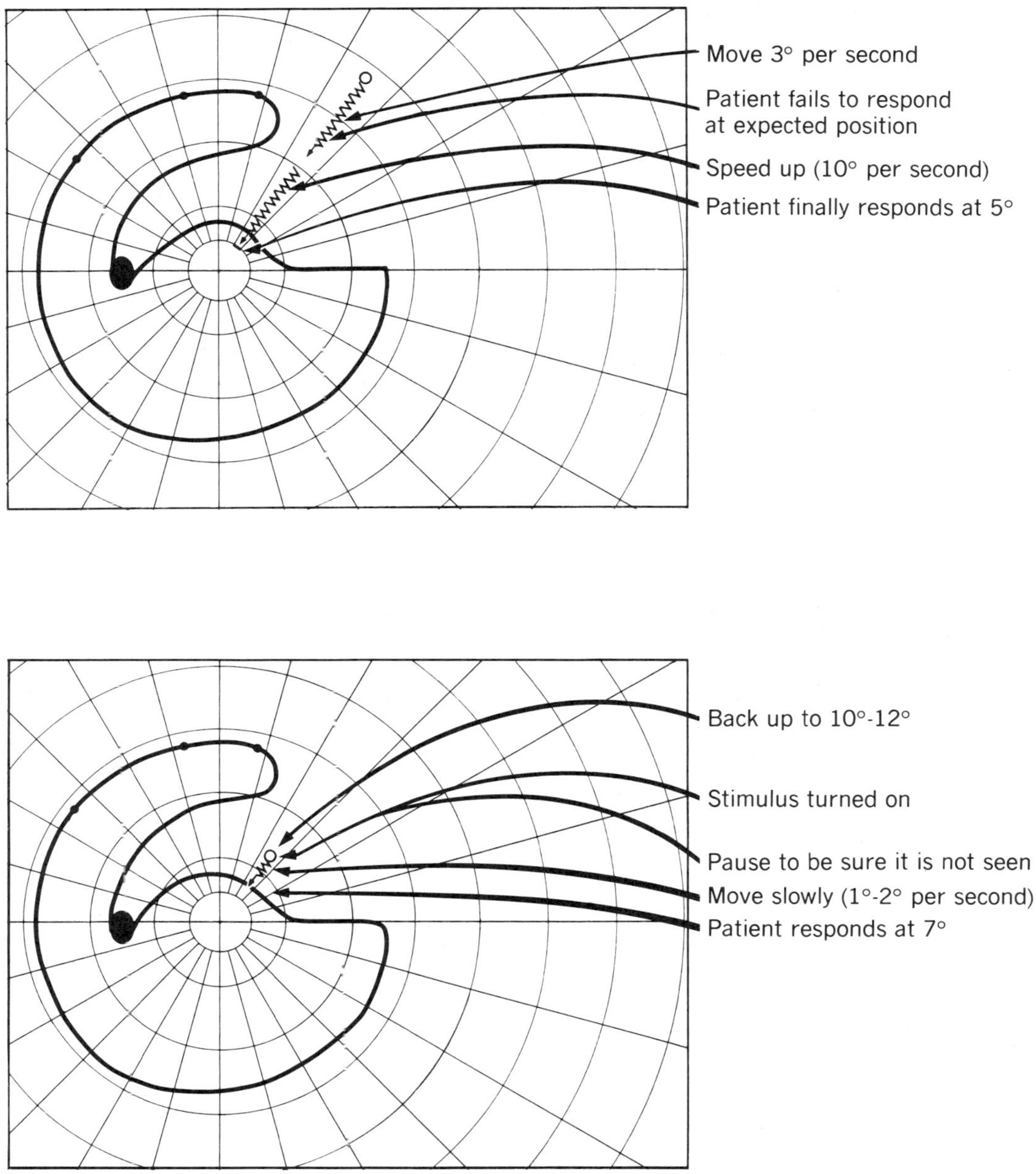
Move 3° per second
Patient fails to respond at expected position
Speed up (10° per second)
Patient finally responds at 5°
Back up to 10°-12°
Stimulus turned on
Pause to be sure it is not seen
Move slowly (1°-2° per second)
Patient responds at 7°

FIG. 23-3

CROSSING THE ISOPTER PERPENDICULARLY

In Chapter 14 a zone of inconsistent responses around isopters was described. Because of this zone, it is important that the movement of a kinetic stimulus be perpendicular to the isopter.

FIG. 23-4. Effect of a nonperpendicular crossing on patient response. If the stimulus passes through the threshold zone perpendicular to the isopter, there is only a short distance over which it goes from definitely invisible to definitely visible. In fact, the patient may give a response within a narrow 2- to 3-degree zone rather consistently.

However, if the stimulus passes through the threshold zone at an angle and if the patient might respond any time while it is still in the threshold zone (after it leaves the definite nonseeing area but before it enters the definite seeing area), it is easy to see how the responses would be at varying locations.

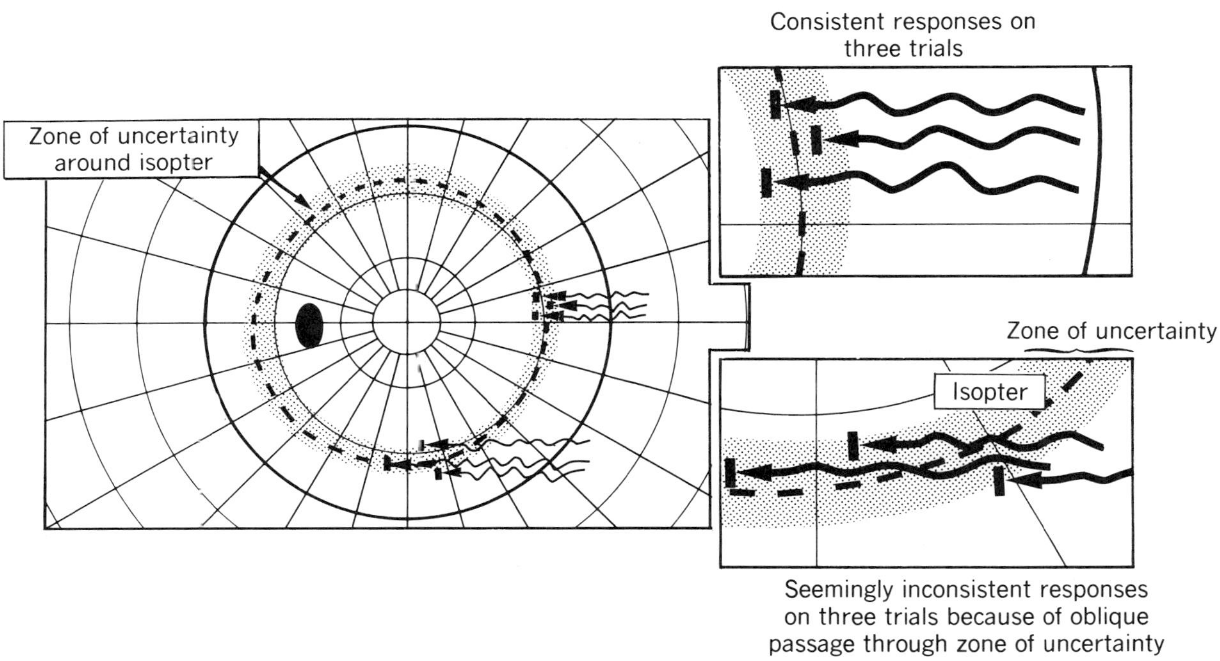
Consistent responses on three trials
Zone of uncertainty around isopter
Zone of uncertainty
Isopter
Seemingly inconsistent responses on three trials because of oblique passage through zone of uncertainty

FIG. 23-4

The responses are thus more consistent when the kinetic stimulus crosses into a seeing zone perpendicular to the isopter. Obviously the best tactic in outlining an isopter is to move the kinetic stimulus perpendicular to the isopter; but, of course, the problem is that you do not know exactly where the isopter is until after it is plotted.

FIG. 23-5. Examples of irregular isopters that may not be crossed perpendicularly.
A, A nasal step may cause responses at 22, 32, and 42 degrees when the stimulus is passed along the horizontal meridian three times.
B, Imagine your confusion if the stimulus is passed along a path three times and three different locations of response are obtained.

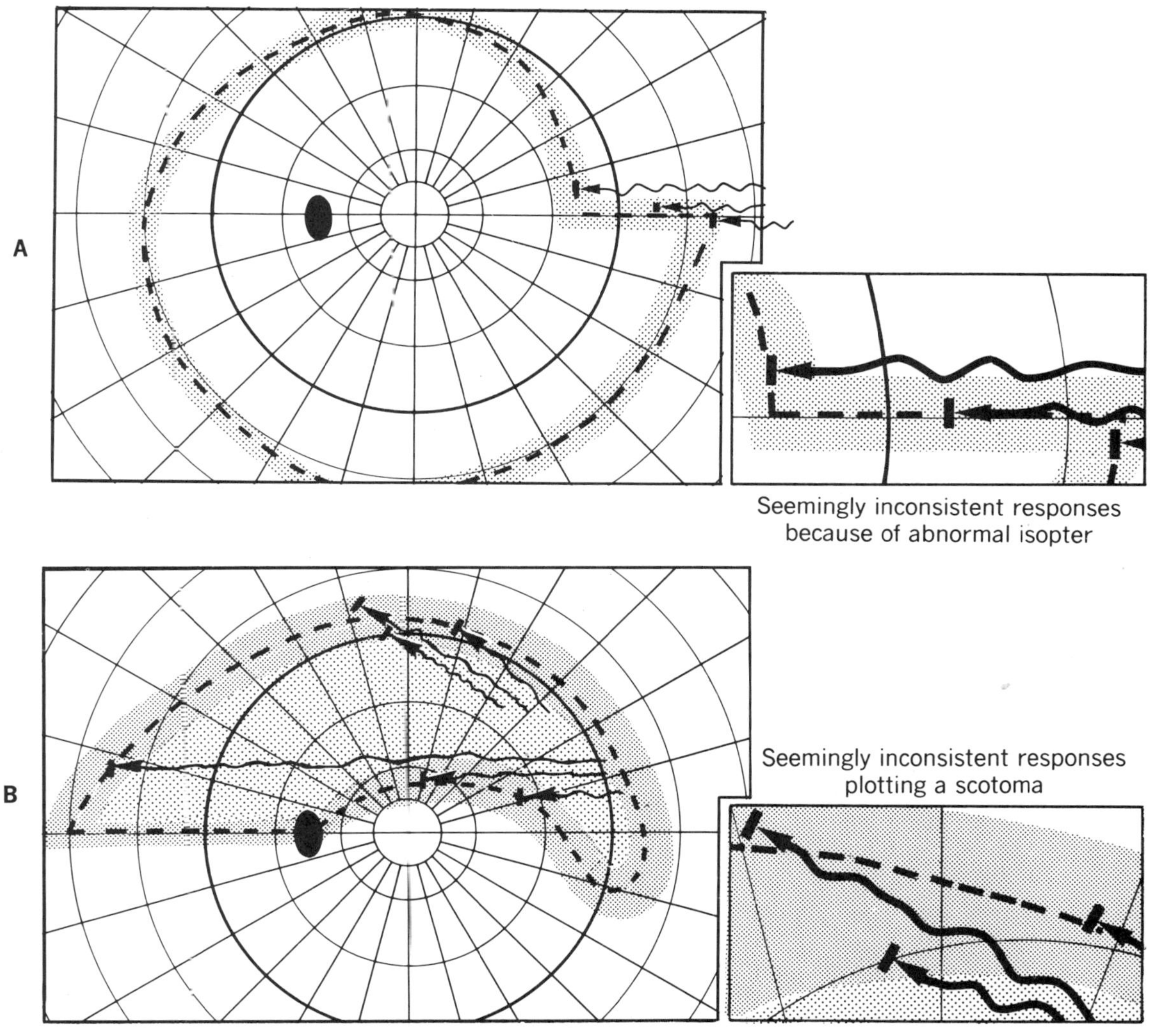
A
Seemingly inconsistent responses because of abnormal isopter
B
Seemingly inconsistent responses plotting a scotoma

FIG. 23-5

To achieve a perpendicular crossing of the isopter, the path of the stimulus should be toward fixation for the usual isopters. If a step is suspected because of responses that are different on the two sides of a meridian, the path should be in an arc around fixation in the suspected location of the step, as was utilized to confirm the nasal step in glaucoma (p. 412).

In plotting scotomas, move the stimulus away from the center of a round scotoma, perhaps in eight meridians, as illustrated for plotting the blind spot (p. 379). For arcuate scotomas the paths can be away from fixation, toward fixation, or in an arc pointing toward or away from the physiologic blind spot.

For plotting irregular isopters and scotomas whose outlines are not yet unfolded in the course of an examination, there is a trick that is helpful in achieving a nearly perpendicular approach to the isopter.

FIG. 23-6. An efficient way to find the contour of an abnormal isopter. The trick is to imagine a line connecting two previous response points and to aim the next path midway between the two points perpendicular to the imaginary line. Any time a region seems abnormal or there is a wide separation between two points on the isopter, plot more points following this rule between each pair of previous points until the exact shape of the isopter is determined. Note that the method to confirm the presence of a nasal step is essentially the principle of going perpendicular to a line connecting two points already plotted.

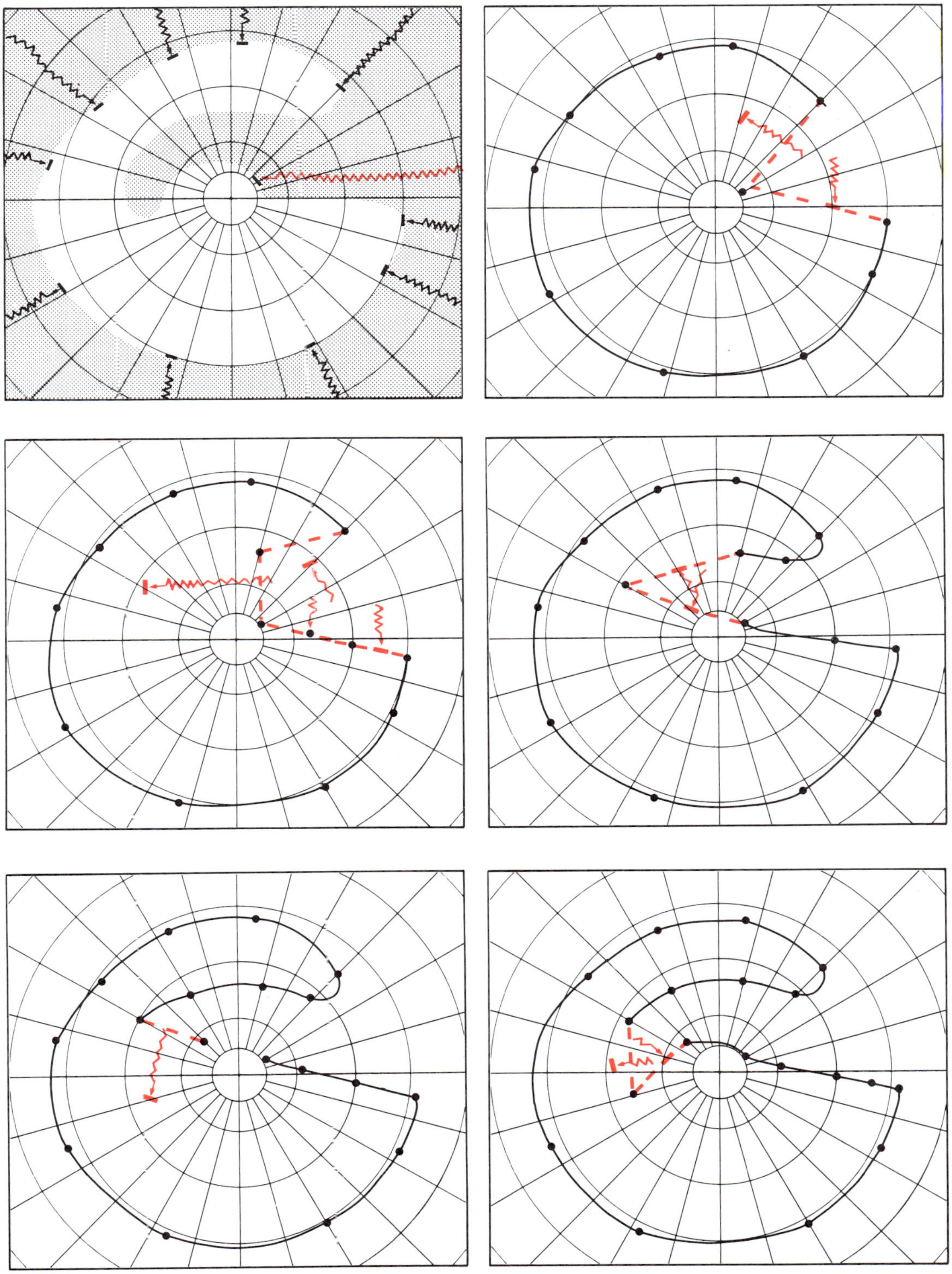

FIG. 23-6

SLOPE OF THE HILL OF VISION

We have just seen that there is a ''zone of uncertainty'' around the isopter and that in kinetic perimetry a stimulus may become visible at any point within this zone. If there is a long path through the zone, there will be a long segment over which the stimulus may become visible and the results will seem inconsistent. The segment of the path within the zone of uncertainty is shortest, and the responses are most consistent, if the path is perpendicular to the isopter.

The breadth of the zone of uncertainty depends in part on the slope of the hill of vision at the isopter.

FIG. 23-7. Influence of the slope on the width of the zone of uncertainty. In the profile plot the zone of uncertainty (shaded area) is the same height everywhere. In the isopter plot the *I-2e* isopter in this example has a narrower zone of uncertainty than the *I-3e* isopter because the slope of the profile is steep near the *I-2e* isopter and flat near the *I-3e* isopter.

The slope influences the consistency of responses in both normal and abnormal regions of the visual field. Generally, the responses during kinetic perimetry are more consistent with a steep slope (isopters crowded together) than with a flat region (isopters widely separated).

In some instances of a generalized depression (e.g., from cataracts or uncorrected refractive error) the hill of vision also becomes flatter. It also becomes flatter under mesopic or scotopic (dark-adapted) conditions instead of the photopic (light adapted) conditions of background illumination used for Goldmann perimetry. In these instances, isopters will be separated and the patient's responses will be somewhat inconsistent, with the exact location of the isopters more difficult to determine.

Of course, this is not the only reason for inconsistent patient responses. If the responses are inconsistent throughout all the visual field with all test stimuli, it could indicate that the patient is not a good subject for this kind of testing or that you have done a poor job of educating him in what is expected.

However, it is good to keep in mind that a flat hill of vision will produce inconsistent responses and inconsistency should be expected when isopters are widely separated (indicating a flat hill of vision). (See Fig. 23-14.)

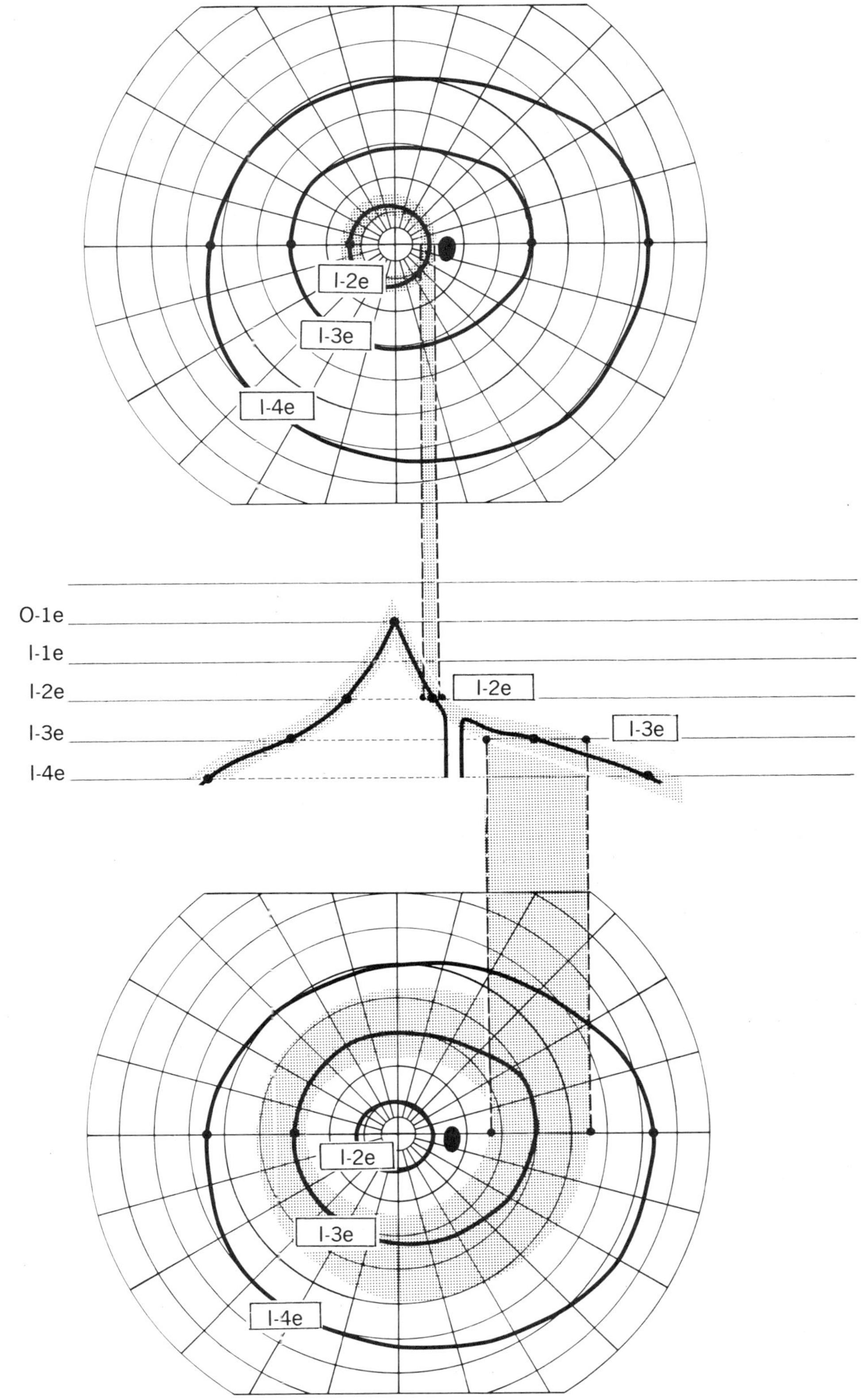

FIG. 23-7

LOCALIZED AREAS OF INCONSISTENT RESPONSES

If a patient has inconsistent responses to a stimulus only in a particular region of the visual field, this may indicate that the stimulus is right in the threshold zone for that region. Often it is due to the presence of a subtle abnormality.

FIG. 23-8. Localized inconsistent responses.
A, Kinetic plotting. The responses are not the same above and below the horizontal meridian, suggesting an abnormality. You should label such an area *inconsistent* even though you do not draw an exact isopter. The plotting of additional isopters (in this example, 0.2 log-unit above and below the threshold indicated by the inconsistent responses) may or may not confirm that the region is abnormal by showing a nasal step.
B, Static spot-checking. In an apparent scotoma the *I-3e* is seen only half the time or with a much slower response in this particular location. Again, what makes this abnormal is that in surrounding areas the stimulus *is* definitely seen. You can confirm the boundary of the abnormal region with a slightly weaker stimulus, *I*-3c, that forms an isopter closer to the region of inconsistent responses and with this stimulus plot the boundary of the scotoma. Moreover, an even weaker stimulus (I-3a) might show a deviation around the shallow scotoma.

The principle illustrated here is that localized inconsistent responses are a clue to the possibility of a subtle abnormality. Inconsistent responses in kinetic plotting and in static spot-checking are each quantified by plotting additional isopters. If the unusual area is far from the original isopter, the new isopter should be just *outside* this region so the weaker stimulus can be used for static spot-checking—perhaps to define a scotoma. If, on the other hand, the area of inconsistent responses is nearer the original isopter, a new isopter that would normally pass *through* the region should be plotted—possibly indicating a localized depression and confirming that the area is, indeed, abnormal. In both cases you need to indicate the region of inconsistent responses on the field diagram as suspicious even if you cannot define it as a genuine defect.

Another method for defining an area of inconsistent responses is discussed on p. 470.

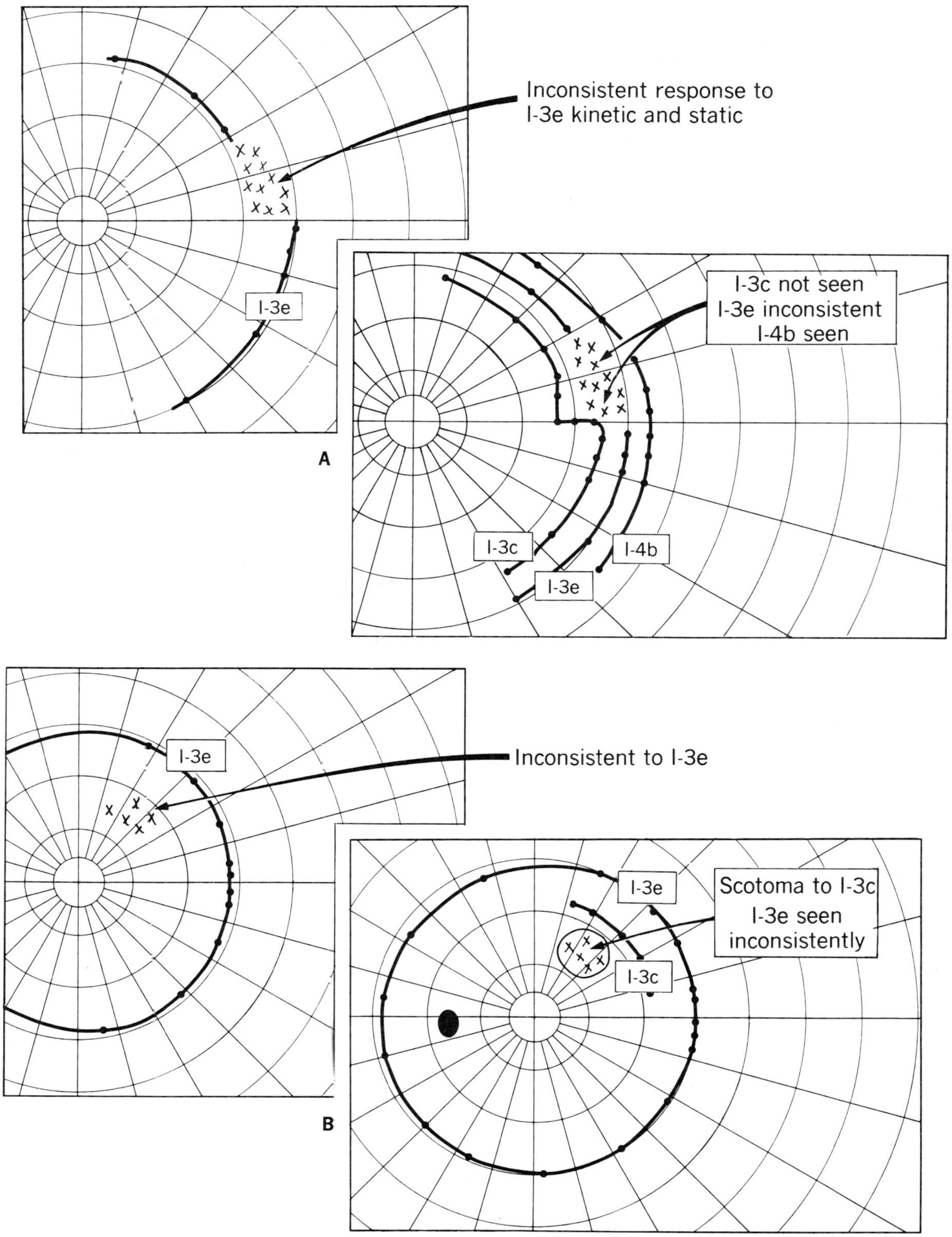
Inconsistent response to
I-3e kinetic and static
I-3e
I-3c not seen
I-3e inconsistent
I-4b seen
I-3c
I-4b
I-3e
A
I-3e
Inconsistent to I-3e
I-3e
Scotoma to I-3c
I-3e seen
inconsistently
I-3c
B

FIG. 23-8

THE DIM AREA

During static spot-checking to look for scotomas, you may note that a patient comments on how the stimulus seems dimmer in a certain region. This area needs to be explored just as an area of inconsistent responses would.

To understand the reason for localized dimness, recall that the stimulus is barely visible near its isopter but is subjectively brighter (more above threshold) in the region nearer fixation. Conceivably, in a shallow scotoma nearer fixation (such as the one in Fig. 21-7, *A*) the object may seem dimmer than in the surrounding region but still be visible. In this instance, the patient will respond with the buzzer because he does see it and thus the scotoma usually goes undetected. However, if the patient spontaneously comments that the object seems dimmer in a certain spot, you need to be aware that this has the same significance as a slow and inconsistent response. It should alert you to the possible presence of a scotoma, which can then be investigated by plotting a new isopter just outside the abnormal region and spot-checking with the weaker stimulus to uncover any defect that may exist.

The principle is that identical stimuli of the same intensity may seem to have different brightnesses inside and outside an area of reduced vision. A stimulus may be suprathreshold in both areas, but its apparent brightness will depend on how much more intense it is than threshold in that particular region.

As an analogy, consider the patient who has 20/20 vision in the right eye and 20/50 in the left. When asked to read the 20/80 line of letters, he can do so with either eye but will tell you that the letters are blurred with the left eye and sharp with the right eye. Thus he can see the letters with each eye but he can also tell you that the quality of vision is not equal. It is this difference in the quality of vision in areas with different thresholds that makes confrontation testing by the comparison method so useful (Chapter 3).

THE UPPER EYELID

A frequent problem is that the isopters are flattened more than the normal depression superiorly (p. 84) because of an overhang of the upper eyelid or eyebrow. The field seems depressed superiorly, simulating an altitudinal defect or an upper nasal depression typical of glaucoma (Fig. 13-37). You should be aware of this and whenever there seems to be a visual depression superiorly, especially if the patient has a droopy upper eyelid or eyebrow, recheck isopter(s) with the eyelid elevated. Often the patient can be instructed simply to "open wide" while you check half a dozen points in the upper field to determine how much effect the eyelid is having. This extra effort to open the eyes widely may be tiring for the patient and it need not be maintained while the lower half or lower two thirds of the field is being tested. Nor is it necessary to continue raising the eyelid to test the upper part of the field once you have determined that the eyelid is not producing a problem in this particular patient. However, when the upper eyelid *is* being troublesome and the patient cannot open his eyes widely, you may have to ask an assistant or the patient himself to hold the eyelid up manually (without, of course, obstructing the field of view). Sometimes a small piece of tape will be adequate to hold the eyelid up, but this is uncomfortable and should be used only briefly while you plot the upper segments of one or two isopters. The remainder of the field is tested and any necessary spot-checking is completed without tape on the eyelids.

THE PROMINENT NOSE

In a similar way, the tip of the nose may interfere with the lower nasal quadrant of the visual field. This problem is overcome by having the patient turn his face very slightly to the opposite side, for instance, to the left while you test the right eye (Fig. 12-2). Interestingly, even with the nose well out of the way, there may normally remain a localized contraction of the visual field corresponding to the tip of the nose.

THE CORNEAL REFLECTION

As you look at the cornea through the telescope, you can see a reflection of the test stimulus. If the nose, eyelid, or rim of the corrective lens is obstructing the patient's view of the stimulus, there will be no corneal reflection. However, it reappears as soon as the stimulus moves to a position where its view is not obstructed. If the patient's response coincides with the appearance of the stimulus reflection in the cornea, you are plotting the boundary of the obstructing object and not an isopter of the visual field. When you obtain puzzling responses, observation of the corneal reflection may be reassuring that the projected test stimulus is actually on.

CREATIVE SPOT-CHECKING

In Chapters 6, 18, and 21, static spot-checking to detect scotomas is discussed. However, there are other uses. For example, spot-checking can be used to confirm the exact location of an isopter, especially in puzzling areas. Remember that the isopter separates the region where the stimulus is seen from the region where it is not seen. Therefore you can use static spot-checking to make sure that the stimulus can be seen just inside where you think the isopter is and that it cannot be seen just outside where you think the isopter is. This method may be useful in a number of circumstances.

FIG. 23-9. Uses of static spot-checking.
A, Checking the size of the blind spot. Sometimes if you are moving the stimulus too fast, the blind spot will be plotted larger than it really is as a result of the delay between when the patient sees the stimulus and when he responds. Occasionally, as a matter of routine, it is good to check yourself after plotting the blind spot kinetically by using static spot-checking to see if the blind spot is really as large as you plotted it.
B, Confirming a nasal step. We have already noted (p. 412) that one way to confirm a nasal step is to move the stimulus vertically across the step. Sometimes the situation may still not be clear, especially if the step is not exactly on the horizontal meridian. Then static spot-checking can be used to locate the isopter.
C, Checking ordinary isopters. Once or twice on each patient you should briefly check one or two of the isopters, even if they seem normal, just to be sure that you are not being fooled by a slow response time, a bias in your technique (pp. 444 and 446), or some other quirk. There is no end to possible quirks. For example, when an isopter is plotted kinetically, the patient may see the stimulus as it is first turned on but may think he is not to respond until it moves; he does not respond during the pause before the stimulus moves but does respond after it starts to move, though with delay. You thus may think you are plotting an isopter.

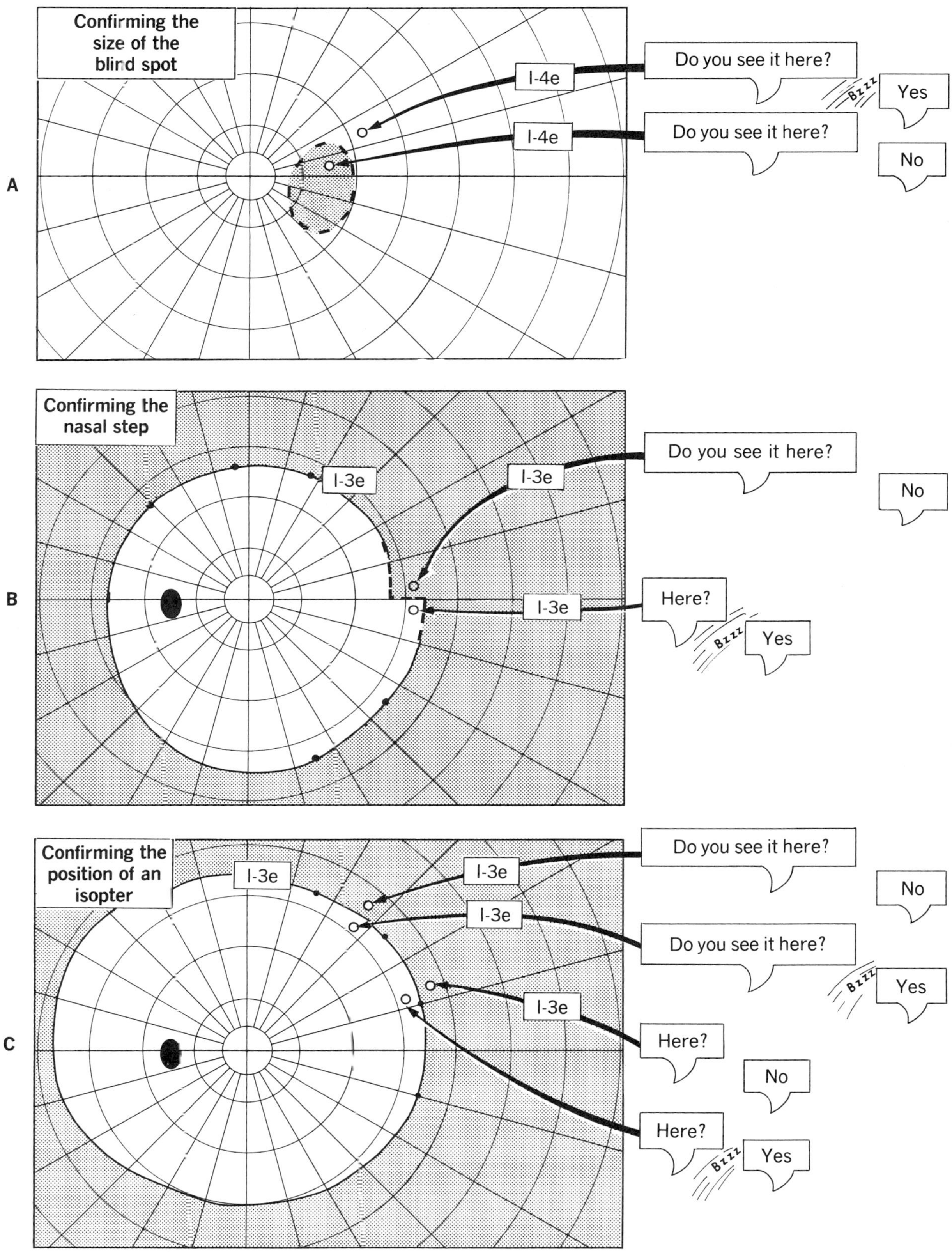
A
Confirming the size of the blind spot
I-4e
Do you see it here?
Bzzz
Yes
I-4e
Do you see it here?
No
B
Confirming the nasal step
I-3e
I-3e
Do you see it here?
No
I-3e
Here?
Bzzz
Yes
C
Confirming the position of an isopter
I-3e
I-3e
Do you see it here?
No
I-3e
Do you see it here?
Bzzz
Yes
I-3e
Here?
No
Here?
Bzzz
Yes

FIG. 23-9

FIG. 23-10. Static spot-checking to confirm the boundary of a scotoma.
A, Based on seven patient responses, including one that was erroneous, an oval scotoma has been outlined instead of the arcuate scotoma actually present.
B, With static spot-checking, the oval boundary is not confirmed and it is discovered that the scotoma is actually larger than had been plotted. Exact boundaries are important in following the progress of scotomas or other abnormalities.

You should not check each point statically—it would take too much time. After all, the reason you use kinetic perimetry to plot the isopters is that it is rapid and for the most part very accurate (if you do not move the stimulus too fast or mark the responses on the chart too sloppily). However, you should do static spot-checking whenever you are uncertain of the boundary, such as in this example in which you might reasonably have wondered if this scotoma had an arcuate shape. Occasional static spot-checking also lets you monitor the patient's reaction time to near-threshold targets, which may be longer than for suprathreshold targets.

MANUAL STATIC THRESHOLD PERIMETRY

Manual static threshold perimetry has been used almost exclusively in specialized institutions, mainly research centers. One reason is that only in these centers can the expensive Tübingen perimeter of Harms and Aulhorn (Oculus), designed with static perimetry in mind, be found. The commonly available Goldmann perimeter, by comparison, is awkward for this purpose. However, there are times when static threshold perimetry is useful to supplement kinetic perimetry with static spot-checking in the everyday ophthalmic practice. Moreover, since most of the automated perimeters now available determine visual threshold statically, it is important to understand the principles, the potential usefulness, and the relationship to kinetic techniques of static threshold perimetry, especially if the newer instruments are to be used intelligently.

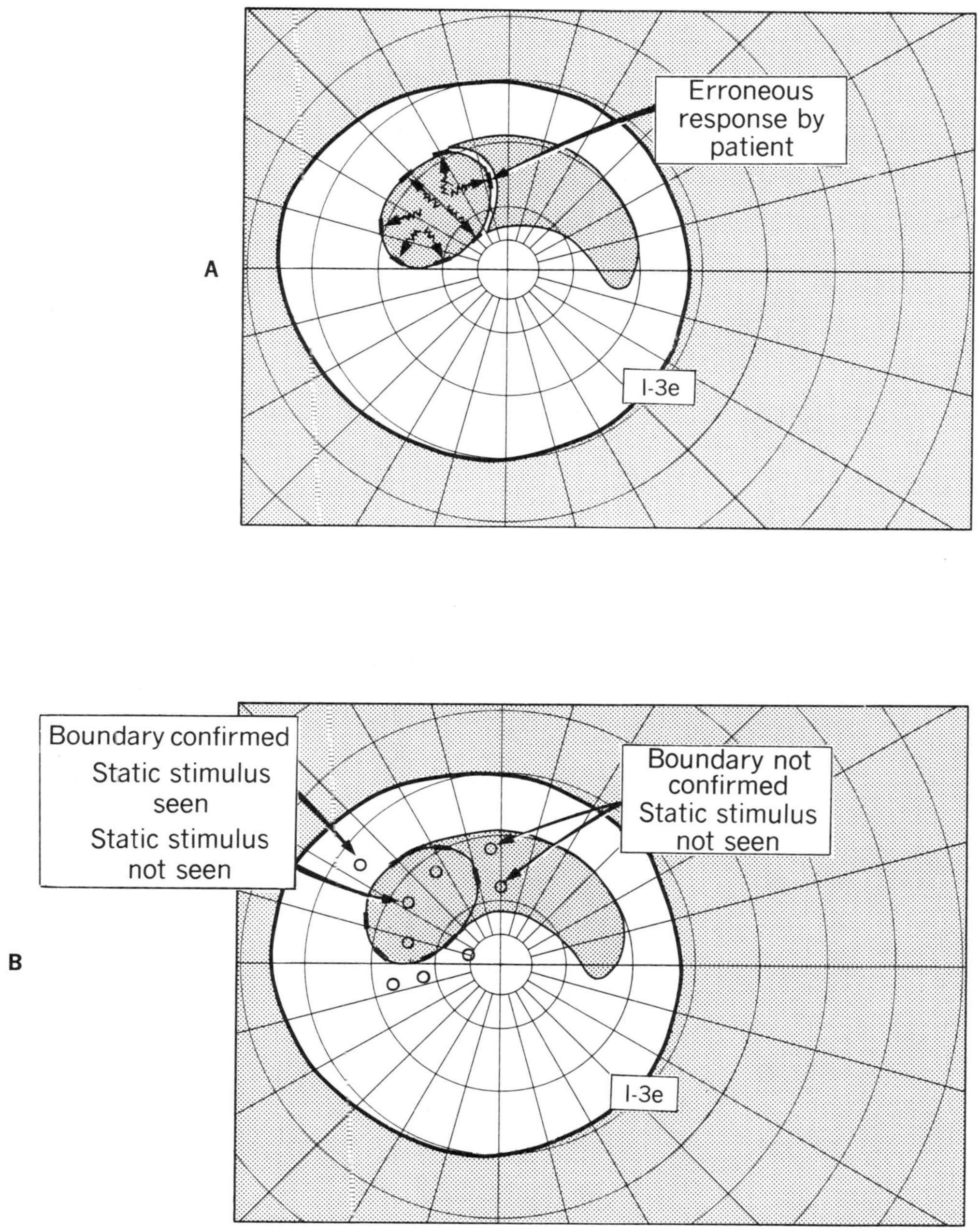
A
Erroneous response by patient
I-3e
B
Boundary confirmed
Static stimulus seen
Static stimulus not seen
Boundary not confirmed
Static stimulus not seen
I-3e

FIG. 23-10

SUPRATHRESHOLD VERSUS THRESHOLD

In static *supra*threshold perimetry, which we have called "spot-checking," an area is explored with a suprathreshold stimulus that is expected to be easily visible. With this method the exact visual threshold is not determined. Rather, what is determined is that in regions where the stimulus is visible the threshold is somewhat weaker than the one being used. By way of analogy, if a person is asked to read the 20/40 visual acuity line when being tested for a driver's license what is being determined is that his visual acuity is either "20/40 or better" or "less than 20/40."

In static threshold perimetry the exact visual threshold is determined at selected points. If these points are along a meridian, we call the technique "static profile perimetry" or a "static cut."

FIG. 23-11. Meridional static cut through a scotoma. Threshold is determined along the 315-degree meridian, from 1 to 33 degrees from fixation at 2-degree intervals.

The static cut along a meridian is but one form of static threshold perimetry. The points tested may be along an arc or circle, or in a grid or other pattern of distribution.

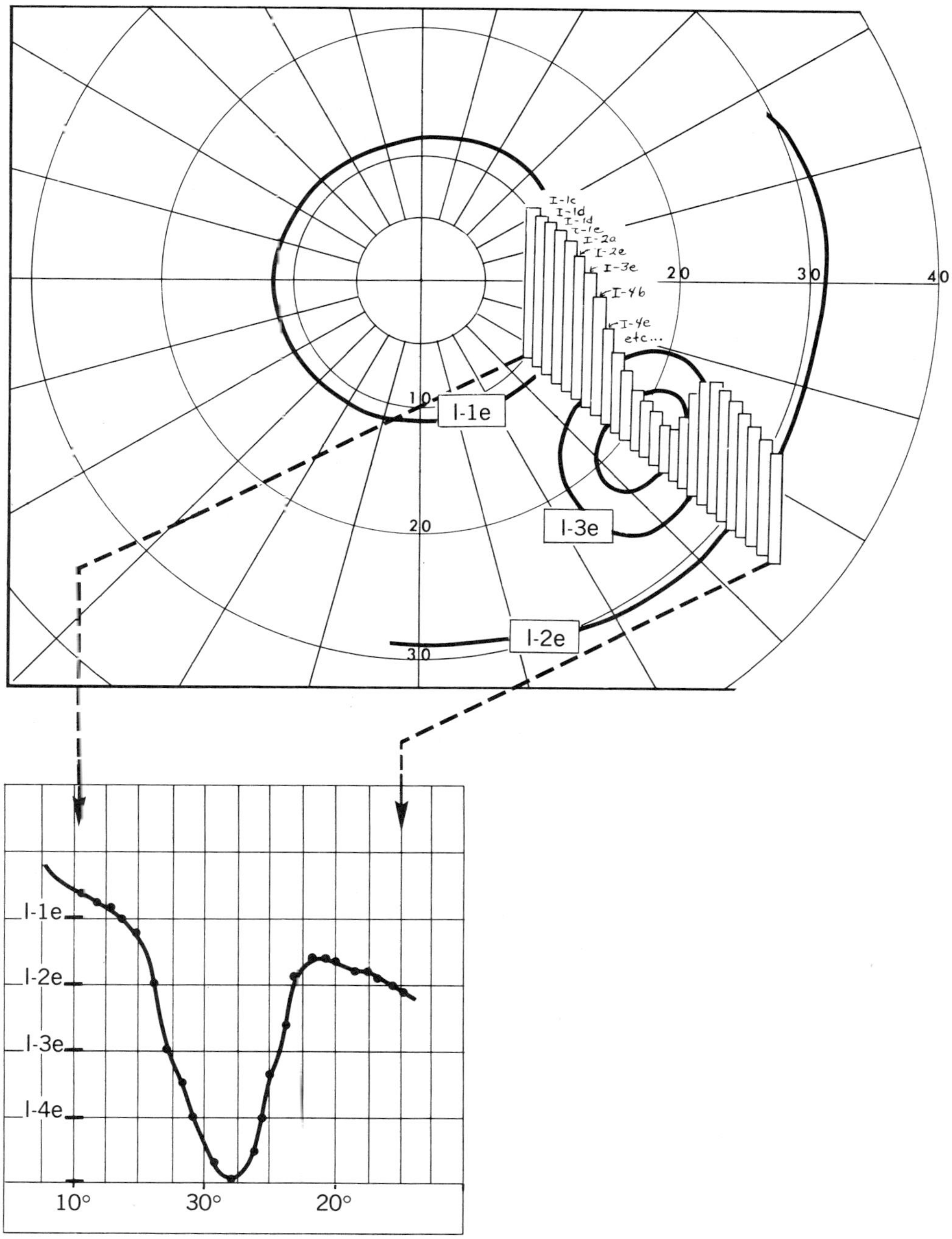

FIG. 23-11

SPECIAL FEATURES OF STATIC PERIMETRY

One helpful feature of static perimetry is that it is not affected by the patient's reaction time. The stimulus is presented, and it does not matter whether the patient responds ½ second later or 3 seconds later. In kinetic perimetry you want to know *when* the patient first sees the stimulus and the reaction time is important.

Static perimetry gives a very accurate threshold determination at each point tested, but the price paid is time and a limited number of points can be tested. It is used to good advantage to quantify very accurately central scotomas or other small scotomas, to explore questionable areas, and to help diagnose other situations (described later in this chapter). However, the technique of kinetic perimetry with static spot-checking is often more efficient in rapidly giving more information about the field in general and outlining the extent of large defects.* Even centers that use static perimetry extensively will use kinetic perimetry to gain general information about a patient's field of vision and to select the locations deserving careful quantitation by static threshold perimetry. Indeed, kinetic perimetry may be required at times to ensure that the static cut is being performed in the right place.†

Once you have decided where in the visual field the static threshold is to be determined, it does not take much skill to perform the static threshold testing. The procedure is rather regimented. By contrast, the technique of kinetic perimetry with static spot-checking requires decisions to be made continually concerning additional points and isopters to be plotted as the nature of the field unfolds. Thus kinetic perimetry relies on the judgment of the perimetrist that comes with experience and skill. Automated perimeters are more easily programmed to examine the field in a regimented fashion by static means.

---

*Aulhorn, E.: Static perimetry, Annee Ther. Clin. Ophtalmol. **25:**164-173, 1974; Aulhorn, E., and Harms, H.: Visual perimetry. In Jameson, D. and Hurvich, L.M., editors: Visual psycophysics, Handbook of sensory physiology, vol. 7, no. 4, New York, 1972, Springer-Verlag, Inc., pp. 102-145; Greve, E.L., et al.: A critical phase in the development of glaucomatous visual field defects, Doc. Ophthalmol. Proc. Ser. **19:**127-136, 1979.

†Aulhorn, E., et al.: The influence of spontaneous eye rotation on the perimetric determination of small scotomas, Doc. Ophthalmol. Proc. Ser. **19:**363-367, 1979.

TECHNIQUE OF DETERMINING THRESHOLD AT A POINT

After the projector arm of the perimeter is positioned at the desired spot, flash a stimulus of standard size (I for the Goldmann perimeter) for ½ to 1 second at a presumed slightly infrathreshold intensity. Provided the patient (as expected) does not respond to the first stimulus, present another of the next brightest intensity for ½ to 1 second. Keep this on for at least ½ second to be sure that maximum temporal summation has occurred (p. 339). The duration should be no longer than 1 second, with a 2-second pause between presentations to avoid light adaptation at the site being tested. Present increasingly intense stimuli until the patient finally does see one. The stimulus first seen can be recorded as threshold. To ensure accuracy, it is best that at least two presentations are invisible (confirming that the initial test stimulus is infrathreshold) before reaching the one that becomes visible.

Usually each location is tested in this manner only once, provided the threshold value obtained is in keeping with what you expected, taking into account the value(s) obtained at adjacent points. However, if there is doubt or if for some reason the visual threshold is to be determined with special care, present the stimulus first seen a second time (double-checking) to confirm that it is visible.* If missed on the second presentation, show it a third and a fourth time, and count it as "visible" when it is seen on both the third and the fourth presentations.

Recall that a stimulus right at threshold (or within the threshold zone) may be seen only a certain percentage of the time. In the double-checking method a stimulus is counted as threshold if it is the weakest seen at all and if it is seen more than half the time, i.e., more than two out of four presentations. If there is doubt, you can present a stimulus one or two steps more intense to confirm that the first was suprathreshold. If there is a wide range of stimuli for which the responses are inconsistent only in a specific area, make a note of this fact. It could be significant.

---

*Burde, R.M.: Static perimetry. In Thompson, H.S., et al.: Topics in neuro-ophthalmology, Baltimore, 1979, The Williams & Wilkins Co., pp. 30-45; Ellenberger, C., Jr.: Perimetry, Int. Ophthalmol. Clin. **17**(1):85-113, 1977.

Greve uses yet another strategy.* He increases the stimulus intensity with each presentation until the patient responds. After the first response, he increases the intensity one more step and presents it again. If the patient also responds to this one, the dimmer one to which the first response occurred is taken as threshold. However, if the patient does not respond to the second stimulus, slightly more intense than the one to which he first responded, then the first is considered to have been a false response. In that case the process of presenting stimuli of increasing intensity is continued until the patient sees two in a row. The first response of a pair is considered the threshold.

Still another strategy is to find rapidly one stimulus that is infrathreshold and one that is suprathreshold (thereby establishing an estimate of threshold) and then to approach in steps from both sides. It is certainly wise to have an estimate of the range in which threshold will be found at a spot. Especially in an abnormal region of the field, estimating may save time by avoiding the presentation of many stimuli far below threshold before finally reaching threshold. While narrowing the estimated range, the presentation of some stimuli above threshold may also reassure the patient (and you) by not having several consecutive presentations that are invisible. However, this is usually not necessary. The normal method is simply to approach threshold from below but to start only slightly below the expected value based on the threshold of an adjacent point or that determined by a quick estimating technique.*

---

*Greve, E.L., and Verduin, W.M.: Detection of early glaucomatous damage. I. Visual field examination, Doc. Ophthalmol. Proc. Ser. **14:**103-114, 1977.

The circumstances will dictate the exactness with which threshold is determined. For example, if you observe that I-1e and I-2e are not seen but I-3e and I-4e are seen in a specific location, you have established to the nearest 0.5 log-unit that I-3e is the visual threshold; actually, the visual threshold is somewhere between I-2e and I-3e, which are stimuli with intensities 0.5 log-unit apart. However, if you note that stimuli I-1e, I-2a, and I-2b are not seen while I-2c, I-2d, etc., are, then you have established that the threshold is I-2c with 0.1 log-unit accuracy (or, better stated, that the visual threshold is somewhere between I-2b and I-2c, which are 0.1 log-unit apart). For convenience, we will simply say that the visual threshold is I-2c, the weakest stimulus visible. Most often in manual perimetry, visual threshold will be determined by using stimuli 0.1 log-unit apart in intensity.

Note the equivalence here between the accuracy of threshold determinations by kinetic and static techniques. If isopters 0.5 log-unit apart (e.g., I-2e and I-3e) are plotted and the region between them is spot-checked with the stronger stimulus, I-3e in this case, it can be known with 0.5 log-unit accuracy that threshold is between I-2e (which is not seen, being outside the I-2e isopter) and I-3e (which is seen, as determined by static spot-checking). However, if isopters 0.2 log-unit apart (e.g., I-2b and I-2d) are plotted and the region between them is spot-checked with the stronger stimulus, threshold in this region can be estimated with 0.2 log-unit accuracy at between I-2b and I-2d.

Typically in static threshold perimetry with the Oculus or Goldmann perimeter, you will determine threshold to an accuracy of 0.1 log-unit. You generally will obtain a gross estimate in steps of 0.5 log-unit (I-2e, I-3e, I-4e). If the I-3e is visible but the I-2e is not, then you will present the sequence I-3a, I-3b, I-3c, and I-3d to determine threshold to the nearest 0.1 log-unit. Sometimes, especially in a normal region, you may have a good idea of what threshold is based on values at adjacent spots or based on knowing where isopters have been plotted. Then you can start 0.2 or 0.3 log-unit below the anticipated threshold, confirm that this stimulus is not seen, and increase it in 0.1 log-unit steps, thereby determining threshold efficiently with only three or four presentations at each location. However, estimating threshold in steps of 0.5 log-unit before refining the determination in 0.1 log-unit steps becomes useful when an unexpected abnormality is encountered.

APPLICATION OF MANUAL STATIC THRESHOLD PERIMETRY

In *kinetic perimetry,* you choose which isopters to plot, how many to plot, and in what region of the field to concentrate. With *static suprathreshold spot-checking,* you select a region in the field to be spot-checked, how many points to spot-check, and the proper stimulus to use in a specific region.

Similarly, in *static threshold perimetry,* there are choices to make. You select which areas of the field to test, how many points to test, with what accuracy to determine threshold at each point, and the distribution of points (e.g., scattered in a grid pattern, along a meridian, or along an arc). Depending on circumstances and the diagnostic information desired, you may test points 1, 2, 3, or 5 degrees apart along a straight line, in a grid pattern, or along an arc. Examples follow.

Scotoma

A static cut can be used to confirm the presence of and to quantify a suspected scotoma, for example, the one in Fig. 23-8.

FIG. 23-12. Static cut through a scotoma. If there is an area of inconsistent responses to static spot checking, it may be faster to perform a single static cut than to plot one or two additional partial isopters plus the boundary of the scotoma, as in Fig. 23-8.

A static cut may determine the depth of a scotoma and the slope of its boundary quite accurately. However, several adjacent cuts may be required to determine the entire boundary or the extent of a defect. If the defect is large, the boundary may be more efficiently determined by kinetic means.

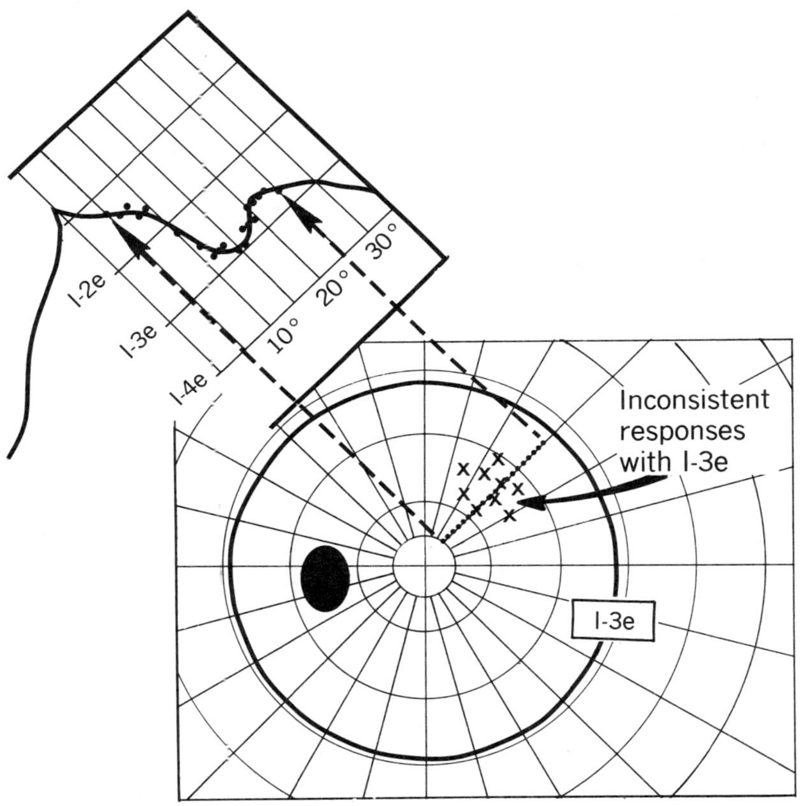

FIG. 23-12

Single point static threshold

You are already familiar with determining static threshold at a single point. When determining the depth of a scotoma, you increase the stimulus strength until it first becomes visible (p. 386) and appropriately label the point to indicate threshold (i.e., "I-2e seen").

There are other occasions when it may be useful to check the threshold of individual points, e.g., in the region of an uncertain nasal step.

FIG. 23-13. Inconsistent responses to kinetic perimetry above the horizontal meridian between 30 and 40 degrees. If the threshold at 35 degrees is *I-4b* above the horizontal meridian but *I-3b* below, the difference in visual threshold is 0.5 log-unit. Note how this is equivalent to Fig. 23-8, but the presence of an abnormality is documented by a different technique.

Threshold testing at selected single points may help clarify the nature of the visual field in other situations. For example, in a flat region of the field with widely separated isopters and difficulty in plotting an exact location of the isopters because of inconsistent responses (p. 454), it may be useful to determine that a somewhat stronger stimulus is seen everywhere.

FIG. 23-14. Flat depressed field with inconsistent response to I-4e. In the inconsistent area, *II-4e* is seen everywhere. This type of field is typical of cataract.

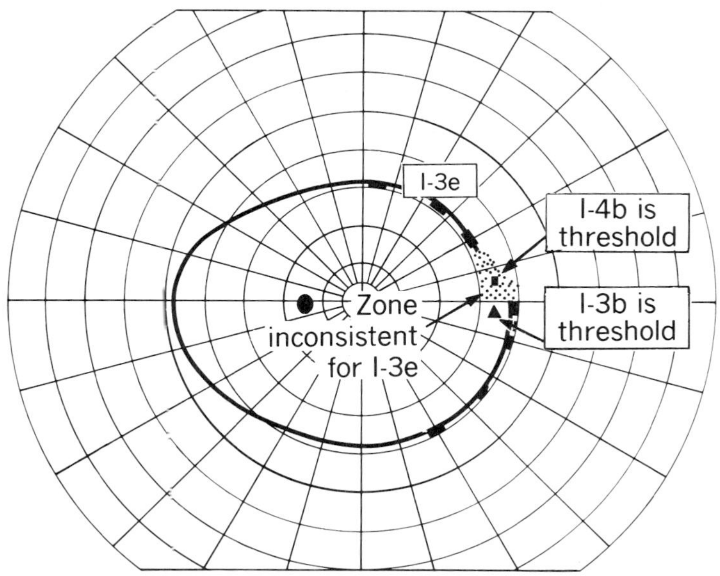

FIG. 23-13

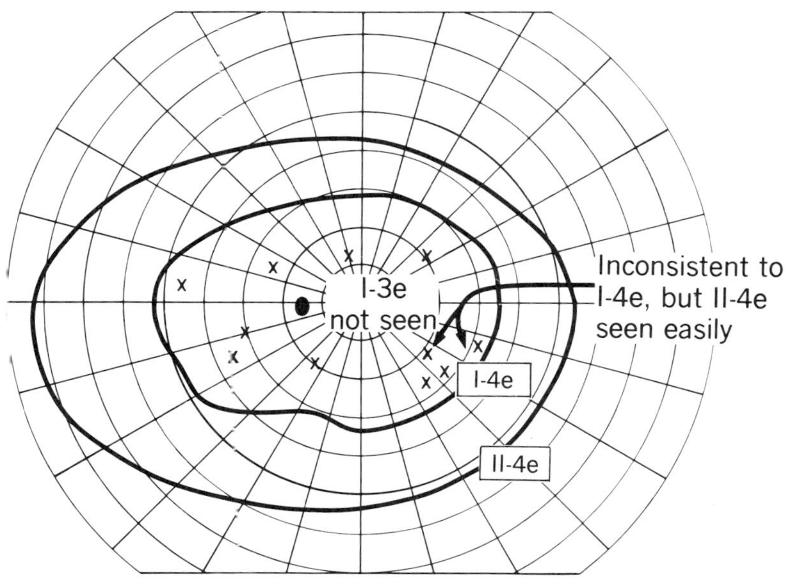

FIG. 23-14

Circular or arc cuts

The static cut need not be along a meridian; it may also be along an arc.

FIG. 23-15. Static cut along an arc through a nasal step. There is a sharply demarcated difference in visual threshold above and below the horizontal meridian, whereas normally there is no such difference. This method is a refinement of the single point static threshold perimetry (Fig. 23-13) and is an alternative to spot-checking (Fig. 23-9, *B*), plotting the isopter kinetically along an arc (Fig. 21-11), or plotting additional isopters (Fig. 23-8). Each method confirms the presence of an abnormality. Artful combination and variation of these methods are useful when there is doubt about the presence or absence of an abnormality such as a nasal step.

Arc cuts can be used in a similar way to confirm or deny the presence of a step along the vertical meridian in the case of a suspected hemianopia (see Fig. 13-44 for an example).

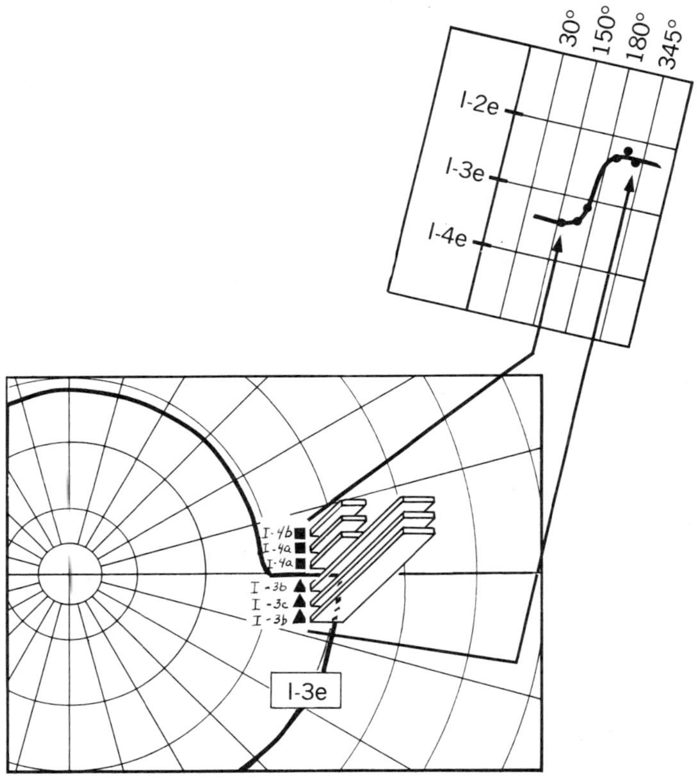

FIG. 23-15

Small island of remaining vision

Because the telescope port occupies 2 degrees around the fixation target, this area of the field cannot be tested with the Goldmann perimeter except by utilizing a special device that projects a fixation target away from the center of the bowl. This device projects a diamond of four red spots, and the patient is told to fixate on the apparent center of the diamond. The visual field chart is slid to one side so its center corresponds to the position of the projected diamond; this is accomplished by aligning the short line on the bottom of the paper in the V-notch.

With this device, the central 2 degrees can be quantified, e.g., by a static cut through the central 5 degrees along the 45- to 225-degree meridian and the 135- to 315-degree meridian. Cuts through the 90- to 270-degree meridian and temporally along the 0- to 180-degree meridian can also be performed, although a cut along the nasal side is best avoided because it may course along a nasal step and produce inconsistent responses.

Equally valid is to plot very carefully two or three isopters to weak stimuli. With any technique, or with a combination, you can afford to be quite accurate since there is so little field area to quantify. When such care is exercised, e.g., for a glaucoma patient, very slight changes over a time can be detected, perhaps allowing more vigorous treatment to be instituted before all is lost.

FIG. 23-16. The small central island. Compare the multiple isopter plot (top) to a static cut through a small severely contracted field.

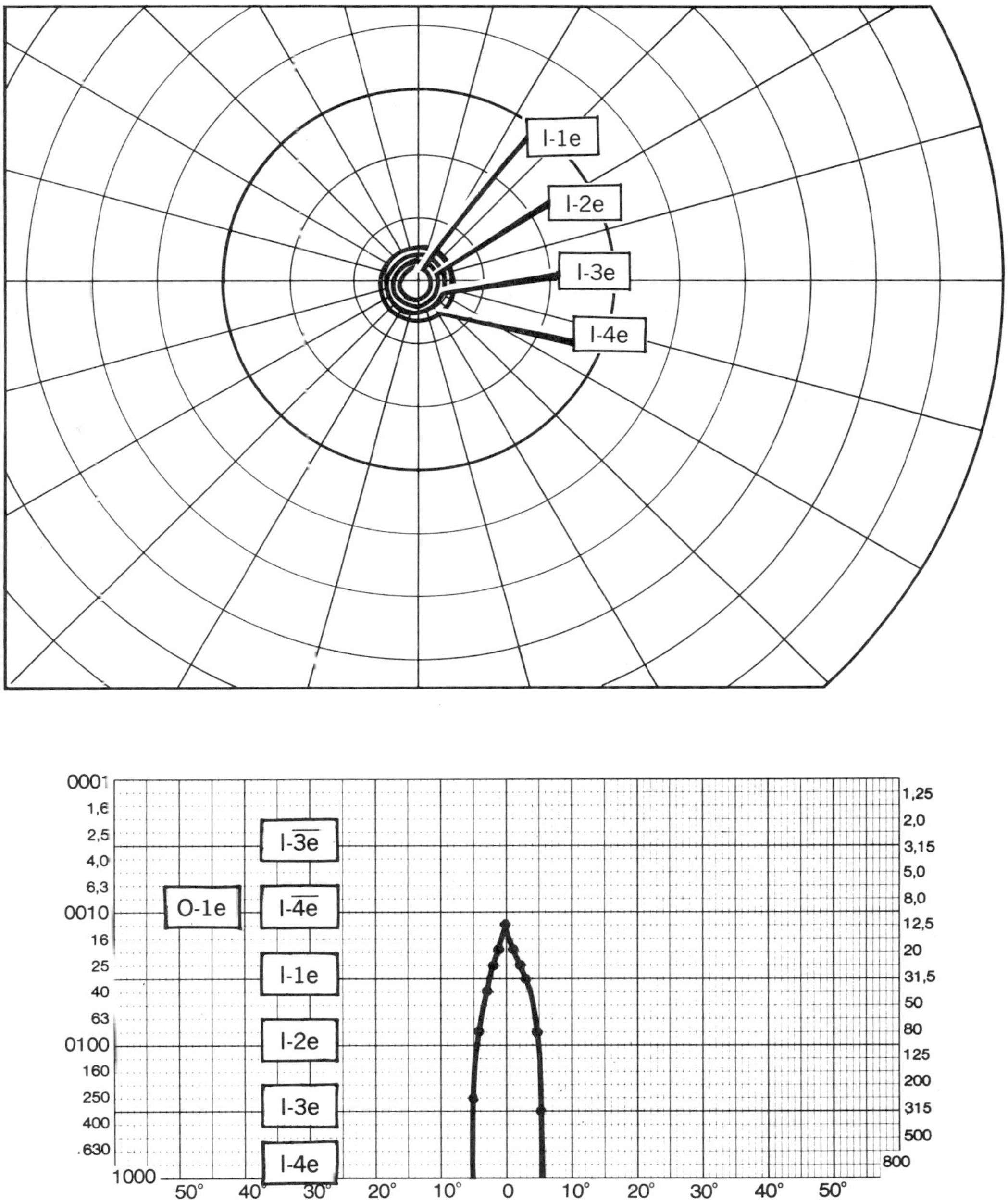
I-1e
I-2e
I-3e
I-4e
0001
1,6
2,5
4,0
6,3
0010
16
25
40
63
0100
160
250
400
630
1000
I-3̄e
O-1e
I-4̄e
I-1e
I-2e
I-3e
I-4e
1,25
2,0
3,15
5,0
8,0
12,5
20
31,5
50
80
125
200
315
500
800
50°
40°
30°
20°
10°
0
10°
20°
30°
40°
50°

FIG. 23-16

"Scatterplot" threshold perimetry

Threshold determinations can be made in any pattern of locations, not only along a single meridian or an arc but also along several adjacent meridians or arcs.

FIG. 23-17. Scattergram threshold perimetry.
A, Visual threshold has been determined at 64 points 1 degree apart, and the results are represented as a series of eight meridional cuts or eight arc cuts.
B, The scattergram is equivalent to the plotting of multiple isopters.
C, Representation of threshold by symbols can give a visual impression of the varying depth in the scotoma.

Such a scatterplot is not a standard procedure with manual perimetry, but could be accomplished. It is illustrated here to show the equivalence of manual methods with automated methods, which routinely use a grid of static threshold determinations. An understanding of this equivalence is required to enable you to compare the results obtained with different instruments or different modes of testing.

The example here also shows how impossible it would be to test thoroughly (with points only 1 degree apart or isopters only 0.1 log-unit different) all parts of the visual field. Just a small segment of the field is covered by the 64 static determinations or the detailed plotting of six isopters. In routine clinical testing the field is not plotted in such detail except in very confined regions of particular clinical importance, such as a small remaining central island of vision in a contracted field.

ADDITIONAL READING

Additional examples of static perimetry's usefulness in clinical practice can be found in the following articles:

Burde, R.M.: Static perimetry. In Thompson, H.S., et al.: Topics in neuro-ophthalmology, Baltimore, 1979. The Williams & Wilkins Co., pp. 38-44.

Ellenberger, C., Jr.: Modern perimetry in neuro-ophthalmic diagnosis, Arch. Neurol. **30:**193-201, 1974.

Greve, E.L.: Visual fields, glaucoma, and cataract, Doc. Ophthalmol. Proc. Ser. **22:**79-88, 1979.

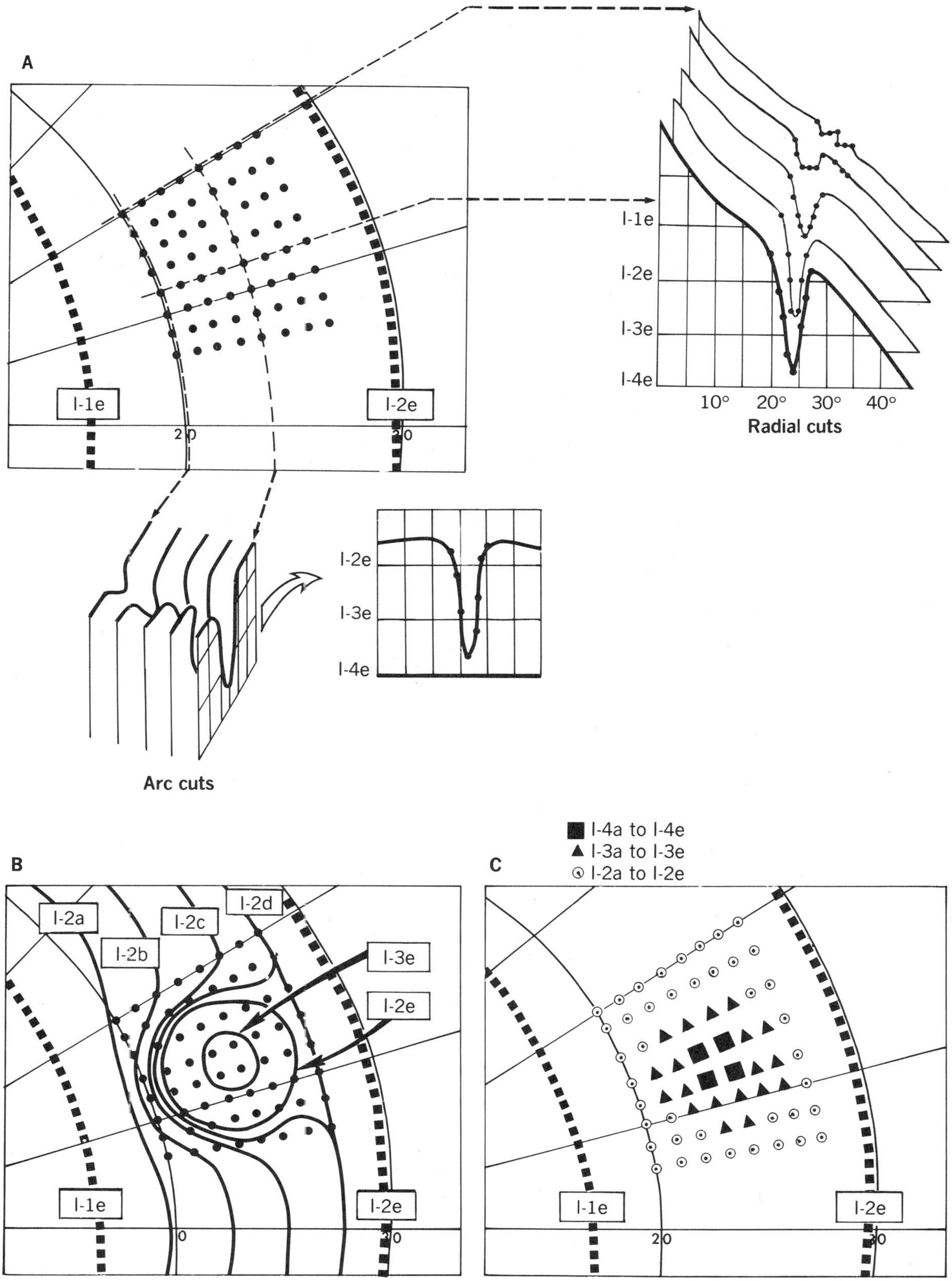
A
I-1e
I-2e
20
30
I-1e
I-2e
I-3e
I-4e
10°
20°
30°
40°
Radial cuts
I-2e
I-3e
I-4e
Arc cuts
B
I-2a
I-2b
I-2c
I-2d
I-3e
I-2e
I-1e
I-2e
C
I-4a to I-4e
I-3a to I-3e
I-2a to I-2e
I-1e
I-2e
20
30

FIG. 23-17

CONFIRMING THE PRESENCE OR ABSENCE OF A DEFECT

With static threshold perimetry or static threshold spot-checking, sometimes the patient may not respond to an individual stimulus presentation simply because you are working near the zone of uncertainty (zone of inconsistent responses) and the stimuli are barely visible. Similarly, there may be a delayed response to a kinetic stimulus, suggesting a localized inward deviation of the isopter that may simply be a response at the innermost portion of the zone of uncertainty. This is particularly a problem when the zone is broad because that region of the field is rather flat. In addition, there may be occasional missed or delayed responses in both static and kinetic perimetry resulting from lapses of attention by the patient.

Thus a missed or delayed response in either kinetic or static perimetry can result from the normal variability of responsiveness but, of course, can also represent a real visual field defect. It is obvious that no real conclusion can be drawn on the basis of one or two presentations to which the patient did not respond when it seemed that he should have. There must be some confirmation of the "defect" before concluding that it really does or does not exist.

This confirmation may take the form of repeated presentations of the kinetic or static stimuli in the region until a more accurate idea of visual sensitivity in the region of suspected defect becomes apparent. An experienced perimetrist does this reflexly: Any time a response is obtained that is out of keeping with the expected response, it is natural to repeat the presentation.

For example, in kinetic perimetry, if a patient responds 10 or 15 degrees closer to fixation than the preceding two or three points that were plotted, you will naturally repeat the presentation to see if the isopter really is deviated inward or if the second response obtained is in keeping with the expected location based on the previous two or three points that were plotted. To judge whether or not there really is a visual field defect, the interpreter of the field, if not the same person who performed the field testing, must consider how many points were plotted in the seemingly abnormal region. If only one point is deviated inward and the perimetrist has not rechecked the finding, the defect may or may not be real.

Similarly, during static threshold perimetry, there is a tendency for an experienced perimetrist to retest the threshold at a spot if, and only if, the response is out of keeping with the expected response, based on the previously plotted adjacent point (p. 467). If the region is *not* retested, usually the interpreter will not accept a "defect" as genuine unless it is 0.5 log-unit deep. Essentially this 0.5 log-unit requirement allows 0.3 log-unit for a normal variability of responsiveness and requires that at least one more stimulus (0.1 log-unit brighter) was not seen before finally a response was obtained. Obviously, if there is a genuine defect 0.3 or 0.4 log-unit deep, it might be ignored when the 0.5 log-unit criterion is used. A defect only 0.2 to 0.4 log-unit deep can be documented only by testing the location in question repeatedly and comparing the average or usual value obtained with a similarly obtained average or usual value in the adjacent regions.

When accuracy is desired, the principle of performing repeated measurments is certainly a valid one. Any kind of measurement is more accurate if it is checked several times, taking the most frequent value or the average value to be the correct one. The average location of a response during kinetic perimetry will be at the center of the zone of uncertainty (the isopter) and not toward the edges. The average response will thus be a more reliable indication of the position of the isopters than any of the individual responses.

Ordinarily you do not retest every point. Only when the response is out of keeping with the expected response will you retest a given location. It would be very time-consuming to repeat every determination (kinetic or static) three to five times to obtain an average at each point. Therefore a single response is usually accepted as representative without retesting if it is as expected, i.e., in keeping with the responses at adjacent points. In this manner the confirmation that an individual response is valid is its congruence with the responses at adjacent points rather than the fact that it was obtained by repeat presentations of the stimulus.

The principle of repeat measurements has been mentioned elsewhere in this book in several situations:

For example, in an effort to determine nasal steps, presentations are performed kinetically—three just above and three just below the horizontal meridian nasally. This maneuver essentially constitutes six repeat exposures around horizontal and increases the accuracy at each location. The method both improves the chances of discovering a nasal step and reduces the risk of a false response that might suggest a defect that did not exist.

The Armaly-Drance suprathreshold testing technique is another example. If there is a missed response, the validity of the "defect" is confirmed only if the stimulus is not seen on the second presentation in the same location or if there are missed responses in adjacent locations (see pp. 46 and 418). The same principle should be applied, with the various modifications of technique, when using the Friedmann Visual Field Analyser or an automated perimeter that makes suprathreshold static presentations. Missed points must be retested manually if they are not retested automatically.

Another example is the procedure used in static threshold perimetry. It has been advocated that threshold be confirmed in each instance by (1) insisting that at least two stimuli be *not* seen (confirming that they are infrathreshold) before accepting a positive response and (2) presenting the stimulus first seen on a second occasion to ensure that it is seen before it is considered visible (p. 467). In Greve's method (p. 468) the validity of a response is confirmed by the patient's signaling that he saw a stimulus 0.1 log-unit brighter. The criteria devised by Greve that a defect must be 0.5 log-unit deep and 3 degrees wide are, in essence, demanding that each missed response must be confirmed by a second missed response before the two can be accepted and also that the apparent defect must be confirmed in an adjacent location.

In addition to rechecking the response in the area of suspected abnormalities, you may decide to use other means to confirm the presence of an abnormality, such as plotting a smaller isopter close to the region and using a weaker stimulus to spot-check (p. 456) or doing a static cut through the suspected area (p. 470).

The accuracy of the test will be influenced by the closeness of the test points (e.g., every 1, 2, or 3 degrees) along a meridian. Another factor will be whether successive presentations at each point were 0.1, 0.2, 0.3, or 0.5 log-unit apart. Only by knowing the intervals of brightness between stimuli and the strategy of repeating or not repeating stimuli can you judge whether a specific suggested defect is likely real or is within the range of expected response variability. Of course, greater accuracy (testing many points 1 degree apart with 0.1 log-unit brightness intervals and a strategy of repeat testing) is obtained at the expense of a longer test time. The expenditure may not be worth the improved accuracy depending on the clinical situation. The only point here is that the interpreter of the field test results must know exactly how accurately the examination was performed if the certainty of its results is to be judged accurately.

By deciding when to perform repeat measurements, where to draw the isopter, and what the threshold is on a static cut, you are making an interpretive judgment. Obviously there is an opportunity to introduce bias. On the one hand, you may be too zealous and indicate as a defect every little area of inconsistent responses that normally occurs in a field test. On the other hand, you may be strongly inclined to accept or encourage responses that indicate normalcy, slowing down to encourage a response in the expected region (p. 444), or overlooking areas where there are several abnormal responses because the patient had also given a few normal responses. You should be looking for areas in which the responses are more inconsistent than elsewhere. A specific region where they are particularly inconsistent while in other regions there is no great variability can certainly indicate the presence of a mild visual field defect.* Such a localized area in which the response is repeatedly inconsistent should be noted. In reaching the decision to indicate as abnormal a certain area of inconsistent responses, you again are making an interpretation that takes into account the responsiveness of the patient in the other regions of the field. Of course, such a judgment will be difficult when the patient is inconsistent in all areas of the field.

In kinetic perimetry it is wise to mark each point where the patient responds so the exactness of the test and the degree of variability in patient responses can be judged by another person who looks at the diagram subsequently. In clinics where it is a practice to show only representative points, the isopter is drawn with or without a nasal step according to the perimetrist's impression as to whether or not there is a demonstrable nasal step. In essence, an interpretive judgment is being made by the person performing the examination. If no nasal step is shown, a sufficient number of representative points should be indicated so another person later looking at the chart will feel confident that a sufficient number of points were plotted to have detected a nasal step if one was present. The field diagram must indicate the areas spot-checked and the stimulus used ("O.K. to I-3e"), the steadiness of fixation, and the perimetrist's overall confidence in the examination's reliability. All these factors enter into the judgment of the diagnostic quality of the examination.

---

*Werner, E.B., and Drance, S.M.: Increased scatter of responses as a precursor of visual field changes in glaucoma, Can. J. Ophthalmol. **12:**140-142, 1977; Werner, E.B., and Drance, S.M.: Early visual field disturbances in glaucoma, Arch. Ophthalmol. **95:**1173-1175, 1977; Holmin, C., and Krakau, C.E.T.: Variability of glaucomatous visual field defects in computerized perimetry, Albrecht von Graefes Arch. Klin. Ophthalmol. **210:**235-250, 1979.

FRIEDMANN VISUAL FIELD ANALYSER

The Friedmann Analyser* is fundamentally different from other instruments in common use. It consists of a strobe light (discharge tube) that flashes for about half a millisecond and evenly illuminates a translucent screen (diffuser). The intensity of the flash is attenuated by filters in 0.2 log-unit steps. A pair of opaque black plates with 98 holes (46 holes in the original model) sits in front of the screen as the patient sees it. An external light source evenly illuminates the front plate surface and represents the "background illumination." The test is conducted in the mesopic, almost scotopic, range of background illumination.

A lever controlling the rear plate can be placed in 31 positions (designated *A* through *Z* and *a* through *h*). In each position two, three, or four of the holes are open; thus two, three, or four spots of light can be seen when the strobe is flashed.

FIG. 23-18. The Friedmann Analyser.

The holes are larger toward the edge of the plate and smaller near fixation. Therefore a specific stimulus intensity that is threshold at 20 degrees will also be threshold (not suprathreshold) at 5 degrees because the size of the spot is smaller by an appropriate amount. When a given stimulus intensity is determined to be 0.4 log-unit suprathreshold at one location, it should be approximately 0.4 log-unit suprathreshold at all locations. Therefore it can be used for static spot-checking throughout the entire central field without fear that it will be too strong for the detection of shallow scotomas near fixation.

The combination of several stimuli presented simultaneously (making it a rapid test) and gradations in size of the hole (making it sensitive to detecting shallow scotomas) enable the Analyser to be used as a quick and accurate screener for glaucomatous visual field defects and for all other defects detectable by static spot-checking. It is even possible to spot-check the point of fixation as the ninety-ninth location. The 98 positions for spot testing are quite adequate, but with a device for eccentric fixation the number of positions can actually be increased to 490 or more. Only the central 25 degrees is tested, however, and in some cases when there is a defect only in the periphery (but none in the central field), the field test may falsely yield normal results. Fortunately, the instrument is so sensitive that it rarely finds a peripheral defect without *any* central defect; and if the Friedmann Analyser does not reveal a defect, you can be reasonably certain that the entire field really is normal.

---

*Clement-Clark International Ltd., 16 Wigmore Street, London W1H ODH, England.

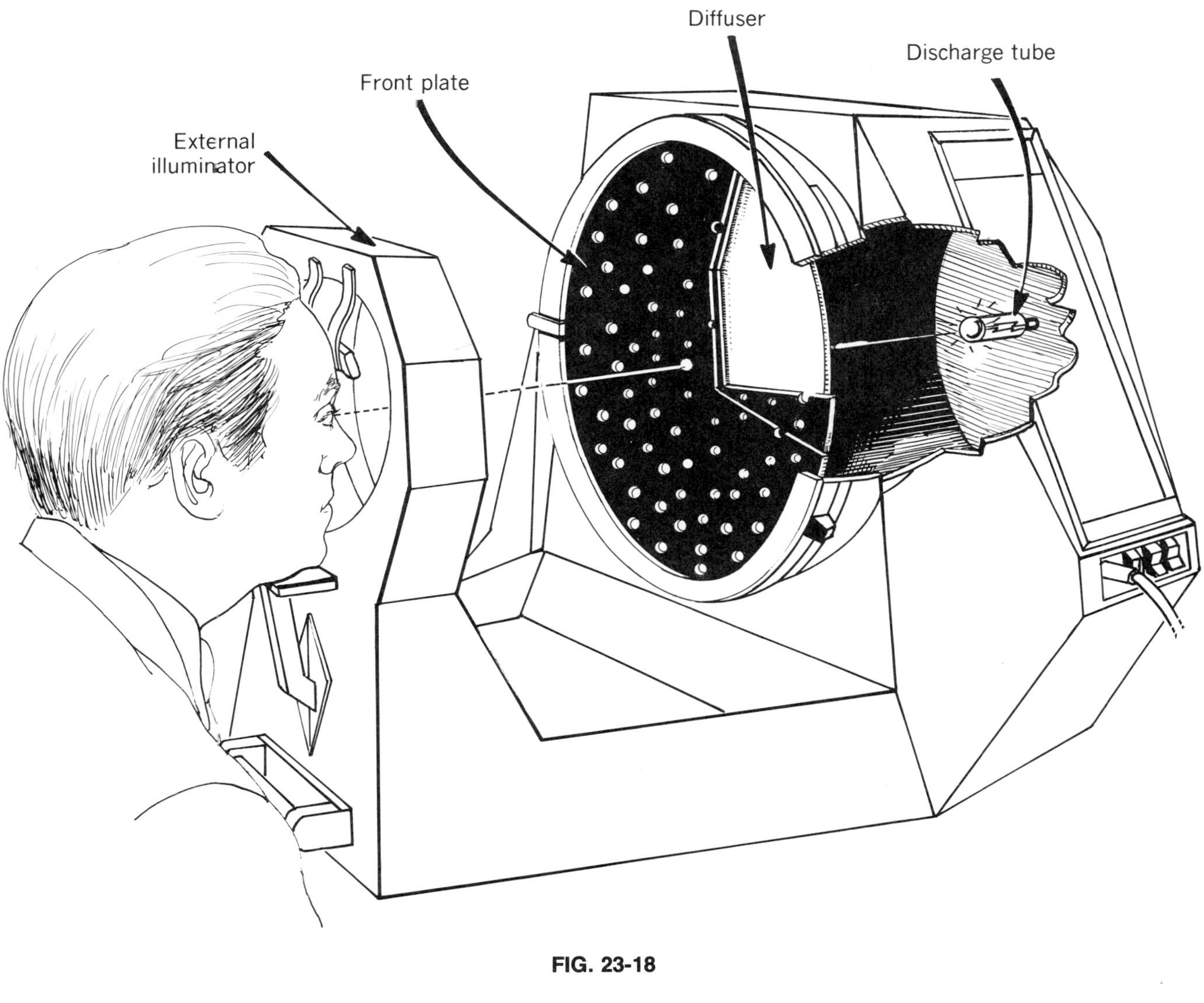
Diffuser
Discharge tube
Front plate
External illuminator

FIG. 23-18

Screening with the Friedmann Analyser

The Analyser (Mark II model) can be used in a number of ways. For screening, the following may be a useful approach. First, determine the patient's best distance correction and use a +4.00 D near add or less according to age. It is important that you accurately center the eye being tested by adjusting the chin rest—a step easy to overlook. You may have to allow a few minutes for the eye to adapt to the low illumination level, especially if the patient has been in a brightly lit waiting area. With the lever in position *h,* determine the weakest stimulus that allows any or all four spots to be seen (threshold stimulus). For a visual field screening test, set the filters so the stimulus is 0.4 log-unit more intense than the threshold stimulus and use this to screen at all 31 lever positions. For example, if the threshold stimulus at *h* is the 2.0 log-unit filter, the test is run with the 1.6 log-unit filter (0.4 log-unit more intense than the threshold at *h*). Ask the patient with each flash to state how many spots he saw. Sometimes scratches on the front of the plate will give reflections that are perceived by the patient and may cause confusion.

Any time the patient reports seeing fewer spots than there actually are, flash the same spots a second time and do not count the miss if he gives the correct number the second time. On the other hand, if he again sees only some of the spots, ask in which quadrants he did see spots and record those he did not see.

As a screening test, nothing more is done except to record the regions where a defect is found. It is possible to quantify the threshold at all missed spots, increasing the intensity (reducing the filters) until each of the missed spots becomes visible. Quantitation is achieved nicely if the defect is small, but threshold determination at many spots is tedious and recording it at each spot in an easily readable format may be a problem.

ADDITIONAL READING

Bedwell, C.H.: Recent developments in investigations of visual fields, Am. J. Optom. Physiol. Opt. **55:**681-699, 1978.

Friedmann, A.I.: Serial analysis of changes in visual field defects, employing a new instrument, to determine the activity of diseases involving the visual pathways, Ophthalmologica **152:**1-12, 1966.

Friedmann, A.I.: Experiences with a prototype 100-hole front plate for the visual field analyser in glaucoma, Doc. Ophthalmol. Proc. Ser. **14:**87-92, 1977.

Friedmann, A.I.: Outline of visual field analyser Mark II, Doc. Ophthalmol. Proc. Ser. **22:**65-67, 1979.

Greve, E.L., and Verduin, W.M.: Mass visual field investigation of 1834 subjects with supposedly normal eyes, Albrecht von Graefes Arch. Klin. Exp. Ophthalmol. **183:**266-293, 1972.

Pashley, J.C.: Assessment of the Friedmann Visual Field Analyser, Annee Ther. Clin. Ophthalmol. **25:**536-541, 1974.

APPENDIX A

Teaching perimetry

This book can be used as a text for a course in manual perimetry. The first phase is an intensive introduction over several days, which might be done as follows:

I	Lecture 1	Chapter 1 (introduction)
	Demonstration	Chapter 15 (Goldmann perimeter)
	Reading homework	Chapter 4 (anatomy of the eye)
	Practice on another student	Chapter 17 (plotting isopters kinetically)
II.	Lecture 2	Chapters 5 and 6 (normal field and scotomas)
	Reading homework	Chapter 5 (normal field) Chapters 6, 18, and 19 (scotomas)
	Practice on another student	Chapter 18 (plotting scotomas)
III.	Lecture-demonstration 3	Chapter 12 (practical techniques)
	Optional demonstration	Chapter 2 (other instruments)
	Reading homework	Chapter 2 (instrumentation)
	Begin practice in clinical setting	
IV.	Lecture 4	Chapter 7 (localized depressions)
	Demonstration	Pages 194-204 (corrective lenses)
	Reading homework	Chapter 2 (anatomy of the eye) and Chapters 7 and 20 (localized depressions)
V.	Lecture 5	Chapters 10 and 21 (field loss in glaucoma)
	Demonstration	Chapter 16 (calibration of Goldmann perimeter)
	Reading homework	Chapters 10 and 21 (visual field loss in glaucoma)
VI.	Lecture 6	Chapter 8 (generalized depressions)
	Reading homework	Review Chapters 12, 15, and 16

The second phase consists of gaining actual practical experience—performing perimetry under supervision in a clinical setting. After a certain amount of practical experience, and while continuing to gain more, the student should review to be sure that no details of technique are being overlooked without realizing it. For this purpose, the following chapters should be read again, one or two per week, in the following sequence: Chapters 15, 12, 16, 1, 5, 6, 7, 8, 18, 19, 20, 10, and 21. The idea is that both the chapters dealing with practical points and those dealing with the theoretical principles are reviewed at a time when they may have more meaning, after the student has some experience encountering field defects in the clinical setting. The outside readings cited in various chapters could also be tackled at this time.

At some point Chapter 9 (on topographic classification of visual field defects) should be introduced, either as a lecture or as a reading assignment. After several patients with hemianopias are encountered, this chapter should be reviewed.

Once the preceding material has been mastered, the third phase of formal teaching should include a review and a refinement of technique (Chapter 23), details of glaucoma evaluation (Chapter 22), supplemental methods (Chapter 3), and an understanding of technique selection (Chapter 11), including the examination of the patient with poor visual acuity and neurologic fields. These topics can be covered at weekly or biweekly intervals as lectures or as reading assignments with the opportunity for questions and discussion.

The subjects of psychophysics (Chapter 14) and interpretation (Chapter 13) can be introduced when they are appropriate, depending on the nature of the group being taught. The basic principles in these three chapters maybe should be studied by every student of perimetry, even if they will not be in a position to perform static perimetry, choose instrumentation, or be responsible for diagnostic interpretation. Understanding the principles involved will be important to anyone who wants to perform a high-quality perimetric examination.

APPENDIX B

Bibliography

GENERAL

Bedwell, C.H.: Visual fields. A basis for efficient investigation, London, 1982, Butterworth Scientific.

Dubois-Poulsen, A.: Le champ visuel; topographie normale et pathologique de ses sensibilités, Paris, 1952, Masson & Cie. *A lengthy and complete textbook and reference book for those who read French.*

Ellenberger, C., Jr.: Perimetry: principles, techniques, and interpretation, New York, 1980, Raven Press.

Harrington, D.O.: The visual fields: a textbook and atlas of clinical perimetry, ed. 5, St. Louis, 1981. The C.V. Mosby Co. *Current standard textbook by one of Traquair's first students on the uses of clinical perimetry based largely on the tangent screen examination. Much of the book deals with the characteristic field defects of various clinical entities.*

Reed, H., and Drance, S.M.: The essentials of perimetry, static and kinetic, London, 1972, Oxford University Press. *Another current primer on clinical visual field testing, briefer than Harrington. Drance was one of Traquair's last students.*

Scott, G.I.: Traquair's clinical perimetry, ed. 7, St. Louis, 1957, The C.V. Mosby Co. *Final edition of Traquair's classic; no longer in print.*

Traquair, H.M.: An introduction to clinical perimetry, ed. 6, St. Louis, 1949, The C.V. Mosby Co. *A classic, filled with valuable information; no longer in print.*

PERIMETRIC TECHNIQUE

Readers who want more practical hints for the performance of field testing or brief reviews of basic principles may be interested in the references cited on pp. 74, 141, 466, 467, and 468 as well as the following:

Burde, R.M.: Static perimetry. In Thompson, H.S., et al., editors: Topics in neuro-ophthalmology, Baltimore, 1979, The Williams & Wilkins Co., pp. 30-45. *This chapter is instructive reading as a brief introduction for anyone who is contemplating performing static perimetry with the Goldmann perimeter. It covers the principles, technique, and examples of its usefulness.*

Ellenberger, C., Jr.: Perimetry international, Int. Ophthalmol. Clin. **17**:85-113, 1977. *Short, didactic, general review emphasizing static perimetry with examples of its use, especially in a neurology practice.*

Frisén, L.: The cornerstones of perimetric strategy. In Thompson, H.S., et al., editors: Topics in neuro-ophthalmology, Baltimore, 1979. The Williams & Wilkins Co., pp. 5-19.

Frisén, L.: Kinetic perimetry: techniques and strateges. In Thompson, H.S., et al., editors: Topics in neuro-ophthalmology, Baltimore, 1979, The Williams & Wilkins Co., pp. 20-29. *This and the previous article by Frisén contain considerable information about details of very compulsive quantitative field testing technique and contain a nice list of references. Many of the details are valuable technical hints that will sharpen the skills of those who have mastered the contents of this book, but some details are nit-picking for the usual clinical purpose and will be of interest mainly to specialized perimetry centers. The information is difficult to find elsewhere and every person who will perform perimetry in a clinical setting will find these two articles instructive.*

Havener, W.H., and Gloeckner, S.L.: Introductory atlas of perimetry, St. Louis, 1972, The C.V. Mosby Co. *This manual was written for the training of an ophthalmologist's office assistant. It contains many practical hints, particularly for the tangent screen. It is no longer in print but may be found in some libraries. A somewhat revised version is being printed by the Continuing Education Department of the Ohio State University School of Medicine, Columbus, Ohio, for use in their visual field course.*

Trobe, J.D., and Glaser, J.S.: The visual fields manual, Gainesville, Fla., 1983, Triad Publishing Co.

Index